Management of Complex Treatment-Resistant Psychotic Disorders

Management of Complex Treatment-Resistant Psychotic Disorders

Edited by

Dr. Michael A. Cummings

Clinical Associate Professor of Psychiatry, University of California,
Irvine and Clinical Professor of Psychiatry, University of California,
Riverside, USA

Dr. Stephen M. Stahl

Clinical Professor of Psychiatry and Neuroscience, University of California, Riverside,
and Adjunct Professor of Psychiatry, University of California, San Diego, USA

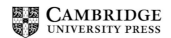

CAMBRIDGE
UNIVERSITY PRESS

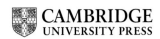

Shaftesbury Road, Cambridge CB2 8EA, United Kingdom

One Liberty Plaza, 20th Floor, New York, NY 10006, USA

477 Williamstown Road, Port Melbourne, VIC 3207, Australia

314–321, 3rd Floor, Plot 3, Splendor Forum, Jasola District Centre, New Delhi – 110025, India

103 Penang Road, #05–06/07, Visioncrest Commercial, Singapore 238467

Cambridge University Press is part of Cambridge University Press & Assessment,
a department of the University of Cambridge.

We share the University's mission to contribute to society through the pursuit of
education, learning and research at the highest international levels of excellence.

www.cambridge.org
Information on this title: www.cambridge.org/9781108965682

DOI: 10.1017/9781108963923

First published 2021

A catalogue record for this publication is available from the British Library

Library of Congress Cataloging-in-Publication data
Names: Cummings, Michael A. (Michael Allen), 1951– editor. | Stahl, Stephen M., 1951– editor.
Title: Management of complex treatment-resistant psychotic disorders / edited by Dr. Michael A. Cummings,
Dr. Stephen M. Stahl. Description: Cambridge, United Kingdom ; New York : Cambridge University
Press, 2021. | Includes bibliographical references and index. Identifiers: LCCN 2020055181 (print) |
LCCN 2020055182 (ebook) | ISBN 9781108965682 (paperback) | ISBN 9781108963923 (ebook) Subjects:
MESH: Psychotic Disorders – drug therapy | Psychotic Disorders – complications | Antipsychotic Agents –
therapeutic use | Antipsychotic Agents – pharmacology | Psychopharmacology – methods | Drug Resistance
Classification: LCC RM333.5 (print) | LCC RM333.5 (ebook) | NLM WM 200 | DDC 615.7/882–dc23
LC record available at https://lccn.loc.gov/2020055181
LC ebook record available at https://lccn.loc.gov/2020055182

ISBN   978-1-108-96568-2   Paperback

....

Disclosures: Dr. Arguello, Dr. Arias, Dr. Cummings, Dr. O'Day, Dr. Schwartz, Dr. Striebel, and Dr. Warburton
declare that they have nothing to disclose. Dr. Meyer reports having received speaking or advising fees
from Alkermes, Forum, Merck, Otsuka-USA and Sunovion. Dr. Stahl reports having received advising fees,
consulting fees, speaking fees and/or research grants from Acadia, Alkermes, Biomarin, Clintara, Eli-Lilly,
EnVivo, Forest, Forum, GenoMind, JayMac, Lundbeck, Merck, Novartis, Orexigen, Otsuka-USA, PamLabs,
Pfizer, RCT Logic, Servier, Shire, Sprout, Sunovion, Sunovion-UK, Taisho, Takeda, Teva, Tonix and Trius.

Contents

Contributors

Dr. Juan C. Arguello Associate Clinical Professor of Psychiatry and Adjunct Associate Clinical Professor, University of California, Riverside and Touro University College of Osteopathic Medicine, Sacramento, California, USA

Dr. Ai-Li W. Arias Assistant Clinical Professor of Psychiatry, University of California, Irvine and Riverside, California, USA

Dr. Michael A. Cummings Clinical Professor of Psychiatry and Associate Clinical Professor of Psychiatry, University of California, Irvine and Riverside, California, USA

Dr. Jonathan M. Meyer Clinical Professor of Psychiatry, University of California, San Diego, California, USA

Dr. Jennifer A. O'Day Assistant Clinical Professor of Psychiatry, University of California, Riverside, California, USA

Dr. George J. Proctor Associate Clinical Professor of Psychiatry, Loma Linda University School of Medicine, California, USA

Dr. Eric H. Schwartz Department of Psychiatry, California Department of State Hospitals, Napa, California, USA

Dr. Stephen M. Stahl Professor of Psychiatry, University of California, San Diego, USA and University of Cambridge, UK

Dr. Joan M. Striebel Assistant Clinical Professor of Psychiatry, University of California, Los Angeles, California, USA

Dr. Katherine Warburton Associate Clinical Professor of Psychiatry, University of California, Davis, California, USA

Acknowledgements

The editors and contributors wish to acknowledge Ms. Tina Lache for her assistance in preparing the manuscript for this book.

Abbreviations

AChE	acetylcholinesterase
Ach-EIs	acetylcholinesterase inhibitors
AD	Alzheimer's disease
ADHD	attention deficit hyperactivity disorder
AED	antiepileptic drugs
AHR	adjusted hazard ratio
AL_{NCD}	aripiprazole lauroxil nanocrystal
ANC	absolute neutrophil count
ASD	autism spectrum disorder
AV	atrioventricular block
BDNF	brain derived neurotrophic factor
BEN	benign ethnic neuropenia
BLT	bright light therapy
BMI	body mass index
BPH	benign prostatic hypertrophy
BPRS	Brief Psychiatric Rating Scale
BuChE	butylcholinesterase
CBT	cognitive behavioral therapy
CGI	clinical global impression
CI	confidence interval
CMA	chromosomal microarray
CNS	central nervous system
CNV	copy number variants
COPD	chronic obstructive pulmonary disease
COS	childhood-onset schizophrenia
CPAP	continuous positive airway pressure
CR	controlled release
CYP	cytochrome P450
DBS	deep brain stimulation
DLB	dementia with Lewy bodies
DLPFC	dorsolateral prefrontal cortex
DN-RIRe	dopamine and norepinephrine reuptake inhibitor and releaser
DRESS	drug reaction with eosinophilia and systemic symptoms
D-RI	dopamine reuptake inhibitor
ECT	electroconvulsive therapy
EOS	early-onset schizophrenia
EPS	extrapyramidal adverse effects
ER	extended-release
FDA	US Food and Drug Administration

FGA	first-generation antipsychotic
GABA	gamma-aminobutyric acid
GABA-PAM	gamma-aminobutyric acid positive allosteric modulator
GAD	generalized anxiety disorder
GC	gas chromotography
GI	gastrointestinal
HR	hazard ratio
HTN	hypertension
IM	intramuscular
IR	immediate-release
LAI	long-acting injectable
LVD	left ventricular dysfunction
LVH	left ventricular hypertrophy
MAOI	monoamine oxidase inhibitor
MCCB	MATRICS Consensus Cognitive Battery
MOAS	Modified Objective Aggression Scale
MS	mass spectroscopy
NAMI	National Alliance on Mental Illness
NDD	neurodevelopmental disorders
NMDA	N-methyl-D-aspartate
NMS	neuroleptic malignant syndrome
NNH	number needed to harm
N-RA	norepinephrine receptor agonist
NSAID	nonsteroidal anti-inflammatory drug
OCD	obsessive-compulsive disorder
ODD	oppositional-defiant disorder
OR	odds ratio
OSAHS	obstructive sleep apnea/hypopnea syndrome
PANSS	Positive and Negative Symptoms Scale
PDMP	prescription drug monitoring program
PFC	prefrontal cortex
PGP	P-glycoprotein
PM	poor metabolizers
PMDD	primary major depressive disorder
PT	protime
PTSD	post-traumatic stress disorder
RAS	reticular activating system
RCT	randomized controlled trial
RTMS	repetitive transcranial magnetic stimulation
SAD-BT	schizoaffective disorder, bipolar type
SANS	Scale for the Assessment of Negative Symptoms
SGA	second-generation antipsychotic
SIADH	syndrome of inappropriate antidiuretic hormone secretion

SJS	Stevens-Johnson syndrome
SNP	single-nucleotide polymorphisms
SNRI	selective serotonin-norepinephrine reuptake inhibitor
SR	sustained-release
SSRI	selective serotonin reuptake inhibitor
TBI	traumatic brain injury
TCA	tricyclic antidepressant
TDCS	transcranial direct current stimulation
TEN	toxic epidermal necrolysis
TEOSS	Treatment of Early Onset Schizophrenia Spectrum Disorders
TGA	third-generation antipsychotic
THC	tetra-hydro-cannabidiol
TMN	tuberomammillary nucleus
TPC	temporoparietal cortex
TRS	treatment-resistant schizophrenia
TSH	thyroid stimulating hormone
tVNS	transcutaneous vagal nerve stimulation
VHA	Veterans Health Administration
VNS	vagal nerve stimulation
VPA	valproic acid

List of Icons

 Clinical pearls of information based on the clinical expertise of the author

 References

 Basic Information

 Classifications

 How the drug works, mechanism of action

 Plasma Concentrations and Treatment Response

 Typical Treatment Response

 Pre-Treatment Workup and Initial Laboratory Testing

 Monitoring

 Dosing and Kinetics

 Warnings and precautions regarding use of the drug

 Drug interactions that may occur

 Medical Precautions and Contraindications

 Do Not Use in patients with

 Recommended Absolute Neutrophil Count Monitoring

Introduction

Increasingly, individuals living with psychotic illnesses are experiencing homelessness, incarceration and associated trauma. Forensic populations are exploding. As people cycle through jails, prisons and the streets, their disorders are going untreated while social stress exacerbates their conditions. As a result of these social determinants, clinical presentations are growing more complex, less categorical and harder to treat. Current guidelines capture the ideal treatment of straightforward presentations in clinically sterile settings. Caretakers working on the front lines often have to move beyond these extant guidelines, an exercise that can feel risky and isolating. This is a book for prescribers on the front lines of treating complex, often treatment-resistant patients.

To address the uncertainty of working with refractory patients in our large forensic hospital system, the California Department of State Hospitals created a psychopharmacology resource network. This network of prescribers, led by the authors of this book, has overcome the isolation experienced by clinicians in our system by developing and communicating best practices beyond previous guidelines. This team has evolved a process of education and consultation by blending the practical application of sophisticated evidence-based knowledge with vast experience in the pharmacological treatment of a very complex and difficult patient population.

The ideal trajectory for an individual who develops a schizophrenia spectrum disorder is early intervention with medication and psychoeducation, followed by close monitoring of optimal psychopharmacology, housing support and vocational therapy. The reality we see is a course of inability to access care, worsening psychotic symptoms, substance abuse, homelessness, and repeated criminal justice contacts as a result of the aforementioned factors. From criminal justice involvement flows trauma, inconsistent psychopharmacology and acquisition of criminogenic risk factors [1]. From these factors flows aggression, alienation and a deepening of the disenfranchisement that began the cycle. Today's complex, treatment-resistant patients require interventions at the level of most of these factors. But the cycle can only be broken with appropriate and effective psychopharmacology.

The goal of the authors is to further widen the network of prescribers working in the most challenging psychiatric environments with the most challenging patients. The authors attempt this by presenting systematic treatment strategies based on current evidence and extensive experience. The focus will be on those medications and strategies they've found especially useful in treating treatment-resistant, severe psychotic illness.

In Chapter 1, approaches to positive psychotic symptoms are explored with straightforward algorithms. In Chapter 2, the authors share the necessity and utility of plasma drug levels in guiding psychopharmacological intervention. Chapter 3 discusses the advantages of using long-acting injectable antipsychotic medication and provides useful initiation strategies. Chapter 4 takes a deep dive into the concept of treatment resistance and reviews the evidence for various strategies. Chapter 5 discusses strategies for working with depressed or suicidal patients who are also living with schizophrenia spectrum disorders. Chapter 6 is an overview of how to address aggression in this population. Chapter 7 addresses the approach to bipolar diathesis in schizophrenia. Chapter 8 provides guidance when an individual living with schizophrenia is also suffering from anxiety. Chapter 9 focuses on sleep disturbances. Psychosis in children and adolescents is addressed in Chapter 10. Chapter 11 is an exploration of electroconvulsive therapy, along with other non-pharmacological treatments in this select patient population. Chapter 12 describes how to approach substance use disorders among these patients. Part I rounds out with strategies to mitigate behavioral disturbances, as well as how to address dementia and traumatic brain injury.

Part II of this book provides a practical and easy to follow prescribers guide for the agents discussed throughout the book based upon the well-known format used in Dr. Stahl's best-selling psychopharmacology prescribers guide [2]. Part III of the book provides further reference material on everything from how to manage constipation to how to load medications.

I am humbled and grateful for the work our psychopharmacology team has done to standardize and improve the care of our most complex, treatment-resistant patients. They have found methodologies to approach patients previously thought to be impossible to treat. I am confident the reader will benefit from the knowledge and experience reflected in this book and will join our network of clinical expertise.

Katherine Warburton, D.O.

Deputy Director (Medical Director)
Clinical Operations Division
California Department of State Hospitals

 References

1. Warburton, K. (2016). *Violence in Psychiatry*. New York: Cambridge University Press.
2. Stahl, S. M. (2020). *Stahl's Essential Psychopharmacology Prescribers Guide*. 7th ed. New York: Cambridge University Press.

Part I
Treatment Strategies

1.01 Approaches to Positive Psychotic Symptoms

📖 **Introduction** In community settings, the most common barriers to independent living, employment, and stable interpersonal relationships for patients suffering from schizophrenia spectrum disorders or other psychotic disorders are negative symptoms and cognitive deficits [1]. In contrast, severely mentally ill individuals, often incarcerated or chronically institutionalized, more frequently experience substantial barriers related to positive psychotic symptoms leading to problematic behaviors such as aggression or violence [2]. This is not to say that among the chronically institutionalized severely mentally ill population that positive psychotic symptoms are the only, or even majority, source of problematic behaviors. A survey conducted within the California Department of State Hospitals, a circa 7000-bed system dedicated to the treatment of conserved and forensically committed patients, reviewed 839 episodes of aggression or violence by 88 persistently aggressive inpatients and found that 54% of such episodes were impulsive, 39% were predatory or instrumental, and 17% were psychotically driven [3]. Nevertheless, amelioration or control of positive psychotic symptoms commonly forms the initial treatment focus among the severely mentally ill [4].

Ⓐ **Dopamine and Positive Symptoms** Elevated dopamine signal transduction in the meso-limbic dopamine pathway (ventral tegmentum to temporal lobe) and/or inadequate top-down glutamate modulation of dopamine signaling in the meso-limbic dopamine circuit by frontal lobe structures is thought to underlie the expression of such positive psychotic signs and symptoms as illusions, hallucinations, delusions and psychomotor agitation. Respectively, these views of the roles of dopamine and glutamate have been termed the dopamine and glutamate hypotheses of psychosis [5, 6].

Ⓑ **Evaluation of Problem Behaviors** As in all of medicine, the initial step in treatment is evaluation. Table 1.1 below outlines the initial evaluation of patients in whom preliminary data point to positive psychotic signs and symptoms as a principle source of problematic behaviors and impairment of psychosocial functioning.

Table 1.1 Initial Review and Treatment of Severely Ill Psychotic Patients [13–17]

Decisions	Assessments	Brief Comments

Problem behaviors arise from psychosis
• Yes, continue
• No, alternate treatment approaches
	Review prior history and assessments
	• Frequency of problem behaviors
	• Severity of problem behaviors
	• Patient factors associated with problem behaviors
	• Environmental factors associated with problem behaviors
	• Cause of latest decompensation
	• Comorbid violence factor
	  - Substance abuse
	  - Impulse dyscontrol
	  - Predatory violence	

Patient poses an immediate risk • Yes, then decide level of control • No, then repeat risk assessment as clinically indicated	Evaluate need for segregation or restraint • Clinical observation • Clinical interview • Use of rating scale, e.g. DASA	Be familiar with relevant regulations/procedures governing seclusion or use of physical restraints
Physical conditions contribute to behavior risk • No, continue • Yes, treat physical condition	Physical evaluations • Psychomotor agitation • Evaluate for akathisia • Evaluate for pain or physical discomfort • Evaluate for delirium • Evaluate for intoxication or withdrawal • Evaluate for complex partial seizures • Evaluate sleep	
Abnormal labs contribute to problem behaviors • Yes, correct underlying abnormality • No, continue	Evaluation of laboratory data • Plasma glucose • Plasma calcium • WBC to rule out sepsis • Infectious disease screens as clinically indicated • Plasma sodium to rule out hyponatremia or hypernatremia • Oxygen saturation if suspect • Serum ammonia if suspect • Thyroid status • Sedimentation rate and C-reactive protein if history of inflammatory disease	Serum ammonia useful only if elements of delirium clinically present

A second important element in approaching the treatment of positive psychotic symptoms is evaluation of past treatment responses and of elements that may affect medication responses such as nonadherence to oral medications, altered medication kinetics or past pharmacodynamic issues. A systematic approach is described below in Table 1.2.

Table 1.2 Evaluation of Psychopharmacology for Severe Psychosis [4, 18, 19]

Decisions	Assessments	Brief Comments
Inadequate treatment contributes • Yes, adjust treatment • No, observe treatment response	Evaluate adequacy of current treatment • Duration (four to six weeks) • Dose (at least standard) • Dosing (e.g. with food if needed) • Adherence • Plasma concentrations • Hepatic inducers, e.g. carbamazepine or phenytoin	See Chapter 2 regarding use of plasma concentrations
Adverse medication effects present • Yes, adjust treatment or treat adverse effect • No, continue	Presence of adverse antipsychotic effects • Neurological ⇒ Akathisia ⇒ Dystonia ⇒ Parkinsonism • Sedation • Orthostasis Presence of adverse anticonvulsant effects • Ataxia • Tremor • Cognitive impairment Presence of adverse lithium effects • Polyuria • Nausea, vomiting, diarrhea • Tremor • Cognitive impairment Presence of adverse beta blocker effects • Hypotension • Bronchospasm • Bradycardia	• Many adverse effects respond to time or gradual dose reduction
Patient is responding to treatment • Yes, optimize and continue • No, alter treatment approach	Evaluate response to current treatment • Partial response • No response	• A partial response (< 20% to 30% improvement on the PANSS or BPRS) with minimal or no adverse effects argues for a higher-dose trial of the present antipsychotic • Failure of ≥ 2 adequate trials with at least one being a second-generation antipsychotic, argues for a clozapine trial • A partial response (small decline in BIS-11) with adequate anticonvulsant plasma concentrations argues for the addition of an anticonvulsant or other medication with distinct mechanism of action

1.01 Approaches to Positive Psychotic Symptoms (Continued)

❻ Treatment of Psychosis After evaluation of the patient and of the patient's pharmacotherapy, the next step is to design the primary pharmacological approach to the patient's illness. In this context, it should be remembered that all medication trials have one of three endpoints: (1) the patient's illness improves; (2) intolerable adverse effects occur which cannot be adequately addressed to permit continuation of the medication trial; or (3) a point of futility is reached. An example of reaching a point of futility would be a patient whose olanzapine plasma concentration has reached circa 150 ng/ml without improvement over four to six weeks. By a plasma concentration of circa 200 ng/ml, olanzapine's receptor occupancy curve for dopamine D_2 receptors has become very flat, such that doubling the drug's plasma concentration would increase receptor occupancy by only an additional 2–3%. An approach to a choice of a principle medication trial is outlined below in Table 1.3.

Table 1.3 Principal Medication Choice (Excluding Elderly Demented) [4, 20, 21]

Decisions	Assessments	Brief Comments
Patient responding to optimal treatment • Yes, continue • No, adjust treatment	Patient's frequency and severity of problem behaviors are improving with adequate dose and plasma concentration, then continue present treatment	Note that although no response by weeks four to six of adequate to high-dose treatment portends a poor outcome, many patients show ongoing improvement for many weeks to months following a favorable, albeit partial, response to early treatment
Patient response absent • Yes, check adherence • No, consider alternate treatment	Patient has demonstrated an inadequate response in problem behavior's frequency or severity to present antipsychotic treatment • Adherent to oral medications • Not adherent to oral medications	• Preferred oral agents: olanzapine; fluphenazine; haloperidol • Preferred long-acting injectable agents: fluphenazine; haloperidol; paliperidone
Plasma concentrations are adequate • Yes, continue • No, adjust dosing or switch to depot	Dosing and plasma concentrations (oral medications)	• Olanzapine: 40–60 mg/d with plasma concentration 120–150 ng/ml • Fluphenazine: 20–60 mg/d with plasma concentration of 0.8–2.0 ng/ml • Haloperidol: 20–80 mg/d with plasma concentration of 5–18 ng/ml
Plasma concentrations are adequate • Yes, continue • No, adjust dosing	Dosing and plasma concentrations (depot medications)	• Fluphenazine: 25–100 mg/14d with plasma concentration of 0.8–2.0 ng/ml • Haloperidol: 200–300 mg/28d after loading with 200–300 mg weekly times three with steady state plasma concentrations 5–18 ng/ml • Paliperidone: 234 mg followed one week by 156 mg then continuing at 117–234 mg every 28d

Note that some patients may require higher than cited antipsychotic plasma concentrations to achieve stabilization, e.g. haloperidol up to 18 ng/ml or fluphenazine up to 4.0 ng/ml.

① Geriatric Patients Due to risks of increased mortality among elderly patients suffering from neurocognitive disorders on antipsychotic exposure, starting with less dangerous alternatives and progressing toward antipsychotic treatment only as forced by failure of safer treatments is prudent [7]. An approach to the elderly demented patient who develops problematic behaviors related to positive psychotic symptoms is shown below in Table 1.4.

Table 1.4 Principal Medication Choice in Major Neurocognitive Disorder with Severe Psychosis [4]

Decisions	Assessments	Brief Comments
Antipsychotic precautions • Yes, consider alternatives • No, treatment with antipsychotic	Patient has increased risk with antipsychotics • Elderly • Vascular disease • Dementia with Lewy bodies • Parkinson's disease • Huntington's disease	
Increased risk with antipsychotics • Yes, select alternative • No, continue	Pharmacological alternatives to antipsychotics in patients with major cognitive disorders • Lithium • Valproic acid • Clonidine • Guanfacine • Memantine • Prazosin • SSRI antidepressant • Trazodone	
Alternative effective • Yes, continue • No, choose recommended antipsychotic	Evidence-based antipsychotics • Aripiprazole • Clozapine • Olanzapine • Quetiapine • Risperidone	• Antipsychotics increase mortality risk by 1.5- to 2.0-fold among elderly demented patients but may be worthwhile if alternative choices to control problem behaviors or violence are ineffective • For major cognitive disorder with Lewy bodies or Parkinson's disease, aripiprazole, clozapine and quetiapine appeared to be the best tolerated antipsychotics if pimavanserin is ineffective

SSRI: selective serotonin reuptake inhibitors.

Some authors have suggested tapering and discontinuing antipsychotic medications after major neurocognitive disorders have stabilized or progressed and/or to periodically test whether the prior antipsychotic dose is required to maintain stability. Given mortality risks in elderly demented patients, begin with the least dangerous options and progress to more dangerous options only as forced by treatment failure.

⑬ Adjunctive Medications In many cases of severe psychotic illness even optimal antipsychotic treatment may not adequately address all the patient's target symptoms. In this context, while the effect sizes of adjunctive treatments are modest, they may exert important effects on specific illness domains [8]. An outline of the approach to the use of adjunctive medications is given below in Table 1.5.

Table 1.5 Adjunctive Medications [20, 22]

Decisions	Assessments	Brief Comments
Mood stabilizers	• Irritability • Mood lability • Suicidality (lithium)	• VPA can be loaded at 20–30 mg/kg, reaching steady state at circa three days. • Lithium can be initiated at 600 mg once per day and titrated by 300 mg every other day to 900–1200 mg once per day. Lithium also can be loaded at 30 mg/kg up to 3000 mg by giving three ER doses at 1600, 1800 and 2000 hours on day one and then measuring a plasma concentration the following morning. If the plasma concentration is < 1.0 meq/l, then give 1200 mg IR q bedtime. If the plasma concentration is > 1.0 meq/l, then give 900 mg IR q bedtime. Once per day dosing spares renal function. Plasma concentrations should be 0.6–1.0 meq/l. • Lamotrigine may be helpful for dysphoric or negative symptoms but may promote hypomania or mania.
Clonazepam	• Agitation or anxiety incompletely responsive to primary treatment	Dose at 0.5–2.0 mg TID and then taper as the patient stabilizes. Avoid use in major neurocognitive disorders.
Selective serotonin reuptake inhibitor antidepressants	• Residual negative symptoms • Impulsive behavior or suicidality	Avoid use in patients in whom bipolarity may be present. May increase irritability in brain injured or autism patients. Avoid use of fluvoxamine with clozapine or olanzapine, as fluvoxamine may increase clozapine or olanzapine plasma concentrations five- to ten-fold.
Sedatives	• Insomnia worsens irritability, dysphoria, agitation and mood lability in many patients • Consider trials of zolpidem 5–10 mg at bedtime, eszopiclone 1–8 mg at bedtime, hydroxyzine 100 mg at bedtime, diphenhydramine 25–50 mg at bedtime or trazodone 25–100 mg at bedtime until the patient stabilizes	Note that antihistamines may cause idiosyncratic excitation and agitation and that diphenhydramine, but not hydroxyzine, will add to anticholinergic burden
Beta blockers	• Propranolol has excellent CNS penetration and the most evidence for response • ECT	Propranolol contraindicated in those with asthma. Monitor blood pressure to avoid hypotension. If adjunctive medications fail, then ECT should be considered. This is especially true if the patient is taking clozapine and continues to have inadequate response

CNS: central nervous system; ECT: electroconvulsive therapy.

⑤ Pro Re Nata Medications While a patient's routine treatment regimen is expected to be the mainstay of pharmacological treatment, fluctuations in symptom severity or behavior may require as needed or PRN medications. This is especially true early in treatment prior to achieving an optimal response from the patient's routine psychopharmacological treatment. Principles and practice in using PRN or STAT medications are described below in Table 1.6.

Table 1.6 PRN and STAT Medications [23]

Decisions	Assessments	Brief Comments
Patient unstable • No, continue • Yes, provide frequent PRN or STAT treatment	Estimate severity of agitation • Mild • Moderate • Severe	• For mild agitation, give lorazepam 1–2 mg or hydroxyzine 25–50 mg PO or IM every two hours not to exceed four doses per 24 hours. Titrate against agitation based on observation, not patient complaint. • For moderate to severe agitation, give antipsychotic ± lorazepam 2 mg ± diphenhydramine 25–50 mg or hydroxyzine 25–50 mg PO or IM not to exceed four doses per 24 hours. (See caveats following table.)
Stability improved • No, continue frequent PRN or STAT medications and adjust primary treatment • Yes, simplify PRN and STAT treatment and eventually discontinue	Estimate frequency of breakthrough agitation • Seldom • Moderately frequent • Very frequent	As determined by frequency and severity of breakthrough psychomotor agitation, gradually increase PRN dose interval and reduce the number of medications or doses prescribed. Once agitation is controlled, discontinue PRN orders for agitation.

Caveats: Whenever possible choose an antipsychotic that also is being used as part of the primary treatment. Available dose forms may limit this option.

The most commonly prescribed PRN and STAT antipsychotics are haloperidol, fluphenazine, chlorpromazine, olanzapine and risperidone. Of these, haloperidol, fluphenazine, chlorpromazine, olanzapine and ziprasidone are available in oral and injectable formulations.

Haloperidol and fluphenazine carry the highest risks of acute neurological adverse effects, especially given parenterally. Chlorpromazine carries a risk of orthostasis. Olanzapine is not effective orally due to an absorption time to peak plasma concentration of six to nine hours. Olanzapine, especially at higher parenteral doses, is prone to cause severe orthostasis if combined with a benzodiazepine, usually lorazepam. Intramuscular ziprasidone should be limited to two doses of 20 mg per 24 hours, especially if given in addition to oral ziprasidone.

Diphenhydramine, but not hydroxyzine, adds to anticholinergic burden.

Limit doses of potent dopamine antagonists in Parkinson's disease and major cognitive disorder with Lewy bodies. Limit benzodiazepine and anticholinergic use in all major neurocognitive disorders.

⊕ Treatment Resistance An important issue among individuals suffering from psychotic severe mental illness is that a substantial portion of such patients are treatment resistant [9]. John Kane et al. defined treatment-resistant schizophrenia according to very stringent criteria. These included failures of three antipsychotic trials of at least six weeks duration at doses of at least 1000 mg chlorpromazine equivalents, absence of any period of good functioning during the prior five years, and failure of a prospective high-dose (haloperidol 60 mg per day or greater) trial to produce a significant reduction in psychotic signs and symptoms [10]. Because the criteria created by Kane et al. are difficult to complete outside a research setting, treatment resistance has more recently been redefined as failure of two six-week trials of antipsychotic medications from two different classes at least 600 mg chlorpromazine equivalents. If one of the antipsychotics was a long-acting injectable formulation, then the trial duration should have been four months. One check of plasma concentration, as well as two other measures of medication adherence were defined as a minimal requirement. Optimal assurance of medication adherence was held to include two measurements of plasma concentration separated by at least two weeks without informing the patient prior to laboratory sampling [6].

The development of treatment resistance is of critical importance because the vast majority of antipsychotic medications become largely ineffective in this context. That is, response rates to almost all antipsychotic medications are 0–5% in treatment-resistant psychosis. High plasma concentration olanzapine does slightly better at 7%. Fortunately, in treatment-resistant psychotic patients clozapine at plasma concentrations of 350 ng/ml to circa 1000 ng/ml produces a decrease in psychotic signs and symptoms of at least 20–30% in up to 60% of such patients [10, 11]. Even clozapine, however, begins to show a decline in efficacy after resistant psychosis has been ongoing for > 2.8 years, arguing strongly for not delaying clozapine treatment among patients determined to be treatment resistant [12].

⊚ Summary Points

- Positive psychotic symptoms are frequently the cause of institutionalization or incarceration for complex severely mentally ill psychotic patients.
- Positive psychotic symptoms are driven by dopaminergic overactivity in the meso-limbic circuit, making dopamine antagonist antipsychotics the first step in treatment.
- Failure to respond to two adequate dopamine antagonist antipsychotic trials should strongly prompt consideration of treatment with clozapine.
- Even clozapine's superior antipsychotic efficacy begins to fade after about 2.8 years of treatment-resistant status, indicating that use of clozapine should not be delayed in such cases.

References

1. Kaneko, K. (2018). Negative symptoms and cognitive impairments in schizophrenia: two key symptoms negatively influencing social functioning. *Yonago Acta Med*, 61, 91–102.
2. Dack, C., Ross, J., Papadopoulos, C., et al. (2013). A review and meta-analysis of the patient factors associated with psychiatric in-patient aggression. *Acta Psychiatr Scand*, 127, 255–268.
3. Quanbeck, C. D., McDermott, B. E., Lam, J., et al. (2007). Categorization of aggressive acts committed by chronically assaultive state hospital patients. *Psychiatr Serv*, 58, 521–528.
4. Stahl, S. M., Morrissette, D. A., Cummings, M., et al. (2014). California State Hospital Violence Assessment and Treatment (Cal-VAT) guidelines. *CNS Spectr*, 19, 449–465.
5. Merritt, K., McGuire, P., Egerton, A. (2013). Relationship between glutamate dysfunction and symptoms and cognitive function in psychosis. *Front Psychiatry*, 4, 151.
6. Howes, O. D., McCutcheon, R., Agid, O., et al. (2017). Treatment-resistant schizophrenia: treatment response and resistance in psychosis (TRRIP) working group consensus guidelines on diagnosis and terminology. *Am J Psychiatry*, 174, 216–229.
7. Maust, D. T., Kim, H. M., Seyfried, L. S., et al. (2015). Antipsychotics, other psychotropics, and the risk of death in patients with dementia: number needed to harm. *JAMA Psychiatry*, 72, 438–445.
8. Galling, B., Roldan, A., Hagi, K., et al. (2017). Antipsychotic augmentation vs. monotherapy in schizophrenia: systematic review, meta-analysis and meta-regression analysis. *World Psychiatry*, 16, 77–89.
9. Nucifora, F. C., Jr., Woznica, E., Lee, B. J., et al. (2018). Treatment resistant schizophrenia: clinical, biological, and therapeutic perspectives. *Neurobiol Dis*, 131, 104–257.
10. Kane, J., Honigfeld, G., Singer, J., et al. (1988). Clozapine for the treatment-resistant schizophrenic. a double-blind comparison with chlorpromazine. *Arch Gen Psychiatry*, 45, 789–796.
11. Stroup, T. S., Gerhard, T., Crystal, S., et al. (2016). Comparative effectiveness of clozapine and standard antipsychotic treatment in adults with schizophrenia. *Am J Psychiatry*, 173, 166–173.
12. Yoshimura, B., Yada, Y., So, R., et al. (2017). The critical treatment window of clozapine in treatment-resistant schizophrenia: secondary analysis of an observational study. *Psychiatry Res*, 250, 65–70.
13. Ogloff, J. R., Daffern, M. (2006). The dynamic appraisal of situational aggression: an instrument to assess risk for imminent aggression in psychiatric inpatients. *Behav Sci Law*, 24, 799–813.
14. Hankin, C. S., Bronstone, A., Koran, L. M. (2011). Agitation in the inpatient psychiatric setting: a review of clinical presentation, burden, and treatment. *J Psychiatr Pract*, 17, 170–185.
15. Vaaler, A. E., Iversen, V. C., Morken, G., et al. (2011). Short-term prediction of threatening and violent behaviour in an Acute Psychiatric Intensive Care Unit based on patient and environment characteristics. *BMC Psychiatry*, 11, 44.
16. Volavka, J., Citrome, L. (2011). Pathways to aggression in schizophrenia affect results of treatment. *Schizophr Bull*, 37, 921–929.
17. Joshi, A., Krishnamurthy, V. B., Purichia, H., et al. (2012). "What's in a name?" Delirium by any other name would be as deadly. A review of the nature of delirium consultations. *J Psychiatr Pract*, 18, 413–418.
18. Ruberg, S. J., Chen, L., Stauffer, V., et al. (2011). Identification of early changes in specific symptoms that predict longer-term response to atypical antipsychotics in the treatment of patients with schizophrenia. *BMC Psychiatry*, 11, 23.
19. Lopez, L. V., Kane, J. M. (2013). Plasma levels of second-generation antipsychotics and clinical response in acute psychosis: a review of the literature. *Schizophr Res*, 147, 368–374.
20. Meyer, J. M., Cummings, M. A., Proctor, G., et al. (2016). Psychopharmacology of persistent violence and aggression. *Psychiatr Clin North Am*, 39, 541–556.
21. Siskind, D., Siskind, V., Kisely, S. (2017). Clozapine response rates among people with treatment-resistant schizophrenia: data from a systematic review and meta-analysis. *Can J Psychiatry*, 62, 772–777.
22. Lally, J., Tully, J., Robertson, D., et al. (2016). Augmentation of clozapine with electroconvulsive therapy in treatment resistant schizophrenia: a systematic review and meta-analysis. *Schizophr Res*, 171, 215–224.
23. Stein-Parbury, J., Reid, K., Smith, N., et al. (2008). Use of pro re nata medications in acute inpatient care. *Aust N Z J Psychiatry*, 42, 283–292.

1.02 Use of Plasma Levels in Antipsychotic and Mood Stabilizer Treatment

📖 **Introduction** Antipsychotic medications represent the pharmacological foundation for the treatment of psychosis and psychomotor agitation. While antipsychotics may be prescribed based on accepted dose ranges, as well as patient response and tolerability, measuring plasma concentrations of antipsychotic medications now represents the standard of care [1].

Ⓐ **Uses of Plasma Concentrations** There are several stages of treatment when steady state plasma antipsychotic levels may be most useful: when the patient has an optimal drug response to benchmark the drug level(s); when adverse effects arise at low doses (e.g. as might be seen with poor metabolizers); when no adverse effects or efficacy are seen at standard doses to help rule out kinetic failure (due to ultrarapid metabolism) or adherence issues; or when there is decompensation or behavior change in a previously stable patient.

Ⓑ **Principles for Using Plasma Concentrations** There are several important principles to consider when using antipsychotic plasma level measurements [2]. The minimum level defines a response threshold below which one is unlikely to find adequate response, although there are always exceptions. If there is inadequate response and no tolerability issues once the minimum level is exceeded, the antipsychotic should be titrated until one of three endpoints is reached: intolerability; maximum level; or positive treatment response.

If levels above the maximum plasma level cited here (of the upper limit of the laboratory range) are obtained, do not reflexively reduce medication doses; first document whether the patient is tolerating the particular plasma level. If there is suspicion of laboratory error, the level should be repeated. If the repeat level remains above the maximum level, one should investigate whether the patient needs this high level for response. If the patient does not need such a high serum level, the dose should be reduced by no more than 5% per month to prevent unmasking super-sensitivity psychosis or other rebound effects. Please see Table 2.1 below regarding optimal antipsychotic plasma concentration ranges [3].

Table 2.1 Antipsychotic Levels and Expected Plasma Levels (in ng/ml) for Given Oral Doses [5]

Medication	Minimum Response Threshold	Point of Futility
Aripiprazole expected level = 11 x oral dose (mg/d)	110 ng/ml	500 ng/ml
Clozapine male nonsmoker – expected level = 1.08 x oral dose (mg/d) female nonsmoker – expected level = 1.32 x oral dose (mg/d)	350 ng/ml	1000 ng/ml
Fluphenazine nonsmoker – expected level = 0.8–1.0 x oral dose (mg/d)	0.8 ng/ml	4.0 ng/ml

Table 2.1 (Cont.)

Medication	Minimum Response Threshold	Point of Futility
Haloperidol expected level = 0.78 x oral dose (mg/d)	2.0 ng/ml	18 ng/ml
Olanzapine nonsmoker – expected level = 2.0 x oral dose (mg/d)	23 ng/ml	150 ng/ml
Paliperidone expected level = 4.09 x oral dose (mg/d)	20 ng/ml	90 ng/ml
Risperidone + 9-OH Risperidone expected level = 7.0 x oral dose (mg/d)	28 ng/ml	112 ng/ml
Perphenazine expected level = 0.04 x oral dose (mg/d)	0.8 ng/ml	5.0 ng/ml

❸ **Mood Stabilizers** Mood stabilizer medications represent the pharmacological foundation for treatment of bipolar disorders and additional indications, such as impulsivity and affective lability, may be found in patients across diagnoses. Analogous to antipsychotic use above, there are principles to consider when using mood stabilizer level measurements.

For lithium and divalproex, different plasma concentration levels are used for acute symptoms versus for maintenance. For sicker patients, it is recommended that maintenance levels be no lower than the midpoint of the maintenance range cited in the literature. For lithium: chronic maintenance lithium levels greater than 1.0 meq/l incur greater risk for renal dysfunction and should only be used transiently. For acute mania, levels up to 1.4 meq/l may be necessary. Once the patient is euthymic and stable, the level can be gradually lowered [4]. For divalproex: because valproic acid is > 90% protein-bound, chronic maintenance VPA levels should fall between 80–120 mcg/ml. For acute mania, VPA levels in the upper portion of the therapeutic range (100–120 mcg/ml) may be necessary. Once mood stabilization is achieved, the level can be gradually lowered [5].

The use of carbamazepine is strongly discouraged for several reasons: it will lower plasma antipsychotic levels by 50–80%, thereby endangering the patient and others if antipsychotic levels are not appropriately adjusted within 10–14 days of starting carbamazepine [5]. Moreover, it is less effective than lithium or VPA, and it carries a risk of hyponatremia [6].

Importantly, oxcarbazepine should never be used as a mood stabilizer for several reasons: it is ineffective for acute mania and for inpatient aggression. There is no long-term data on suicidality reduction or risk for mania relapse; there is no defined dose or serum level range; and it carries a greater risk for hyponatremia than carbamazepine [7]. Please see Table 2.2 regarding optimal plasma concentrations for selected mood stabilizers.

Table 2.2 Plasma Levels of Effective Mood Stabilizers [5]

| Mood Stabilizer | Plasma concentration of mood stabilizer | |
	Acute Mania	Maintenance
Lithium	1.0–1.4 meq/l	0.8–1.2 meq/l (see #2 under Mood Stabilizers)
Divalproex valproic acid	100–120 mcg/ml	80–120 mcg/ml
Carbamazepine	9–12 mcg/ml	6–12 mcg/ml

Importantly, chronic exposure to maintenance lithium plasma concentrations > 1.0 meq/l may increase the long-term risk of renal insufficiency.

⊚ Summary Points

• Use of plasma antipsychotic and mood stabilizer levels which correlate much more tightly with relevant receptor occupancies than the prescribed dose of a medication could afford an individual approach for each patient, resulting in better control of symptoms.
• Lithium and divalproex are excellent mood stabilizers for both acute mania and maintenance. Lithium also exerts modest antidepressant properties.
• Oxcarbazepine is not a mood stabilizer.

1.02 Use of Plasma Levels in Antipsychotic and Mood Stabilizer (Continued)

References

1. Schoretsanitis, G., Kane, J. M., Correll, C. U., et al. (2020). Blood levels to optimize antipsychotic treatment in clinical practice: a joint consensus statement of the American Society of Clinical Psychopharmacology and the Therapeutic Drug Monitoring Task Force of the Arbeitsgemeinschaft für Neuropsychopharmakologie und Pharmakopsychiatrie. *J Clin Psychiatry*, 81(3), 19CS13169.
2. Meyer, J. M. (2014). A rational approach to employing high plasma levels of antipsychotics for violence associated with schizophrenia: case vignettes. *CNS Spectr*, 19, 432–438.
3. Meyer, J. M., Cummings, M. A., Proctor, G., et al. (2016). Psychopharmacology of persistent violence and aggression. *Psychiatr Clin North Am*, 39, 541–556.
4. Castro, V. M., Roberson, A. M., McCoy, T. H., et al. (2016). Stratifying risk for renal insufficiency among lithium-treated patients: an electronic health record study. *Neuropsychopharmacol*, 41, 1138–1143.
5. Meyer, J. M. (2018). *Gilman: The Pharmacological Basis of Therapeutics. Pharmacotherapy of Psychosis and Mania.* New York: McGraw-Hill.
6. Letmaier, M., Painold, A., Holl, A. K., et al. (2012). Hyponatraemia during psychopharmacological treatment: results of a drug surveillance programme. *Int J Neuropsychopharmacol*, 15, 739–748.
7. Kim, Y-S., Kim, D. W., Jung, K-H., et al. (2014). Frequency of and risk factors for oxcarbazepine-induced severe and symptomatic hyponatremia. *Seizure*, 23, 208–212.

1.03 Advantages of Long-Acting Injectable Antipsychotics

🔖 **Introduction** Schizophrenia spectrum and other psychotic disorders afflict the bulk of chronically mentally ill individuals [1]. Thus, antipsychotic medications form the core of pharmacological treatment in complex treatment-resistant populations [2].

Unfortunately, adherence to oral antipsychotics in outpatient settings, even when defined as taking only 80% of prescribed doses, is consistently less than 50% [3, 4]. Due to enhanced adherence, long-acting injectable (LAI) antipsychotics have proven superior to their oral counterparts in reducing crime and violence, as well as in increasing longevity [5–8].

Despite their demonstrated superiority to oral antipsychotics in several areas relevant to chronically mentally ill populations (e.g. improving treatment adherence with a consequential decrease in violence), LAI antipsychotics remain underutilized [9, 10].

Ⓐ **Long-Acting Injectable Initiation** Key to successful employment of LAI antipsychotics are strategies for their initiation [11]. Please see Table 3.1 below regarding initiation strategies for LAI antipsychotics.

Table 3.1 Long-Acting Injectable Antipsychotic Initiation Strategies [11]

Medication	Comments on Initiation
Aripiprazole	Dosing of aripiprazole monohydrate is initiated at either 300 mg or 400 mg intramuscularly every 28 days with continuation of oral aripiprazole 10–20 mg for the first 14 days after the initial injection. Aripiprazole monohydrate 300 mg q 28 days produces on average plasma concentrations comparable to aripiprazole 15 mg per day orally, while 400 mg q 28 days produces plasma concentrations on average comparable to 20 mg orally per day. Aripiprazole lauroxil is initiated at 441 mg q four weeks, 662 mg q four weeks, 882 mg q four or six weeks, or 1064 mg q eight weeks, with the three higher doses requiring gluteal administration. In lieu of oral coverage, patients can be given a single 30 mg dose of oral aripiprazole and a 675 mg IM injection of aripiprazole lauroxil nanocrystal suspension on the same day (or up to 10 days thereafter) the first dose of aripiprazole lauroxil is administered. If the patient refuses the aripiprazole lauroxil nanocrystal injection, then oral aripiprazole must be continued for the first 21 days of aripiprazole lauroxil treatment. Aripiprazole monohydrate and aripiprazole lauroxil have different half-lives, so consult the package insert for the missed dose guidelines. These formulations also have different rules for adjustments based on use of cyp P450 2D6 or 3A4 inhibitors. Aripiprazole monohydrate cannot be used with CYP3A4 inducers, but aripiprazole lauroxil can. For either formulation, response to oral aripiprazole at a dose of 20 mg per day should be established by a clear history of response or a prospective six- to eight-week trial.

Fluphenazine	For each 10 mg of oral fluphenazine per day, prescribe 12.5–25 mg of fluphenazine decanoate IM q week times three and then continue every two weeks at 12.5 mg to a maximum of 100 mg as guided by plasma concentration measurements. Optimal for most patients is 0.8–2.0 ng/ml. Some more treatment-resistant patients may require plasma concentrations of 2.0–4.0 ng/ml. Note that fluphenazine decanoate exhibits both an immediate and delayed release from its vehicle, requiring initial reduction or discontinuation of oral dosing in some individuals to avoid post-injection emergence of neurologic adverse effects.
Haloperidol	Because haloperidol decanoate has little immediate-release phase, a loading dose strategy is required to avoid the need for prolonged co-administration of an oral antipsychotic. That is, administration at a fixed dose would require three to five months to reach steady state. Give 100–300 mg IM q one-week times two to three doses. For each 100 mg used in loading the average steady state plasma concentration is 7.75 ng/ml. Measurement of a plasma concentration before the third loading dose will assist in determining whether the third loading dose is needed. Measurement of a plasma concentration shortly before the first maintenance dose will be helpful in fine tuning ongoing dosing. Optimal for most patients is 5 ng/ml to 15 ng/ml. A few more treatment-resistant patients may require plasma concentrations of 30 to up to 18 ng/ml to 30 ng/ml. Adverse neurological effects become more frequent at plasma concentrations > 20 ng/ml. Maintenance dosing should begin 14 days after the last loading injection. For maintenance, give on average 100 mg q four weeks per 5 mg of the prior oral haloperidol daily dose. If the maintenance dose exceeds 300 mg, then divide the dose and administer every 14 days, as the maximum injectable volume is 3 ml.
Olanzapine	Long-acting injectable olanzapine is available in 150 mg, 210 mg, 300 mg and 405 mg doses. Oral equivalents have not been established. There is no need for oral cross-over or loading. Note, however, that there is a circa 0.1% risk of delirium, obtundation and coma follows each dose. Direct nursing observation is required for a minimum of three hours following each injection.
Paliperidone	Give an initial dose of 234 mg followed by a second initiation dose of 156 mg after one week. The initial two doses should be deltoid. Maintenance doses may be deltoid or gluteal. The modal maintenance dose is 117 mg q 4 weeks, with a dose range of 39 mg to 234 mg. A dose of 234 mg per month produces 9-hydroxy risperidone plasma concentrations comparable to 4–5 mg of oral risperidone per day (risperidone + 9-hydroxy risperidone). Oral risperidone or paliperidone is not required after the initiation phase. Paliperidone palmitate three-month extended-release is restricted to patients who have received effective and stable treatment with paliperidone palmitate monthly formulation for a minimum of four months. At the time the next dose of paliperidone palmitate monthly formulation would be due, give the equivalent dose of paliperidone palmitate extended-release.

Table 3.1 (Cont.)

Medication	Comments on Initiation
Risperidone	Initiate risperidone microspheres at 25–50 mg IM q two weeks, while continuing oral risperidone treatment. After three weeks have passed since the initial injection, taper and discontinue oral risperidone treatment. Each 25 mg of risperidone microspheres produces plasma concentrations of risperidone + 9-hydroxy risperidone comparable to 2–3 mg of oral risperidone. Risperidone is also available in a subcutaneous LAI formulation that can be given in abdominal subcutaneous injections of 90 mg (0.6 ml) or 120 mg (0.8 ml), achieving plasma concentrations comparable to 3 mg or 4 mg of oral risperidone, respectively, at about one week, obviating the need for oral cross-over. Injections of this formulation are monthly. A higher dose of risperidone subcutaneous LAI equivalent to 6 mg oral risperidone is being studied.

Derived from the 2019 California DSH Psychotropic Medication Policy, Chapter 9, "Depot Antipsychotics", and from package inserts for: Abilify Maintena, Aristada, Aristada Initio, Risperdal Consta, Invega Sustenna, Invega Trinza, Perseris and Relprevv.

❸ Long-Acting Injectable Antipsychotic Kinetics Partial dopamine agonists such as aripiprazole may be more effective in patients in whom the negative and cognitive domains of psychosis are more prominent, while dopamine antagonist antipsychotics may be more effective in controlling positive psychotic symptoms [10, 12, 13]. As positive psychotic symptoms are often the gateway (e.g. via persecutory delusion associated with anger) to arrest and criminalization or chronic institutionalization for the mentally ill, utilization of LAI dopamine antagonist antipsychotics should be considered as the first-line option [2, 10].

Beyond initiation, understanding the pharmacokinetics of each formulation in relation to its optimal plasma concentration and receptor occupancy is critical to effective use of LAI antipsychotics [11, 14, 15]. Table 3.2 provides kinetic information on LAI antipsychotics.

Table 3.2 Kinetics of Long-Acting Injectable Antipsychotics [16–19]

Drug	Vehicle	Dosage	T_{max}	$T_{1/2}$ Multiple Dosing	Able to Be Loaded
Fluphenazine decanoate	Sesame oil	12.5–100 mg/2 weeks	0.3–1.5 days	14 days	Yes
Haloperidol decanoate	Sesame oil	25–600 mg/4 weeks	3–9 days	21 days	Yes
Risperidone subcutaneous (Perseris®)	Water	90–120 mg/ 4 weeks	4–6 hours ~ 8 days	9–11 days	Not needed
Risperidone microspheres (Risperdal Consta®)	Water	12.5–50 mg/2 weeks	21 days	3–6 days	No (21–28 days oral overlap)

Paliperidone palmitate (Invega Sustenna®)	Water	39–234 mg/4 weeks	13 days	25–49 days	Yes
Paliperidone palmitate (3 months) (Invega Trinza®)*	Water	273–819 mg/12 weeks	84 – 95 days (deltoid) 118–139 days (gluteal)	30–33 days	No
Olanzapine pamoate (Zyprexa Relprevv®)**	Water	150–300 mg/2 weeks 300–405 mg/4 weeks	7 days	30 days	Yes
Aripiprazole monohydrate (Abilify Maintena®)	Water	300–400 mg/4 weeks	6.5–7.1 days	29.9–46.5 days	Maybe (14 days oral overlap)
Aripiprazole lauroxil (Aristada®)***	Water	441 mg, 662 mg 882 mg/4 weeks 882 mg/6 weeks 1064 mg/8 weeks	41 days (single dose) [18] 24.4–35.2 days (repeated dosing) [18]	53.9–57.2 days	No (Start with AL$_{NCD}$ 675 mg IM+30 mg oral OR 21 days oral overlap)
Aripiprazole lauroxil nanocrystal (Aristada Initio®)****	Water	675 mg once	27 days (range: 16–35 days)	15–18 days (single dose)	no

* Only for those on paliperidone palmitate monthly for four months.

** See US FDA bulletin, available at: https://www.accessdata.fda.gov/drugsatfda_docs/label/2009/022173lbl.pdf

*** Twenty-one days oral overlap unless starting with aripiprazole lauroxil nanocrystal + single 30 mg oral dose.

**** Aripiprazole lauroxil nanocrystal (AL$_{NCD}$) is only used for initiation of treatment with aripiprazole lauroxil, or for resumption of treatment. It is always administered together with aripiprazole lauroxil, although the latter can be given up to 10 days after the aripiprazole lauroxil nanocrystal injection.

ⓔ Use of Plasma Concentrations As noted, the second element to optimal use of LAI antipsychotics is understanding use of plasma concentrations of the prescribed medication. Please see Table 3.3 regarding core concepts in using plasma concentrations, as well as Chapter 2 regarding monitoring of medication plasma concentrations.

Table 3.3 Core Concepts in Using Plasma Concentrations [19]

Concept	Definition
Therapeutic Threshold	The plasma level below which response rates are low (but not zero).
	Example: In a clinical trial of haloperidol, the response rate for levels < 2 mg/ml was 9% compared to 73% for levels 5–12 ng/ml [16].
Tolerability Threshold	The plasma level at which 80% of patients have intolerable adverse effects.
	Example: In a clinical trial of fluphenazine, 80% of subjects with a plasma level of 2.72 ng/ml manifested intolerable adverse effects [16].
Point of Futility	Some schizophrenia patients may not develop parkinsonism, akathisia, dystonia or other dose-limiting adverse effects despite doses that significantly exceed the tolerability threshold.
	Example: Based on clinical trials data and clinical experience, the chances of responding to a plasma fluphenazine level > 4.0 ng/ml are virtually nil, yet plasma levels as high as 16 ng/ml have been reported in the literature [17, 20].

ⓒ Summary Points
- Dopamine antagonist antipsychotics form the basis of treatment for those afflicted with illness dominated by positive psychotic signs and symptoms.
- Adherence to oral antipsychotics is < 50%, such that corresponding LAI antipsychotics are more effective than their oral counterparts, improving survival by circa 30%.
- The key to using LAI antipsychotics lies in understanding their kinetics and using plasma concentrations to guide treatment.

References

1. Gottfried, E. D., Christopher, S. C. (2017). Mental disorders among criminal offenders: a review of the literature. *J Correct Health Care*, 23, 336–346.
2. Cummings, M. A., Proctor, G. J., Arias, A. W. (2020). Dopamine antagonist antipsychotics in diverted forensic populations. *CNS Spectr*, 25, 128–135.
3. de Haan, L., Lavalaye, J., van Bruggen, M., et al. (2004). Subjective experience and dopamine D2 receptor occupancy in patients treated with antipsychotics: clinical implications. *Can J Psychiatry*, 49, 290–296.
4. Garcia, S., Martinez-Cengotitabengoa, M., Lopez-Zurbano, S., et al. (2016). Adherence to antipsychotic medication in bipolar disorder and schizophrenic patients: a systematic review. *J Clin Psychopharmacol*, 36, 355–371.
5. Ostuzzi, G., Barbui, C. (2016). Comparative effectiveness of long-acting antipsychotics: issues and challenges from a pragmatic randomised study. *Epidemiol Psychiatr Sci*, 25, 21–23.
6. Stevens, G. L., Dawson, G., Zummo, J. (2016). Clinical benefits and impact of early use of long-acting injectable antipsychotics for schizophrenia. *Early Interv Psychiatry*, 10, 365–377.
7. Mohr, P., Knytl, P., Vorackova, V., et al. (2017). Long-acting injectable antipsychotics for prevention and management of violent behaviour in psychotic patients. *Int J Clin Pract*, 71, 1–7.
8. Taipale, H., Mittendorfer-Rutz, E., Alexanderson, K., et al. (2018). Antipsychotics and mortality in a nationwide cohort of 29,823 patients with schizophrenia. *Schizophr Res*, 197, 274–280.
9. Marcus, S. C., Zummo, J., Pettit, A. R., et al. (2015). Antipsychotic adherence and rehospitalization in schizophrenia patients receiving oral versus long-acting injectable antipsychotics following hospital discharge. *J Manag Care Spec Pharm*, 21, 754–768.
10. Cummings, M. A., Proctor, G. J., Arias, A. W. (2019). Dopamine antagonist antipsychotics in diverted forensic populations. *CNS Spectr,* in press. doi: 10.1017/S1092852919000841
11. Meyer, J. M. (2017). Converting oral to long-acting injectable antipsychotics: a guide for the perplexed. *CNS Spectr*, 22, 14–28.
12. Lieberman, J. A. (2004). Dopamine partial agonists: a new class of antipsychotic. *CNS Drugs*, 18, 251–267.
13. Stip, E., Tourjman, V. (2010). Aripiprazole in schizophrenia and schizoaffective disorder: a review. *Clin Ther*, 32, S3–20.
14. Park, E. J., Amatya, S., Kim, M. S., et al. (2013). Long-acting injectable formulations of antipsychotic drugs for the treatment of schizophrenia. *Arch Pharm Res*, 36, 651–659.
15. Spanarello, S., La Ferla, T. (2014). The pharmacokinetics of long-acting antipsychotic medications. *Curr Clin Pharmacol*, 9, 310–317.
16. Midha, K. K., Hubbard, J. W., Marder, S. R., et al. (1994). Impact of clinical pharmacokinetics on neuroleptic therapy in patients with schizophrenia. *J Psychiatry Neurosci*, 19, 254–264.
17. Nyberg, S., Dencker, S. J., Malm, U., et al. (1998). D(2)- and 5-HT(2) receptor occupancy in high-dose neuroleptic-treated patients. *Int J Neuropsychopharmacol*, 1, 95–101.
18. Hard, M. L., Mills, R. J., Sadler, B. M., et al. (2017). Aripiprazole lauroxil: pharmacokinetic profile of this long-acting injectable antipsychotic in persons with schizophrenia. *J Clin Psychopharmacol*, 37, 289–295.
19. Meyer, J. M. (2019). Monitoring and improving antipsychotic adherence in outpatient forensic diversion programs. *CNS Spectr*, 25(2), 136–144.
20. Meyer, J. M. (2014). A rational approach to employing high plasma levels of antipsychotics for violence associated with schizophrenia: case vignettes. *CNS Spectr*, 19, 432–438.

1.04 Approach to Treatment-Resistant Schizophrenia Spectrum Patients

📖 **Introduction** Inadequate treatment contributes not only to poor quality of life but also to an increase in disease-related societal burdens. A small subset (20–30%) of the schizophrenia patient population are treatment-resistant and financially cost approximately ten-fold more than non-treatment-resistant schizophrenia patients [1]. Numerous ineffective antipsychotic trials continue to be prescribed while clozapine, which has widespread compelling efficacy data, continues to be underutilized in treatment-resistant schizophrenia. This chapter addresses clozapine efficacy in not only treatment-resistant psychosis but also comorbid suicidality and aggression, as well as treatment-resistant mania. Further, initiation and maintenance of clozapine treatment is summarized.

A Treatment Resistance Defined Kane Criteria were initially used to define treatment resistance [2]. These were:

- At least three periods of treatment in the preceding five years with antipsychotics from at least two different chemical classes at dose equivalents ≥ 1000 mg of chlorpromazine daily for six weeks without significant symptomatic relief
- No period of good functioning within the preceding five years
- Failure to respond to a prospective high-dose trial of a typical antipsychotic (haloperidol at doses of ≥ 60 mg daily administered with benztropine 6 mg daily).

Response was defined as a 20% decrease in BPRS total score plus either a post-treatment CGI severity rating of ≤ 3 (mildly ill) or a post-treatment BPRS ≤ 35. Studies omitting criterion three of the Kane Criteria resulted in overestimation of the efficacy of other antipsychotics due to inclusion of non-resistant cases. This led to the development of the **Consensus Criteria for Treatment Resistance** [3].

These are:
- Six weeks or greater at a therapeutic dosage (dose equivalents to ≥ 600 mg of chlorpromazine per day)
- Two or more past adequate treatment episodes for a duration of six weeks each with different antipsychotic medications. If a long-acting injectable (LAI) antipsychotic was used, the trial was at least four months in duration
- Eighty percent or more of prescribed doses must have been taken (adherence measured with at least two sources such as pill counts, medication administration record and/or patient/caregiver report)
- At minimum, there should be at least one measured antipsychotic plasma level to ascertain for treatment adherence
- Optimally, trough antipsychotic serum levels should be obtained without notifying the patient prior to the blood draws on at least two occasions, which are separated by at least two weeks

❸ Efficacy of Antipsychotic Combination Regimens Tiihonen et al. did a nationwide cohort study in Finland where they found that rational antipsychotic polypharmacy with two different mechanisms of action appears feasible even though current treatment guidelines state that antipsychotic monotherapy should be preferred, and polypharmacy avoided if possible [4]. Additionally, they found that although clozapine monotherapy is associated with the best outcomes in schizophrenia patients, clozapine plus aripiprazole was significantly superior to clozapine monotherapy. This study also indicated that there is double-blind/high-quality evidence supporting efficacy for negative symptom reduction with aripiprazole augmentation of clozapine therapy.

❸ The Gold Standard Failure to achieve a 20–30% reduction in psychotic symptoms in response to adequate dopamine antagonist trials indicates that the patient is treatment-resistant and hence, exhibits a pharmacodynamic failure in response to adequate dopamine antagonism [3].

Most first- and second-generation antipsychotic medications show a response rate of 0–5% among such patients, while high plasma concentration olanzapine (120–200 ng/ml) produces a response rate of about 7% [5]. In contrast, the response rate of treatment-resistant schizophrenia to clozapine is 40–60% [6].

Importantly, as disease course progresses, even clozapine begins to lose its potency after 2.8 years of treatment-resistant status; thus, clozapine treatment should begin as soon as treatment resistance is identified [7]. Hence, clozapine is the gold standard for treatment-resistant schizophrenia. These points are illustrated below in Table 4.1 and Figure 4.1.

Table 4.1 Response Rate to Antipsychotics in Treatment-Resistant Psychosis

ANTIPSYCHOTIC MEDICATION	RESPONSE RATE OF TREATMENT-RESISTANT PSYCHOSIS
FGA, SGA, TGA*	0–5%
Olanzapine	7%
Clozapine	40–60%

* First-, second-, third-generation antipsychotic.

Figure 4.1 Delaying the time to starting clozapine reduces the likelihood of response in resistant schizophrenia [7].

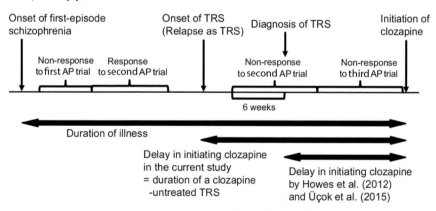

(Example of multiple-episodes patient)

TRS: treatment-resistant schizophrenia.

(Adaptation from Yoshimura, B., Yada, Y., So, R., et al. (2017). The critical treatment window of clozapine in treatment-resistant schizophrenia: secondary analysis of an observational study. *Psychiatry Res*, 250, 65–70.)

ⓓ Suicidality in Schizophrenia Although clozapine and olanzapine had similar reductions in total PANSS scores in 980 non-treatment-resistant patients who were at high risk for suicide in a 24-month prospective, randomized study (InterSePT), clozapine had a superior impact on suicidality; hence, clozapine's effect on suicidality is independent of its antipsychotic effect [8].

Fewer schizophrenia patients treated with clozapine attempted suicide, required hospitalization or rescue interventions as a suicide precaution, or required concomitant antidepressant or anxiolytic/ hypnotic medications. For both Type 1 (significant suicide attempt/hospitalization for imminent suicide risk) and Type 2 (worsening suicidality as measured on the Clinical Global Impression Severity of Suicidality Scale with a rating of "much worse" or "very much worse"), clozapine delayed the time to suicidal event occurrence more than olanzapine; this effect was increasingly magnified over time. Clozapine reduces suicidality in schizophrenia patients. Time to suicidal events is illustrated below in Figure 4.2.

Figure 4.2 Time to suicidal events in the InterSePT Study [1].

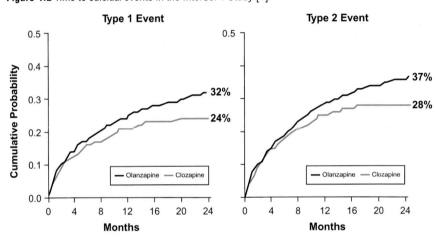

(Adaptation from Meyer, J. M. (2019). *The Clozapine Handbook: Stahl's Handbooks*. New York: Cambridge University Press, pp. 126–127.)

ⓔ Categories of Violence Based on a review of videotaped assaults supplemented with assailant and victim interviews, the New York State Hospital system identified three categories of violence based on the motivation for each act: psychotic, impulsive and predatory [9, 10]. Predatory violence is spurred by secondary gain and requires custodial care rather than pharmacotherapy. Psychotic violence is driven by persistent delusions or hallucinations and is treated with optimized antipsychotic medication regimens, including clozapine for those with treatment-resistant psychosis. Impulsive violence results from inappropriate, disproportionate responses to misperceived, real-world stimuli and may not respond to non-clozapine antipsychotics. Based on a survey of the California Department of State Hospitals, a circa 7000-bed forensic hospital system, the most common category of assault is impulsive (54%); 29% are classified as predatory, while 17% are characterized as psychotic.

ⓕ Aggression in Schizophrenia Standard pharmacological interventions for aggression in untreated or undermedicated schizophrenia patients include antipsychotics without or with mood stabilizers (in the presence of a bipolar diathesis) [9]. A comprehensive 2009 review notes that the risk for violence is elevated in both male and female patients with schizophrenia and is increased by 3.7- to 4.2-fold with concomitant substance use [11, 12]. A 12-week-long randomized, double-blind, parallel-group study of chronically physically assaultive male inpatients with schizophrenia or schizoaffective disorder in the New York State Hospital system were prescribed either clozapine, olanzapine or haloperidol with no significant differences in change in PANSS scores across all three groups; however, clozapine significantly reduced verbal, physical and total aggression scores (Modified Objective Aggression Scale, MOAS) compared to haloperidol or olanzapine due to related improvements in executive functions likely stemming from glutamate modulation in the prefrontal cortex [13]. Because of its anti-aggressive property independent of its effect on psychosis, clozapine is the preferred agent for schizophrenia patients treated with optimal non-clozapine antipsychotics who continue to have impulsive aggression [14]. Studies demonstrating clozapine's anti-aggressive properties and comparative effects on psychotic symptoms are shown below in Table 4.2.

Table 4.2 Summary of Randomized Studies of Clozapine for Aggression in Schizophrenia [1]

	COMMENTS
(Niskanen et al., 1974)	**SAMPLE**: Randomized, double-blind, 40-day trial of clozapine vs. chlorpromazine in 48 patients with chronic schizophrenia, 75% of whom were experiencing acute symptoms or exacerbation of chronic symptoms. **OUTCOMES OF INTEREST**: Change in BPRS score. **RESULTS**: Improvements in tension, hostility and excitement were seen in the clozapine group compared to baseline, with no between group differences in BPRS scores.
(Chow et al., 1996)	**SAMPLE**: Open-label 14-week randomized trial in aggressive inpatients with schizophrenia (n = 12), schizoaffective disorder (n = 2) or dementia with psychotic features (n = 1). Subjects were randomized to clozapine or remaining on their current antipsychotic (i.e. TAU). **OUTCOMES OF INTEREST**: Change in total score on the MOAS. Secondary outcome was change in PANSS total score. **RESULTS**: Aggression scores improved in the clozapine group at week 10 and at week 14 compared to baseline. PANSS total scores did not improve for either group.
(Citrome et al., 2001) (Volavka et al., 2002) (Volavka et al., 2004)	**SAMPLE**: Randomized, double-blind, 14-week trial of clozapine, olanzapine, risperidone or haloperidol in 157 adult inpatients (ages 18–60) with total PANSS ≥60, suboptimal response to treatment and poor functioning over the prior two years. **OUTCOMES OF INTEREST**: Change in PANSS total score, and total aggression severity score. **RESULTS**: Atypical antipsychotics were superior to haloperidol for symptom reduction, and clozapine was superior to haloperidol in reducing the number and severity of aggressive incidents. Risperidone and olanzapine had less antipsychotic efficacy in aggressive patients; the opposite was true for clozapine.

Table 4.2 (Cont.)

	COMMENTS
(Krakowski et al., 2006)	**SAMPLE**: Randomized, double-blind, parallel-group, 12-week trial. Subjects were physically assaultive inpatients with schizophrenia or schizoaffective disorder in New York State psychiatric facilities randomly assigned to clozapine (n = 37), olanzapine (n = 37) or haloperidol (n = 36).
	OUTCOMES OF INTEREST: Changes in total score on the MOAS-30, and the three MOAS-30 subscales (physical aggression against other people, verbal aggression and physical aggression against objects). Nursing staff reported all behaviors on a monitoring form with 30- to 60-minute intervals. Research personnel interviewed the nursing staff after each event.
	RESULTS: There were no significant between-group differences for mean change in PANSS total score. Clozapine was superior to olanzapine for change in MOAS-30, for physical aggression against other people and for verbal aggression. Clozapine was superior to haloperidol for MOAS-30 total score, and for physical aggression against other people, verbal aggression and physical aggression against objects.

BPRS: Brief psychiatric rating scale.

MOAS: Modified overt aggression scale.

PANSS: Positive and negative syndrome scale.

TAU: Treatment as usual.

(Courtesy of Meyer, J. M. (2019). *The Clozapine Handbook. Stahl's Handbooks*. New York: Cambridge University Press, pp. 126–127.)

Table 4.3 Comparison of Changes in Positive and Negative Syndrome Scale Scores among Clozapine, Haloperidol and Olanzapine

PANSS Variable	Medication Group	Analysis	
		Mean ± SD	F (*P* Value)
Total score	Clozapine	2.39 ± 14.2	
	Olanzapine	4.83 ± 9.7	1.23 (.30)
	Haloperidol	0.58 ± 15.2	
Positive symptoms	Clozapine	1.54 ± 5.0	
	Olanzapine	1.41 ± 3.6	2.30 (.11)
	Haloperidol	−0.50 ± 5.3	
Negative symptoms	Clozapine	−0.56 ± 4.9	
	Olanzapine	0.72 ± 3.0	1.65 (.20)
	Haloperidol	0.44 ± 4.6	
General psychopathology	Clozapine	1.43 ± 7.0	
	Olanzapine	2.69 ± 5.5	1.21 (.30)
	Haloperidol	0.64 ± 8.2	

(Adaptation from Krakowski M., et al. (2006). Atypical antipsychotic agents in the treatment of violent patients with schizophrenia and schizoaffective disorder. *Arch Gen Psych*, 63, 622–629.)

Figure 4.3 Clozapine's superiority for aggression compared to olanzapine and haloperidol among schizophrenia patients with cognitive dysfunction.

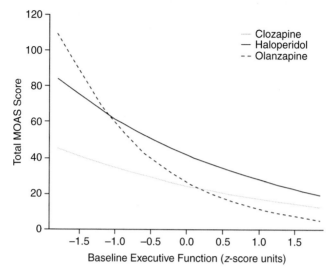

(Courtesy of Meyer, J. M. (2019). *The Clozapine Handbook. Stahl's Handbooks.* New York: Cambridge University Press, pp. 126–127.)

Ⓖ Approaching Treatment-Resistant Mania Treatment-resistant mania was first defined in 1994 as a documented response failure or intolerance to lithium, an anticonvulsant, and at least two typical antipsychotics [1]. The presence of antidepressant medication in the context of a bipolar diathesis risks destabilization of a patient with bipolar mood disorder or schizoaffective disorder, bipolar type despite optimization of mood stabilizer(s); hence, it is critical that antidepressants be avoided in patients who have a bipolar diathesis. In long-term bipolar I patient studies of one year or more, mean clozapine endpoint doses range from 234–305 mg daily (see Figure 4.5).

For schizoaffective disorder, bipolar type patients, higher doses (and plasma levels) typically used in schizophrenia spectrum disorders are usually warranted (see Figure 4.5). As shown below, clozapine is equally effective as an adjunct in treatment-resistant nonpsychotic bipolar disorder and schizoaffective disorder, bipolar type.

Figure 4.4 Adjunctive clozapine treatment in bipolar diathesis.

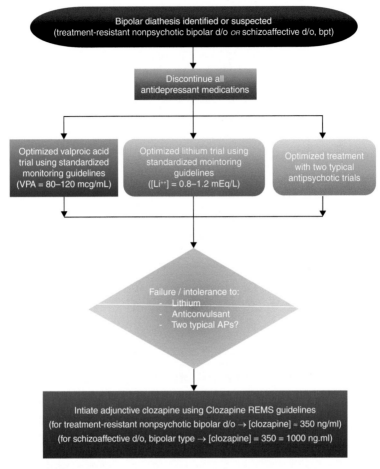

AP: antipsychotic.

⊕ Initiation of Clozapine Treatment Pre-treatment evaluation requirements include:

• ANC (per Clozapine REMS guidelines)
• ECG (if there is a positive history of unstable cardiovascular disease)
• fasting blood sugar and Hgb A1c
• lipid panel (or total cholesterol and triglycerides)
• blood pressure
• BMI, abdominal girth
• AIMS examination

Pre-treatment absolute neutrophil counts (ANC) are mandatory and ideally should be > 1500 cells/mm^3 for non-benign ethnic neutropenia (non-BEN) patients or >1000 cells/mm^3 for those with BEN. Pre-treatment evaluation is summarized in Table 4.4 below.

Table 4.4 Pre-Treatment Monitoring for Clozapine Treatment

Monitoring Points	Monitoring Tests	
Pre-treatment **requirements** (30 days <u>prior</u> to treatment)	✓ ANC* (preferably 1 week prior) ✓ FBS & Hgb A1c ✓ PE/BMI/abdominal girth	✓ lipid panel ✓ blood pressure ✓ ECG*, AIMS
Pre-treatment recommendations (30 days <u>prior</u> to treatment)	✓ female – pregnancy test ✓ KUB (if clinically indicated)**	
Pre-treatment **requirements** (within 12 months <u>prior</u> to treatment)	✓ complete physical exam*** ✓ ECG, AIMS	✓ CMP ✓ urinalysis
Pre-treatment **requirements** (within 24 hours <u>prior</u> to first dose)	VS + orthostatics twice (separated by at least one hour)	

* Clozapine REMS requires measured ANC one week prior to clozapine initiation.

** Findings or history of constipation, paralytic ileus, partial bowel obstruction; bowel or related surgery; abdominal adhesions; diverticulitis/diverticulosis; dehydration; anorexia; unreliability reporting bowel movements.

*** Including pulmonary/cardiovascular/abdominal exam, as well as breast exam in females with history of medications that elevate prolactin.

Once pre-treatment evaluation is complete, administer an initial dose of clozapine 125 mg at bedtime. If this is tolerated, increase the dose the following day to 25 mg twice per day. Thereafter, titrate the dose by 25–50 mg twice per week such that the target dose by the end of the second week is 200 mg daily.

In patients vulnerable to orthostasis, the initiation and titration of clozapine is gentler and more gradual beginning with clozapine 12.5 mg at bedtime. If this is tolerated, increase the dose the following day to 12.5 mg twice per day. Thereafter, titrate the dose by 12.5–25 mg twice per week such that the target dose by the end of the second week is 100 mg daily. Initiation is summarized in Figure 4.5 below.

Figure 4.5 Initiating clozapine treatment.*

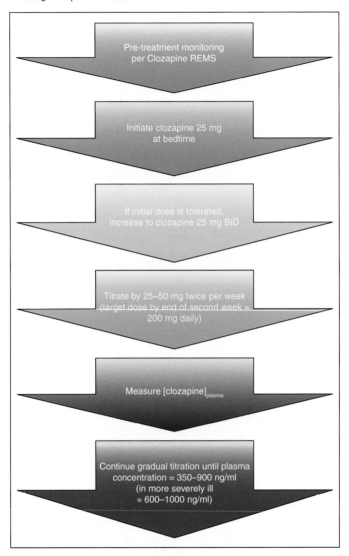

*In patients with orthostatic issues, titrate with 50% lower doses.

After treatment is initiated, monitoring of ANC is required. The monitoring requirements are summarized in Table 4.5 below.

Table 4.5 Monitoring of Absolute Neutrophil Count during Treatment with Clozapine

Normal Absolute Neutrophil Count Level	Treatment Recommendations	Absolute Neutrophil Count Monitoring
General non-BEN patients (ANC >1500/mm³)	• Initiate treatment • If treatment interrupted for <30 days, continue monitoring as before • If treatment interrupted for >30 days, monitor as if new patient	• Weekly for months 1–6 • Q-2 weeks for months 7–12 • Q-4 weeks after 1 year
BEN patients (established baseline ANC >1000/mm³)	• Obtain at least two baseline ANC levels before initiating treatment • If treatment interrupted for <30 days, continue monitoring as before • If treatment interrupted for >30 days, monitor as if new patient	• Weekly for months 1–6 • Q-2 weeks for months 7–12 • Q-4 weeks after 1 year

❶ **Maintenance of Clozapine Treatment** Absolute neutrophil count is checked weekly for the first six months, then every two weeks for the next six months. If all continues to be well, ANC is checked monthly thereafter. According to Clozapine REMS, the pharmacy will not dispense clozapine if ANC data are not received.

Maintenance monitoring requirements include:
• ANC (per Clozapine REMS guidelines)
• vital signs and orthostatic measurements
• fasting blood sugar and Hgb A1c
• BMI
• lipid panel (or total cholesterol and triglycerides)
• ECG (if there is a positive history of unstable cardiovascular disease)
• AIMS
• prolactin level

After reaching a total daily dose of 200 mg, check a plasma clozapine level to help guide dosing.

Using monitoring guidelines as delineated in Clozapine REMS, continue gradual titration by 25–50 mg twice weekly until the plasma concentration is in the 350–600 ng/ml range. (For patients whose psychosis continues to be inadequately treated at these levels, consideration could be given to increasing serum clozapine levels further to the 600–1000 ng/ml range.) Maintenance monitoring requirements are summarized in Table 4.6 below.

1.04 Approach to Treatment-Resistant Schizophrenia Patients (Continued)

Table 4.6 Maintenance Monitoring for Clozapine Treatment

Monitoring Points	Monitoring Tests	
First two weeks of treatment	✓ Daily VS + orthostatic measurements	
Monthly	✓ Fasting blood sugar^A (for first three months only) ✓ BMI	
Quarterly	✓ Hgb A1c^ ✓ Fasting lipid panel^^	✓ KUB (if ↑ risk) ✓ AIMS* [if (+), until (−) twice]
Biannually	✓ ECG (if on other medications that may prolong QTc as per the package insert)	
Annually	✓ ECG, AIMS, prolactin level	

^ If FBS >110 gm/dl or Hgb A1c ≥6.5% → repeat FBS and medical consultation.

^^ Dyslipidemia →medical and dietary consultation + lipid-lowering medications (e.g. statins).

* If (+) AIMS → neurological consultation.

❶ Motivational Interviewing in Adherence to Clozapine Treatment According to Reimer et al., motivational interviewing could have a positive impact on insight into schizophrenia and medication adherence. Vanderwaal did a literature review to address the efficacy of motivational interviewing on improving medication adherence in schizophrenia patients and found that while most did not provide any evidence for this, one study presented evidence supporting a direct relationship between the two. However, some studies found evidence supporting a relationship between motivational interviewing and other relevant outcomes (e.g. improved psychotic symptomatology and decreased re-hospitalization rates) [15, 16]. Despite slight positive data, motivational interviewing should not be considered first-line therapy for patients with schizophrenia.

ⓒ Summary Points

- Using consensus criteria, it is critical to identify treatment resistance as soon as possible.
- With the exception of aripiprazole augmentation of clozapine, various combinations of antipsychotics are largely ineffective.
- The gold standard for treatment-resistant schizophrenia is clozapine, which has a 40–60% response rate compared to <7% for other antipsychotics.
- It is critical to begin clozapine treatment as soon as treatment resistance is identified because delaying clozapine initiation may reduce clozapine's efficacy.
- Clozapine reduces suicide and violence risk in patients suffering from schizophrenia.
- Clozapine also exhibits efficacy in bipolar spectrum disorders and schizoaffective disorders.
- Achieving optimal plasma concentrations is vital to successful clozapine treatment.

1.04 Approach to Treatment-Resistant Schizophrenia Patients (Continued)

References

1. Meyer, J. M. (2019). *The Clozapine Handbook. Stahl's Handbooks*. New York: Cambridge University Press.
2. Kane, J., Honigfeld, G., Singer, J., et al. (1988). Clozapine for the treatment-resistant schizophrenic: a double-blind comparison with chlorpromazine. *Arch Gen Psychiatry*, 45, 789–796.
3. Howes, O. D., McCutcheon, R., Agid, O., et al. (2016). Treatment-resistant schizophrenia: treatment response and resistance in psychosis (TRRIP) working group consensus guidelines on diagnosis and terminology. *Am J Psychiatry*, 174, 216–229.
4. Galling, B., Roldan, A., Hagi, K., et al. (2017). Antipsychotic augmentation vs. monotherapy in schizophrenia: systematic review, meta-analysis and meta-regression analysis. *World Psychiatry*, 16, 77–89.
5. Stroup, T. S., Gerhard, T., Crystal, S., et al. (2015). Comparative effectiveness of clozapine and standard antipsychotic treatment in adults with schizophrenia. *Am J Psychiatry*, 173, 166–173.
6. Siskind, D., Siskind, V., Kisely, S. (2017). *Clozapine Response Rates among People with Treatment-resistant Schizophrenia: Data from a Systematic Review and Meta-analysis*. Los Angeles, CA: SAGE Publications.
7. Yoshimura, B., Yada, Y., So, R., et al. (2017). The critical treatment window of clozapine in treatment-resistant schizophrenia: secondary analysis of an observational study. *Psychiatry Res*, 250, 65–70.
8. Meltzer, H. Y., Alphs, L., Green, A. I., et al. (2003). Clozapine treatment for suicidality in schizophrenia: international suicide prevention trial (InterSePT). *Arch Gen Psychiatry*, 60, 82–91.
9. Quanbeck, C. D., McDermott, B. E., Lam, J., et al. (2007). Categorization of aggressive acts committed by chronically assaultive state hospital patients. *Psychiatr Serv*, 58, 521–528.
10. Meyer, J. M., Cummings, M. A., Proctor, G., et al. (2016). Psychopharmacology of persistent violence and aggression. *Psychiatr Clin North Am*, 39, 541–556.
11. Fazel, S., Gulati, G., Linsell, L., et al. (2009). Schizophrenia and violence: systematic review and meta-analysis. *PLoS Med*, 6, e1000120.
12. Fazel, S., Långström, N., Hjern, A., et al. (2009). Schizophrenia, substance abuse, and violent crime. *JAMA*, 301, 2016–2023.
13. Krakowski, M. I., Czobor, P., Citrome, L., et al. (2006). Atypical antipsychotic agents in the treatment of violent patients with schizophrenia and schizoaffective disorder. *Arch Gen Psychiatry*, 63, 622–629.
14. Frogley, C., Taylor, D., Dickens, G., et al. (2012). A systematic review of the evidence of clozapine's anti-aggressive effects. *Int J Neuropsychopharmacol*, 15, 1351–1371.
15. Vanderwaal, F. M. (2015). Impact of motivational interviewing on medication adherence in schizophrenia. *Issues Ment Health Nurs*, 36, 900–904.
16. Reimer, J., Kuhn, J., Wietfeld, R., et al. (2019). Motivational interviewing: a possibility for doctor-patient communication in schizophrenia? *Der Nervenarzt*, 90(11), 1144–1153.

1.05 Approach to Depressed or Suicidal Schizophrenia Spectrum Patients

📖 **Introduction** Negative symptoms and cognitive deficits are major barriers to employment, stable interpersonal relationships and independent living for persons afflicted with schizophrenia in the community [1]. Negative symptoms, such as blunting of affect, impaired behavioral initiation, decreased motivation, ambivalence and social withdrawal, interact on a continuum with illness features such as impaired executive functions, decreased verbal fluency and emotional dyscontrol [2, 3]. Moreover, deficits in emotional control coupled with deficits in impulse control place the schizophrenic individual at elevated risk for suicide. The overall suicide rate in schizophrenia has been estimated to be circa 10%, with suicide being a primary factor involved in shortening the expected life span of schizophrenic patients [4]. Thus, negative symptoms, dysphoric mood states and suicidality should be considered major treatment targets among complex treatment-resistant patients with schizophrenia.

Ⓐ **Antipsychotic Treatment** As noted, psychotic illness interacts with emotional dyscontrol and impulsivity to increase risk of dysphoric mood states and suicide. A critical element to decreasing this interaction is assuring the patient is receiving adequate antipsychotic medication exposure. This point is illustrated by the observation that long-acting injectable antipsychotics, owing to greater adherence, reduce hospitalizations and also reduce suicide risk [5, 6]. Beyond improving survival by enhancing antipsychotic adherence, clozapine has demonstrated a robust five-fold reduction in suicide risk among patients suffering from schizophrenia or schizoaffective disorders independently of its superior antipsychotic effects, resulting in a US Food and Drug Administration (FDA) indication for suicide [7]. Moreover, clozapine has been found to reduce all-cause mortality despite its adverse effect profile [8].

Ⓑ **Lithium Reduces Suicide** Like clozapine, lithium reduces the risk of suicide independently of its mood stabilizing properties and also carries an FDA indication [9]. For suicide prevention, lithium plasma concentrations do not correlate tightly with effectiveness, however, observational data suggest that higher concentrations (e.g. >0.6 meq/l) are more protective [10]. It is worth noting that some animal data suggest that clozapine may be more effective than lithium at preventing suicidal behavior in persons suffering from a schizophrenia spectrum disorder [11].

Ⓒ **Antidepressants Reduce Suicide Risk** For psychotic patients not vulnerable to bipolar diathesis, antidepressants reduce suicide risk and overall mortality. This was clearly illustrated by epidemiological studies that compared schizophrenia spectrum disordered patients taking two antipsychotics to no antipsychotic treatment, taking an antipsychotic plus an antidepressant, or an antipsychotic plus a benzodiazepine.

Moreover, the significant reduction in death due to suicide during treatment with an antipsychotic and an antidepressant observed in the initial study (2012) and reflected in Table 5.1 below was confirmed by later follow-up studies.

Table 5.1 Polypharmacy Effects on Mortality in Schizophrenia [19–21]

Medication Combination	Suicide Risk (HR, 95% CI)	Overall Mortality Risk (HR, 95% CI)
Two antipsychotics	0.41, 0.25–0.68 (significant decrease over no antipsychotic)	0.86, 0.51–1.44 (nonsignificant)
Antipsychotic plus antidepressant	0.15, 0.03–0.77 (significant decrease)	0.57, 0.28–1.16 (nonsignificant)
Antipsychotic plus benzodiazepine	3.83, 1.45–10.12 (significant increase)	1.91, 1.13–3.22 (significant increase)

D Bipolar Depression In contrast to schizophrenic patients suffering from depression not associated with vulnerability to a bipolar diathesis, those with a history of hypomania or mania show little beneficial response to antidepressants [12]. Further, even with mood stabilizer treatment, antidepressants may increase the risks of switches into hypomania or mania, as well as an increase in mood cycling rate [13, 14]. Thus, antidepressants should be used with caution in patients prone to a bipolar diathesis and never in patients actively exhibiting hypomanic, manic or mixed mood symptoms.

E Alternatives for Bipolar Depression For patients with psychosis who are vulnerable to a bipolar diathesis, pharmacological treatments are limited, but not absent. Data-supported options are shown in Table 5.2 below.

Table 5.2 Pharmacological Treatments for Bipolar Depression [22–24]

Medication	Comments
Lamotrigine	Offers antidepressant benefits but no protection against mood elevation. Typical doses are 200–400 mg at bedtime. Plasma concentrations do not correlate with effectiveness because the drug is rapidly cleared from the plasma compartment.
Lithium	Offers protection against both mood elevation and depression, however, effects against mood elevation are more robust. When used as an augmenting agent, plasma concentrations do not correlate with effectiveness but should be >0.6 meq/l.
Lurasidone	Offers robust treatment for bipolar depression at modest doses (20–60 mg per day). Note that lurasidone must be given proximate to a meal of at least 500 kcal to be effectively absorbed. Evening dosing mitigates against akathisia.
Pramipexole	May be especially effective for dysphoria or depression with prominent anergic features. Typical effective dose range is 1–2 mg at bedtime.
Quetiapine	The active metabolite, Nor-quetiapine or desmethyl-quetiapine, likely provides antidepressant effects via inhibition of the norepinephrine reuptake transporter. The optimal dose range has not been clearly established.

A variety of nutritional agents, e.g. S-adenosylmethionine (SAM-E), St. John's Wort, omega-3 fatty acids, also have been suggested and used, however, adequate controlled data in the context of schizophrenia are lacking [15]. Recently, nonpharmacological approaches, such as direct current stimulation and rapid transcranial magnetic stimulation have been explored, however, investigations of these technologies to treat schizophrenia associated with dysphoria or depression are preliminary at this time [16, 17]. Finally, electroconvulsive therapy is well supported as an effective treatment for those patients who fail pharmacological interventions [18].

ⓒ Summary Points

- Negative symptoms, dysphoria and depression exist on a continuum in schizophrenia and pose a major barrier to occupational functioning, stable interpersonal relationships and independent living.
- Individuals suffering from schizophrenia spectrum disorders are at elevated risk for suicide.
- Assuring adequate antipsychotic treatment reduces suicide risk.
- Clozapine and lithium exert anti-suicide effects independent of their respective antipsychotic and mood stabilizing properties.
- Antidepressants should be avoided in patients vulnerable to bipolar diathesis.

References

1. Kaneko, K. (2018). Negative symptoms and cognitive impairments in schizophrenia: two key symptoms negatively influencing social functioning. *Yonago Acta Med*, 61, 91–102.
2. Liu, J., Chan, T. C. T., Chong, S. A., et al. (2019). Impact of emotion dysregulation and cognitive insight on psychotic and depressive symptoms during the early course of schizophrenia spectrum disorders. *Early Interv Psychiatry*, 14(6), 691–697.
3. Barch, D. M., Pagliaccio, D., Luking, K. (2016). Mechanisms underlying motivational deficits in psychopathology: similarities and differences in depression and schizophrenia. *Curr Top Behav Neurosci*, 27, 411–449.
4. Sher, L., Kahn, R. S. (2019). Suicide in schizophrenia: an educational overview. *Medicina (Kaunas)*, 55(7), 361.
5. Pompili, M., Orsolini, L., Lamis, D. A., et al. (2017). Suicide prevention in schizophrenia: do long-acting injectable antipsychotics (LAIs) have a role? *CNS Neurol Disord Drug Targets*, 16, 454–462.
6. Taipale, H., Mittendorfer-Rutz, E., Alexanderson, K., et al. (2018). Antipsychotics and mortality in a nationwide cohort of 29,823 patients with schizophrenia. *Schizophr Res*, 197, 274–280.
7. Ertugrul, A. (2002). Clozapine and suicide. *Am J Psychiatry*, 159, 323; author reply 324.
8. Kane, J. M. (2017). Clozapine reduces all-cause mortality. *Am J Psychiatry*, 174, 920–921.
9. Roberts, E., Cipriani, A., Geddes, J. R., et al. (2017). The evidence for lithium in suicide prevention. *Br J Psychiatry*, 211, 396.
10. Kanehisa, M., Terao, T., Shiotsuki, I., et al. (2017). Serum lithium levels and suicide attempts: a case-controlled comparison in lithium therapy-naive individuals. *Psychopharmacology (Berl)*, 234, 3335–3342.
11. Deslauriers, J., Belleville, K., Beaudet, N., et al. (2016). A two-hit model of suicide-trait-related behaviors in the context of a schizophrenia-like phenotype: distinct effects of lithium chloride and clozapine. *Physiol Behav*, 156, 48–58.
12. Sachs, G. S., Nierenberg, A. A., Calabrese, J. R., et al. (2007). Effectiveness of adjunctive antidepressant treatment for bipolar depression. *N Engl J Med*, 356, 1711–1722.
13. Gitlin, M. J. (2018). Antidepressants in bipolar depression: an enduring controversy. *Int J Bipolar Disord*, 6, 25.
14. Cheniaux, E., Nardi, A. E. (2019). Evaluating the efficacy and safety of antidepressants in patients with bipolar disorder. *Expert Opin Drug Saf*, 18, 893–913.
15. Marx, W., Moseley, G., Berk, M., et al. (2017). Nutritional psychiatry: the present state of the evidence. *Proc Nutr Soc*, 76, 427–436.
16. Dougall, N., Maayan, N., Soares-Weiser, K., et al. (2015). Transcranial magnetic stimulation for schizophrenia. *Schizophr Bull*, 41, 1220–1222.
17. Moffa, A. H., Brunoni, A. R., Nikolin, S., et al. (2018). Transcranial direct current stimulation in psychiatric disorders: a comprehensive review. *Psychiatr Clin North Am*, 41, 447–463.
18. Pompili, M., Lester, D., Dominici, G., et al. (2013). Indications for electroconvulsive treatment in schizophrenia: a systematic review. *Schizophr Res*, 146, 1–9.
19. Tiihonen, J., Suokas, J. T., Suvisaari, J. M., et al. (2012). Polypharmacy with antipsychotics, antidepressants, or benzodiazepines and mortality in schizophrenia. *Arch Gen Psychiatry*, 69, 476–483.
20. Tiihonen, J., Mittendorfer-Rutz, E., Torniainen, M., et al. (2016). Mortality and cumulative exposure to antipsychotics, antidepressants, and benzodiazepines in patients with schizophrenia: an observational follow-up study. *Am J Psychiatry*, 173, 600–606.
21. Rubio, J. M., Correll, C. U. (2017). Reduced all-cause mortality with antipsychotics and antidepressants compared to increased all-cause mortality with benzodiazepines in patients with schizophrenia observed in naturalistic treatment settings. *Evid Based Ment Health*, 20, e6.
22. Loebel, A., Xu, J., Hsu, J., et al. (2015). The development of lurasidone for bipolar depression. *Ann N Y Acad Sci*, 1358, 95–104.
23. Post, R. M. (2016). Treatment of bipolar depression: evolving recommendations. *Psychiatr Clin North Am*, 39, 11–33.
24. Szmulewicz, A. G., Angriman, F., Samame, C., et al. (2017). Dopaminergic agents in the treatment of bipolar depression: a systematic review and meta-analysis. *Acta Psychiatr Scand*, 135, 527–538.

1.06 Approach to Persistent Aggression and Violence in Schizophrenia Spectrum Psychotic Disorders

🔲 **Introduction** The first step to addressing persistent aggression in patients with schizophrenia spectrum disorders is to categorize the nature of the aggression to help inform the approach to treatment strategies [1]. There is evidence that understanding violence as a dimension of psychiatric illness, by identifying the underlying etiology, is an effective approach to treatment [2–4]. Based on studies within the New York and California State Hospital Systems [2, 3], three categories of aggression can be utilized to help focus treatment: psychotic, impulsive and predatory (also called organized or instrumental).

• Psychotic aggression derives from the positive symptoms of schizophrenia such as command hallucinations or persecutory delusional beliefs about a threat of harm from the victim. This type of aggression often appears to be unprovoked and some evidence indicates that it is the least common type of aggression in inpatient settings but also the most treatable.

• Impulsive aggression is thought to be the most common form of inpatient aggression and is usually provoked in reaction to undesirable external stimuli, e.g. intrusive or threatening peer, denial of privilege by staff, etc. It occurs without due consideration of the consequences of the behavior and is often associated with an aroused emotional state, e.g. excited, angry or agitated [4].

• Predatory aggression is planned, goal-oriented behavior not obviously related to threat or provocation that is often driven by retaliation and intimidation. These instrumental aggressors often present with little autonomic arousal. Predatory aggression is the second most common type of aggression and the least amenable to psychopharmacological interventions.

A Persistent Aggression Persistent aggressive behavior in patients with schizophrenia spectrum disorders is often due to insufficient psychopharmacological treatment or failure to adjust treatment over time. A complicating factor in the treatment of the violent patient is that many acts of aggression may be multifactorial – that is, patients may be driven to act by more than one of the three characterized forms of violence. Furthermore, once a patient's positive psychotic symptoms are reduced, impulsive or predatory aggression may emerge as the primary forms of violence requiring different approaches to treatment [5]. Conventional use of psychotropic medications is often insufficient in adequately controlling violence [6], or there is hesitation on the part of treating psychiatrists to use recommended treatments such as clozapine. This hesitation may be due to concerns about patient cooperation with blood draws, lack of familiarity with use of the medication and discomfort with side-effect management [7].

B Treatment Approach This chapter focuses on a simplified model of psychopharmacological approaches within the three described aggression types as a foundation, with acknowledgement that psychiatric violence is often driven by a complex interaction of biological, psychological, environmental and social factors. While pharmacological approaches may be very useful, and necessary for certain types of violence, it must be noted that environmental variables, staffing ratios and expertise, and psychosocial stressors play an important role in aggressive behavior. These areas must also be addressed to obtain the maximum benefit from medication options.

Before embarking on new courses of psychopharmacological treatment, it is important to consider the following issues that could lead to persistent aggression:

- Suboptimal antipsychotic plasma levels due to poor adherence or rapid metabolism can lead to undertreated psychosis. Recommendations include frequent antipsychotic plasma level monitoring combined with strategies to help ensure increased adherence (e.g. long-acting injectable (LAI) antipsychotic, liquid/dissolvable formulations, increased periods of observation, etc.) [8–10].
- Rule out akathisia as an underappreciated cause of aggression [11–14].
- Patients with a bipolar component to their illness can become destabilized by antidepressants leading to agitation and aggression without accruing long-term benefits toward depression. It is important to also add a mood stabilizer such as lithium or valproate [15, 16].
- It is important to consider the adverse contributions of benzodiazepines to persistent aggression. There is an absence of convincing evidence to support the chronic use of adjunctive benzodiazepines in patients with schizophrenia spectrum disorders [17–21] and benzodiazepines are associated with increased aggression and impulsivity that often arises through disinhibition [22].

❸ Psychotic Aggression Aggression in undertreated schizophrenia spectrum patients is best approached with dopamine antagonist antipsychotics as the cornerstone treatment to reduce dopamine overactivity in the meso-limbic dopamine circuit. There is evidence that long-acting injectable dopamine antagonist antipsychotics are superior to their oral counterparts in decreasing aggression and violence. Patients with schizoaffective disorder, bipolar type require consistent optimized plasma levels of a mood stabilizer, i.e. lithium or a valproic acid, for mood stabilization to help prevent destabilization with subsequent worsening psychosis [15, 16].

A clozapine trial is indicated following failure of two adequate antipsychotic trials because the probability of response to additional dopamine antagonist trials is <7%. Furthermore, adjunctive medications offer only modest added benefit, and partial dopamine agonist antipsychotics may help more with negative symptoms rather than positive symptoms of psychosis. Dopamine partial agonists can even worsen psychosis and aggression in patients who require full dopamine antagonism [23, 24].

In contrast, clozapine produces a beneficial response in up to 60% of treatment-resistant patients as well as providing decreases in violence and suicide risks [25].

Evidence for adjunctive pharmacologic treatments to clozapine is weak, consisting primarily of open-label trials and case series. Strategies with evidence of reductions in aggression and violence include adjunctive dopamine antagonist antipsychotics, aripiprazole, valproic acid, centrally acting β-adrenergic antagonists, and selective serotonin reuptake inhibitor antidepressants. Lithium has robust data supporting its capacity to reduce violence and suicide in mood disorders; however, the data in schizophrenia are relatively weak [1]. If lithium or valproate are employed for patients without a bipolar diathesis, they should be used at high therapeutic serum levels with appropriate safety monitoring, and should be withdrawn after eight weeks unless there is compelling evidence of response in order to avoid the additive weight gain seen when combined with antipsychotic therapy [1]. Psychiatrists at a California State Hospital reported enhancement of inhibition of impulsive violence in five women treated with stimulants after psychosis was well controlled with clozapine. Finally, electroconvulsive therapy is an effective and well-tolerated adjunct to clozapine for treatment-resistant schizophrenia [25].

❹ Impulsive Aggression Clozapine again emerges as the preferred agent because of its anti-aggressive properties apart from antipsychotic efficacy. This is especially prominent in those with low baseline neurocognitive functioning [1]. Retrospective analysis indicates that clozapine's aggression reduction is due to improvements in executive functions that are likely secondary to clozapine's impact on the prefrontal cortex [1]. The initiation of treatment with clozapine for patients demonstrating impulsive aggression should be considered early in the course of treatment due to its demonstrated efficacy [5]. As noted above, evidence for adjunctive pharmacologic treatments to clozapine is weak with mood stabilizers and antipsychotics showing efficacy in treating impulsive aggression among patients prone to bipolar diathesis or intense mood lability.

❸ Predatory Aggression For the most part, treatment of predatory aggression and violence has relied upon behavioral treatments with limited success. However, clozapine emerges as a viable pharmacological intervention based on evidence that clozapine's anti-aggression effect is independent of its antipsychotic properties [1], including a small case series of clozapine therapy for impulsive aggression among nonpsychotic patients with antisocial personality disorders [1]. Not only did clozapine significantly decrease rates of impulsive aggression and violence in this cohort, it did so at serum levels below 350 ng/ml, with level mean 171 ng/ml. Finally, the reader is referred to the California State Hospital Violence Assessment and Treatment (Cal-VAT) guidelines for further discussion of psychosocial treatment of predatory violence [4].

ⓒ Summary Points

- The initial step in addressing persistent aggression and violence is to determine if it is driven by psychosis, impulsivity or predation.
- Persisting aggression and violence often results from insufficient psychopharmacological treatment, i.e. either pharmacokinetic or pharmacodynamic failures.
- All pharmacological trials should pursue three endpoints: (1) the target signs and symptoms improve; (2) intolerable adverse effects emerge which cannot be reasonably mitigated or managed; or (3) a point of futility is reached, e.g. plasma concentrations which saturate relevant receptors are reached without adequate benefit.
- Akathisia must be considered as an underappreciated cause of aggression and violence.
- Antidepressants may drive aggression and violence in patients vulnerable to a bipolar diathesis. Patients with a bipolar component may benefit greatly from treatment with a mood stabilizer.
- Benzodiazepines may promote disinhibition and impulsive violence in some patients.
- Finally, clozapine is effective for aggression and violence across psychotic and impulsive violence, with at least some uncontrolled data also suggesting efficacy for predatory aggression.

📖 References

1. Meyer, J. M., Cummings, M. A., Proctor, G., et al. (2016). Psychopharmacology of persistent violence and aggression. *Psychiatr Clin North Am*, 39, 541–556.
2. Nolan, K. A., Czobor, P., Roy, B. B., et al. (2003). Characteristics of assaultive behavior among psychiatric inpatients. *Psychiatr Serv*, 54, 1012–1016.
3. Quanbeck, C. D., McDermott, B. E., Lam, J., et al. (2007). Categorization of aggressive acts committed by chronically assaultive state hospital patients. *Psychiatr Serv*, 58, 521–528.
4. Stahl, S. M., Morrissette, D. A., Cummings, M., et al. (2014). California State Hospital Violence Assessment and Treatment (Cal-VAT) guidelines. *CNS Spectr*, 19, 449–465.
5. Dardashti, L., O'Day, J., Barsom, M., et al. (2015). Illustrative cases to support the Cal-VAT guidelines. *CNS Spectr*, 20, 311–318.
6. Morrissette, D. A., Stahl, S. M. (2014). Treating the violent patient with psychosis or impulsivity utilizing antipsychotic polypharmacy and high-dose monotherapy. *CNS Spectr*, 19, 439–448.
7. Nielsen, J., Dahm, M., Lublin, H., et al. (2010). Psychiatrists' attitude towards and knowledge of clozapine treatment. *Psychopharmacol*, 24, 965–971.
8. Meyer, J. M. (2014). A rational approach to employing high plasma levels of antipsychotics for violence associated with schizophrenia: case vignettes. *CNS Spectr*, 19, 432–438.
9. McCutcheon, R., Beck, K., Bloomfield, M. A., et al. (2015). Treatment resistant or resistant to treatment? Antipsychotic plasma levels in patients with poorly controlled psychotic symptoms. *J Psychopharmacol*, 29, 892–897.
10. Meyer, J. M. (2019). Monitoring and improving antipsychotic adherence in outpatient forensic diversion programs. *CNS Spectr*, 25(2), 1–9.
11. Keckich, W. (1978). Neuroleptics: violence as a manifestation of akathisia. *JAMA*, 240, 2185.
12. Schulte, J. (1985). Homicide and suicide associated with akathisia and haloperidol. *Am J Forensic Psychiatry*, 6, 3–7.
13. Galynker, I., Nazarian, D. (1997). Akathisia as violence. *J Clin Psychiatry*, 58, 31–32.
14. Stubbs, J. H., Hutchins, D. A., Mountjoy, C. Q. (2000). Relationship of akathisia to aggressive and self-injurious behaviour: a prevalence study in a UK tertiary referral centre. *Int J Psychiatry Clin Pract*, 4, 319–325.
15. Antosik-Wojcinska, A., Stefanowski, B., Swiecicki, L. (2015). Efficacy and safety of antidepressant's use in the treatment of depressive episodes in bipolar disorder – review of research. *Psychiatr Pol*, 49, 1223–1239.
16. Lähteenvuo, M., Tanskanen, A., Taipale, H., et al. (2018). Real-world effectiveness of pharmacologic treatments for the prevention of rehospitalization in a Finnish nationwide cohort of patients with bipolar disorder. *JAMA Psychiatry*, 75, 347–355.
17. Volz, A., Khorsand, V., Gillies, D., et al. (2007). Benzodiazepines for schizophrenia. *Cochrane Database Syst Rev*, 11, CD006391.
18. Dold, M., Li, C., Tardy, M., et al. (2012). Benzodiazepines for schizophrenia. *Cochrane Database Syst Rev*, 11, CD006391.
19. Tiihonen, J., Suokas, J. T., Suvisaari, J. M., et al. (2012). Polypharmacy with antipsychotics, antidepressants, or benzodiazepines and mortality in schizophrenia. *Arch Gen Psychiatry*, 69, 476–483.
20. Dold, M., Li, C., Gillies, D., et al. (2013). Benzodiazepine augmentation of antipsychotic drugs in schizophrenia: a meta-analysis and Cochrane review of randomized controlled trials. *Eur Neuropsychopharmacol*, 23, 1023–1033.
21. Gillies, D., Sampson, S., Beck, A., et al. (2013). Benzodiazepines for psychosis-induced aggression or agitation. *Cochrane Database Syst Rev*, 9, CD003079.
22. Dodds, T. J. (2017). Prescribed benzodiazepines and suicide risk: a review of the literature. *Prim Care Companion CNS Disord*, 19(2).
23. Takeuchi, H., Remington, G. (2013). A systematic review of reported cases involving psychotic symptoms worsened by aripiprazole in schizophrenia or schizoaffective disorder. *Psychopharmacology (Berl)*, 228, 175–185.
24. Stahl, S. (2014). Antipsychotic agents. In *Stahl's Essential Psychopharmacology* (ed.). New York: Cambridge University Press, p. 169.
25. Meyer, J. M., Stahl, S. M. (2019). *The Clozapine Handbook*. New York: Cambridge University Press.

1.07 Approach to Bipolar Diathesis in Schizophrenia Spectrum Patients

📖 Introduction

ⓐ Management of Acute Manic Episodes in Schizoaffective Disorder, Bipolar Type Patients

The mainstay of acute mania treatment for schizoaffective disorder, bipolar type (SAD-BT) patients includes the use of antipsychotic therapy combined with one of the two first-line mood stabilizers, lithium or a form of valproic acid (VPA) (e.g. divalproex) [1, 2]. In controlled acute mania studies with bipolar I patients, response rates to monotherapy with antipsychotics, lithium or VPA are comparable and roughly 50% [2]. While carbamazepine can be used for maintenance treatment, and has been studied in acute mania, rapid titration is poorly tolerated due to central nervous system (CNS) adverse effects such as sedation, dizziness, ataxia and nausea, and thus should be avoided unless treatment with lithium or VPA is contraindicated [3]. As an inducer of cytochrome P450 (cyp) enzymes and the drug transporter P-glycoprotein (PGP), carbamazepine may reduce antipsychotic levels by 30–80% and thus presents a source of kinetic interaction that can be problematic during acute and maintenance treatment [4]. Carbamazepine is also associated with hyponatremia [1]. Other anticonvulsants have been studied for acute mania and have been found to be ineffective, including gabapentin, lamotrigine, licarbazepine, oxcarbazepine and topiramate [2].

Most antipsychotics have compelling data for mania, and many have completed registrational trials leading to indications for acute mania. As will be noted, both lithium and VPA can be loaded to hasten the achievement of therapeutic CNS levels, but neither of these agents exist in parenteral forms limiting use to those who are cooperative enough to take oral medication and are willing to do so on a daily basis. The value of antipsychotic treatment lies in the availability of acute intramuscular preparations that can be used in the early hours and days of mania treatment. The antipsychotic chosen for acute mania treatment will not necessarily be the agent used in combination with lithium or VPA for maintenance. In particular, those antipsychotics with marked propensity for weight gain (e.g. olanzapine, quetiapine, risperidone/paliperidone) should be eschewed in lieu of other options (e.g. high potency first-generation antipsychotics, aripiprazole, cariprazine) due to the additive weight gain posed by use with lithium or VPA [5]. Also, the antipsychotic dose used to control acute mania may be much greater than that used for maintenance treatment especially if the patient initially refuses mood stabilizer therapy. Once a mood stabilizer is started, the antipsychotic dose should be adjusted to control the target psychotic symptoms that persisted in the past during periods of euthymia (e.g. hallucinations, delusions, disorganized speech or behavior).

As will be discussed in Chapter 1.08, some patients who are labeled with a diagnosis of schizophrenia may present with persistent anxiety, recurrent aggression or treatment-resistant psychotic symptoms despite antipsychotic therapy. Before coming to conclusions regarding the next approach for pharmacotherapy, one should entertain the hypothesis that these symptoms might represent inadequate mood stabilization in a patient whose bipolar diathesis was overlooked due to the fact that the antipsychotic addressed the more florid aspects of mania. A detailed search of prior records or discussions with providers or caregivers might elucidate clues to a history of mania. When in doubt, one could consider a trial of lithium under the presumed hypothesis that this is a SAD-BT patient whose mood component has not been optimally treated with antipsychotic monotherapy. Lithium has no demonstrable value in treatment-resistant schizophrenia, so marked improvement with an adjunctive lithium trial should be considered *prima facie* evidence that the underlying diagnosis is SAD-BT [6].

Table 7.1 Antipsychotic Doses for Agents with Oral and Acute Intramuscular Preparations

Medication	Oral Dosing in Acute Mania	Intramuscular Dosage	Acute Adverse Effects
Fluphenazine	5 mg every 4–6 hours. Usually given together with diphenhydramine 50 mg for EPS prophylaxis and sedation.	2.5 mg IM every 4–6 hours. IM doses must be given together with diphenhydramine 50 mg.	Extrapyramidal
Haloperidol	5 mg every 4–6 hours. Usually given together with diphenhydramine 50 mg for EPS prophylaxis and sedation.	5 mg IM every 4–6 hours. IM doses must be given together with diphenhydramine 50 mg.	Extrapyramidal
Olanzapine	Start 10 or 15 mg. Max daily dose 20 mg.	10 mg (5 mg or 7.5 mg when warranted). Assess for orthostasis prior to subsequent dosing. Daily max: three doses 2–4 hours apart [30].	Sedation, orthostasis
Ziprasidone	40 mg BID on day 1, increasing to 80 mg BID on day 2. Mean endpoint dosing in acute mania trials 129–136 mg/d. (Note: oral doses must be given with 500 kcal food.)	Recommended dose: 10–20 mg IM, max 40 mg/d. 10 mg doses can be given every two hours; 20 mg can be given every four hours.	QT prolongation for two IM doses given four hours apart (20 mg, then 30 mg was comparable to that for haloperidol IM (7.5 mg, then 10 mg) [31].

The mood stabilizers of choice for treatment of acute mania are lithium and VPA due to the ability to be loaded, and superior long-term efficacy data than carbamazepine [2, 7]. As noted previously, there are no double-blind controlled trials demonstrating the acute or long-term effectiveness of other anticonvulsants such as gabapentin, licarbazepine, oxcarbazepine or topiramate, and these agents should not be used [8–10]. Oxcarbazepine, like carbamazepine, also presents a risk for hyponatremia. Many are unfamiliar with lithium loading and wrongly assume that lithium must be started slowly. However, a group at Los Angeles County-USC Medical Center developed a 30 mg/kg loading formula predicted to achieve 12-hour trough levels in the range of 0.9–1.1 meq/l. Critical to the success of their approach was to administer lithium in three divided doses of approximately 10 mg/kg each (4 pm, 6 pm and 8 pm), and to use an extended-release lithium preparation for the loading phase to minimize gastrointestinal (GI) adverse effects. The resulting 12-hour trough levels ranged from 0.45–1.29 meq/l, demonstrating that patients with an estimated glomerular filtration rate (eGFR) >60 ml/min can be safely loaded with extended-release lithium at 30 mg/kg in three divided doses. A lithium level should be obtained the morning after the loading doses are administered, and that evening lithium can be started at bedtime with the dose based on the 12-hour trough level. If the trough level is <1.0 meq/l, then give 1500 mg lithium q bedtime. If the level is >1.0, then give 1200 mg q bedtime. A sustained-release preparation or multiple daily doses should be avoided during maintenance therapy for two reasons: a) lithium has a brain half-life >28 hours, so there is no greater efficacy from use of sustained-release formulations or from multiple daily dosing [11]; b) dosing lithium more than once daily increases the risk for long-term renal insufficiency [12]. Sustained-release formulations are used (again given once daily at bedtime) only for those who have GI adverse effects from regular lithium preparations. It should be noted that in routine clinical practice one might avoid starting lithium in those with eGFR <70 ml/min as some in this group might experience renal dysfunction and need to be removed from lithium relatively soon. For those with adequate renal function, lithium has superior anti-suicide and neuroprotective data than VPA, and should be the first option [13–16].

Valproate can be loaded using a similar weight-based formula of 30 mg/kg, usually given in two divided doses within the same day [17]. The target serum levels for acute and maintenance lithium and VPA treatment are in Table 7.2 below. As noted above, carbamazepine loading is poorly tolerated although it can be used for maintenance treatment bearing in mind the kinetic interactions with antipsychotics. Lamotrigine can be used for bipolar maintenance only, as slow titration is needed to minimize the risk for Stevens-Johnson Syndrome (SJS) [2].

Table 7.2 Doses, Loading Regimens and Levels for Acute Mania and Bipolar Maintenance for Mood Stabilizers [1] (Note: See Part II Chapters 1–4 for Detailed Information on These Medications)

Medication	Loading Regimen in Acute Mania	Trough Serum Levels in Acute Mania	Trough Maintenance Serum Levels	Monitoring Labs
Lithium	Three doses of ~ 10 mg/kg of extended-release lithium given at 4 pm, 6 pm and 8 pm (the total dose amount should be 30 mg/kg) [32]. A 12-hour trough level is drawn the next morning and regular lithium started qhs.	1.0–1.5 meq/l*	0.6–1.0 meq/l**	Six months: lithium level, creatinine (for eGFR), serum calcium, TSH
Valproate/ Divalproex	30 mg/kg, usually in two divided doses over 24 hours. Divalproex is preferred to valproic acid for tolerability reasons (less GI adverse effects).	100–120 µg/ml***	60–100 µg/ ml	Six months: VPA level, liver function tests, complete blood count
Carbamazepine	Cannot be loaded. Before starting, must obtain testing for HLA-B*1502 in patients of Asian heritage, as there is a ten-fold greater risk of SJS in these individuals.****	10–12 µg/ml	6–12 µg/ml	Complete blood count, serum sodium. Consider checking plasma antipsychotic levels due to kinetic interaction

| Lamotrigine | Cannot be loaded. Must use mandated dose adjustment if added to existing VPA therapy. | Not used for acute mania due to prolonged titration to avoid SJS.**** | Levels not used for bipolar disorder. | None |

* Lithium has a 28-hour half-life in the CNS and should be dosed once daily at bedtime [11]. Dosing more than once per day significantly increases the risk for long-term renal dysfunction and does not improve efficacy [12].

** Any trough maintenance levels >1.2 meq/l significantly increases the risk for long-term renal dysfunction [12].

*** Although the trough value for Depakote ER is 24 hours post-dose, this is impractical in many settings. A sample drawn 12–15 hours post-dose yields a VPA level only 18–25% higher on average than the 24-hour trough value [33].

**** SJS = Stevens-Johnson Syndrome.

Ⓑ Antipsychotic and Mood Stabilizer Therapy during Maintenance Phase in Schizoaffective Disorder, Bipolar Type Patients For bipolar I patients the optimal duration of antipsychotic treatment adjunctive to lithium or valproate is not well established in the literature [5, 18]; however, for the SAD-BT patient, combination mood stabilizer and antipsychotic therapy is needed to cover all aspects of the psychiatric illness. Among bipolar I patients, antipsychotic monotherapy is associated with higher all-cause treatment failure, and failure due to medication switching [18]. Even in bipolar I patients, a group who lack the persistent psychotic symptoms seen in SAD-BT patients, naturalistic data show that the risks for overall treatment failure are significantly lower for combination antipsychotic and mood stabilizer therapy [18]. Importantly, one study showed that treatment failure among bipolar I patients was 20% lower when associated with the use of a long-acting injectable (LAI) antipsychotic [18]. Since nonadherence is common among schizophrenia spectrum patients [19], strong consideration should be given to the use of an LAI antipsychotic, with the basic properties of those available in the US covered in Table 7.3 below. The choice of LAI agent depends greatly on prior history of response and tolerability and must address both provider and patient concerns about specific adverse effects such as weight gain, hyperprolactinemia and extrapyramidal adverse effects (EPS). Some antipsychotics (e.g. aripiprazole, olanzapine) have indications for bipolar I maintenance as monotherapy, but this should not be the primary reason for choosing these agents.

Table 7.3 Kinetic Properties of Depot Antipsychotics Available in the United States [34]

Drug	Vehicle	Dosage	T_{max}	$T_{1/2}$ Multiple Dosing	Able to Be Loaded
Fluphenazine decanoate	Sesame oil	12.5–75 mg/2 weeks	0.3–1.5 days	14 days	Yes
Haloperidol decanoate	Sesame oil	25–300 mg/4 weeks	3–9 days	21 days	Yes
Risperidone subcutaneous (Perseris®)	Water	90–120 mg/ 4 weeks	4–6 hours (first peak) ~ 8 days (second peak)	9–11 days	Not needed
Risperidone microspheres (Risperdal Consta®)	Water	12.5–50 mg/2 weeks	21 days	3–6 days	No (21–28 days oral overlap)

Table 7.3 (Cont.)

Drug	Vehicle	Dosage	T$_{max}$	T$_{1/2}$ Multiple Dosing	Able to Be Loaded
Paliperidone palmitate (Invega Sustenna®)	Water	39–234 mg/4 weeks	13 days	25–49 days	Yes
Paliperidone palmitate (3 mo) (Invega Trinza®)*	Water	273–819 mg/12 weeks	84–95 days (deltoid) 118–139 days (gluteal)	30–33 days	No
Olanzapine pamoate (Zyprexa Relprevv®)**	Water	150–300 mg/2 weeks 300–405 mg/4 weeks	7 days	30 days	Yes
Aripiprazole monohydrate (Abilify Maintena®)	Water	300–400 mg/4 weeks	6.5–7.1 days	29.9–46.5 days	No (14 days oral overlap)
Aripiprazole lauroxil (Aristada®)***	Water	441 mg, 662 mg, 882 mg/4 weeks 882 mg/6 weeks 1064 mg/8 weeks	41 days (single dose) [35] 24.4–35.2 days (repeated dosing) [36]	53.9–57.2 days	No (start with AL$_{NCD}$ 675 mg IM+30 mg oral *OR* 21 days oral overlap)
Aripiprazole lauroxil nanocrystal (Aristada Initio®)****	Water	675 mg once	27 days (range: 16–35 days)	15–18 days (single dose)	No

IM = intramuscular.

* Only for those on paliperidone palmitate monthly for four months; cannot be converted from oral medication.

** See US FDA bulletin, available here: https://www.accessdata.fda.gov/drugsatfda_docs/label/2009/022173lbl.pdf

*** Twenty-one days oral overlap unless starting with aripiprazole lauroxil nanocrystal + single 30 mg oral dose.

**** Aripiprazole lauroxil nanocrystal (AL$_{NCD}$) is only used for initiation of treatment with aripiprazole lauroxil, or for resumption of treatment. It is always administered together with the clinician-determined dose of aripiprazole lauroxil, although the latter can be given ≤10 days after the aripiprazole lauroxil nanocrystal injection.

Unfortunately there is no method for assuring adherence with oral mood stabilizer therapy, and studies of bipolar I and SAD-BT patients indicate high rates of nonadherence for both diagnostic groups (bipolar I: 32%; SAD-BT: 44%) [20]. Psychoeducation regarding the need to persist with mood stabilizer treatment during periods of euthymia has been proven useful [21, 22], along with implementation of objective measures to track adherence including pill counts and serum levels [2, 23]. While levels need not be obtained more often than every six months in stable patients on unchanging doses of lithium, VPA or carbamazepine, one can use random level determination as a means to ascertain the degree of adherence based on the known levels obtained during a period of stability, especially when that level was drawn in a controlled setting. Although serum levels are not employed to manage efficacy for lamotrigine, these levels are available and can be used to monitor adherence. Decreases >30% from baseline levels obtained at roughly the same time post-dose (±2 hours) indicate an adherence issue and should prompt further discussions with the patient and a repeat level.

There is considerable debate about the value and safety of antidepressants in bipolar disorder patients, but antidepressant use in the SAD-BT population is little studied [24]. Cross-sectional data indicate that clinicians are more wary about the use of antidepressants in SAD-BT patients that nonpsychotic variants of bipolar disorder [24], but some reviews suggest consideration of traditional antidepressants [25]. As of 2019, there are four approved antipsychotics for bipolar depression that represent opportunities to manage the depressive phase of the illness with less concern for mania induction: quetiapine, lurasidone, cariprazine and the combination product olanzapine/fluoxetine (see Table 7.4). Ideally one would prefer to treat both the depressive component and the chronic psychotic aspect of SAD-BT with one antipsychotic, but this may not always be possible. Moreover, none of the four approved antipsychotics for bipolar depression have LAI forms with the exception of olanzapine, but olanzapine by itself has no efficacy data for bipolar depression, only the combination with oral fluoxetine. Optimizing mood stabilizer treatment, especially lithium, may be helpful in some patients, but it is worth noting that there are limited data to support that switching from non-lithium mood stabilizers to lithium is an effective strategy for acute depression in SAD-BT patients [26]. Lamotrigine has a bipolar maintenance indication and appears to reduce the risk of depressive recurrence, but there is a paucity of data about its use in acute bipolar depression. As noted previously, use of lamotrigine for any acute mood state is limited by the prolonged titration to mitigate SJS risk, but once the patient is euthymic may be very helpful [2]. Repetitive transcranial magnetic stimulation (RTMS), ketamine preparations and electroconvulsive therapy (ECT) have abundant evidence in bipolar depression and some positive data in schizophrenia [27]. These should be considered despite the lack of studies in SAD-BT patients, especially ECT and RTMS which have a significant body of data for their use in schizophrenia spectrum patients. Pramipexole has modest data supporting use in unipolar and bipolar depression but no data in SAD-BT patients [28]. Pramipexole has been studied in adult patients with schizophrenia or schizoaffective disorder as an augmenting strategy, typically to target residual negative symptoms. In a 12-week, placebo-controlled trial (n = 24), mean pramipexole doses of 4.25 mg/d appeared to be well tolerated with reductions in both positive and negative psychotic symptoms [29]. While the study subjects were not chosen on the basis of depressive symptomatology, this study demonstrates the feasibility of using pramipexole in otherwise stable schizophrenia spectrum patients.

Table 7.4 Considerations in Choice of Antipsychotic for Management of Bipolar Depression in Schizoaffective Disorder, Bipolar Type Patients*

Medication	Advantages	Disadvantages	Dosages in Bipolar I Depression
Quetiapine	Promotes sleep. Can be added to other antipsychotics without increasing risk for EPS.	Sedation, weight gain.	300 mg qhs

Table 7.4 (Cont.)

Medication	Advantages	Disadvantages	Dosages in Bipolar I Depression
Lurasidone	Non-sedating. Lower risk for metabolic adverse effects.	Should be taken with 350 kcal of food. Usually ordered 30 minutes after dinner. If taken on an empty stomach (i.e. at bedtime), absorption is decreased by 50%, so dose must be doubled (up to the FDA maximum of 160 mg).	Starting: 20 mg given 30 minutes after dinner Max: 120 mg given 30 minutes after dinner
Cariprazine	Non-sedating. Lower risk for metabolic adverse effects.	Has very high affinity for the D_2 receptor and may displace other antipsychotics whose efficacy is highly related to D_2 occupancy resulting in decompensation in some patients. (The weak D_2 antagonists clozapine, lumateperone and quetiapine are exceptions.)	Starting: 1.5 mg qhs Max: 3.0 mg qhs
Olanzapine/ fluoxetine combination	Promotes sleep.	Metabolic adverse effects. Fluoxetine is a strong cyp 2D6 inhibitor and may interact with other medications. Fluoxetine's active metabolite norfluoxetine has a 1–2-week half-life which may prove problematic if mania develops.	Starting: 6 mg (olanzapine)/25 mg (fluoxetine) Max: 12 mg (olanzapine)/50 mg (fluoxetine)

* The dosages recommended for bipolar depression may be insufficient to manage the psychotic symptoms in SAD-BT patients. Higher doses consistent with schizophrenia treatment should be utilized if the antipsychotic listed above will not be used adjunctively with another antipsychotic, or in the case of cariprazine which should not be combined with most antipsychotics (clozapine, lumateperone and quetiapine being notable exceptions).

☺ Summary Points
- Schizoaffective disorder, bipolar type (SAD-BT) is an illness composed of two distinct components that typically demands combination antipsychotic/mood stabilizer therapy.
- The choice of antipsychotic during the acute manic phase may be driven more by availability of acute intramuscular formulations, while that used in the maintenance phase may be driven more by long-term tolerability concerns such as avoidance of weight gain.
- Lithium is preferred over VPA due to superior neuroprotective and anti-suicide properties. Lithium can be loaded.
- Measures to maximize and track adherence, including use of long-acting injectable antipsychotics, pill counts and frequent determination of mood stabilizer serum levels are important.
- Treatment of the depressive phase should focus on the use of agents that have low risk for mania induction (quetiapine, lurasidone, cariprazine, olanzapine/fluoxetine) and avoidance of traditional antidepressants.

References

1. Meyer, J. M. (2018). Pharmacotherapy of psychosis and mania. In Brunton, L. L., Hilal-Dandan, R., and Knollmann, B. C. (eds.). *Goodman & Gilman's The Pharmacological Basis of Therapeutics*, 13th ed. Chicago, IL: McGraw-Hill, pp. 279–302.
2. Baldessarini, R. J., Tondo, L., Vazquez, G. H. (2019). Pharmacological treatment of adult bipolar disorder. *Mol Psychiatry*, 24, 198–217.
3. Post, R. M., Ketter, T. A., Uhde, T., et al. (2007). Thirty years of clinical experience with carbamazepine in the treatment of bipolar illness: principles and practice. *CNS Drugs*, 21, 47–71.
4. Zaccara, G., Perucca, E. (2014). Interactions between antiepileptic drugs, and between antiepileptic drugs and other drugs. *Epileptic Disord*, 16, 409–431.
5. Yatham, L. N., Beaulieu, S., Schaffer, A., et al. (2016). Optimal duration of risperidone or olanzapine adjunctive therapy to mood stabilizer following remission of a manic episode: a CANMAT randomized double-blind trial. *Mol Psychiatry*, 21, 1050–1056.
6. Leucht, S., Helfer, B., Dold, M., et al. (2015). Lithium for schizophrenia. *Cochrane Database Syst Rev*, 10, CD003834.
7. Jochim, J., Rifkin-Zybutz, R. P., Geddes, J., et al. (2019). Valproate for acute mania. *Cochrane Database Syst Rev*, 10, CD004052.
8. Vasudev, A., Macritchie, K., Watson, S., et al. (2008). Oxcarbazepine in the maintenance treatment of bipolar disorder. *Cochrane Database Syst Rev*, 10, CD005171.
9. Vasudev, A., Macritchie, K., Vasudev, K., et al. (2011). Oxcarbazepine for acute affective episodes in bipolar disorder. *Cochrane Database Syst Rev*, 10, CD004857.
10. Kim, Y. S., Kim, D. W., Jung, K. H., et al. (2014). Frequency of and risk factors for oxcarbazepine-induced severe and symptomatic hyponatremia. *Seizure*, 23, 208–212.
11. Malhi, G. S., Tanious, M. (2011). Optimal frequency of lithium administration in the treatment of bipolar disorder: clinical and dosing considerations. *CNS Drugs*, 25, 289–298.
12. Castro, V. M., Roberson, A. M., McCoy, T. H., et al. (2016). Stratifying risk for renal insufficiency among lithium-treated patients: an electronic health record study. *Neuropsychopharmacology*, 41, 1138–1143.
13. Gerhard, T., Devanand, D. P., Huang, C., et al. (2015). Lithium treatment and risk for dementia in adults with bipolar disorder: population-based cohort study. *Br J Psychiatry*, 207, 46–51.
14. Hayes, J. F., Pitman, A., Marston, L., et al. (2016). Self-harm, unintentional injury, and suicide in bipolar disorder during maintenance mood stabilizer treatment: a UK population-based electronic health records study. *JAMA Psychiatry*, 73, 630–637.
15. Song, J., Sjolander, A., Joas, E., et al. (2017). Suicidal behavior during lithium and valproate treatment: a within-individual 8-year prospective study of 50,000 patients with bipolar disorder. *Am J Psychiatry*, 174, 795–802.
16. Van Gestel, H., Franke, K., Petite, J., et al. (2019). Brain age in bipolar disorders: effects of lithium treatment. *Aust N Z J Psychiatry*, 53(12), 1179–1188.
17. Hirschfeld, R. M., Allen, M. H., McEvoy, J. P., et al. (1999). Safety and tolerability of oral loading divalproex sodium in acutely manic bipolar patients. *J Clin Psychiatry*, 60, 815–818.
18. Wingard, L., Brandt, L., Boden, R., et al. (2019). Monotherapy vs. combination therapy for post mania maintenance treatment: a population based cohort study. *Eur Neuropsychopharmacology*, pii, S0924-977X(19)30234-2. doi: 10.1016/j.euroneuro.2019.04.003
19. Remington, G., Teo, C., Mann, S., et al. (2013). Examining levels of antipsychotic adherence to better understand nonadherence. *J Clin Psychopharmacol*, 33, 261–263.
20. Murru, A., Pacchiarotti, I., Amann, B. L., et al. (2013). Treatment adherence in bipolar I and schizoaffective disorder, bipolar type. *J Affect Disord*, 151, 1003–1008.
21. Even, C., Thuile, J., Kalck-Stern, M., et al. (2010). Psychoeducation for patients with bipolar disorder receiving lithium: short and long term impact on locus of control and knowledge about lithium. *J Affect Disord*, 123, 299–302.
22. Butler, M., Urosevic, S., Desai, P., et al. (2018). AHRQ comparative effectiveness reviews. In *Treatment for Bipolar Disorder in Adults: A Systematic Review* (eds.). Rockville, MD: Agency for Healthcare Research and Quality.
23. Meyer, J. M. (2020). Monitoring and improving antipsychotic adherence in outpatient forensic diversion programs. *CNS Spectr*, 25, 136–144.
24. Murru, A., Pacchiarotti, I., Nivoli, A. M., et al. (2011). What we know and what we don't know about the treatment of schizoaffective disorder. *Eur Neuropsychopharmacol*, 21, 680–690.
25. Vieta, E. (2010). Developing an individualized treatment plan for patients with schizoaffective disorder: from pharmacotherapy to psychoeducation. *J Clin Psychiatry*, 71 Suppl. 2, 14–19.
26. Koola, M. M., Fawcett, J. A., Kelly, D. L. (2011). Case report on the management of depression in schizoaffective disorder, bipolar type focusing on lithium levels and measurement-based care. *J Nerv Ment Dis*, 199, 989–990.
27. Bartova, L., Papageorgiou, K., Milenkovic, I., et al. (2018). Rapid antidepressant effect of S-ketamine in schizophrenia. *Eur Neuropsychopharmacol*, 28, 980–982.
28. Tundo, A., de Filippis, R., De Crescenzo, F. (2019). Pramipexole in the treatment of unipolar and bipolar depression. A systematic review and meta-analysis. *Acta Psychiatr Scand*, 140, 116–125.
29. Kelleher, J. P., Centorrino, F., Huxley, N. A., et al. (2012). Pilot randomized, controlled trial of pramipexole to augment antipsychotic treatment. *Eur Neuropsychopharmacol*, 22, 415–418.
30. Eli Lilly and Company (2019). *Zyprexa Package Insert*. Indianapolis.
31. Pfizer Inc. (2018). *Geodon Package Insert*. New York, New York.
32. Kook, K. A., Stimmel, G. L., Wilkins, J. N., et al. (1985). Accuracy and safety of a priori lithium loading. *J Clin Psychiatry*, 46, 49–51.
33. Reed, R. C., Dutta, S. (2006). Does it really matter when a blood sample for valproic acid concentration is taken following once-daily administration of divalproex-ER? *Ther Drug Monit*, 28, 413–418.

1.07 Approach to Bipolar Diathesis in Schizophrenia Patients (Continued)

34. Meyer, J. M. (2019). Monitoring and improving antipsychotic adherence in outpatient forensic diversion programs. *CNS Spectr*, in press. doi: 10.1017/S1092852919000865
35. Hard, M. L., Mills, R. J., Sadler, B. M., et al. (2017). Aripiprazole lauroxil: pharmacokinetic profile of this long-acting injectable antipsychotic in persons with schizophrenia. *J Clin Psychopharmacol*, 37, 289–295.
36. Hard, M. L., Mills, R. J., Sadler, B. M., et al. (2017). Pharmacokinetic profile of a 2-month dose regimen of aripiprazole lauroxil: a phase i study and a population pharmacokinetic model. *CNS Drugs*, 31, 617–624.

1.08 Approach to Anxiety in Schizophrenia Spectrum Patients

Introduction Large studies and meta-analyses have noted that anxiety symptoms can occur in up to 65% of patients with schizophrenia, and the prevalence of any anxiety disorder (at the syndromal level) is estimated to be up to 38% [1, 2]. Anxiety symptoms are thus commonly encountered when treating patients with chronic psychotic disorders; however, of equal importance is the conclusion that more than 40% of schizophrenia spectrum patients who report an anxiety symptom are suffering from a cause other than a primary anxiety disorder or depression with anxiety. The differential diagnosis of anxiety symptoms is quite broad among patients with chronic psychotic disorders, but the correct action depends greatly on the underlying etiology. Reflexive use of a benzodiazepine or a selective serotonin reuptake inhibitor (SSRI) to treat anxiety is not appropriate in many instances and can be associated with deleterious outcomes such as increased mortality (benzodiazepines), or antidepressant-induced destabilization of patients with a bipolar diathesis (i.e. patients with a diagnosis of schizoaffective disorder, bipolar type). The issues to consider in documenting a treatment rationale are outlined in Table 8.1. A thoughtful review of the anxiety symptom evolution in relationship to medication changes or other factors should enable the clinician to arrive at a testable hypothesis and plot a course of action.

Table 8.1 Differential Diagnosis of Anxiety Symptoms in Schizophrenia Patients

1.	Is the anxiety related to undertreated psychotic symptoms?
2.	Is the anxiety due to akathisia?
3.	Is the anxiety related to lack of (or undertreated) mood stability in someone with a bipolar diathesis on no mood stabilizer or on an antidepressant?
4.	Is the anxiety associated with depressive symptoms in the absence of worsening or undertreated positive psychotic symptoms?
5.	Is there a primary anxiety disorder?

A Association with Psychosis and Relapse It is well established that patients with acute exacerbations of positive psychotic symptoms have a high prevalence of depressive and anxiety complaints [3, 4]. However, as a predictor of relapse, anxiety emerges as a more useful sign. In a longitudinal study of schizophrenia patients, 267 of whom experienced a relapse, only seven of the 30 items in the Positive and Negative Syndrome Scale (anxiety, delusions, suspiciousness, hallucinations, excitement, tension and conceptual disorganization) increased in the seven to ten days before relapse [4]. Anxiety is now considered important enough as a predictor of relapse that it is a core component of a new self-report screening tool: Relapse Risk Assessment for Schizophrenia Patients [5]. The anxiety complaint may be intimately tied to hallucinations or the content of a delusion, but in many instances is simply a nonspecific symptom. The clinical imperative is to discern whether undertreated psychotic symptoms are present, and, critically, if akathisia is the cause. As noted below, as akathisia becomes more severe it can be distressing enough to worsen the positive symptoms of psychosis, and rarely has been cited as a cause of suicide [6]. If akathisia is driving the psychotic exacerbation, an increase in antipsychotic dosages will only worsen the underlying problem of akathisia and its secondary manifestations of anxiety and positive symptoms of psychosis. When there is no suspicion of akathisia, then the differential is narrowed down to causes of persistent or exacerbated psychotic symptoms including antipsychotic undertreatment or nonadherence, substance use or psychosocial stressors [7]. In instances where anxiety is related to undertreated psychosis, increasing antipsychotic dosages, or assuring adherence with previously effective doses is indicated.

B Akathisia The pathophysiology of akathisia is less well understood than that for parkinsonism and acute dystonia, although it is often related to the degree of dopamine D_2 antagonism [6, 8]. Akathisia responds to medications not useful for parkinsonism or acute dystonia (e.g. centrally acting beta-adrenergic antagonists, clonazepam), and responds incompletely to antimuscarinic anticholinergic medications, features that point to pathways outside of the nigrostriatal dopaminergic system [6, 8]. The classic presentation of akathisia involves a subjective complaint of restlessness that may be objectively observable when more severe; however, the complaint may be solely one of anxiety in certain individuals [1]. Differentiating akathisia-induced anxiety from other etiologies can be challenging, but the clinical clues outlined in Table 8.2 provide a roadmap. The time course of the evolving complaint can be particularly instructive, bearing in mind that for oral antipsychotics with long half-lives (e.g. cariprazine) or for long-acting injectable antipsychotics, akathisia may not emerge for several weeks after a dosage increase. While undertreated psychosis is associated with anxiety, akathisia can induce not only anxiety symptoms, but also exacerbate psychotic symptoms [6]. In its more severe forms, akathisia can be distressing enough to not only worsen psychopathology but also result in suicide attempts [9–11].

Table 8.2 Clinical Features Suggesting Akathisia as a Source of Anxiety Symptoms

1.	There may be classical akathisia-related complaints (e.g. restlessness)
2.	The complaint of anxiety arose or increased after a recent antipsychotic dosage increase
3.	There are other D_2-related adverse effects noted (e.g. parkinsonism)
4.	There is no evidence for a bipolar diathesis

When akathisia is suspected, the correct approach involves antipsychotic dose reduction, and urgent use of propranolol, clonazepam or mirtazapine (if there is no bipolar diathesis) to manage the acute distress [12–14]. Anticholinergics appear less effective and should be avoided, especially since they also carry the burden of cognitive impairment [15–17]. As discussed in Section D, clonazepam is effective for akathisia but should not be used for long-term treatment due to the association between benzodiazepine use and increased mortality in schizophrenia spectrum patients [18, 19]. The value of mirtazapine lies primarily in its $5HT_{2A}$ antagonist properties, and the placebo-controlled literature indicates that it is effective even when added to atypical antipsychotics [14]. As mirtazapine is an antidepressant, it must be avoided in schizoaffective disorder, bipolar type patients. The long-term strategy is to decrease antipsychotic exposure and thereby eliminate the akathisia complaint. In some instances, switching from a typical to an atypical antipsychotic, or to clozapine may be necessary [8].

ⓒ Association with Bipolar Diathesis in Schizoaffective Disorder Bipolar Type In

a large cohort of outpatients (n = 631) carefully screened for anxiety comorbidity using the Structured Clinical Interview for the Diagnostic and Statistical Manual of Mental Disorders, the rates of anxiety disorders in those with schizoaffective disorder (30.1%) were nearly twice that for those with schizophrenia (16.7%), and also higher than in bipolar disorder patients (22.4%) [20]. The high rates of anxiety in bipolar and schizoaffective disorder bipolar type (SAD-BT) patients relate to the concept that anxiety can be a manifestation of inadequately treated mania or hypomania [21]. When the diagnosis (or history) support that this patient has SAD-BT, the usual steps should be taken to ensure that mood instability is not the cause of anxiety. In those circumstances any antidepressants must be stopped (if being used), and mood stabilizer levels optimized into the high end of the maintenance therapeutic range (see Chapter 1.07).

Some SAD-BT patients on antipsychotic monotherapy without a mood stabilizer may have a working diagnosis of schizophrenia because the more florid neurovegetative aspects of mania are not evident due to the antimanic effects of D_2 antagonism. In certain instances, there may be clues from prior records of a history of mania, or there may be indications that the recent addition of an antidepressant actually induced anxiety instead of alleviating it. When there is any suspicion that this patient might suffer from SAD-BT and not schizophrenia, antidepressants must be stopped if being used. Improvement in the level of anxiety after antidepressant discontinuation is sufficient to replace the schizophrenia diagnosis with SAD-BT, and for this patient to be started on a mood stabilizer (e.g. lithium). For those patients in whom the SAD-BT diagnosis is entertained on the basis of prior history but who are not on antidepressants and also not on a mood stabilizer, the hypothesis is that the anxiety complaint is a residual symptom of a partially treated mixed or manic state. In these instances the next course of action is to add a mood stabilizer (e.g. lithium). If the patient indeed has schizophrenia and not SAD-BT, lithium should produce no benefit (there is some low-quality evidence that augmentation of antipsychotics with lithium is effective, but the effects are not significant when more prone-to-bias open RCTs are excluded) [22]. In that circumstance, one must seek other etiologies for the anxiety complaint.

ⓓ Emerging Concerns about Benzodiazepines and Increased Mortality in Schizophrenia Spectrum Disorder Patients A high potency benzodiazepine will address

akathisia, and might transiently improve psychotic anxiety or anxiety as a symptom of a bipolar mixed state or hypomania, so why not try this first?

There are two compelling reasons to avoid reflexive use of a benzodiazepine when a schizophrenia spectrum patient complains of anxiety:

1. An initial positive response to a benzodiazepine gets one no closer to understanding the underlying cause and pursuing a more specific treatment.
2. The use of benzodiazepines in schizophrenia is increasingly associated with higher rates of mortality, especially suicide mortality. The first signal of this association emerged from an analysis of mortality trends in a sample of 2588 Finnish first episode schizophrenia patients followed on average for 4.2 years. Compared with antipsychotic monotherapy, concomitant use of two or more antipsychotics or an antidepressant was not associated with increased mortality; moreover, antidepressant use was associated with a markedly decreased hazard ratio (HR) for suicide deaths (HR, 0.15; 95% CI, 0.03–0.77). Conversely, benzodiazepine use was associated with a substantial increase in all-cause mortality (HR, 1.91; 95% CI, 1.13–3.22), and this was attributable to suicidal deaths (HR, 3.83; 95% CI, 1.45–10.12) not to non-suicidal deaths (HR, 1.60; 95% CI, 0.86–2.97) [18]. A subsequent Swedish retrospective study of 21,492 schizophrenia patients, aged 16–65, with median follow-up of five years also noted the association between benzodiazepine use and increased mortality [19]. In this predominantly chronic population (only 6% were first episode patients), both high-dose and moderate dose benzodiazepine use was associated with an elevated adjusted hazard ratio (AHR) for all-cause mortality: high-dose AHR 1.74 [95% CI,1.50–2.03]; moderate dose AHR 1.23 [95% CI, 1.06–1.42]. Moreover, high-dose benzodiazepine exposure doubled suicide mortality 2.16 [95% CI, 1.29–3.64]; moderate or low-dose exposure did not significantly increase suicide risk.

Aside from very short-term use in unmedicated patients, benzodiazepines confer no demonstrable benefit on the course of schizophrenia [23, 24]. The value in management of psychosis-induced aggression is also questionable in patients who are already on some form of antipsychotic therapy [24, 25]. The only evidence-based use for benzodiazepines rests in the treatment of acute antipsychotic-associated akathisia [12]. Clonazepam, mirtazapine and propranolol are effective for akathisia management, but the preferred long-term strategy for akathisia is antipsychotic dose reduction or switching to a less offending antipsychotic [8]. In patients without a bipolar diathesis, mirtazapine can be used for its $5HT_{2A}$ antagonist properties to manage akathisia [14] (see Section B above).

ⓔ Treatment of Primary Anxiety Disorders or Depression with Anxiety in Schizophrenia Spectrum Patients

Many anxiety disorders respond to agents that promote serotonergic neurotransmission, with the SSRI antidepressants considered standard initial treatment [1]. An SSRI is an appropriate choice for the group of stable patients with schizophrenia for whom other anxiety-related etiologies have been ruled out and who are diagnosed with panic disorder, social phobia, post-traumatic stress disorder (PTSD), obsessive compulsive disorder (OCD), or who have depression with associated anxiety [1]. As noted previously and in Chapter 1.07, the use of an antidepressant in SAD-BT patients should be approached cautiously, even when such patients have therapeutic levels of a primary mood stabilizer (lithium or valproate/divalproex). The concern is that any antidepressant, even an SSRI, can destabilize such individuals [26]. For SAD-BT type patients with anxiety due to depressive symptoms, other options exist that do not possess the risk for induction of mania/hypomania or a mixed state, and are discussed in Chapter 1.07. When the SAD-BT patient has a primary anxiety disorder (e.g. panic disorder), the SSRI should be titrated slowly so that any sign of mood instability can be addressed rapidly by discontinuation. Fluoxetine should be avoided due to the long half-life of the metabolite norfluoxetine (one to two weeks). For those patients with obsessive-compulsive symptoms, the differential diagnosis is OCD or obsessive symptoms related to the psychotic symptoms [27]. In the latter group, optimal management of the psychotic symptoms should decrease the frequency and severity of the obsessional symptoms. When the patient clearly has obsessions or compulsions that are unrelated to the psychotic disorder (e.g. hand washing that is not driven by delusions or hallucinatory content), clinicians should first assess whether the OCD symptoms arose after the use of an atypical antipsychotic. In some instances, the serotonin $5HT_{2A}$ antagonist properties of atypical antipsychotics have been associated with new onset OCD symptoms [1]. Where no such temporal relationship exists an SSRI can be introduced, but with the same caveats as noted before if the patient has a bipolar diathesis. Where an SSRI is contraindicated or not tolerated due to a bipolar diathesis one could consider exposure and response prevention, although the literature for its use in schizophrenia spectrum patients is virtually nonexistent [28].

ⓒ Summary Points

- Clinicians must carefully consider several possible etiologies of anxiety complaints in schizophrenia spectrum patients.
- Emergence of anxiety in relationship to an antipsychotic dosage increase points to akathisia as the cause of anxiety.
- Emergence or worsening of anxiety following addition of an antidepressant implicates a bipolar diathesis.

1.08 Approach to Anxiety in Schizophrenia Spectrum Patients (Continued)

📖 References

1. Temmingh, H., Stein, D. J. (2015). Anxiety in patients with schizophrenia: epidemiology and management. *CNS Drugs*, 29, 819–832.
2. Bosanac, P., Mancuso, S. G., Castle, D. J. (2016). Anxiety symptoms in psychotic disorders: results from the Second Australian National Mental Health Survey. *Clin Schizophr Relat Psychoses*, 10, 93–100.
3. Van der Heiden, W., Konnecke, R., Maurer, K., et al. (2005). Depression in the long-term course of schizophrenia. *Eur Arch Psychiatry Clin Neurosci*, 255, 174–184.
4. Wang, D., Gopal, S., Baker, S., et al. (2018). Trajectories and changes in individual items of positive and negative syndrome scale among schizophrenia patients prior to impending relapse. *NPJ Schizophr*, 4, 10.
5. Velligan, D., Carpenter, W., Waters, H. C., et al. (2018). Relapse Risk Assessment for Schizophrenia Patients (RASP): a new self-report screening tool. *Clin Schizophr Relat Psychoses*, 11, 224–235.
6. Lohr, J. B., Eidt, C. A., Abdulrazzaq Alfaraj, A., et al. (2015). The clinical challenges of akathisia. *CNS Spectr*, 20 Suppl. 1, 1–14; quiz 15–16.
7. Porcelli, S., Bianchini, O., De Girolamo, G., et al. (2016). Clinical factors related to schizophrenia relapse. *Int J Psychiatry Clin Pract*, 20, 54–69.
8. Salem, H., Nagpal, C., Pigott, T., et al. (2017). Revisiting antipsychotic-induced akathisia: current issues and prospective challenges. *Curr Neuropharmacol*, 15, 789–798.
9. Shear, M. K., Frances, A., Weiden, P. (1983). Suicide associated with akathisia and depot fluphenazine treatment. *J Clin Psychopharmacol*, 3, 235–236.
10. Drake, R. E., Ehrlich, J. (1985). Suicide attempts associated with akathisia. *Am J Psychiatry*, 142, 499–501.
11. Sachdev, P., Loneragan, C. (1992). Reported association of akathisia with suicide. *J Nerv Ment Dis*, 180, 339.
12. Lima, A. R., Soares-Weiser, K., Bacaltchuk, J., et al. (2002). Benzodiazepines for neuroleptic-induced acute akathisia. *Cochrane Database Syst Rev*, 1999(1), CD001950.
13. Lima, A. R., Bacalcthuk, J., Barnes, T. R., et al. (2004). Central action beta-blockers versus placebo for neuroleptic-induced acute akathisia. *Cochrane Database Syst Rev*, 2004, CD001946.
14. Praharaj, S. K., Kongasseri, S., Behere, R. V., et al. (2015). Mirtazapine for antipsychotic-induced acute akathisia: a systematic review and meta-analysis of randomized placebo-controlled trials. *Ther Adv Psychopharmacol*, 5, 307–313.
15. Lima, A. R., Weiser, K. V., Bacaltchuk, J., et al. (2004). Anticholinergics for neuroleptic-induced acute akathisia. *Cochrane Database Syst Rev*, 2004, CD003727.
16. Vinogradov, S., Fisher, M., Warm, H., et al. (2009). The cognitive cost of anticholinergic burden: decreased response to cognitive training in schizophrenia. *Am J Psychiatry*, 166, 1055–1062.
17. Borghans, L., Sambeth, A., Blokland, A. (2020). Biperiden selectively impairs verbal episodic memory in a dose- and time-dependent manner in healthy subjects. *J Clin Psychopharmacol*, 40, 30–37.
18. Tiihonen, J., Suokas, J. T., Suvisaari, J. M., et al. (2012). Polypharmacy with antipsychotics, antidepressants, or benzodiazepines and mortality in schizophrenia. *Arch Gen Psychiatry*, 69, 476–483.
19. Tiihonen, J., Mittendorfer-Rutz, E., Torniainen, M., et al. (2016). Mortality and cumulative exposure to antipsychotics, antidepressants, and benzodiazepines in patients with schizophrenia: an observational follow-up study. *Am J Psychiatry*, 173, 600–606.
20. Young, S., Pfaff, D., Lewandowski, K. E., et al. (2013). Anxiety disorder comorbidity in bipolar disorder, schizophrenia and schizoaffective disorder. *Psychopathology*, 46, 176–185.
21. Serafini, G., Gonda, X., Aguglia, A., et al. (2019). Bipolar subtypes and their clinical correlates in a sample of 391 bipolar individuals. *Psychiatry Res*, 281, 112528.
22. Leucht, S., Helfer, B., Dold, M., et al. (2015). Lithium for schizophrenia. *Cochrane Database Syst Rev*, 2015, CD003834.
23. Dold, M., Li, C., Tardy, M., et al. (2012). Benzodiazepines for schizophrenia. *Cochrane Database Syst Rev*, 11, CD006391.
24. Zaman, H., Sampson, S. J., Beck, A. L., et al. (2017). Benzodiazepines for psychosis-induced aggression or agitation. *Cochrane Database Syst Rev*, 12, CD003079.
25. Dold, M., Li, C., Gillies, D., et al. (2013). Benzodiazepine augmentation of antipsychotic drugs in schizophrenia: a meta-analysis and Cochrane review of randomized controlled trials. *Eur Neuropsychopharmacol*, 23, 1023–1033.
26. Murru, A., Pacchiarotti, I., Nivoli, A. M., et al. (2011). What we know and what we don't know about the treatment of schizoaffective disorder. *Eur Neuropsychopharmacol*, 21, 680–690.
27. Tezenas du Montcel, C., Pelissolo, A., Schurhoff, F., et al. (2019). Obsessive-compulsive symptoms in schizophrenia: an up-to-date review of literature. *Curr Psychiatry Rep*, 21, 64.
28. Scotti-Muzzi, E., Saide, O. L. (2017). Schizo-obsessive spectrum disorders: an update. *CNS Spectr*, 22, 258–272.

1.09 Approach to Insomnia and Sleep Disturbance in Schizophrenia Spectrum Disorders

📖 **Introduction** Nature is replete with cyclic biological rhythms ranging in periodicity from much less than a day (ultradian) to months or years (infradian) [1]. For humans, however, biological rhythms that are about 24 hours in duration (circadian) are critical to healthy functioning. Among the most important of these is the sleep-wake cycle [2]. A recent review, meta-analysis and moderator analysis of 31 polysomnographic studies (n = 574) conducted between 1968 and 2014 found that patients suffering from schizophrenia spectrum disorders have significantly shorter total sleep time, longer sleep onset latency, more wake time after sleep onset, lower sleep efficiency, and decreased stage 4 sleep, slow wave sleep, and duration and latency of rapid eye movement sleep compared to healthy controls. The findings regarding delta waves and sleep spindles were inconsistent. Moderator analysis could not find any abnormalities in sleep architecture [3]. Among healthy sleep-deprived individuals subclinical psychotic experiences are increased. While data are less clear, insomnia also may increase psychotic signs and symptoms among schizophrenic patients, suggesting a possible bidirectional pathologic effect [4]. In particular, patients vulnerable to a bipolar diathesis may have their clinical stability decompensated and driven by insomnia [5]. Thus, maintenance of adequate sleep may be a critical element in the treatment of some patients with schizophrenia spectrum disorders.

Ⓐ **Background** Historically, many substances and medications have been used to induce sedation, e.g. ethyl alcohol, opium, paraldehyde, chloral hydrate, barbiturates and benzodiazepines [6, 7]. Classical benzodiazepine sedatives have fallen out of favor for several reasons, including risk of dependence or addiction, rapid tolerance to sedative properties when taken chronically, and increased mortality risk [8, 9, 10]. Currently, the most commonly prescribed sedatives include selective benzodiazepine receptor agonists (a.k.a. Z-drugs), circadian modulators (i.e. melatonin and its synthetic analogs), low-dose doxepin (tricyclic antidepressant) and the orexin receptor antagonist suvorexant [11].

Ⓑ **Z-Drugs** Three drugs are available in the US that show relative selectivity for benzodiazepine receptors in the reticular activating system (RAS). As a group, these hypnotics produce less complete tolerance and less withdrawal when used routinely than classic benzodiazepine hypnotics. They also cause less disturbance of sleep architecture. These medications are briefly described in Table 9.1 below.

Table 9.1 Z-Drug Hypnotics [24–27]

Medication	Half-Life	Dose Range	Comments
Zaleplon	1–1.5 hours	5–10 mg	Effective for initial insomnia but does not maintain sleep in patients with middle or late insomnia due to short half-life.

Zolpidem	2–3 hours	5–10 mg	Effective for initial and early middle insomnia. May cause dissociation if the patient remains awake after dosing.
Zolpidem CR	2–4 hours	6.25–12.5 mg	More effective than zolpidem for middle to late insomnia due to later release of a controlled-release layer, but also is more prone to cause morning drowsiness.
Eszopiclone	4–6 hours	1–8 mg	Sleep duration is proportional to bedtime dose. Effective for both short-term and chronic insomnia. It may cause an unpleasant metallic aftertaste in some patients.

⊙ Circadian Dysregulation In addition to insomnia, persons suffering from schizophrenia spectrum disorders are prone to sleep fragmentation and shifts in sleep phase up to day-night reversal [4, 12]. The neurohormone melatonin and two synthetic analogs are available to act as sedatives/circadian rhythm modulators. Melatonin and its synthetic analogs act at melatonin receptors (MT_1 and MT_2) in the suprachiasmatic nucleus to provide the brain with a neurohormonal signal of dusk. The evening rise in melatonin or rising melatonin/analog plasma concentrations from evening doses act to phase advance (move to an earlier clock time) the onset of the sleep-wake cycle [13]. These medications, especially when used to modulate sleep-wake cycle phase, should be given routinely (Table 9.2).

Table 9.2 Circadian Modulators [28–30]

Medication	Dose Range	Comments
Melatonin	3–10 mg	As a nutritional product, a critical element is ensuring that the patient receives an accurately labeled product. Melatonin has been reported to increase reactive aggression in healthy individuals.
Ramelteon	8 mg	Ramelteon should be avoided in moderate to severe hepatic impairment. Efficacy may be limited by low bioavailability.
Tasimelteon	20 mg	Tasimelteon should be avoided in severe hepatic impairment.

① Orexin Antagonist Autoimmune loss of the small hypothalamic population of neurons that synthesize and secrete the peptide neurotransmitter, orexin (a.k.a. hypocretin) causes narcolepsey [14]. Suvorexant is an orexin receptor antagonist that is active at both OR_1 and OR_2 receptors located on neurons in the brainstem reticular activating system. Antagonism at these G-protein linked receptors changes the second messenger populations of the neurons of the reticular activating system such that activity levels fall and less stimulation is provided to forebrain areas [15]. At doses of 10–20 mg taken within 30 minutes of bedtime, suvorexant produces initiation and maintenance of sleep comparable to that of the longer-acting Z-drug hypnotics, albeit by a different mechanism [16, 17]. A second nonselective orexin receptor antagonist, lemvorexant, was approved at doses of 5–10 mg at bedtime for treatment of insomnia in adults by the US Food and Drug Administration in December 2020 [18]. Its utility beyond its prerelease trials largely remains to be explored. That is, both available orexin antagonists have yet to be extensively evaluated in the context of insomnia in schizophrenia spectrum patients. Also, both orexin antagonists should be given routinely, as opposed to pro renata.

⊕ Other Commonly Used Medications A variety of medications that are antagonists or inverse agonists at histamine H_1 receptors have been used for their sedating properties. Commonly prescribed medications include sedating antipsychotics, e.g. chlorpromazine or quetiapine, sedating antidepressants, e.g. doxepin and trazodone, and first-generation antihistamines, e.g. diphenhydramine and hydroxyzine [19]. Rarely, especially in children and the elderly, antihistaminic medications may cause psychomotor agitation [20]. Two additional important caveats need to be raised with respect to such medications. First, medications with antidepressant properties should be used with caution in patients vulnerable to a bipolar diathesis and avoided among those presenting with signs and symptoms consistent with hypomania or mania [21, 22]. Second, it is worth noting that diphenhydramine adds to anticholinergic burden, while hydroxyzine does not [23].

Table 9.3 below describes a systematic approach to the assessment and treatment of insomnia in the context of complex treatment-resistant psychotic disorders.

Table 9.3 Systematic Approach to Insomnia in Schizophrenia [31, 32]

Issue	Approach to Treatment
Insomnia complaint	Assess whether daytime fatigue/sedation are present, if not consider normal short-term sleeper (sleep < 6 hours per night) or hypomania/mania. Consider environmental issues, e.g. irregular sleep hours, noisy nocturnal environment, afternoon or evening intake of stimulants (e.g. caffeine, nicotine, etc.), vigorous exercise before bedtime, activities in bed incompatible with sleep (e.g. television, electronic games, reading, etc.).
Assessment of medical or other psychiatric conditions	Consider whether medical or psychiatric conditions such as pain syndromes, apnea, inadequately controlled positive psychotic symptoms, anxiety, phobias, post-traumatic stress disorder, hypomania or mania, parasomnias, seizures, REM-associated behavior disorder, etc. may be disrupting sleep. If identified, treatment should be directed toward the underlying disorder or condition.
Characterize insomnia	Consider whether insomnia is chronic, transient or sporadic. Also identify whether insomnia is early, middle and/or global.
Step I	Encourage good sleep hygiene, i.e. routine hours of sleep, quiet environment, avoidance of late intake of stimulating substances or activities, avoidance of in-bed activities that conflict with sleep, etc.
Step II	Move stimulating medications, e.g. noradrenergic or dopaminergic, toward morning as much as is feasible. Also, as much as possible, consolidate sedating medications to evening.
Step III	If insomnia is characterized by phase advance or phase delay of the sleep-wake cycle, then treat initially with melatonin, ramelteon or tasimelteon. If not, then initiate treatment with a Z-drug, using controlled-release zolpidem or eszopiclone if middle or global insomnia is present.
Step IV	If Z-drug or circadian modulator monotherapy isn't adequately effective, then consider a combined trial.
Step V	If Z-drug or circadian modulator treatment isn't effective, then consider a combined trial of Z-drug plus suvorexant or circadian modulator plus suvorexant.
Step VI	If clinical assessment and the described interventions aren't adequately effective, then consider referral for polysomnographic sleep studies. Also note that cognitive-behavioral therapy has been shown to be effective in improving sleep in schizophrenia spectrum disorders.

⊛ Summary Points

- Sleep abnormalities and insomnia are common in schizophrenia spectrum disorders.
- Sleep abnormalities and insomnia in schizophrenia likely promote psychosis and are likely to induce hypomania or mania in patients vulnerable to a bipolar diathesis.
- Selective Z-drugs and circadian modulators have become first-line treatments for insomnia in schizophrenia.
- If insomnia is chronic, treatment should be routine rather than PRN.
- Suvorexant is about as effective as the Z-drugs but offers an alternative mechanism of action for sedation.
- Psychiatric medications used for sedation provide hypnosis by antagonism at histamine H_1 receptors. This may result in idiosyncratic agitation, especially in children and the elderly.
- Sedating antidepressants should be used with caution in patients prone to bipolar diathesis and must be avoided in cases of active hypomania, mania or mixed mood states.

1.09 Approach to Insomnia and Sleep Disturbance in Schizophrenia (Continued)

📖 References

1. Kuhlman, S. J., Craig, L. M., Duffy, J. F. (2018). Introduction to chronobiology. *Cold Spring Harb Perspect Biol*, 10(9), a033613.
2. Capezuti, E. A. (2016). The power and importance of sleep. *Geriatr Nurs*, 37, 487–488.
3. Chan, M. S., Chung, K. F., Yung, K. P., et al. (2017). Sleep in schizophrenia: a systematic review and meta-analysis of polysomnographic findings in case-control studies. *Sleep Med Rev*, 32, 69–84.
4. Cosgrave, J., Wulff, K., Gehrman, P. (2018). Sleep, circadian rhythms, and schizophrenia: where we are and where we need to go. *Curr Opin Psychiatry*, 31, 176–182.
5. Altena, E., Micoulaud-Franchi, J. A., Geoffroy, P. A., et al. (2016). The bidirectional relation between emotional reactivity and sleep: from disruption to recovery. *Behav Neurosci*, 130, 336–350.
6. Bollu, P. C., Kaur, H. (2019). Sleep medicine: insomnia and sleep. *Mo Med*, 116, 68–75.
7. Sargant, W. (1958). Sedatives and tranquillizers. I. *Br Med J*, 2, 1031–1032.
8. Ashton, H. (1994). Guidelines for the rational use of benzodiazepines. When and what to use. *Drugs*, 48, 25–40.
9. de la Iglesia-Larrad, J. I., Barral, C., Casado-Espada, N. M., et al. (2019). Benzodiazepine abuse, misuse, dependence, and withdrawal among schizophrenic patients: a review of the literature. *Psychiatry Res*, 284(1), 12660.
10. Tiihonen, J., Mittendorfer-Rutz, E., Torniainen, M., et al. (2016). Mortality and cumulative exposure to antipsychotics, antidepressants, and benzodiazepines in patients with schizophrenia: an observational follow-up study. *Am J Psychiatry*, 173, 600–606.
11. Matheson, E., Hainer, B. L. (2017). Insomnia: pharmacologic therapy. *Am Fam Physician*, 96, 29–35.
12. Monti, J. M., Monti, D. (2005). Sleep disturbance in schizophrenia. *Int Rev Psychiatry*, 17, 247–253.
13. Pavlova, M. (2017). Circadian rhythm sleep-wake disorders. *Continuum (Minneap Minn)*, 23, 1051–1063.
14. Liblau, R. S., Vassalli, A., Seifinejad, A., et al. (2015). Hypocretin (orexin) biology and the pathophysiology of narcolepsy with cataplexy. *Lancet Neurol*, 14, 318–328.
15. Coleman, P. J., Gotter, A. L., Herring, W. J., et al. (2017). The discovery of suvorexant, the first orexin receptor drug for insomnia. *Annu Rev Pharmacol Toxicol*, 57, 509–533.
16. Kuriyama, A., Tabata, H. (2017). Suvorexant for the treatment of primary insomnia: a systematic review and meta-analysis. *Sleep Med Rev*, 35, 1–7.
17. Herring, W. J., Connor, K. M., Ivgy-May, N., et al. (2016). Suvorexant in patients with insomnia: results from two 3-month randomized controlled clinical trials. *Biol Psychiatry*, 79, 136–148.
18. Murphy, P., Moline, M., Mayleben, D., et al. (2017). Lemborexant, a dual orexin receptor antagonist (DORA) for the treatment of insomnia disorder: results from a bayesian, adaptive, randomized, double-blind, placebo-controlled study. *J Clin Sleep Med*, 13, 1289–1299.
19. Dujardin, S., Pijpers, A., Pevernagie, D. (2018). Prescription drugs used in insomnia. *Sleep Med Clin*, 13, 169–182.
20. Yanai, K., Rogala, B., Chugh, K., et al. (2012). Safety considerations in the management of allergic diseases: focus on antihistamines. *Curr Med Res Opin*, 28, 623–642.
21. Antosik-Wojcinska, A. Z., Stefanowski, B., Swiecicki, L. (2015). Efficacy and safety of antidepressant's use in the treatment of depressive episodes in bipolar disorder – review of research. *Psychiatr Pol*, 49, 1223–1239.
22. Mendelson, W. B. (2005). A review of the evidence for the efficacy and safety of trazodone in insomnia. *J Clin Psychiatry*, 66, 469–476.
23. Chew, M. L., Mulsant, B. H., Pollock, B. G., et al. (2008). Anticholinergic activity of 107 medications commonly used by older adults. *J Am Geriatr Soc*, 56, 1333–1341.
24. Rosenberg, R. P. (2006). Sleep maintenance insomnia: strengths and weaknesses of current pharmacologic therapies. *Ann Clin Psychiatry*, 18, 49–56.
25. Zammit, G. K., Corser, B., Doghramji, K., et al. (2006). Sleep and residual sedation after administration of zaleplon, zolpidem, and placebo during experimental middle-of-the-night awakening. *J Clin Sleep Med*, 2, 417–423.
26. Huedo-Medina, T. B., Kirsch, I., Middlemass, J., et al. (2012). Effectiveness of non-benzodiazepine hypnotics in treatment of adult insomnia: meta-analysis of data submitted to the Food and Drug Administration. *BMJ*, 345, e8343.
27. Atkin, T., Comai, S., Gobbi, G. (2018). Drugs for insomnia beyond benzodiazepines: pharmacology, clinical applications, and discovery. *Pharmacol Rev*, 70, 197–245.
28. Williams, W. P., 3rd, McLin, D. E., 3rd, Dressman, M. A., et al. (2016). Comparative review of approved melatonin agonists for the treatment of circadian rhythm sleep-wake disorders. *Pharmacotherapy*, 36, 1028–1041.
29. Liu, J., Zhong, R., Xiong, W., et al. (2017). Melatonin increases reactive aggression in humans. *Psychopharmacology (Berl)*, 234, 2971–2978.
30. Tordjman, S., Chokron, S., Delorme, R., et al. (2017). Melatonin: pharmacology, functions and therapeutic benefits. *Curr Neuropharmacol*, 15, 434–443.
31. Asnis, G. M., Thomas, M., Henderson, M. A. (2015). Pharmacotherapy treatment options for insomnia: a primer for clinicians. *Int J Mol Sci*, 17(1), 50.
32. Joober, R., Cole, K., Tabbane, K., et al. (2017). An algorithmic approach to the management of insomnia in patients with schizophrenia. *Ann Clin Psychiatry*, 29, 133–144.

1.10 Approach to Psychosis in Children and Adolescents

Introduction Psychotic symptoms in children and adolescents are common especially in the context of anxiety and mood disorders. The prevalence is higher in younger children than in adolescents [1]. Assessing, diagnosing and treating young people presenting with psychotic symptoms is challenging. Children have psychotic experiences that may or may not indicate a psychotic spectrum disorder or other psychopathology. In fact, there is evidence that 40–60% of youth with bipolar illness and 15–35% with depression have psychotic symptoms [2]. One must establish a systematic approach when trying to determine the underlying cause of psychosis in children and adolescents. Moreover, it is vital to understand the presentations of schizophrenia that occur in children and adolescents, the psychiatric and medical conditions that have psychotic features, the drugs and medications that can induce a psychotic state, the recommended parameters when assessing and diagnosing youth with psychotic disorders, the recommended parameters when using antipsychotic medications in youth, the effectiveness of different antipsychotics when treating this population, the medications that are currently approved by the US Food and Drug Administration (FDA) for use in children and adolescents and the psychosocial interventions that may ameliorate psychotic symptoms. While no fail-safe approach exists to correctly identify children and adolescents with psychotic disorders, utilizing a systematic structure can increase accuracy, and therefore support development of an appropriate and comprehensive plan of care that will benefit the youth. An African proverb says that it takes a village to raise a child. The same applies when assessing, diagnosing and treating youth with psychosis. It takes collaboration with different disciplines, systems, organizations and working closely with guardians and family members.

Ⓐ Childhood-Onset Schizophrenia Childhood-onset schizophrenia (COS) is described as developing prior to 12 years of age [3]. COS is extremely rare and the differential diagnoses for a child this young should always include medical and neurological etiologies including genetic disorders [3]. Another important factor to consider is normal developmental experience such as having vivid fantasies and imaginary friends, although imaginary friends are usually controlled by the child and remain within age-appropriate bounds of reality testing [3–5]. Neurodevelopmental disability disorders, especially those involving language, can be difficult to distinguish from symptoms of schizophrenia [4]. Psychotic symptoms, unlike schizophrenia, are common in children aged 9–12 years [1]. Once a medical/neurological condition or toxic exposure has been ruled out (please see the differential diagnosis section), psychotic symptoms should suggest mood disorders, such as bipolar spectrum disorder, depressive disorders or anxiety disorders including obsessive-compulsive disorder (OCD) and developmental syndromes. In this age group the prevalence for schizophrenia is greater for males [3], the child is isolative and withdrawn and disruptive behavior is usually present at home and school. Academic performance is commonly affected. Cognitive problems such as difficulty with verbal reasoning, working memory, attention and processing speed are common [6]. Correctly identifying the diagnosis can be difficult since the presentation may be confused with depression or Oppositional-Defiant Disorder (ODD) [4]. The younger the onset of schizophrenia-related psychotic symptoms, the more severe the illness, the poorer the prognosis and the more resistant to medication therapy [7]. COS represents a more severe form of the disorder that includes more structural brain abnormalities and genetic risk factors [8]. Children with COS have been found to have a significant decrease in gray matter volume, less cortical folding and more cortical abnormalities [9].

Ⓑ Early-Onset Schizophrenia Early-onset schizophrenia (EOS) is described as developing between the ages of 13–18 years. In this age group the prodromal period typically includes a significant decrease in function, changes in behavior, decline in school performance, deficits in cognition, social withdrawal, preoccupation, suspiciousness, unusual behaviors and decrease in self-care. Just as in COS, these symptoms can also be associated with depression, anxiety, conduct problems and substance abuse [3]. Some limited data suggest that prodromal symptoms treated with selective serotonin reuptake inhibitors (SSRI) antidepressants, omega-3 fatty acids or psychosocial interventions may prevent these sub-syndromal symptoms from progressing to a psychotic disorder [10–12]. Risk factors that predict progression to overt psychotic illness include familial risk, recent deterioration in function, unusual suspicious or paranoid thought content, greater social impairment and/or history of substance abuse [13]. Treating youth diagnosed with schizophrenia promptly and aggressively with antipsychotic medications and psychosocial interventions may improve outcomes such as limiting impairment in their development and decreasing impacts on learning [14]. Compared to adults, EOS youth have fewer delusions, they experience less catatonia and their hallucinations are more multimodal (auditory, visual and tactile) [2, 4]. Their auditory hallucinations often contain comments or commands [4]. Hallucinations experienced by adolescents with more severe symptomatology, along with comorbid behavioral disturbance and lower functioning, more often exhibit progression to psychotic disorder [15]. Suicidality is common in youth experiencing psychotic symptoms. For example, in one study, 86% of youth interviewed with psychotic symptoms and suicidal ideation had planned or attempted suicide, which is a 20-fold greater rate than youth with suicidal ideation without psychosis [4]. Approximately 5% of EOS youth died by suicide [3].

The goals of treatment are to improve symptoms, limit impairment and prevent delay in learning. Prompt diagnosis of schizophrenia and aggressive treatment are necessary because repeated and prolonged psychotic episodes have harmful neuropsychological, neurophysiological and brain structural effects in patients diagnosed with a first psychosis [14, 16]. Psychotic symptoms during childhood are linked to psychotic disorder in adults [17]. Adult schizophrenia patients that had psychosis in childhood show greater social deficits, less employment history and less independent living than those schizophrenia patients who developed symptoms later in life [5].

Figure 10.1 Etiologies of psychosis in youth

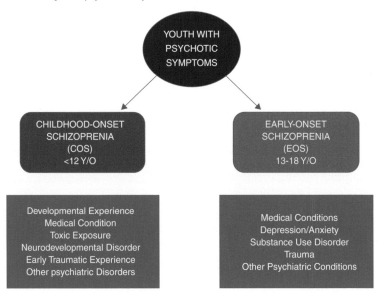

⊙ Differential Diagnosis: Psychiatric Conditions It is of great importance to determine if the symptoms experienced by a child or adolescent are secondary to a psychotic process or to a different psychopathology. This is easier said than done, especially in younger children, as the symptoms are nonspecific. When assessing any youth for possible psychosis, an in-depth history, observation, collateral information, direct questioning, use of rating scales and comprehensive workup are crucial to assist in narrowing the differential diagnosis. As stated earlier, it is common in childhood and adolescence to have psychotic experiences. Careful attention to details and diagnostic criteria can enhance ability to develop a working diagnosis. Psychiatric illnesses in children and adolescents that may present with psychotic symptoms include Affective Disorders (Depressive Disorders/Bipolar Disorders), Anxiety Disorders, Autism Spectrum Disorders, Trauma-Related Disorders, Obsessive-Compulsive Disorders, Neurodevelopmental Disorders and Substance Use Disorders.

Affective Disorders are very difficult to differentiate from psychosis since both can present with nonspecific psychotic experiences including hallucinations [2–5]. Using rating scales can be useful in identifying psychotic symptoms and other psychiatric or behavioral disorders [18–60]. See Table 10.1 below for commonly used tools.

Table 10.1 Commonly Used Evaluation Instruments

GENERAL PSYCHIATRIC SYMPTOMS
Child Behavior Checklist (CBCL)
Behavioral Assessment System for Children (BASC)
Brief Psychiatric Report for Children (BPRS-C)
Pediatric System Checklist (PSC)
Child System Inventory (CSI)
Child and Adolescent Psychiatric Assessment (CAPA)
Diagnostic Interview Schedule for Children (DISC)

PSYCHIATRIC SYMPTOMS
Kiddie Schedule for Affective Disorders and Schizophrenia Present and Lifetime Version (K-SAD-PL)
Schizophrenia Proneness Instrument – Child and Youth Version (SPI-CY)
Positive and Negative Symptoms Scale (PANSS)
Scale for Assessing Positive Symptoms (SAPS)
Scale for Assessing Negative Symptoms (SANS)
Washington University in St. Louis Kiddie Schedule for Affective Disorders and Schizophrenia (Wash-UKSADS)

ANXIETY DISORDER
Pediatric Anxiety Rating Scale (PARS)
Screen for Child Anxiety-Related Disorders (SCARED)
Spence Children's Anxiety Rating Scale (SCAS)

DEPRESSION
Children's Depression Inventory (CDI)
Beck Depression Inventory (BDI)
Modified Patient Health Questionnaire (PHQ-9)
Kutcher Adolescent Depression Scale (KADS)

BIPOLAR
Young Mania Rating Scale (YMRS)
Mood Disorder Questionnaire (MDQ)

PTSD
UCLA PTSD Reaction Index for Children (PTDS-RI)
Trauma Symptoms Checklist for Children (TSCC)
Children's Revised Impact of Event Scale (CRIES)

OCD
Children's Yale-Brown Obsessive-Compulsive Scale (CY-BOCS)

AUTISM SPECTRUM
Child Autism Rating Scale (CARS)
Vineland Adaptive Behavioral Scale (VABS)
Social Communication Questionnaire (SCQ)
Autism Spectrum Screening Questionairre (ASSQ)

ADHD
Conners' Rating Scales (CRS)
Strength and Weakness of ADHD Symptoms and Normal Behavior (SWAN)
Vanderbilt Diagnostic Rating Scale (VDRS)
ADHD Rating Scale (ARS)
Autism Spectrum Rating Scales (ASRS)

Table 10.1 (Cont.)

SUBSTANCE USE DISORDER
Crafft Screen
Personal Experience Screening Questionnaire (PESQ)
Global Appraisal of Indivudal Needs (GAIN)
Teen Addiction Severity Index (T-ASI)

Anxiety disorders are the most common mental health disorders in children and adolescents [61]. In anxiety, psychosis is highly prevalent [5]. In younger children phobias and separation anxiety are common, while in older children social anxiety and panic disorder are more prevalent. Youth that experience panic attacks may experience brief hallucinations at the peak of an attack. The psychotic symptoms in anxiety disorders are not typically as long-lasting as in psychotic illness [62].

Traumatic events experienced by children and adolescents include abuse (emotional, physical and sexual), neglect, witnessing domestic violence, being bullied plus a myriad of other possible traumatic events. Post-traumatic stress disorder (PTSD) is a major consequence of childhood abuse [63]. Children and adolescents diagnosed with PTSD often experience psychotic symptoms. Childhood trauma has been associated with the development of an array of psychiatric illnesses in adults including mood disorders, anxiety disorders, eating disorders, personality disorders and substance use disorders [63].

Obsessive-compulsive disorder (OCD) in children and adolescents can appear to be psychosis, while conversely schizophrenia can have obsessive and compulsive symptoms [64]. In children, obsessions are challenging to diagnose because despite the distress and impairment experienced it is difficult for a child to describe what is happening. Compulsions are less difficult because they can be observed.

① Differential Diagnosis: Neurodevelopmental Disorders Neurodevelopmental disorders (NDD) similarly present with a wide array of symptoms that include impairment in cognition, emotional dysregulation, behavioral problems, developmental delays, self-control difficulties, learning disabilities, memory and concentration problems [65]. Intellectual disabilities, communication disorders, autistic spectrum disorder, attention deficit hyperactivity disorder, genetic disorders and schizophrenia are included in the umbrella of neurocognitive disorders [66]. The overlap of symptoms in these disorders can confuse nosology and treatment. Autism spectrum disorder (ASD) symptoms include atypical social communication, decreased social interaction and restricted, repetitive patterns of behavior. Usually the lack of development of communication skills is present by the age of two years [67]. One possible way to differentiate ASD from psychotic disorders is that children who develop schizophrenia have had a normal period of development. In addition, in schizophrenia, restricted unusual interests and motor clumsiness are not typically present. Genetic disorders that may have associated psychotic symptoms include Down syndrome, acute intermittent porphyria, 22q11 Deletion Syndrome (Velocardiofacial deletion syndrome or DiGeorge syndrome), Marfan syndrome and Huntington's disease. Of all the genetic syndromes, 22q11 Deletion Syndrome is the most important to differentiate because 25% of these individuals will develop psychosis during adolescence [4]. The genetic defects that produce NDD range from large chromosomal deletions to single-nucleotide polymorphisms (SNPs). Several chromosomal deletions are associated with ASD and schizophrenia including 1q21.1, 16p11.2 and 22q11.2. Several NDDs share SNP [66].

Karyotyping examines the number of chromosomes and looks at structural changes. Karyotyping may indicate Down's syndrome, Klinefelter syndrome, Trisomy 18 and Turner syndrome among other conditions. Chromosomal microarray (CMA) looks for duplicated or deleted chromosomal segments called copy number variants (CNV). Microdeletions and microduplications can be detected with CMA and can test for 22q11.2, Fragile-X syndrome and Klinefelter [68]. When considering genetic testing, it is important to closely collaborate with the youth's pediatrician and consult a geneticist during the diagnostic evaluation.

ⓔ Differential Diagnosis: Substance Use Disorders Substance abuse is a common cause of psychosis especially in adolescents.

1. MDMA, GHB and methamphetamine are considered club drugs.
    a. MDMA or 3,4-methylenedioxymethamphetamine is also called Ecstasy/Molly/Mandy. MDMA produces altered sensations such as hallucinations, empathy, increased energy and pleasure. In addition, MDMA causes dangerously high body temperatures, muscle cramping, involuntary teeth clenching, chills and sweating.
    b. GHB or gamma-hydroxybutyrate is also called easy lay, Georgia home boy, G, scoop. GHB is commonly referred to as a "date rape drug" along with Rohypnol. GHB causes memory lapses, drowsiness, hallucinations, clumsiness, dizziness, low body temperature and nausea. If taken with alcohol the effect intensifies and overdose can be fatal.
    c. Methamphetamine is also called blue, crystal, ice, meth and speed. It causes increased wakefulness and physical activity, hallucinations, increased heart rate, decreased appetite, increased blood pressure, increased body temperature and increased breathing rate. Long-term use causes paranoia, hallucinations, severe dental problems, extreme weight loss, memory loss, violent behavior, confusion and sleeping problems. About 80% of the psychotic symptoms resolve within one month but some may last for years. Antipsychotics are highly effective in treating psychotic symptoms in amphetamine users [69].
2. Ketamine is also called special K, Dorothy, vitamin K and Kit-Kat. Ketamine is a dissociative anesthetic. It produces out-of-body experiences (k-hole), hallucinations, relaxation, numbness, euphoria, paranoia, increased heart rate, nystagmus, hyperthermia, increased blood pressure, muscle rigidity, and long-term cognitive deficits. About 3% of heavy ketamine users experience persisting psychotic symptoms [70].
3. Dextromethorphan (DXM) is a cough suppressant found in many over-the-counter cold medications. DXM is commonly abused by adolescents to experience hallucinations and psychedelic effects like ketamine and phencyclidine (PCP). The hallucinogenic high experienced with DXM is known as "robotripping" and is characterized by a distorted sense of reality, confusion, visual hallucinations, diaphoresis, tachycardia, hyperthermia, euphoria and restlessness. The effects usually last six hours but depend on the amount used [71].
4. LSD (lysergic acid diehtylamide) also known as acid, blotter, dots, mellow yellow and yellow sunshine is a powerful hallucinogen. LSD can be made in small tablets, gelatin squares or added to absorbent paper. The experience during use is called a "trip" and is characterized by changes in perception, sensory enhancement, diaphoresis, dry mouth, panic, dissociation, visual hallucinations, delusions, intense bliss usually mistaken for enlightenment and synesthesia (e.g. hearing colors and seeing sounds). The effects usually last approximately 8–12 hours. One can experience "bad trips" that are terrifying thoughts and feelings. Flashbacks of the LSD "trip" or drug-free hallucinogenic experiences are common and may last for years [72].
5. Phencyclidine is a hallucinogen and an anesthetic. PCP is also known as angel dust, hog, amoeba, super grass, belladonna and zoom. PCP produces euphoria, false perception of clear thinking, delusion, hallucinations, exaggerated strength, increased heart rate, numbness, paranoia, ideas of invulnerability and aggression. The drug causes painful withdrawal ("coming down") that includes confusion, agitation, increased appetite, depression, hallucinations, hyperthermia, muscle twitching and seizures. Recovery can take months. Other hallucinogens include Psilocybin (magic mushrooms, shrooms), Peyote or mescaline (buttons, cactus and mesc), Salvia divinorum (salvia, divine's sage, Maria Pastora, sally-d, Magic mint) [73].
6. Cannabis (THC – tetra-hydro-cannabinol) also known as marijuana, ganja, grass, pot, weed and reefer. Cannabis can be hand rolled in paper (joints) and smoked, smoked in pipes, bongs and by using electronic cigarettes (vaping) when in liquid or wax form. Cannabis can also be eaten (edibles) when combined with bake products or candy. Cannabis causes altered senses, relaxation, drowsiness, bloodshot eyes, increased appetite, paranoia, changes in mood, difficulty with thinking, problem solving difficulties, impaired memory, and when taken

in high doses or via regular use can cause hallucinations and delusions. In 2018, more than 11.8 million youths had used marijuana in the past year. The number of senior high-school students that reported vaping THC during the past month increased from 7.5% in 2018 to 14% in 2019 [74]. Synthetic cannabinoids (K2, Spice, fake weed) are man-made chemicals that are like those found in the marijuana plant. These chemicals are sprayed on plant material such as dried leaves so that it can be smoked or are made into liquid to be able to vaporize and inhale. Synthetic cannabinoids are falsely advertised as a safe and legal alternative to cannabis. Synthetic cannabinoids are in fact more powerful and dangerous than cannabis [75].

7. Synthetic cathinones, also known as bath salts, flakka, bliss, boom, cloud nine and vanilla sky, cause paranoia, hallucinations, increased friendliness, distorted reality, nose bleeds, increased blood pressure, increased sex drive, panic, agitation and violent behavior. It is sold as a white powder and is usually snorted or swallowed. The user can experience delirium, myocardial infarction, seizures, stroke, dehydration, muscle breakdown and kidney failure. The use is increasing in adolescents in the US [76].

8. Other drugs that can cause psychotic symptoms include anticholinergic plants (jimson weed, moonflower, angel's trumpet), barbiturates and opioids. Medications that can cause bizarre behaviors, delusions or hallucinations in children and adolescents are shown in Table 10.2 below.

Table 10.2 Commonly Abused Substances in Youth

Drug Name/Class	Common Street Names	Typical Characteristics
Club Drugs		
MDMA 3,4-methylenedioxymethamphetamine	Ectasy, Molly, Mandy	Hallucinations, increased empathy, high energy, euphoria, hyperthermia, muscle cramps, teeth clenching, chills and diaphoresis
GHB Gammahydroxybutyrate	Easy lay, Georgia home boy, G and scoop	Hallucinations, memory lapses, drowsiness, dizziness, ataxia, hyperthermia and nausea
Methamphetamine	Blue, crystal, ice, meth and speed	Hallucinations, paranoia, euphoria, increased physical activity, wakefulness, hypertension, tachycardia, anorexia, hyperthermia, tachypnea, dental loss, violence, confusion and insomnia
Other Drugs		
Ketamine	Special K, Dorothy, vitamin K and Kit-Kat	Hallucinations, depersonalization, paranoia, numbness, euphoria, relaxation, tachycardia, nystagmus, hyperthermia, muscle rigidity and cognitive deficits

DMX Dextromethorphan	Cough medication	Robotripping, hallucinations, distorted reality, confusion, diaphoresis, tachycardia, hyperthermia, euphoria and restlessness
LSD Lysergic acid diethylamide	Acid, blotter, dots, mellow yellow and yellow sunshine	Hallucinations, illusions, sensory enhancement, diaphoresis, dry mouth, panic, dissociation, delusions, intense bliss and synesthesia
PCP Phencyclidine	Angel dust, hog, amoeba, super grass, bella donna and zoom	Hallucinations, paranoia, delusions, euphoria, false perception of clear thinking, exaggerated strength, tachycardia, numbness, ideas of invulnerability and aggression
THC/Cannabis Tetrahydrocannabinol	Marijuana, ganja, grass, pot, weed and reefer	Hallucinations, delusions, paranoia, altered senses, relaxation, drowsiness, conjunctivitis, increased appetite, mood lability, slowed thinking and impaired memory
Synthetic Cannabinoids	Spice, K2, fake weed	Similar to cannabis but more potent
Synthetic Cathinones	Bath salts, flakka, bliss, boom, cloud nine and vanilla sky	Hallucinations, paranoia, increased friendliness, distorted reality, nose bleeds, increase blood pressure, increased sex drive, panic, agitation and violence

❼ Differential Diagnosis: Medication-Related Psychosis Several medications that are commonly used in children and adolescents can cause psychotic symptoms [77, 78]. These are summarized in Table 10.3 below.

Table 10.3 Medications That Can Cause Psychosis in Youth

Amphetamine-like drugs	Methylphenidate, dexmethylphenidate, amphetamine salts, dextroamphetamine, lisdexamfetamine
Corticosteroids	Prednisone, prednisolone
Antiepileptic drugs	Carbamazepine, phenobarbital, phenytoin, oxcarbazepine, valproic acid, lamotrigine
Anticholinergics	Diphenhydramine, atropine, oxybutynin, scopolamine, dextromethorphan, chlorpromazine

Table 10.3 (Cont.)

Beta-adrenergic blockers	Propranolol, atenolol, esmolol
Cephalosporin antibiotics	Cephalexin, cefadroxil, cefaclor, cefixime
Sulfonamide antibiotics	Sulfamethoxazole/trimethoprim, sulfadiazine, erythromycin/sulfisoxazole
Fluroquinolone antibiotics	Ciprofloxacin, moxifloxacin, levofloxacin
Procaine penicillin	Penicillin G
Antihistamines	Diphenhydramine, hydroxyzine, promethazine, chlorpheniramine, cyproheptadine, loratadine
Nonsteroidal anti-inflammatory drugs	Ibuprofen, naproxen
Salicylates	Aspirin
Benzodiazepines	Clonazepam, lorazepam, diazepam, alprazolam
SSRI antidepressants	Fluoxetine, sertraline, paroxetine, fluvoxamine, citalopram, escitalopram
Tricyclic antidepressants	Amitriptyline, clomipramine, mirtazapine, desipramine, nortriptyline, imipramine

Ⓖ **Differential Diagnosis: Medical Conditions** Narrowing down the medical differential in a child presenting with psychosis, one must keep in mind the age of the child and how rapidly the symptoms developed. The younger the child, the higher the chances of genetic syndromes or developmental neurocognitive disorders causing the psychotic symptoms. Sudden or acute presentation points toward infection, medication side effects or electrolyte imbalance. Table 10.4 presents a list of medical conditions that can induce psychosis [2, 4, 5, 77, 78].

Table 10.4 Medical Conditions That Can Induce Psychosis

Condition	Example
Central nervous system infections	Meningitis
	Encephalitis
Infections	Epstein-Barr virus
	Lyme disease
	Mycoplasma pneumonia
Delirium	Infection
	Drug-induced trauma
Neoplasms	Frontal lobe
	Temporal lobe
	Pituitary
	Neoplasm
Endocrine disorders	Lupus

Genetic syndromes	22q11 (velo-cardio-facial syndrome, DiGeorge syndrome) Down syndrome Marfan syndrome Prader-Willi syndrome, Neiman-Pick disease Fabry's disease Huntington disease
Autoimmune disorders	Anti-N-methyl-D-aspartate receptor encephalitis Cerebral lupus
Toxic exposures	Mercury Lead
Seizures	Temporal lobe epilepsy Interictal psychosis
Traumatic brain injury (TBI)	Usually around age 4–5 years with loss of consciousness over 30 minutes
Anticholinergic toxicity	Diphenhydramine Atropine Other anticholinergics
Metabolic disorders	Wilson's disease Acute intermittent porphyria Tay-Sachs disease Homocystinuria Juvenile metachromatic leukodystrophy
Electrolyte imbalances	Hyponatremia Hypernatremia Hypocalcemia Hypercalcemia Hypomagnesemia Hypermagnesemia Hypophosphatemia Hypokalemia
Other conditions	Syphilis HIV Cushing's disease Migraines Hypoglycemia Narcolepsy Vitamin B12 deficiency Pellagra (vitamin B6 deficiency) Hypothyroidism (Hashimoto's) Hyperthyroidism (thyroid storm) Parathyroid disease

⊕ Evaluation and Workup of Children and Adolescents Presenting with

Psychosis Evaluation of children and adolescents presenting with psychotic symptoms should start with a thorough history and physical examination that includes hearing and visual testing. Collaboration with a pediatrician and neurologist is key when ruling out medical/neurological conditions. A neurological examination can provide clues that may indicate the possibility of a brain lesion, a genetic disorder, CNS infection, seizure disorder, metabolic disorders and delirium secondary to toxic ingestion. Mental status examination can help assess for thought content, thought process, perception, cognition and bizarre behaviors. Vital signs can point to infection or toxic ingestion. Electrocardiogram can be useful if anticholinergic poisoning is suspected.

Tests that can aid in determining what is the cause of a positive finding on the neurological exam are listed below [2, 4, 77, 78, 79, 80, 81].

1. Neuroimaging or MRI with contrast should be ordered when suspecting brain-occupying lesions.
2. Genetic consult and testing (microarray/karyotype) for genetic disorders.
3. Lumbar puncture for CNS infections. Vital signs can provide information for possible infections or substance-induced psychosis.
4. Sleep-deprived EEG if complex partial seizures are suspected.

The following Table 10.5 contains the laboratory tests that can help identify the etiology of the psychotic symptoms in youth [2, 4, 78, 79, 80, 81].

Table 10.5 Laboratory Tests Relevant to Psychosis Evaluation

Laboratory Tests	
Sodium	Level decreased
Calcium	Level decreased
Magnesium	Level decreased
Phosphorus	Level decreased
Glucose	Level decreased
Complete Blood Count (CBC)	Infection/antibiotic use
Thyroid Stimulating Hormone (TSH) and Free T4	Hyperthyroidism
Urine Toxicology	Substance-induced psychosis
Urinalysis	Urea cycle disorders, non-ketotic hyperglycemia
Erythrocyte Sedimentation Rate (ESR)	Infection, autoimmune disorders
Ceruloplasmin	Wilson's Disease
Vitamin B12	Deficiency
Vitamin B9 (Folate)	Deficiency
Vitamin D	Deficiency
FTA-Abs	Syphilis
HIV	Encephalopathy, delirium, opportunistic infections
Heavy Metals	Lead, mercury

❶ Psychosis in Children and Adolescents Assessment Recommendations The

American Academy of Child and Adolescent Psychiatry has ten recommendations (shown in Table 10.6 below) when assessing children and adolescents with schizophrenia [3].

Table 10.6 Assessment Recommendations in Childhood Psychosis

• A psychiatric assessment for children and adolescents should always include questions for psychosis
• The DSM-5 diagnostic criteria for schizophrenia are the same for youth and for adults
• Evaluate for other pertinent clinical conditions and associated problems such as suicidality, comorbid disorder, substance abuse, developmental disabilities and medical conditions
• The primary treatment for children and adolescents with schizophrenia is antipsychotic medication
• Medication therapy should be continued in children and adolescents with schizophrenia to improve functioning and to prevent relapse
• Adjunctive treatment with medication may be beneficial to address associated symptoms such as side effects, depression, bipolar disorder, etc.
• Clozapine should be considered for youth with treatment-resistant illness after failure of two adequate trials of antipsychotics. A second opinion should be obtained prior to the clozapine trial
• Baseline and follow-up monitoring of symptoms and laboratory test should be performed including metabolic function, weight, fasting glucose, blood pressure and lipid profile
• Psychotherapeutic interventions should be provided in combination with medication therapy
• Electroconvulsive therapy (ECT) may be used in cases with severe impairment if medications have not been effective or are not tolerated

❶ Practice Parameter for Atypical Antipsychotic Use in Children and Adolescents The American Academy of Child and Adolescent Psychiatry has provided parameters for the use of atypical antipsychotic medications in children and adolescents [82]. Metabolic changes such as weight gain and diabetes are greater in youth than in adults. The cardiovascular side effects, such as increased QTc, hypotension and tachycardia, are greater in youths than adults. Severe neutropenia induced by clozapine is greater in youths than adults. Seizures are more frequent with clozapine. Hepatic dysfunction and steatohepatitis in youths is more weight-related than in adults. Long-term effects in youths of elevated prolactin are unknown. Antipsychotic-induced movement disorders are more common in youths than in adults. Neuroleptic malignant syndrome (NMS) is rare in youths taking antipsychotics.

Atypical antipsychotics are mainly used in youth for nonpsychotic conditions including aggression and dysfunctional behaviors for autism, disruptive mood dysregulation disorder, manic and mixed episodes in bipolar disorders, OCD, eating disorders, depression, sleep problems and impulse control associated with personality disorders.

Specific recommendations for screening and assessment of children and adolescents taking atypical antipsychotics are listed below in Table 10.7 [82].

Table 10.7 Antipsychotic Parameters in Childhood Psychosis

• Prior to prescribing an atypical antipsychotic medication to children and adolescents, and during treatment, guidelines such as performing a careful diagnostic assessment, attention to comorbid medical conditions and reviewing the drugs that the patient is already taking should be given attention. A multidisciplinary plan should be developed. Psychoeducation should be provided to the patient and family. Monitor the progress of the treatment and assess for improvement. Discuss the risk and benefits of the atypical antipsychotic medication with the youth and the guardian.

Table 10.7 (Cont.)

- When selecting an atypical agent for youth, consult the most current available evidence in the scientific literature.

- Obtain a personal and family history of diabetes, hyperlipidemia, seizure, cardiac conditions as well as familial adverse effects to atypical antipsychotic medication.

- Start at low doses and increase slowly to reach the lowest effective dose.

- Dosing should be supported by current literature and will vary depending on the condition treated, side effects and tolerability.

- If side effects develop, lower the dose or change to another agent. If side effects subside with decreasing the dose of the offending agent, slowly increase the dose to target the symptoms.

- The use of multiple psychotropics may be necessary, especially in refractory patients. Polypharmacy should be avoided if possible.

- Avoid using multiple atypical antipsychotic medications when treating youth.

- After failing one atypical medication select an alternative since another atypical medication may be effective. A different type of agent may be tried. An adequate trial of a medication prior to switching is four to six weeks of treatment at a therapeutic plasma concentration. If a medication fails, re-evaluate and reassess for comorbid conditions.

- Short- and long-term safety in youth has not been fully studied. Frequent monitoring for side effects is warranted.

- Body mass index (BMI) should be obtained at baseline and monitored regularly. It is recommended that weight is taken initially, at four weeks, at eight weeks, at 12 weeks and then annually. If the youth exceeds the 90th percentile of BMI for age or if increases 5 BMI units if obese at baseline, consider weight management interventions and increase frequency of obtaining regular fasting glucose and lipid levels.

- Fasting plasma glucose should be monitored regularly. Levels should be taken at baseline, at 12 weeks and annually. If abnormal obtaining a hemoglobin A1c may be warranted. There is evidence that the development of diabetes in youth taking atypical antipsychotics is not directly related to weight gain.

- In youth with weight gain and a family history of hyperlipidemia, lipid levels should be monitored regularly. Obtain lipid levels at baseline, at 12 weeks and annually. Elevated lipid levels even in childhood may have a role in developing cardiovascular disease later in life. Weight management and dietary interventions may be effective.

- Monitor for movement disorders induced by antipsychotic medication using structured measures such as the Abnormal Involuntary Movement Scale (AIMS) and the Neurological Rating Scale (NRS) at regular intervals and when tapering off medication.

- Due to possible impact on the cardiovascular system, heart rate, blood pressure and ECG changes should be monitored on a regular basis. Obtain a family history of sudden death, cardiovascular disease and personal history of palpitation or syncope. If heart rate reaches over 130 beats per minute, the PR interval over 200 milliseconds, the QRS greater than 120 milliseconds or QTc over 460 milliseconds consider an alternative therapy. ECG may not be needed for all patients. Consider obtaining an initial and subsequent monitoring ECGs if patient has a family history, history of palpitations or syncope.

- Although atypical antipsychotics increase prolactin, regular levels are not necessary unless prolactin-related side effects develop. If prolactin-related side effects develop, lower the dose, change to a different antipsychotic or discontinue medication.

- Drug-specific risks of specific atypical antipsychotics include:
  - Clozapine hematological parameters are the same for youths as for adults. Due to seizure risk with clozapine obtain a pre-treatment EEG and another to compare when optimal drug level is reached. If a youth on clozapine develops acute behavioral changes obtain an EEG.
  - Quetiapine is associated with developing cataracts in animal-based studies. The manufacturer recommends an ophthalmologic examination (slit lamp) at baseline and periodically.
  - Ziprasidone is associated with prolongation of QTc. Obtain an ECG at baseline and once the patient reaches a stable dose.

- Limited data on the long-term safety and efficacy of atypical antipsychotics in youths requires regular reassessments of the continued need for medication.

- Abrupt discontinuation of atypical antipsychotics is not recommended. Abrupt discontinuation can cause withdrawal dyskinesia and may destabilize the patient.

Ⓚ Antipsychotic Medication Comparisons

1. Atypical antipsychotics are typically initially taken orally in divided doses. They can, however, often be consolidated to a single daily dose after titration [2].
2. For studies of antipsychotic medication use in children and adolescents see: [83–102].
3. One pivotal study that deserves special attention is the Treatment of Early Onset Schizophrenia Spectrum Disorders (TEOSS) study conducted by Dr. Lin Sikich, Dr. Robert Findling and others [94, 97]. The first phase or acute phase of the study examined 116 patients aged 8–19 years diagnosed with early-onset schizophrenia that were randomly assigned to molindone plus benztropine, risperidone or olanzapine for eight weeks. Approximately 50% responded to treatment. There were differences in side effects with molindone having more akathisia, and risperidone and olanzapine having more weight gain, especially olanzapine. There were no significant efficacy differences among the three medications. These findings were similar to those from the CATIE study that concluded that first-generation antipsychotics may be as effective as atypical antipsychotic medications [103]. The second or maintenance phase of the study continued the patients that were doing well on their assigned medication until 44 weeks. Only 14 patients completed the trial period and there was no significant difference in effectiveness among the three medications and the side-effect profile was similar. This study was the first double-blind study in youngsters diagnosed with early-onset schizophrenia that received antipsychotic treatment for 12 months. This study underscored the possibility that other antipsychotics could be effective long-term in children and adolescents and set the stage for more studies to be conducted with different medications.

Table 10.8 Key Studies in Childhood Psychosis

Medication Trials	
Randomized clinical trials showing decrease in positive and negative symptoms in youth	Olanzapine
	Aripiprazole
	Quetiapine
	Risperidone
	Lurasidone
Comparative trials in youth with schizophrenia that have shown efficacy	Paliperidone and aripiprazole
	Risperidone, haloperidol and olanzapine
	Clozapine and haloperidol
	Clozapine and olanzapine
	Molindone, olanzapine and risperidone
	Fluphenazine and haloperidol

Table 10.8 (Cont.)

Medication Trials	
First-generation antipsychotics that have shown efficacy in youth	Chlorpromazine
	Loxapine
	Haloperidol
	Fluphenazine
Clozapine has shown superior efficacy for treatment-resistant psychosis in randomized clinical trials in youth compared to other agents	Haloperidol
	Olanzapine
Long-acting injectable (LAI) antipsychotics studies The use of LAI antipsychotics is generally restricted to youth over the age of 16 years due to lack of rigorous testing and because the optimal dosing of LAI for pediatric use is unknown. Nevertheless, LAI antipsychotics should be considered if lack of compliance is an issue in late adolescence	• Paliperidone extended release vs. aripiprazole showed that both groups had positive effects in youth ages 12–17 years of age • Open trials of LAI risperidone vs. paliperidone palmitate showed clinical improvement • Open trial of fluphenazine decanoate vs. aripiprazole extended-release injectable showed efficacy • Open trial of fluphenazine decanoate vs. aripiprazole extended-release injectable showed efficacy • Open trial of zuclopenthixol decanoate vs. olanzapine extended-release injectable improved symptoms

🄛 2019 Food and Drug Administration-Approved Atypical Antipsychotics for Children and Adolescents [2, 104]

Medication	Age in Years
Aripiprazole	>13
Asenapine	>10
Chlorpromazine	>6 months
Lurasidone	>13
Olanzapine	>13
Paliperidone	>12
Pimozide	>12
Prochlorperazine	>2
Quetiapine	>13
Risperidone	>13

🅜 **Psychosocial Interventions** Antipsychotic medications are the cornerstone of treatment of schizophrenia in children and adolescence and should be augmented by psychosocial treatments. Medication treatment along with other services provided within two years of onset of the first psychotic episode reduce the risk of recurring episodes by 50%. In addition, 52% of those youths with first episode psychosis make a full or partial recovery with early intervention in comparison to 15% of those receiving typical treatment [61].

1. Psychosocial interventions reduce environmental stressors at home and especially in school that may induce clinical deterioration in the youth. Making the surroundings less stimulating

may decrease agitation, decrease distress, increase socialization and help youthful patients understand what is real vs. unreal [105]. Skill training helps with attention problems, working memory and poor affect regulation.

2. Psychosocial intervention must be customized to fit the patient's age, developmental age, social setting, family and risk factors. Youth outcomes are tied to stability of parental mental health and extended support systems [105]. Psychoeducation should be provided to the youth and family on information about illness, medication and additional interventions that may help improve function [106]. An excellent resource to provide the family with is the National Alliance on Mental Illness (NAMI). NAMI provides educational programs, advice, groups and support to youth diagnosed with mental illness and their families (www.nami.org).

3. Individual and family therapy should contain a combination of education, support, problem solving and cognitive behavioral therapy (CBT). Cognitive therapy addresses delusional beliefs while behavioral therapy provides social and vocational skills. CBT cognitive techniques look at the youth's irrational beliefs or thinking and through explanation of the youth's perceptions can decrease behavioral dysfunction. The behavioral techniques utilized in CBT provide support to the youth by establishing home and school responses that aim to diminish misperception of daily events [107]. Studies of CBT showing effectiveness in children and adolescents with schizophrenia are limited but when combined with antipsychotic medication the evidence of effectiveness is stronger [108]. Therapeutic schools provide academic assistance, counseling, behavior modification, individual/group therapy, skill training and support children with cognitive and emotional challenges.

4. Cognitive Enhancement and Remediation have been shown to be superior to other psychotherapies in clinical trials of randomized youth [109, 110].

Table 10.10 Cognitive Enhancement and Remediation in Childhood Psychosis

Computer-based exercises	• Slows deterioration of attention, memory, language and executive function
Social-cognitive groups	• Improvement in experimental learning and interpersonal interaction

Ⓒ Summary Points

- Psychotic symptoms in children and adolescents do not immediately indicate a psychotic disorder. First, think about the possibility of other psychiatric disorders including affective disorders and substances that have or induce psychotic symptoms. Also explore medical conditions with psychotic symptoms in their presentation and make sure all the medications prescribed to the youth are reviewed.
- Assessing, evaluating and treating children presenting with psychosis is puzzling and time-consuming. Collaboration with the child's pediatrician is crucial. An extensive history and physical examination must be performed. If focal signs are present an in-depth neurological examination by a neurologist is warranted.
- If the youth presents with dysmorphic features, neurocognitive impairments or neurodevelopmental delays, consultation with a geneticist can inform whether genetic testing should be performed.
- The information obtained by carefully performing a mental status examination and talking with family members, caretakers and teachers can provide clues to help narrow the diagnosis.
- Following the recommended parameters for assessing, diagnosing and using antipsychotics in children and adolescents will assist and inform the clinical process. Significant advances have been made in the last 10–15 years on establishing the effectiveness of new antipsychotic medications and their use in children and adolescents. Keeping updated on the latest scientific information regarding psychosis in youth and studies of antipsychotics for use in children and adolescents is important since it may provide clues to solving the riddle that is the presence of psychosis in young people.
- Lastly, but critically, is to always follow the golden rule, "Start at low doses and increase slowly to reach the lowest effective dose".

1.10 Approach to Psychosis in Children and Adolescents (Continued)

References

1. Kelleher, I., Connor, D., Clarke, M. C., et al. (2012). Prevalence of psychotic symptoms in childhood and adolescence: a systematic review and meta-analysis of population-based studies. *Psychol Med*, 42, 1857–1863.
2. Maloney, A. E., Yakutis, L. J., Frazier, J. A. (2012). Empirical evidence for psychopharmacologic treatment in early-onset psychosis and schizophrenia. *Child Adolesc Psychiatr Clin*, 21, 885–909.
3. McClellan, J., Stock, S. (2013). Practice parameter for the assessment and treatment of children and adolescents with schizophrenia. *J Am Acad Child Adolesc Psychiatry*, 52, 976–990.
4. Sikich, L. (2013). Diagnosis and evaluation of hallucinations and other psychotic symptoms in children and adolescents. *Child Adolesc Psychiatr Clin*, 22, 655–673.
5. McClellan, J. (2018). Psychosis in children and adolescents. *J Am Acad Child Adolesc Psychiatry*, 57, 308–312.
6. Reichenberg, A., Caspi, A., Harrington, H., et al. (2010). Static and dynamic cognitive deficits in childhood preceding adult schizophrenia: a 30-year study. *Am J Psychiatry*, 167, 160–169.
7. Ross, R. G. (2008). New findings on antipsychotic use in children and adolescents with schizophrenia spectrum disorders. *Am J Psychiatry*, 165(11), 1369–1372.
8. Rapoport, J. L., Gogtay, N. (2011). Childhood onset schizophrenia: support for a progressive neurodevelopmental disorder. *Int J Dev Neurosci*, 29, 251–258.
9. Penttilä, J., Paillére-Martinot, M-L., Martinot, J-L., et al. (2008). Global and temporal cortical folding in patients with early-onset schizophrenia. *J Am Acad Child Adolesc Psychiatry*, 47, 1125–1132.
10. Cornblatt, B. A., Lencz, T., Smith, C. W., et al. (2007). Can antidepressants be used to treat the schizophrenia prodrome? Results of a prospective, naturalistic treatment study of adolescents. *J Clin Psychiatry*, 64(4), 546–557.
11. Amminger, G. P., Schäfer, M. R., Papageorgiou, K., et al. (2010). Long-chain ω-3 fatty acids for indicated prevention of psychotic disorders: a randomized, placebo-controlled trial. *Arch Gen Psychiatry*, 67, 146–154.
12. McGorry, P. D., Nelson, B., Markulev, C., et al. (2017). Effect of ω-3 polyunsaturated fatty acids in young people at ultrahigh risk for psychotic disorders: the NEURAPRO randomized clinical trial. *JAMA Psychiatry*, 74, 19–27.
13. Cannon, T. D., Cadenhead, K., Cornblatt, B., et al. (2008). Prediction of psychosis in youth at high clinical risk: a multisite longitudinal study in North America. *Arch Gen Psychiatry*, 65, 28–37.
14. Ienciu, M., Romoşan, F., Bredicean, C., et al. (2010). First episode psychosis and treatment delay – causes and consequences. *Psychiatria Danubina*, 22, 540–543.
15. Rubio, J. M., Sanjuán, J., Flórez-Salamanca, L., et al. (2012). Examining the course of hallucinatory experiences in children and adolescents: a systematic review. *Schizophr Res*, 138, 248–254.
16. Norman, R. M., Mallal, A. K., Manchanda, R., et al. (2007). Does treatment delay predict occupational functioning in first-episode psychosis? *Schizophr Res*, 91, 259–262.
17. Poulton, R., Caspi, A., Moffitt, T. E., et al. (2000). Children's self-reported psychotic symptoms and adult schizophreniform disorder: a 15-year longitudinal study. *Arch Gen Psychiatry*, 57, 1053–1058.
18. Robins, L. N., Helzer, J. E., Croughan, J., et al. (1981). National Institute of Mental Health diagnostic interview schedule: its history, characteristics, and validity. *Arch Gen Psychiatry*, 38, 381–389.
19. Barrera, M., Garrison-Jones, C. V. (1988). Properties of the Beck Depression Inventory as a screening instrument for adolescent depression. *J Abnorm Child Psychol*, 16, 263–273.
20. Jellinek, M. S., Murphy, J. M., Robinson, J., et al. (1988). Pediatric Symptom Checklist: screening school-age children for psychosocial dysfunction. *J Pediatrics*, 112, 201–209.
21. Werry, J. S., McClellan, J. M., Chard, L. (1991). Childhood and adolescent schizophrenic, bipolar, and schizoaffective disorders: a clinical and outcome study. *J Am Acad Child Adolesc Psychiatry*, 30, 457–465.
22. Carlson, G. A., Fennig, S., Bromet, E. J. (1994). The confusion between bipolar disorder and schizophrenia in youth: where does it stand in the 1990s? *J Am Acad Child Adolesc Psychiatry*, 33, 453–460.
23. Kaufman, J., Birmaher, B., Brent, D., et al. (1997). Schedule for affective disorders and schizophrenia for school-age children – present and lifetime version (K-SADS-PL): initial reliability and validity data. *J Am Acad Child Adolesc Psychiatry*, 36, 980–988.
24. Conners, C. K., Sitarenios, G., Parker, J. D., et al. (1998). The revised Conners' Parent Rating Scale (CPRS-R): factor structure, reliability, and criterion validity. *J Abnorm Child Psychol*, 26, 257–268.
25. Angold, A., Costello, E. J. (2000). The child and adolescent psychiatric assessment (CAPA). *J Am Acad Child Adolesc Psychiatry*, 39, 39–48.
26. Muris, P., Schmidt, H., Merckelbach, H. (2000). Correlations among two self-report questionnaires for measuring DSM-defined anxiety disorder symptoms in children: The Screen for Child Anxiety Related Emotional Disorders and the Spence Children's Anxiety Scale. *Pers Individ Differ*, 28, 333–346.
27. Geller, B., Zimerman, B., Williams, M., et al. (2001). Reliability of the Washington University in St. Louis Kiddie Schedule for Affective Disorders and Schizophrenia (WASH-U-KSADS) mania and rapid cycling sections. *J Am Acad Child Adolesc Psychiatry*, 40, 450–455.
28. Lachar, D., Randle, S. L., Harper, R. A., et al. (2001). The brief psychiatric rating scale for children (BPRS-C): validity and reliability of an anchored version. *J Am Acad Child Adolesc Psychiatry*, 40, 333–340.
29. Gracious, B. L., Youngstrom, E. A., Findling, R. L., et al. (2002). Discriminative validity of a parent version of the Young Mania Rating Scale. *J Am Acad Child Adolesc Psychiatry*, 41, 1350–1359.
30. Group, R. U. o. P. P. A. S. (2002). The pediatric anxiety rating scale (PARS): development and psychometric properties. *J Am Acad Child Adolesc Psychiatry*, 41, 1061–1069.
31. Knight, J. R., Sherritt, L., Shrier, L. A., et al. (2002). Validity of the CRAFFT substance abuse screening test among adolescent clinic patients. *Arch Pediatr Adolesc Med*, 156, 607–614.
32. Kroenke, K., Spitzer, R. L. (2002). The PHQ-9: a new depression diagnostic and severity measure. *Psychiatr Ann*, 32, 509–515.
33. Mohamadesmaiel, E., Alipour, A. (2002). A preliminary study on the reliability, validity and cut off points of the disorders of Children Symptom Inventory-4 (CSI-4). *J Except Child*, 2, 239–254.

34. Brooks, S. J., Krulewicz, S. P., Kutcher, S. (2003). The Kutcher Adolescent Depression Scale: assessment of its evaluative properties over the course of an 8-week pediatric pharmacotherapy trial. *J Child Adolesc Psychopharmacol*, 13, 337–349.
35. Pavuluri, M. N., Herbener, E. S., Sweeney, J. A. (2004). Psychotic symptoms in pediatric bipolar disorder. *J Affect Disord*, 80, 19–28.
36. Timbremont, B., Braet, C., Dreessen, L. (2004). Assessing depression in youth: relation between the Children's Depression Inventory and a structured interview. *J Clin Child Adolesc Psychol*, 33, 149–157.
37. Hale III , W. W., Raaijmakers, Q., Muris, P., et al. (2005). Psychometric properties of the Screen for Child Anxiety Related Emotional Disorders (SCARED) in the general adolescent population. *J Am Acad Child Adolesc Psychiatry*, 44, 283–290.
38. Perrin, S., Meiser-Stedman, R., Smith, P. (2005). The Children's Revised Impact of Event Scale (CRIES): validity as a screening instrument for PTSD. *Behav Cog Psychother*, 33, 487–498.
39. Pappas, D. (2006). ADHD Rating Scale-IV: checklists, norms, and clinical interpretation. *J Psychoed Assess*, 24, 172–178.
40. Wagner, K. D., Hirschfeld, R., Emslie, G. J., et al. (2006). Validation of the Mood Disorder Questionnaire for bipolar disorders in adolescents. *J Clin Psychiatry*, 67(5), 827–830.
41. Chandler, S., Charman, T., Baird, G., et al. (2007). Validation of the social communication questionnaire in a population cohort of children with autism spectrum disorders. *J Am Acad Child Adolesc Psychiatry*, 46, 1324–1332.
42. Charman, T., Baird, G., Simonoff, E., et al. (2007). Efficacy of three screening instruments in the identification of autistic-spectrum disorders. *Br J Psychiatry*, 191, 554–559.
43. Polderman, T. J., Derks, E. M., Hudziak, J. J., et al. (2007). Across the continuum of attention skills: a twin study of the SWAN ADHD rating scale. *J Child Psychol Psychiatry*, 48, 1080–1087.
44. Gallant, J., Storch, E. A., Merlo, L. J., et al. (2008). Convergent and discriminant validity of the Children's Yale-Brown Obsessive Compulsive Scale-symptom checklist. *J Anxiety Disord*, 22, 1369–1376.
45. Kaminer, Y. (2008). The teen addiction severity index around the globe: the tower of Babel revisited. *Subst Abuse*, 29, 89–94.
46. Lanktree, C. B., Gilbert, A. M., Briere, J., et al. (2008). Multi-informant assessment of maltreated children: convergent and discriminant validity of the TSCC and TSCYC. *Child Abuse Negl*, 32, 621–625.
47. Winters, K. C., Kaminer, Y. (2008). Screening and assessing adolescent substance use disorders in clinical populations. *J Am Acad Child Adolesc Psychiatry*, 47, 740.
48. Mayes, S. D., Calhoun, S. L., Murray, M. J., et al. (2009). Comparison of scores on the Checklist for Autism Spectrum Disorder, Childhood Autism Rating Scale, and Gilliam Asperger's Disorder Scale for children with low functioning autism, high functioning autism, Asperger's disorder, ADHD, and typical development. *J Aut Dev Disord*, 39, 1682–1693.
49. Nakamura, B. J., Ebesutani, C., Bernstein, A., et al. (2009). A psychometric analysis of the child behavior checklist DSM-oriented scales. *J Psychopathol Behav Assess*, 31, 178–189.
50. Posserud, M-B., Lundervold, A. J., Gillberg, C. (2009). Validation of the autism spectrum screening questionnaire in a total population sample. *J Aut Dev Disord*, 39, 126–134.
51. Chlebowski, C., Green, J. A., Barton, M. L., et al. (2010). Using the childhood autism rating scale to diagnose autism spectrum disorders. *J Aut Dev Disord*, 40, 787–799.
52. Reynolds, C. R. (2010). Behavior assessment system for children. *The Corsini Encyclopedia of Psychology*, 1–2.
53. Becker, S. P., Langberg, J. M., Vaughn, A. J., et al. (2012). Clinical utility of the Vanderbilt ADHD diagnostic parent rating scale comorbidity screening items. *J Dev Behav Pediatr*, 33, 221.
54. Fux, L., Walger, P., Schimmelmann, B. G., et al. (2013). The schizophrenia proneness instrument, child and youth version (SPI-CY): practicability and discriminative validity. *Schizophr Res*, 146, 69–78.
55. Martinez, W., Polo, A. J., Zelic, K. J. (2014). Symptom variation on the Trauma Symptom Checklist for Children: a within-scale meta-analytic review. *J Traumatic Stress*, 27, 655–663.
56. Stucky, B. D., Edelen, M. O., Ramchand, R. (2014). A psychometric assessment of the GAIN General Individual Severity Scale (GAIN-GISS) and Short Screeners (GAIN-SS) among adolescents in outpatient treatment programs. *J Subst Abuse Treat*, 46, 165–173.
57. Sparrow, S., Cicchetti, D. V., Saulnier, C. A. (2016). *Vineland adaptive behavior scales (Vineland-3)*. Antonio: Psychological Corporation.
58. Pagsberg, A. K., Tarp, S., Glintborg, D., et al. (2017). Acute antipsychotic treatment of children and adolescents with schizophrenia-spectrum disorders: a systematic review and network meta-analysis. *J Am Acad Child Adolesc Psychiatry*, 56, 191–202.
59. Craddock, K. E., Zhou, X., Liu, S., et al. (2018). Symptom dimensions and subgroups in childhood-onset schizophrenia. *Schizophr Res*, 197, 71–77.
60. Doric, A., Stevanovic, D., Stupar, D., et al. (2019). UCLA PTSD reaction index for DSM-5 (PTSD-RI-5): a psychometric study of adolescents sampled from communities in eleven countries. *Eur J Psychotraumatology*, 10, 1605282.
61. Child Mind Institute. (2017). Children's Mental Health Report. Available from: https://childmind.org/report/2017-childrens-mental-health-report (last accessed November 3, 2020).
62. Galynker, I., Ieronimo, C., Perez-Acquino, A., et al. (1996). Panic attacks with psychotic features. *J Clin Psychiatry*, 57, 402–406.
63. Schäfer, I., Fisher, H. L. (2011). Childhood trauma and psychosis – what is the evidence? *Dialogues Clin Neurosci*, 13, 360.
64. Rodowski, M. F., Cagande, C. C., Riddle, M. A. (2008). Childhood obsessive-compulsive disorder presenting as schizophrenia spectrum disorders. *J Child Adolesc Psychopharmacol*, 18, 395–401.
65. American Psychiatric Association. (2013). *Diagnostic and Statistical Manual of Mental Disorders*. Arlington: American Psychiatric Association, p. 81.

66. Mullin, A., Gokhale, A., Moreno-De-Luca, A., et al. (2013). Neurodevelopmental disorders: mechanisms and boundary definitions from genomes, interactomes and proteomes. *Transl Psychiatry*, 3, e329–e329.
67. Landa, R. J., Gross, A. L., Stuart, E. A., et al. (2013). Developmental trajectories in children with and without autism spectrum disorders: the first 3 years. *Child Dev*, 84, 429–442.
68. McNamara, D. (2012). Genetic microarrays grow for neurodevelopmental diagnosis. Available from: http://www.mdedge.com/clinicalneurologynews/article/52657/neurology/genetic-microarrays-grow-neurodevelopmental-diagnosis (last accessed November 3, 2020).
69. Fluyau, D., Mitra, P., Lorthe, K. (2019). Antipsychotics for amphetamine psychosis. A systematic review. *Front Psychiatry*, 10, 740.
70. Cheng, W-J., Chen, C-H., Chen, C-K., et al. (2018). Similar psychotic and cognitive profile between ketamine dependence with persistent psychosis and schizophrenia. *Schizophr Res*, 199, 313–318.
71. American Addiction Centers. (2019). Dextromethorphan abuse. Available from: http://www.drugabuse.com/dextromethorphan (last accessed November 3, 2020).
72. Abraham, H. D. (1983). Visual phenomenology of the LSD flashback. *Arch Gen Psychiatry*, 40(8), 884–889.
73. National Institute on Drug Abuse. (2019). Hallucinogens Drug Facts. Available from: http://www.drugabuse.gov/publications/drugfacts/hallucinogens (last accessed November 3, 2020).
74. National Institute on Drug Abuse. (2019). Marijuana Drug Facts. Available from: http://www.drugabuse.gov/publications/drugfacts/marijuana (last accessed November 3, 2020).
75. National Institute on Drug Abuse. (2018). Synthetic Cannabinoids Drug Facts. Avavilable from: http://www.drugabuse.gov/publications/drugfacts/synthetic-cannabinoids-k2spice (last accessed November 3, 2020).
76. National Institute on Drug Abuse. (2018). Synthetic Cathinones Drug Facts. Available from: http://www.drugabuse.gov/publications/drugfacts/synthetic-cathinones-bath-salts (last accessed November 3, 2020).
77. Fohrman, D. A., Stein, M. T. (2006). Psychosis: 6 steps rule out medical causes in kids. *Curr Psychiatr*, 5, 35–47.
78. Stevens, J. R., Prince, J. B., Prager, L. M., et al. (2014). Psychotic disorders in children and adolescents: a primer on contemporary evaluation and management. *Prim Care Companion CNS Disord*, 16, PCC.13f01514.
79. Lowenthal, E. D., Cruz, N., Yin, D. (2010). Neurologic and psychiatric manifestations of pediatric HIV infection. *HIV Curriculum for the Health Professional*, 194–205.
80. Ramsey, D., Muskin, P. R. (2013). Vitamin deficiencies and mental health: how are they linked. *Curr Psychiatr*, 12, 37–43.
81. Firth, J., Carney, R., Stubbs, B., et al. (2018). Nutritional deficiencies and clinical correlates in first-episode psychosis: a systematic review and meta-analysis. *Schizophr Bull*, 44, 1275–1292.
82. American Academy of Child and Adolescent Psychiatry. (2011). Practice parameters for the use of atypical antipsychotics medication in children and adolescents. Available from: https://www.aacap.org/App_Themes/AACAP/docs/practice_parameters/Atypical_Antipsychotic_Medications_Web.pdf
83. Werry, J. S., Weiss, G., Douglas, V., et al. (1966). Studies on the hyperactive child: III. The effect of chlorpromazine upon behavior and learning ability. *J Am Acad Child Psychiatry*, 5, 292–312.
84. Engelhardt, D. M., Polizos, P., Waizer, J., et al. (1973). A double-blind comparison of fluphenazine and haloperidol in outpatient schizophrenic children. *J Aut Child Schizophr*, 3, 128–137.
85. Pool, D., Bloom, W., Mielke, D., et al. (1976). A controlled evaluation of loxitane in seventy-five adolescent schizophrenic patients. *Curr Therapeut Res*, 19(1), 99–104.
86. Spencer, E. K., Kafantaris, V., Padron-Gayol, M. V., et al. (1992). Haloperidol in schizophrenic children: early findings from a study in progress. *Psychopharmacol Bull*, 28(2), 183–186.
87. Kumra, S., Frazier, J. A., Jacobsen, L. K., et al. (1996). Childhood-onset schizophrenia: a double-blind clozapine-haloperidol comparison. *Arch Gen Psychiatry*, 53, 1090–1097.
88. Woods, S. W., Breier, A., Zipursky, R. B., et al. (2003). Randomized trial of olanzapine versus placebo in the symptomatic acute treatment of the schizophrenic prodrome. *Biological Psychiatry*, 54, 453–464.
89. Sikich, L., Hamer, R. M., Bashford, R. A., et al. (2004). A pilot study of risperidone, olanzapine, and haloperidol in psychotic youth: a double-blind, randomized, 8-week trial. *Neuropsychopharmacology*, 29, 133–145.
90. McGlashan, T. H., Zipursky, R. B., Perkins, D., et al. (2006). Randomized, double-blind trial of olanzapine versus placebo in patients prodromally symptomatic for psychosis. *Am J Psychiatry*, 163, 790–799.
91. Shaw, P., Sporn, A., Gogtay, N., et al. (2006). Childhood-onset schizophrenia: a double-blind, randomized clozapine-olanzapine comparison. *Arch Gen Psychiatry*, 63, 721–730.
92. Berger, G. E., Proffitt, T-M., McConchie, M., et al. (2008). Dosing quetiapine in drug-naive first-episode psychosis: a controlled, double-blind, randomized, single-center study investigating efficacy, tolerability, and safety of 200 mg/day vs. 400 mg/day of quetiapine fumarate in 141 patients aged 15 to 25 years. *J Clin Psychiatry*, 69, 1702–1714.
93. Findling, R. L., Robb, A., Nyilas, M., et al. (2008). A multiple-center, randomized, double-blind, placebo-controlled study of oral aripiprazole for treatment of adolescents with schizophrenia. *Am J Psychiatry*, 165, 1432–1441.
94. Sikich, L., Frazier, J. A., McClellan, J., et al. (2008). Double-blind comparison of first- and second-generation antipsychotics in early-onset schizophrenia and schizo-affective disorder: findings from the treatment of early-onset schizophrenia spectrum disorders (TEOSS) study. *Am J Psychiatry*, 165, 1420–1431.
95. Haas, M., Unis, A. S., Armenteros, J., et al. (2009). A 6-week, randomized, double-blind, placebo-controlled study of the efficacy and safety of risperidone in adolescents with schizophrenia. *J Child Adolesc Psychopharmacol*, 19, 611–621.
96. Kryzhanovskaya, L., Schulz, S. C., Mcdougle, C., et al. (2009). Olanzapine versus placebo in adolescents with schizophrenia: a 6-week, randomized, double-blind, placebo-controlled trial. *J Am Acad Child Adolesc Psychiatry*, 48, 60–70.
97. Findling, R. L., Johnson, J. L., McClellan, J., et al. (2010). Double-blind maintenance safety and effectiveness findings from the Treatment of Early-Onset Schizophrenia Spectrum (TEOSS) study. *J Am Acad Child Adolesc Psychiatry*, 49, 583–594.

98. Singh, J., Robb, A., Vijapurkar, U., et al. (2011). A randomized, double-blind study of paliperidone extended-release in treatment of acute schizophrenia in adolescents. *Biological Psychiatry*, 70, 1179–1187.

99. Findling, R. L., McKenna, K., Earley, W. R., et al. (2012). Efficacy and safety of quetiapine in adolescents with schizophrenia investigated in a 6-week, double-blind, placebo-controlled trial. *J Child Adolesc Psychopharmacol*, 22, 327–342.

100. Savitz, A. J., Lane, R., Nuamah, I., et al. (2015). Efficacy and safety of paliperidone extended release in adolescents with schizophrenia: a randomized, double-blind study. *J Am Acad Child Adolesc Psychiatry*, 54, 126–137. e121.

101. Goldman, R., Loebel, A., Cucchiaro, J., et al. (2017). Efficacy and safety of lurasidone in adolescents with schizophrenia: a 6-week, randomized placebo-controlled study. *J Child Adolesc Psychopharmacol*, 27, 516–525.

102. Lytle, S., McVoy, M., Sajatovic, M. (2017). Long-acting injectable antipsychotics in children and adolescents. *J Child Adolesc Psychopharmacol*, 27, 2–9.

103. Lieberman, J. A., Stroup, T. S., McEvoy, J. P., et al. (2005). Effectiveness of antipsychotic drugs in patients with chronic schizophrenia. *N Engl J Med*, 353, 1209–1223.

104. Stahl, S. M. (2019). *Stahl's Essential Psychopharmacology: Prescriber's Guide, Children and Adolescents*. New York: Cambridge University Press.

105. Stevens, J. R., Prince, J. B. (2012). Schooling students with psychotic disorders. *Child Adolesc Psychiatr Clin N Am*, 21(1), 187–200.

106. Xia, J., Merinder, L. B., Belgamwar, M. R. (2011). Psychoeducation for schizophrenia. *Cochrane Database Syst Rev*, 2011(6), CD002831.

107. Turkington, D., Kingdon, D., Turner, T. (2002). Effectiveness of a brief cognitive–behavioural therapy intervention in the treatment of schizophrenia. *Br J Psychiatry*, 180, 523–527.

108. McGorry, P. D., Yung, A. R., Phillips, L. J., et al. (2002). Randomized controlled trial of interventions designed to reduce the risk of progression to first-episode psychosis in a clinical sample with subthreshold symptoms. *Arch Gen Psychiatry*, 59, 921–928.

109. Wykes, T., Newton, E., Landau, S., et al. (2007). Cognitive remediation therapy (CRT) for young early onset patients with schizophrenia: an exploratory randomized controlled trial. *Schizophr Res*, 94, 221–230.

110. Lee, R., Redoblado-Hodge, M., Naismith, S., et al. (2013). Cognitive remediation improves memory and psychosocial functioning in first-episode psychiatric out-patients. *Psychol Med*, 43, 1161–1173.

1.11 Electroconvulsive Therapy and Other Non-Pharmacological Treatments

🗔 **Introduction** Electroconvulsive therapy (ECT) was initially utilized in the treatment of schizophrenia in the 1930s. ECT involves applying an electrical current to the brain to induce a therapeutic seizure [1]. Muscle relaxants were not available early on so adverse effects of ECT included fractures due to vigorous muscle contractions during the seizure. These undesirable effects, stigma, and the availability of alternative antipsychotic medications led to ECT falling out of favor [2].

Ⓐ **Treatment Resistance** Approximately 30% of people with schizophrenia do not respond to antipsychotic therapy and meet criteria for treatment-resistant schizophrenia (TRS) [3–5]. Clozapine remains the most effective treatment for TRS, though 30–40% of patients with TRS fail trials of clozapine treatment [6]. Pharmacologic augmentation strategies including adding another antipsychotic, mood stabilizer, anxiolytic, antidepressant, anti-inflammatory or glutamatergic agent have shown only modest efficacy, i.e. small effect sizes [7–11].

Ⓑ **Electroconvulsive Therapy Indications** Electroconvulsive therapy is recommended for schizophrenia with an acute exacerbation of positive and/or affective symptoms, catatonia, a past history of response to ECT and incomplete response to pharmacotherapy [12]. Antipsychotics are the mainstay for acute treatment and relapse prevention of schizophrenia though ECT can augment psychopharmacologic treatment of schizophrenia, especially if associated with catatonia, aggression and suicide [13, 14].

Ⓒ **Electroconvulsive Therapy for Treatment-Resistant Psychosis** Although studies comparing ECT vs. antipsychotics favor medication, there is evidence that antipsychotics combined with ECT can lead to improvement in mental state [15]. This augmentation strategy may be tried in patients with limited response to medications alone and/or when a more rapid improvement in symptoms or a more rapid global improvement is desired [16, 17].

A 2015 randomized controlled trial (RCT) of 39 patients with clozapine-resistant schizophrenia were observed in a single-blind eight-week study. Twenty were assigned ECT plus clozapine and the rest were assigned clozapine treatment only. Fifty percent of the ECT plus clozapine patients met response criteria. None of the patients in the clozapine only group met response criteria [18].

A 2015 review of the combined use of clozapine and ECT identified 40 reports which included 208 patients. A majority were between the ages of 18–65 years old and diagnosed with either schizophrenia or schizoaffective disorder. Most patients were clozapine resistant and initiated on ECT as an augmentation strategy. Thirty-eight to 100% of the patients improved within three weeks. Sustained long-term improvement, of up to 24 months, was also found in a few studies [19]. A 2016 review and meta-analysis of augmentation of clozapine with ECT showed an overall response to clozapine and ECT of 66%. The mean number of ECT treatments was 11.3. Thirty-two percent of cases relapsed following cessation of ECT over a range of 3–48 weeks. These studies support the use of ECT with clozapine as a safe and effective augmentation strategy in the acute treatment of schizophrenia.

ⓘ Electroconvulsive Therapy for Relapse Prevention Continuing antipsychotic medication alone after the acute course of ECT significantly decreases the rate of relapse in patients with schizophrenia [20, 21]. However, augmentation with continuation (C-ECT) and maintenance ECT (M-ECT) are also used to prevent relapse once remission has been achieved during the acute course of ECT treatment. ECT up to six months after remission is achieved is referred to as C-ECT. ECT administered beyond this time period is termed M-ECT [22]. A 2018 review of maintenance ECT, consisting of 37 studies, found that there was evidence to show that patients who received maintenance ECT benefited from sustained improvement. This review highlighted two RCTs [23]. The Chanpattana study found a 40% relapse rate with ECT and flupentixol vs. 93% for the medication alone and maintenance ECT alone groups [24]. The Yang study revealed a statistically significant decreased likelihood of relapse over 12 months in the ECT and risperidone group compared to the group receiving risperidone alone [25].

ⓔ Repetitive Transcranial Magnetic Stimulation Repetitive Transcranial Magnetic Stimulation (RTMS) is a noninvasive treatment that utilizes repetitive magnetic field pulses, delivered through the scalp by a coil, to inhibit or stimulate underlying brain tissue. RTMS is approved for the treatment of major depressive disorder and has been studied for off-label treatment of other psychiatric illnesses including psychotic disorders [26]. More specifically, studies have looked at using low-frequency (1 Hz) RTMS to inhibit the left temporoparietal cortex (TPC) for positive symptoms, primarily hallucinations [27–29]. Higher-frequency RTMS has been studied in the stimulation of the dorsolateral prefrontal cortex (DLPFC) for negative symptoms including avolition, apathy and cognitive dulling [30–32].

A recent four-week randomized, double-blind, sham-controlled trial of 60 patients with schizophrenia showed adjunctive treatment with 20 Hz of RTMS to the left DLPFC led to a significant decrease in negative symptoms as measured by the Scale for the Assessment of Negative Symptoms (SANS) and the Positive and Negative Symptom Scale (PANSS). However, no significant improvement was found in cognition measured with the MATRICS Consensus Cognitive Battery (MCCB). Authors suggest that more severe baseline positive symptoms predict poorer improvement in negative symptoms after four weeks [33]. Alternatively, a 2019 systematic review of 30 clinical trials found only 12 with evidence to support treatment of positive symptoms with RTMS. Twenty-five of the studies specifically targeted auditory hallucinations. Authors suggested that other positive symptoms such as delusions or thought disorder could be the target of future research of RTMS treatment [34].

Repetitive Transcranial Magnetic Stimulation in general is a well-tolerated treatment. A 2016 expert review of the efficacy and safety of combining clozapine and RTMS in TRS found that high-frequency RTMS over the DLPFC and low-frequency RTMS over the TPC has been safely administered in clozapine patients [35]. Absolute contraindications include: ferromagnetic material in the head, intracardiac lines, increased intracranial pressure and cochlear implants [36].

❻ Transcranial Direct Current Stimulation Transcranial Direct Current Stimulation (TDCS) involves passing a weak electrical current through electrodes from the scalp to the brain. This stimulates neuronal activity but does not produce depolarizing action potentials. The side-effect profile of TDCS is favorable when compared with RTMS. It has been studied for treatment of several neurological and psychiatric conditions [26]. With respect to treatment of schizophrenia, anodal stimulation of the left DLPFC may reduce negative symptoms and cathodal inhibitory stimulation of the left temporoparietal junction may improve auditory hallucinations [37]. In 2017, a review found that anodal and cathodal stimulation may improve deficits in attention, working memory and cognitive abilities [38], although other studies have failed to show any effect or have been unable to show a significant effect vs. placebo [39, 40]. Most recently in 2019, a systematic review and meta-analysis looked at RCTs of TDCS' effect on cognitive deficits in patients with schizophrenia and schizoaffective disorder. Nine studies were reviewed with a total of 270 patients, 133 of which were included in the active stimulation group. The meta-analysis found a significant mean effect of TDCS on working memory (SMD = 0.49, 95% CI, 0.16–0.83) but nonsignificant effects for other cognitive domains [41].

❻ Vagal Nerve Stimulation Vagal Nerve Stimulation (VNS) involves electrical impulses emitted by a generator through the vagus nerve in order to indirectly stimulate the brain. The generator is surgically implanted, or the procedure can be noninvasive with the use of transcutaneous vagal nerve stimulation (tVNS). VNS is approved for the treatment of epilepsy and treatment-resistant depression. There are limited studies evaluating the use of VNS in schizophrenia. A 2015 randomized double-blinded study of 20 patients with schizophrenia received tVNS vs. sham treatment. At the end of the study the treatment was well tolerated but there was no statistically significant outcome between groups [42]. In a 2014 study using a rodent model of schizophrenia, VNS targeting the ventral hippocampus found a reversal of hyperactivity in the ventral hippocampus and meso-limbic dopamine pathway [43]. VNS may also increase cholinergic neurotransmission and serotonin release, thus improving cognitive symptoms of schizophrenia [44]. It should be noted that VNS may lead to psychiatric sequelae in patients with epilepsy. More specifically, Blumer and colleagues found that seven of 81 patients, treated with six months of VNS, ended up with psychiatric complications such as psychosis, dysphoria or both [45, 46].

❿ Deep Brain Stimulation Deep Brain Stimulation (DBS) involves implanting electrodes into targeted brain structures. The battery is implanted into the chest. When activated, electrical impulses are delivered directly into the targeted brain structures. DBS is approved by the FDA for the treatment of movement disorders, obsessive-compulsive disorder and medication refractory epilepsy [26]. Theories in regard to its therapeutic benefit in schizophrenia include targeting the anterior hippocampus to reduce dopaminergic overactivity and targeting the nucleus accumbens to balance the dopaminergic environment. DBS may also normalize neuronal oscillations improving cognitive and attentional deficits [47, 48]. To date, improvement in positive and negative symptoms has only been seen in a few clinical phase I trials [49]. Although DBS appears well tolerated, it can be associated with serious complications including intracerebral hemorrhage and infection [50].

❶ Phototherapy Light therapy or bright light therapy (BLT) is used to treat depressive illnesses and circadian rhythm sleep disorders by exposure to artificial light. Light therapy is thought to affect brain chemicals linked to mood and sleep, easing symptoms associated with these conditions. Depression and negative symptoms in patients with schizophrenia are common and overlap in terms of their symptoms [51].

Bright light therapy was initially studied on negative symptoms in ten patients with schizophrenia in 2007. The study consisted of a single center, open design with no control group. The results showed statistically significant improvement in negative symptoms scores on the PANSS and subjective improvement in drive after four weeks. The improvement in drive persisted after BLT was discontinued and no patients experienced psychotic exacerbation [52]. Conversely, a more rigorous study of BLT in schizophrenia was published in 2016. The aim of the study was to improve negative and depressive symptoms. It included 20 patients in a single center, add-on trial with two control groups. The results indicated no effect on negative or positive symptoms though a general trend in improvement in general psychopathology scales of the PANSS were seen in the BLT group. No change in daily mood ratings were seen with BLT treatment. The authors opined that BLT was an additional burden on the participants and they did not benefit from BLT [53].

Summary Points

- Electroconvulsive therapy use in the acute treatment of psychosis and in relapse prevention is well supported.
- Repetitive Transcranial Magnetic Stimulation has positive, albeit limited supporting data in the treatment of positive and negative symptoms in schizophrenia.
- Both ECT and RTMS have been shown to be safe and effective in combination with clozapine.
- Transcranial Direct Current Stimulation has data suggesting cognitive benefits, but the data are very preliminary.
- There is one failed RCT looking at the use of VNS in patients with schizophrenia-associated symptoms.
- There are early data showing improvement in positive and negative symptoms with DBS though it is associated with rare but serious complications.
- Studies of phototherapy for negative and depressive symptoms in schizophrenia have shown mixed results.

📖 References

1. Kennedy, S. H., Milev, R., Giacobbe, P., et al. (2009). Canadian Network for Mood and Anxiety Treatments (CANMAT) clinical guidelines for the management of major depressive disorder in adults. IV. Neurostimulation therapies. *J Affect Disord*, 117 Suppl. 1, S44–53.
2. Poublon, N. A., Haagh, M., et al. (2011). The efficacy of ECT in the treatment of schizophrenia. A systematic review. *Erasmus J Med*, 2(1), 48.
3. Brenner, H. D., Dencker, S. J., Goldstein, M. J., et al. (1990). Defining treatment refractoriness in schizophrenia. *Schizophr Bull*, 16, 551–561.
4. Conley, R. R., Buchanan, R. W. (1997). Evaluation of treatment-resistant schizophrenia. *Schizophr Bull*, 23, 663–674.
5. Meltzer, H. Y. (1997). Treatment-resistant schizophrenia – the role of clozapine. *Curr Med Res Opin*, 14, 1–20.
6. Meltzer, H. Y. (1992). Treatment of the neuroleptic-nonresponsive schizophrenic patient. *Schizophr Bull*, 18, 515–542.
7. Remington, G., Saha, A., Chong, S. A., et al. (2005). Augmentation strategies in clozapine-resistant schizophrenia. *CNS Drugs*, 19, 843–872.
8. Tranulis, C., Mouaffak, F., Chouchana, L., et al. (2006). Somatic augmentation strategies in clozapine resistance – what facts? *Clin Neuropharmacol*, 29, 34–44.
9. Cipriani, A., Boso, M., Barbui, C. (2009). Clozapine combined with different antipsychotic drugs for treatment resistant schizophrenia. *Cochrane Database Syst Rev*, 8(3), CD006324.
10. Porcelli, S., Balzarro, B., Serretti, A. (2012). Clozapine resistance: augmentation strategies. *Eur Neuropsychopharmacol*, 22, 165–182.
11. Taylor, D. M., Smith, L., Gee, S. H., et al. (2012). Augmentation of clozapine with a second antipsychotic – a meta-analysis. *Acta Psychiatr Scand*, 125, 15–24.
12. American Psychiatric Association. (2001). *The Practice of Electroconvulsive Therapy: Recommendations for Treatment, Training, and Privileging: A Task Force Report of the American Psychiatric Association*. Washington, D.C.
13. Tharyan, P., Adams, C. E. (2005). Electroconvulsive therapy for schizophrenia. *Cochrane Database Syst Rev*, 18(2), CD000076.
14. Pompili, M., Lester, D., Dominici, G., et al. (2013). Indications for electroconvulsive treatment in schizophrenia: a systematic review. *Schizophr Res*, 146, 1–9.
15. Gazdag, G., Kocsis-Ficzere, N., Tolna, J. (2006). The augmentation of clozapine treatment with electroconvulsive therapy. *Ideggyogy Sz*, 59, 261–267.
16. Small, J. G., Milstein, V., Klapper, M., Kellams, J.J., Small, I.F. (1982). ECT combined with neuroleptics in the treatment of schizophrenia. *Psychopharmacol Bull*, 18(2), 34–35.
17. Abraham, K. R., Kulhara, P. (1987). The efficacy of electroconvulsive therapy in the treatment of schizophrenia. A comparative study. *Br J Psychiatry*, 151, 152–155.
18. Petrides, G., Malur, C., Braga, R. J., et al. (2015). Electroconvulsive therapy augmentation in clozapine-resistant schizophrenia: a prospective, randomized study. *Am J Psychiatry*, 172, 52–58.
19. Grover, S., Hazari, N., Kate, N. (2015). Combined use of clozapine and ECT: a review. *Acta Neuropsychiatr*, 27, 131–142.
20. Leucht, S., Tardy, M., Komossa, K., et al. (2012). Maintenance treatment with antipsychotic drugs for schizophrenia. *Cochrane Database Syst Rev*, 2012, CD008016.
21. Zipursky, R. B., Menezes, N. M., Streiner, D. L. (2014). Risk of symptom recurrence with medication discontinuation in first-episode psychosis: a systematic review. *Schizophr Res*, 152, 408–414.
22. Sackeim, H. A., Haskett, R. F., Mulsant, B. H., et al. (2001). Continuation pharmacotherapy in the prevention of relapse following electroconvulsive therapy: a randomized controlled trial. *JAMA*, 285, 1299–1307.
23. Ward, H. B., Szabo, S. T., Rakesh, G. (2018). Maintenance ECT in schizophrenia: a systematic review. *Psychiatry Res*, 264, 131–142.
24. Chanpattana W., Chakrabhand, M. L., Sackeim H. A., et al. (1999). ECT in treatment-resistant schizophrenia: a controlled study. *Journal of ECT*, 15(3), 178–192.
25. Yang, Y., Cheng, X., Xu, Q., et al. (2016). The maintenance of modified electroconvulsive therapy combined with risperidone is better than risperidone alone in preventing relapse of schizophrenia and improving cognitive function. *Arq Neuropsiquiatr*, 10, 823–828.
26. Maley, C. T., Becker, J. E., Shultz, E. K. B. (2019). Electroconvulsive therapy and other neuromodulation techniques for the treatment of psychosis. *Child Adolesc Psychiatr Clin N Am*, 28, 91–100.
27. Freitas, C., Fregni, F., Pascual-Leone, A. (2009). Meta-analysis of the effects of repetitive transcranial magnetic stimulation (rTMS) on negative and positive symptoms in schizophrenia. *Schizophr Res*, 108(1–3), 11–24.
28. Slotema, C. W., Blom, J. D., van Lutterveld, R., et al. (2014). Review of the efficacy of transcranial magnetic stimulation for auditory verbal hallucinations. *Biol Psychiatry*, 76, 101–110.
29. Nieuwdorp, W., Koops, S., Somers, M., et al. (2015). Transcranial magnetic stimulation, transcranial direct current stimulation and electroconvulsive therapy for medication-resistant psychosis of schizophrenia. *Curr Opin Psychiatry*, 28, 222–228.
30. Dlabac-de Lange, J. J., Knegtering, R., Aleman, A. (2010). Repetitive transcranial magnetic stimulation for negative symptoms of schizophrenia: review and meta-analysis. *J Clin Psychiatry*, 71, 411–418.
31. Prikryl, R., Kucerova, H. (2013). Can repetitive transcranial magnetic stimulation be considered an effective treatment option for negative symptoms of schizophrenia? *Journal of ECT*, 29(1), 67–74.
32. Shi, C., Yu, X., Cheung, E., et al. (2014). Revisiting the therapeutic effect of rTMS on negative symptoms in schizophrenia: a meta-analysis. *Psychiatry Res*, 215(3), 505–513.
33. Zhou, K., Tang, Y., Song, Z., et al. (2019). Repetitive transcranial magnetic stimulation as an adjunctive treatment for negative symptoms and cognitive impairment in patients with schizophrenia: a randomized, double-blind, sham-controlled trial. *Neuropsychiatr Dis Treat*, 15, 1141–1150.

34. Marzouk, T., Winkelbeiner, S., Azizi, H., et al. (2019). Transcranial magnetic stimulation for positive symptoms in schizophrenia: a systematic review. *Neuropsychobiology*, 10, 1–13.
35. Arumugham, S. S., Thirthalli, J., Andrade, C. (2016). Efficacy and safety of combining clozapine with electrical or magnetic brain stimulation in treatment-refractory schizophrenia. *Expert Rev Clin Pharmacol*, 9, 1245–1252.
36. Narayana, S., Papanicolaou, A. C., McGregor, A., et al. (2015). Clinical applications of transcranial magnetic stimulation in pediatric neurology. *J Child Neurol*, 30, 1111–1124.
37. Brunelin, J., Mondino, M., Gassab, L., et al. (2012). Examining transcranial direct-current stimulation (tDCS) as a treatment for hallucinations in schizophrenia. *Am J Psychiatry*, 169, 719–724.
38. Mervis, J. E., Capizzi, R. J., Boroda, E., et al. (2017). Transcranial direct current stimulation over the dorsolateral prefrontal cortex in schizophrenia: a quantitative review of cognitive outcomes. *Front Hum Neurosci*, 11, 44.
39. Fitzgerald, P. B., McQueen, S., Daskalakis, Z. J., et al. (2014). A negative pilot study of daily bimodal transcranial direct current stimulation in schizophrenia. *Brain Stimul*, 7, 813–816.
40. Frohlich, F., Burrello, T. N., Mellin, J. M., et al. (2016). Exploratory study of once-daily transcranial direct current stimulation (tDCS) as a treatment for auditory hallucinations in schizophrenia. *Eur Psychiatry*, 33, 54–60.
41. Narita, Z., Stickley, A., DeVylder, J., et al. (2019). Effect of multi-session prefrontal transcranial direct current stimulation on cognition in schizophrenia: a systematic review and meta-analysis. *Schizophr Res*, 216, 367–373.
42. Hasan, A., Wolff-Menzler, C., Pfeiffer, S., et al. (2015). Transcutaneous noninvasive vagus nerve stimulation (tVNS) in the treatment of schizophrenia: a bicentric randomized controlled pilot study. *Eur Arch Psychiatry Clin Neurosci*, 265, 589–600.
43. Perez, S. M., Carreno, F. R., Frazer, A., et al. (2014). Vagal nerve stimulation reverses aberrant dopamine system function in the methylazoxymethanol acetate rodent model of schizophrenia. *J Neurosci*, 34, 9261–9267.
44. Smucny, J., Visani, A., Tregellas, J. R. (2015). Could vagus nerve stimulation target hippocampal hyperactivity to improve cognition in schizophrenia? *Front Psychiatry*, 6, 43.
45. Blumer, D., Davies, K., Alexander, A., et al. (2001). Major psychiatric disorders subsequent to treating epilepsy by vagus nerve stimulation. *Epilepsy Behav*, 2, 466–472.
46. Keller, S., Lichtenberg, P. (2008). Psychotic exacerbation in a patient with seizure disorder treated with vagus nerve stimulation. *Isr Med Assoc J*, 10, 550–551.
47. Mikell, C. B., McKhann, G. M., Segal, S., et al. (2009). The hippocampus and nucleus accumbens as potential therapeutic targets for neurosurgical intervention in schizophrenia. *Stereotact Funct Neurosurg*, 87, 256–265.
48. Kuhn, J., Bodatsch M., Sturm, V., et al. (2014). Deep brain stimulation in schizophrenia. *Act Nerv Super*, 3, 69–78.
49. Gault, J. M., Davis, R., Cascella, N. G., et al. (2018). Approaches to neuromodulation for schizophrenia. *J Neurol Neurosurg Psychiatry*, 89, 777–787.
50. Schermer, M. (2011). Ethical issues in deep brain stimulation. *Front Integr Neurosci*, 5, 17.
51. Benazzi, F. (2006). Various forms of depression. *Dialogues Clin Neurosci*, 8, 151–161.
52. Aichhorn, W., Stelzig-Schoeler, R., Geretsegger, C., et al. (2007). Bright light therapy for negative symptoms in schizophrenia: a pilot study. *J Clin Psychiatry*, 68, 1146.
53. Roopram, S. M., Burger, A. M., van Dijk, D. A., et al. (2016). A pilot study of bright light therapy in schizophrenia. *Psychiatry Res*, 245, 317–320.

1.12 Approach to Substance Use Disorders in Schizophrenia Spectrum Disorders

Introduction For many patients with schizophrenia, substance use predates the first psychotic episode. Patients suffering from their first psychotic break are more likely to be daily cannabis users and have a higher rate of tobacco use [1, 2]. Cannabis appears to exert a dose-dependent effect on the risk of developing a psychotic illness and illness onset is earlier [3]. Methamphetamine may increase the risk of schizophrenia on par with cannabis [4]. Overall, 13–51% of patients entering treatment for their first psychotic episode have a co-occurring substance use disorder [5]. If substance use continues in parallel with a first episode psychosis, patients fare more poorly in both the short and long terms.

In schizophrenia patients the rates of lifetime substance use and substance use disorders are higher than those of the general population (see Table 12.1). Using data from the NIMH Clinical Antipsychotic Trials of Intervention Effectiveness (CATIE) project, 60.3% of subjects had used substances with almost two-thirds fulfilling criteria for a substance use disorder [6]. CATIE data showed that moderate to severe substance use resulted in significantly poorer outcomes in multiple domains (psychosis, depression, quality of life) when compared with patients with mild or no substance use [7].

Table 12.1 Substance and Rates of Use in Schizophrenia Patients Compared with Individuals with No Psychiatric Disorder [18]

Substance	Schizophrenia Patients		General Adult Population	
	Lifetime User (%, 95% CI)	Substance Use Disorder (%, 95% CI)	Lifetime User (%, 95% CI)	Substance Use Disorder (%, 95% CI)
Tobacco	70.1, 64.2–75.9	45.3, 38.9–51.6	43.4, 42.7–44.1	12.4, 11.6–13.2
Cannabis	45.4, 38.6–51.8	7.9, 3.2–12.6	16.4, 15.7–16.7	0.4, 0.3–0.5
Alcohol	89.3, 85.9–92.8	32.8, 26.0–39.7	80.3, 79.8–80.6	7.2, 6.6–7.7

Amphetamines	16.6, 11.8–21.3	2.7, 0.9–4.4	2.1, 2.6–3.1	0.2, 0.1–0.3
Cocaine	20.3, 14.9–25.6	7.7, 4.6–10.8	4.4, 4.1–4.7	0.3, 0.2–0.4
Hallucinogens	22.5, 16.2–28.5	3.4, 0.2–6.6	4.0, 3.7–4.3	0.05, 0.02–0.1
Sedatives	16.4, 11.7–21.0	1.5, 0.1–2.8	2.6, 2.3–2.8	0.05, 0.01–0.1
Opioids	17.6, 12.4–22.8	3.6, 0.4–6.8	3.0, 2.8–3.2	0.1, 0.03–0.1

Figure 12.1 Pathways from Substance Use to Violence in Schizophrenia.

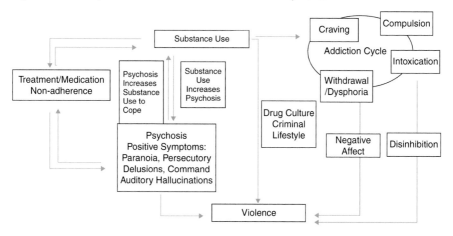

ⓐ Schizophrenia, Substance Use and Violence Among schizophrenia patients, substance use greatly increases the risk of aggression and violence. The general risk of violence in patients with schizophrenia is similar to that of the general population (odds ratio (OR) 1.2, confidence interval (CI) 1.1–1.4). However, for a patient with schizophrenia, the presence of a substance use disorder greatly increases the odds of violent crime (OR 4.4, CI 3.9–5.0) [8]. While in the general population, certain substances (e.g. alcohol) are more associated with violence, this appears not to be the case in patients with psychotic disorders. Two nationwide samples with a total of 1792 patients with psychotic disorders showed that daily and nondaily use of cannabis, stimulants, depressants (sedatives, opioids, inhalants), and hallucinogens all increased violence risk [9]. Figure 12.1 illustrates the pathways from substance use to violence in patients with schizophrenia.

ⓑ Screening and Evaluation Attention to screening is vital in identifying substance use and clinicians should maintain a high index of suspicion with all patients. Ideally, combining the clinical interview with other tools – screening tests, collateral information and objective data – will cast a wide net allowing identification and evaluation of substance use. During the clinical interview, regularly screen all patients with psychosis for use of illicit and other substances including alcohol, cannabis, caffeine and all forms of nicotine. Keep an eye out for misuse of substances such as anticholinergics, cough medicines or other prescription medications (e.g. opioids, benzodiazepines, muscle relaxants). In forensic settings, psychotropic medications such as quetiapine (baby heroin or baby-q), bupropion (wellbies), buspirone, venlafaxine (red dragons), oxcarbazepine, gabapentin and trihexyphenidyl are abused by some patients. Ask about patterns of use, including quantity, frequency, duration and method of use. Knowledge of various substances and methods of use can improve screening. For example, smoking or ingesting cannabis are well-known methods of use. Within the last ten years, "dabbing" has emerged as a means of using "cannabis wax", a high potency cannabis concentrate. Employing special equipment and high temperatures, dabbing allows users to vaporize the concentrate, resulting in a much greater high. Creative approaches, such as using a calendar, can assist with understanding frequency and duration of use. The interview can be used to probe for negative consequences of use including legal problems, interpersonal problems, social and medical consequences, as well as substance-induced psychiatric symptoms.

In certain patients, schizophrenia-related neurocognitive impairments coupled with active psychosis can interfere with effective information gathering during the clinical interview. In these cases, the patient's family members, case managers and other contacts can provide collateral information on substance use and/or behaviors related to substance use. In forensic settings, members of the treatment team, medical providers, state hospital staff or correctional staff all can provide helpful perspectives. For example, unbeknownst to his mental health treatment team, a prisoner had repeatedly visited a primary care provider for treatment of injection drug-related abscesses. Establishing open lines of communication between disciplines can prevent drug use from going unnoticed.

Most states have prescription drug monitoring programs (PDMPs), which are electronic databases that track the prescription of controlled substances. Routinely checking the PDMP database allows the physician to see if the patient is prescribed controlled substances and if there are any irregularities in the pattern of prescriptions that suggest a substance use disorder.

Objective screening tests such as urine or blood toxicology can uncover substance use not reported during the clinical interview and should be regularly incorporated into the evaluation. Breath carbon monoxide (CO) monitors allow approximation of how much smoke an individual inhales from a traditional cigarette, serving as a proxy for nicotine consumption. Note that electronic cigarettes do not involve combustion. Alcohol use can be tested via breathalyzers, saliva, urine, blood and hair. Overall, urine toxicology is the most commonly used type of test; however, there are limitations. These include the specific drug panel employed, the amount of drug used by the patient, the length of time a substance is present in the urine, cut-off values, false positives/negatives, and whether positives are confirmed by more sensitive methods such as gas chromotography/mass spectrometry (GC/MS).

Psychotropic medications can be substances of abuse or can be bartered for illicit drugs in forensic settings. A comprehensive behavioral health urine screen used by one correctional system includes a panel of common illicit substances, comprehensive antidepressant and antipsychotic panels, prescription medications with abuse potentials (gabapentin, cyclobenzaprine, oxcarbazepine, diphenhydramine and others) as well as creatinine, pH, specific gravity and detection of adulterants. Positives are confirmed by liquid or gas chromotography/mass spectrometry. Of note, urine samples can be manipulated via use of either commercial or household product-based urine adulterants, in vivo adulterants or dilution, or urine substitution. Bleach is a widely used and very effective adulterant that can produce false-negative results on immunoassay as well as conceal certain drugs on GC/MS [10]. Table 12.2 lists detection times of some common substances of abuse and notes regarding cross-reactivity.

Table 12.2 Urine Drug Testing Detection Times for Common Drugs of Abuse [31–37]

Substance	Detection Time (Approximate)	Notes
Amphetamine and methamphetamine	48 hours	• False positives: bupropion (structurally related to amphetamines), ranitidine, over-the-counter nasal decongestants (metabolize to l-amphetamine), selegiline (metabolizes to l-amphetamine and l-methamphetamine)

Barbiturates	24–72 hours (short- to intermediate-acting) 2–3 weeks (long-acting)	• Short-acting barbiturates include butalbital, included in headache preparations
Benzodiazepines	72 hours (short-acting, e.g. lorazepam) 30 days (long-acting, e.g. diazepam)	• As a class, benzodiazepines are structurally diverse and benzodiazepine metabolites react variably with immunoassays resulting in a high incidence of false negatives and false positives • Lorazepam and clonazepam are particularly prone to false negatives with point-of-care immunoassay tests • False positive: sertraline
Cannabinoids	48–72 hours (single use) 5–7 days (moderate use, 4x/week) 10–15 days (daily use) >30 days (long-term, heavy use)	• False positives: efavirenz, ibuprofen, naproxen
Cocaine	72 hours	• None
Heroin	24–48 hours	• Rapidly metabolizes to 6-acetylmorphine, which is then metabolized to morphine
3,4-methylenedioxy methamphetamine (MDMA)	24–72 hours	• False positive: trazodone
Phencyclidine (PCP)	8 days	• False positive: venlafaxine and its metabolite o-desmethylvenlafaxine
Prescription opioids (codeine, morphine, oxycodone, and others)	2–4 days	• Prescription opioids can metabolize to other opioids. For example, codeine metabolizes to both hydrocodone and morphine. Review pathways carefully • Rapid cyp 2D6 metabolizers metabolize a greater percentage of codeine to morphine • At lower thresholds, poppy seed consumption can produce positive screening results for morphine and codeine

Note: Detection time is dependent on drug metabolism and half-life, the patient's physical condition, fluid intake, frequency and method of drug use.

In addition to performing a thorough clinical interview, obtaining collateral information from family or treatment team members, reviewing objective evidence and other labs that may indicate use, e.g. infectious disease panels, transaminases, gamma glutamyl transferase and the use of self-report instruments can provide valuable information. Table 12.3 reviews some of the most commonly used self-report instruments.

Table 12.3 Substance Use Screening Instruments [38–45]

Instrument	Populations	Description
Alcohol Use Disorders Identification Test (AUDIT)	Adults, adolescents	• Ten-item screening tool • Identifies harmful or hazardous alcohol consumption • Clinician-administered and self-report versions • Responses scored 0–4, maximum score of 40 • Score of ≥8 indicated hazardous or harmful alcohol use • In adults with severe mental illness, scores of 7 and 8 showed good sensitivity and specificity for substance use disorders
AUDIT-C	Adults	• First three questions of AUDIT • Combines brevity with high performance • Optimal screening thresholds for alcohol misuse are ≥4 men and ≥3 women
CRAFFT	Adolescents	• Six-item screening tool • Covers alcohol and drugs in adolescent-specific contexts • A score of ≥2 identifies problematic use
Fagerström Test for Nicotine Dependence	Adults	• Six-item screening tool for nicotine dependence • Severity rating used for treatment planning • Can be adapted for e-cigarettes
Drug Abuse Screening Test (DAST-10)	Adults	• Ten-item screening test assessing involvement with prescribed, over-the-counter and illicit drugs • Severity rating used for treatment planning • Tested in adults with severe mental illness

❻ Motivation for Change in Patients with Schizophrenia After diagnosing a substance use disorder, the next step is assessing motivation to engage in treatment. Motivation for change is dynamic, depending on many different factors. In contrast to patients without a psychotic disorder, schizophrenia patients are more externally motivated [11]. While motivational enhancement techniques have assisted many patients in progressing through the stages of change, schizophrenia-related cognitive impairments may hinder a patient's ability to set goals and make steps toward them. A flexible approach focused on engagement, coupled with the understanding that motivation may develop gradually over time demonstrates respect for the patient in the early stages of change.

Harm reduction clinical approaches recognize that a patient may not be ready to accept treatment for his or her substance use disorder. This approach focuses on mitigating the harmful effects of substance use without attempting to reduce or treat substance use. Examples of harm reduction strategies include teaching safe injection techniques, providing clean needles and sterile water for injection drug users or providing condoms to patients who trade sex for drugs. Deciding not to treat nicotine use is not an example of harm reduction.

❼ Psychosocial Treatment Approaches Ziedonis and colleagues provide an excellent review of evidence-based psychosocial approaches in their consensus recommendations for improving the care of patients with schizophrenia and substance use disorders [12]. Of the psychosocial approaches, contingency management is effective in not only reducing psychostimulant use but also reducing use of alcohol and smoking in patients with serious mental illness [13, 14].

❸ Pharmacotherapy Treatment Approaches Schizophrenia patients with substance use disorders tend to present with more positive symptoms and demonstrate a decreased response to both first- and second-generation antipsychotics [15]. Bennet and colleagues reviewed open label and randomized controlled trials (RCTs) examining the use of antipsychotic medications to treat psychosis and substance use. Of the five open label and six RCT studies reviewed, olanzapine and clozapine each had two positive studies (one open label and one RCT, each) [16].

Medication-assisted treatment of certain substance use disorders is the standard of care. There are several medications that have demonstrated effectiveness in treating alcohol, tobacco, and opioid use disorders and are FDA-approved for these indications. Only a few trials have studied these treatments in patients with schizophrenia and none of these medications has been specifically approved for patients with schizophrenia and co-occurring substance use. The 2009 Schizophrenia Patient Outcomes Research Team (PORT) found insufficient evidence to recommend specific pharmacological treatments for schizophrenia patients beyond treatments used in the general population [17].

❹ Treatment of Tobacco Use Disorder/Nicotine Use Disorder As described above in Table 12.1, a majority of schizophrenia patients have used tobacco and over 45% have a tobacco use disorder [18]. Although smoking is one of the largest modifiable risk factors for premature all-cause mortality, smokers with schizophrenia are less likely to be advised to quit or receive treatment [19, 20]. Cigarettes – either electronic or combustibles – are the most commonly used methods to rapidly deliver nicotine to the central nervous system. A variety of neurotransmitters are released by nicotine binding, resulting in a myriad of positive effects ranging from a reduction in anxiety to enhancement of learning and memory. While initially it was hoped that electronic cigarettes would assist smokers in quitting, a meta-analysis of 20 controlled studies found that the odds of quitting smoking were 28% lower in those who used e-cigarettes compared with those who did not [21].

The evidence-based, FDA-approved pharmacological treatments for tobacco use disorder are reviewed in Table 12.4. The choice of treatment depends on several factors including history of quit attempts, severity of use, cravings and patient preference. It is recommended that treatment be commenced when the patient is stable. There is a high rate of relapse observed in schizophrenia patients with maintenance treatment. Evidence supports the integration of pharmacological approaches integrated with psychosocial treatments.

Table 12.4 Pharmacotherapy for Tobacco Use Disorder

Treatment	Class	Notes

Nicotine replacement therapy (NRT)[a]	Nicotinic receptor agonist	• Five formulations, two groups:
		  1. Short-acting NRT: gum, lozenge, nasal spray, inhaler
		  2. Long-acting NRT: patch
		• Short-acting NRT assists with acute cravings while the patch provides a steadier stream of nicotine delivery
		• Combination of patch and short-acting NRT is preferred.
		• Match NRT dose to patient's pretreatment level of nicotine.
		
		<10 cigarettes/day = 7–14 mg/day patch
		10–20 cigarettes/day = 14–21 mg/day patch
		21–40 cigarettes/day = 21–42 mg/day patch
		>40 cigarettes/day = >42 mg/day patch
		
		• As monotherapy, the number needed to treat (NNT) with NRT = 15. When NRT is combined with bupropion, the NNT = 5 at three months [46]

Table 12.4 (Cont.)

Treatment	Class	Notes
Bupropion SR[a]	Dopamine and norepinephrine reuptake inhibitor Nicotinic receptor antagonist	- Inhibits nicotine's effect on brain reward centers - Start at 150 mg once daily for three days, then increase to 150 mg twice daily for 7–12 weeks - Works best if combined with NRT - Systematic review and meta-analysis found that bupropion increases abstinence from nicotine without worsening schizophrenia [47] - Bupropion is a strong inhibitor of cytochrome P450 2D6 (cyp 2D6) and certain first- and second-generation antipsychotics are cyp 2D6 substrates
Varenicline[a]	$\alpha_4\beta_2$ nicotinic acetylcholine receptor partial agonist	- Reduces craving, smoking satisfaction and reward - Start one week prior to quit date beginning with 0.5 mg once daily and increasing to 0.5 mg twice daily on day four - The most effective agent in schizophrenia patients with a NNT of six [46] - Maintenance treatment (varenicline + CBT, to 76 weeks) prolonged tobacco abstinence rates in patients with schizophrenia [48] - No significant differences in psychiatric symptoms between varenicline and placebo [47] - Most common side effects are nausea, headache and vomiting

Cytochrome P450 1A2 is induced by polycyclic aromatic hydrocarbons generated by the incomplete combustion of tobacco (and cannabis). A variety of different medications including certain psychotropic medications (e.g. clozapine, olanzapine, chlorpromazine, fluvoxamine and others) are cyp 1A2 substrates. cyp 1A2 induction results in clozapine-treated and olanzapine-treated patients requiring a dose 30–50% greater than that required by a nonsmoker to achieve comparable plasma concentrations [22]. Smoking cessation results in a rapid, exponential decrease in the activity of cyp 1A2. Drug plasma levels will begin to rise within 24 hours of smoking cessation with a mean increase of 57.4% [23]. Side effects of higher clozapine plasma levels may include sedation, hypersalivation, seizures and other neurological effects. Clozapine patients should be monitored carefully and a step-wise dose reduction of 30–50% should be considered.

Ⓖ Treatment of Alcohol Use Disorder Like tobacco use disorder, alcohol use disorder occurs at a much higher rate in patients with psychotic disorders than it does in the general population. There are three FDA-approved medications to treat alcohol use disorder and gabapentin has emerged as a novel treatment, though not FDA-approved. Although few studies have examined these treatments in patients with psychotic disorders, in patients with severe mental illness (including schizophrenia), the three FDA-approved treatments were found to reduce psychiatric hospitalizations, emergency department visits, and improve adherence to medications [24]. These treatments are reviewed in Table 12.5.

Table 12.5 Pharmacotherapy for Alcohol Use Disorder

Medication	Class	Notes
Acamprosate[a]	NMDA receptor modulator	• Reduces glutamatergic hyperactivity that occurs after cessation of heavy drinking • Start as soon as possible after alcohol cessation • Increases abstinence from alcohol • Recommended dose is 666 mg three times daily. No titration is required • One RCT in schizophrenia patients showed no difference on any drinking outcome [49] • Seems to induce relatively higher risk of suicidal ideation and attempts (2.4%) when compared with placebo (0.8%) [50] • The incidence of completed suicide was 0.13% in acamprosate group and 0.10% in placebo group in controlled clinical trials [51]
Disulfiram[a]	Acetyl aldehyde dehydrogenase inhibitor	• Deterrent to alcohol use • Starting dose is 500 mg/day for 1–2 weeks, tapering to a maintenance dose of 250 mg daily • Twelve-week RCT in schizophrenia patients showed significantly fewer drinking days with disulfiram compared with placebo. No significant changes in positive or negative symptoms [52] • Disulfiram blocks dopamine β-hydroxylase, the enzyme that converts dopamine to norepinephrine. High disulfiram doses (1000 mg/day) could theoretically worsen psychosis. Low doses have little or no effect on psychosis • Catatonia is a rare side effect of disulfiram therapy
Gabapentin	Calcium channel/γ-aminobutyric acidmodulator	• Reduces postsynaptic neuronal excitability and decreases release of excitatory neurotransmitters • Dose-dependent effect on reducing alcohol use, ameliorates acute withdrawal and reduces post-acute withdrawal • No studies in patients with psychotic disorders • Gabapentinoids are medications of abuse in forensic populations

Naltrexone[a]	μ-opioid receptor antagonist	• Reduces reinforcing effects of alcohol
		• Two formulations:
		  ◦ Oral formulation – start with 25 mg and titrate to 50 mg daily
		  ◦ Intramuscular injection – 380 mg IM (gluteal muscle) every four weeks
		• Twelve-week RCT in schizophrenia patients demonstrated significantly fewer drinking days with naltrexone compared with placebo. No significant changes in positive or negative symptoms [52]
		• Should not be used in patients with an active opioid use disorder or patients on chronic opioid therapy

[a] FDA approved for the treatment of alcohol use disorder.

⊕ Treatment of Opioid Use Disorder Given the degree of organization required to maintain a constant supply of opioids to avoid withdrawal, opioid use disorders are not commonly seen in patients with treatment-resistant schizophrenia. When present, opioid use disorders in patients with complex, serious mental illness are more likely to result in homelessness, disability, frequent hospitalization and involvement in the criminal justice system. Treatment with any one of the three FDA-approved medications reduces mental health service utilization in patients with schizophrenia [25]. However, there is a paucity of controlled trials specifically examining treatment employing these medications in patients with psychotic disorders. Table 12.6 reviews the three FDA-approved treatments for opioid use disorder.

Table 12.6 Pharmacotherapy for Opioid Use Disorder

Medication	Class	Notes
Buprenorphine[a]	μ-opioid receptor partial agonist and κ-opioid antagonist	• Long-acting synthetic opioid • Administered on an outpatient basis • Available as buprenorphine alone or as combination of buprenorphine and naloxone, which is designed to prevent misuse/diversion • Three formulations: sublingual tablet, sublingual film and implant • No controlled trials in patients with psychotic disorders • Buprenorphine is a controlled substance with abuse potential
Methadone[a]	μ-opioid receptor agonist	• Long-acting synthetic opioid • Administered daily at a clinic with long-term, adherent patients able to take home a 30-day supply • Gold standard for treatment of opioid use disorder during pregnancy • No controlled trials in patients with psychotic disorders • Monitor QTc in patients co-prescribed methadone and antipsychotics that tend to prolong the QTc

Naltrexone[a]	μ-opioid receptor antagonist	• Blocks the effects of opioids
		• Two formulations:
		  ○ Oral formulation – start with 25 mg and titrate to 50 mg daily
		  ○ Intramuscular injection – 380 mg IM (gluteal muscle) every four weeks
		• Cannot be started until opioid withdrawal has ended or administration will precipitate opioid withdrawal
		• No controlled efficacy studies in patients with psychotic disorders

[a] FDA approved for the treatment of opioid use disorder.

❶ Treatment of Cannabis Use Disorder Cannabis, specifically tetra-hydro-cannabidiol (THC), is one of the top three substances used by patients with psychotic disorders. Motivations for use range from use to cope with unpleasant aspects of mental illness, enhancement of positive feelings, and increasing social interactions and social acceptance [26]. The legalization of cannabis in many states has reduced perception of harm; nevertheless, schizophrenia patients who are heavy cannabis users suffer from a greater burden of both positive and negative symptoms while those who have reduced their use show a decrease in symptom severity [27].

In terms of pharmacological treatment of cannabis use disorder, there are no FDA-approved medications, nor are there any promising drugs with trials in this population. One small retrospective study found that over the short-term, abstinence rates were higher in clozapine-treated schizophrenia patients with alcohol and cannabis use disorders than in patients treated with risperidone [28].

❿ Stimulant Use Disorder (Cocaine, Methamphetamine) Owing to the enormous release of dopamine resulting from the use of psychostimulants, these substances are particularly problematic when used by patients with schizophrenia spectrum disorders. Despite a multitude of trials, most drugs have not shown a statistically significant effect on reducing use in nonpsychotic individuals [29, 30]. Transcranial magnetic stimulation is showing early promise in reducing stimulant craving.

❿ Other Substances Unfortunately, there are not yet any FDA-approved medications or medications with a solid evidence base to treat other illicit drugs of abuse.

❿ Conclusion Substance use may predate a patient's first psychotic episode and if not treated, continued use after a schizophrenia spectrum disorder has developed, complicates and negatively affects the patient's mental health, physical health and social functioning. Substance use in patients with schizophrenia exceeds that seen in individuals without psychosis. Tobacco or nicotine, alcohol and cannabis are the most commonly used substances, with polysubstance use being the rule rather than the exception. The increased violence risk observed in patients with psychotic disorders is largely attributable to substance use. Assessment of substance use disorder is multi-pronged including a clinical interview, collateral information and objective measures. Once a disorder is uncovered, treatment proceeds with the flexible integration of pharmacological and psychosocial approaches. Evidence-based medications exist for tobacco, alcohol and opioid use disorders. While they have demonstrated benefit and are recommended by the Schizophrenia PORT, they are underutilized in schizophrenia patients.

ⓒ Summary Points

- Over half of schizophrenia spectrum disorder patients have used substances and the severity of substance use is positively correlated with poorer clinical outcomes and an increased risk of violence.
- Integrated treatment, using a flexible combination of pharmacotherapy and psychosocial approaches targeting both disorders, is the standard of care for these patients.
- Evidence-based pharmacotherapy targeting substance use disorders in patients with psychotic disorders is understudied and underutilized.
- Schizophrenia patients with substance use disorders should be engaged in medication-assisted treatment targeting the substance use disorder(s).

References

1. Myles, N., Newall, H. D., Curtis, J., et al. (2012). Tobacco use before, at, and after first-episode psychosis: a systematic meta-analysis. *J Clin Psychiatry*, 73, 468–475.
2. Myles, H., Myles, N., Large, M. (2016). Cannabis use in first episode psychosis: meta-analysis of prevalence, and the time course of initiation and continued use. *Aust N Z J Psychiatry*, 50, 208–219.
3. Hasan, A., von Keller, R., Friemel, C. M., et al. (2019). Cannabis use and psychosis: a review of reviews. *Eur Arch Psychiatry Clin Neurosci*, 270(4), 403–412.
4. Callaghan, R. C., Cunningham, J. K., Allebeck, P., et al. (2012). Methamphetamine use and schizophrenia: a population-based cohort study in California. *Am J Psychiatry*, 169, 389–396.
5. Substance Abuse and Mental Health Services Administration. (2019). *First-episode psychosis and co-occurring substance use disorders*. Rockville, MD: National Mental Health and Substance Use Policy Laboratory. Publication no. PEP19-PL-Guide-3.
6. Swartz, M. S., Wagner, H. R., Swanson, J. W., et al. (2006). Substance use in persons with schizophrenia: baseline prevalence and correlates from the NIMH CATIE study. *J Nerv Ment Dis*, 194, 164–172.
7. Kerfoot, K. E., Rosenheck, R. A., Petrakis, I. L., et al. (2011). Substance use and schizophrenia: adverse correlates in the CATIE study sample. *Schizophr Res*, 132, 177–182.
8. Fazel, S., Långström, N., Hjern, A., et al. (2009). Schizophrenia, substance abuse, and violent crime. *JAMA*, 301, 2016–2023.
9. Lamsma, J., Cahn, W., Fazel, S. (2019). Use of illicit substances and violent behaviour in psychotic disorders: two nationwide case-control studies and meta-analyses. *Psychol Med*, 50(12), 2028–2033.
10. Jaffee, W. B., Trucco, E., Levy, S., et al. (2007). Is this urine really negative? A systematic review of tampering methods in urine drug screening and testing. *J Subst Abuse Treat*, 33, 33–42.
11. DiClemente, C. C., Nidecker, M., Bellack, A. S. (2008). Motivation and the stages of change among individuals with severe mental illness and substance abuse disorders. *J Subst Abuse Treat*, 34, 25–35.
12. Ziedonis, D. M., Smelson, D., Rosenthal, R. N., et al. (2005). Improving the care of individuals with schizophrenia and substance use disorders: consensus recommendations. *J Psychiatr Pract*, 11, 315.
13. McDonell, M. G., Srebnik, D., Angelo, F., et al. (2013). Randomized controlled trial of contingency management for stimulant use in community mental health patients with serious mental illness. *Am J Psychiatry*, 170, 94–101.
14. McPherson, S., Orr, M., Lederhos, C., et al. (2018). Decreases in smoking during treatment for methamphetamine-use disorders: preliminary evidence. *Behav Pharmacol*, 29, 370–374.
15. Green, A. I., Tohen, M. F., Hamer, R. M., et al. (2004). First episode schizophrenia-related psychosis and substance use disorders: acute response to olanzapine and haloperidol. *Schizophr Res*, 66, 125–135.
16. Bennett, M. E., Bradshaw, K. R., Catalano, L. T. (2017). Treatment of substance use disorders in schizophrenia. *Am J Drug Alcohol Abuse*, 43, 377–390.
17. Buchanan, R. W., Kreyenbuhl, J., Kelly, D. L., et al. (2012). The 2009 schizophrenia PORT psychopharmacological treatment recommendations and summary statements. *FOCUS*, 10, 194–216.
18. Martins, S. S., Gorelick, D. A. (2011). Conditional substance abuse and dependence by diagnosis of mood or anxiety disorder or schizophrenia in the U.S. population. *Drug Alcohol Depend*, 119, 28–36.
19. Wildgust, H. J., Beary, M. (2010). Are there modifiable risk factors which will reduce the excess mortality in schizophrenia? *J Psychopharmacol*, 24, 37–50.
20. Cather, C., Pachas, G. N., Cieslak, K. M., et al. (2017). Achieving smoking cessation in individuals with schizophrenia: special considerations. *CNS Drugs*, 31, 471–481.
21. Kalkhoran, S., Glantz, S. A. (2016). E-cigarettes and smoking cessation in real-world and clinical settings: a systematic review and meta-analysis. *Lancet Respir Med*, 4, 116–128.
22. Tsuda, Y., Saruwatari, J., Yasui-Furukori, N. (2014). Meta-analysis: the effects of smoking on the disposition of two commonly used antipsychotic agents, olanzapine and clozapine. *BMJ Open*, 4, e004216.
23. Meyer, J. M. (2001). Individual changes in clozapine levels after smoking cessation: results and a predictive model. *J Clin Psychopharmacol*, 21, 569–574.
24. Robertson, A. G., Easter, M. M., Lin, H., et al. (2018). Medication-assisted treatment for alcohol-dependent adults with serious mental illness and criminal justice involvement: effects on treatment utilization and outcomes. *Am J Psychiatry*, 175, 665–673.
25. Robertson, A. G., Easter, M. M., Lin, H. J., et al. (2018). Associations between pharmacotherapy for opioid dependence and clinical and criminal justice outcomes among adults with co-occurring serious mental illness. *J Subst Abuse Treat*, 86, 17–25.
26. Spencer, C., Castle, D., Michie, P. T. (2002). Motivations that maintain substance use among individuals with psychotic disorders. *Schizophr Bull*, 28, 233–247.
27. Toftdahl, N. G., Nordentoft, M., Hjorthoj, C. (2016). The effect of changes in cannabis exposure on psychotic symptoms in patients with comorbid cannabis use disorder. *J Dual Diagn*, 12, 129–136.
28. Green, A. I., Burgess, E. S., Dawson, R., et al. (2003). Alcohol and cannabis use in schizophrenia: effects of clozapine vs. risperidone. *Schizophr Res*, 60, 81–85.
29. Chan, B., Freeman, M., Kondo, K., et al. (2019). Pharmacotherapy for methamphetamine/amphetamine use disorder – a systematic review and meta-analysis. *Addiction*, 114, 2122–2136.
30. Chan, B., Kondo, K., Freeman, M., et al. (2019). Pharmacotherapy for cocaine use disorder – a systematic review and meta-analysis. *J Gen Intern Med*, 34, 2858–2873.
31. Sena, S. F., Kazimi, S., Wu, A. H. (2002). False-positive phencyclidine immunoassay results caused by venlafaxine and O-desmethylvenlafaxine. *Clin Chem*, 48, 676–677.
32. Heit, H. A., Gourlay, D. L. (2004). Urine drug testing in pain medicine. *J Pain Symptom Manage*, 27, 260–267.
33. Moeller, K. E., Lee, K. C., Kissack, J. C. (2008). Urine drug screening: practical guide for clinicians. *Mayo Clin Proc*, 83(1), 66–76.

34. Nasky, K. M., Cowan, G. L., Knittel, D. R. (2009). False-positive urine screening for benzodiazepines: an association with sertraline? A two-year retrospective chart analysis. *Psychiatry (Edgmont)*, 6, 36.
35. Reisfield, G. M., Goldberger, B. A., Bertholf, R. L. (2009). "False-positive" and "false-negative" test results in clinical urine drug testing. *Bioanalysis*, 1, 937–952.
36. Mikel, C., Pesce, A. J., Rosenthal, M., et al. (2012). Therapeutic monitoring of benzodiazepines in the management of pain: current limitations of point of care immunoassays suggest testing by mass spectrometry to assure accuracy and improve patient safety. *Clin Chim Acta*, 413, 1199–1202.
37. Saitman, A., Park, H-D., Fitzgerald, R. L. (2014). False-positive interferences of common urine drug screen immunoassays: a review. *J Anal Toxicol*, 38, 387–396.
38. Bohn, M., Babor, T., Kranzler, H. (1991). Validity of the Drug Abuse Screening Test (DAST-10) in inpatient substance abusers. *Problems of Drug Dependence*, 119, 233–235.
39. Heatherton, T. F., Kozlowski, L. T., Frecker, R. C., et al. (1991). The Fagerström test for nicotine dependence: a revision of the Fagerstrom Tolerance Questionnaire. *Br J Addict*, 86, 1119–1127.
40. Saunders, J. B., Aasland, O. G., Babor, T. F., et al. (1993). Development of the Alcohol Use Disorders Identification Test (AUDIT): WHO collaborative project on early detection of persons with harmful alcohol consumption – II. *Addiction*, 88, 791–804.
41. Bush, K., Kivlahan, D. R., McDonell, M. B., et al. (1998). The AUDIT alcohol consumption questions (AUDIT-C): an effective brief screening test for problem drinking. *Arch Intern Med*, 158, 1789–1795.
42. Knight, J. R., Shrier, L. A., Bravender, T. D., et al. (1999). A new brief screen for adolescent substance abuse. *Arch Pediatr Adolesc Med*, 153, 591–596.
43. Maisto, S. A., Carey, M. P., Carey, K. B., et al. (2000). Use of the AUDIT and the DAST-10 to identify alcohol and drug use disorders among adults with a severe and persistent mental illness. *Psychol Assess*, 12, 186–192.
44. Knight, J. R., Sherritt, L., Shrier, L. A., et al. (2002). Validity of the CRAFFT substance abuse screening test among adolescent clinic patients. *Arch Pediatr Adolesc Med*, 156, 607–614.
45. Bradley, K. A., DeBenedetti, A. F., Volk, R. J., et al. (2007). AUDIT-C as a brief screen for alcohol misuse in primary care. *Alcohol Clin Exp Res*, 31, 1208–1217.
46. Pearsall, R., Smith, D. J., Geddes, J. R. (2019). Pharmacological and behavioural interventions to promote smoking cessation in adults with schizophrenia and bipolar disorders: a systematic review and meta-analysis of randomised trials. *BMJ Open*, 9, e027389.
47. Tsoi, D. T-Y., Porwal, M., Webster, A. C. (2010). Efficacy and safety of bupropion for smoking cessation and reduction in schizophrenia: systematic review and meta-analysis. *Br J Psychiatry*, 196, 346–353.
48. Evins, A. E., Cather, C., Pratt, S. A., et al. (2014). Maintenance treatment with varenicline for smoking cessation in patients with schizophrenia and bipolar disorder: a randomized clinical trial. *JAMA*, 311, 145–154.
49. Ralevski, E., O'Brien, E., Jane, J. S., et al. (2011). Treatment with acamprosate in patients with schizophrenia spectrum disorders and comorbid alcohol dependence. *J Dual Diagn*, 7, 64–73.
50. Paz, R. D., Tardito, S., Atzori, M., et al. (2008). Glutamatergic dysfunction in schizophrenia: from basic neuroscience to clinical psychopharmacology. *Eur Neuropsychopharmacol*, 18, 773–786.
51. Forest Pharmaceuticals, I. (2004). *Highlights of prescribing information for acamprosate sodium*. New York.
52. Petrakis, I. L., Nich, C., Ralevski, E. (2006). Psychotic spectrum disorders and alcohol abuse: a review of pharmacotherapeutic strategies and a report on the effectiveness of naltrexone and disulfiram. *Schizophr Bull*, 32, 644–654.

1.13 Approaches to Behavioral Disturbances in Dementia and Traumatic Brain Injury Patients

Introduction Of the many behavioral disturbances associated with severe mental and neurocognitive disorders, impulsive behaviors, including agitation and aggression, present unique challenges. Frontal inhibition, cognitive impairments and executive dysfunction commonly combine to promote behavioral disturbances in severe mental and neurocognitive disorders, and the interplay between structures and circuits may explain a mechanism for the impulsive behaviors, agitation and aggression. A circuit of periaqueductal gray matter, hippocampus, amygdala and hypothalamus mediates threat response, a bottom-up impulse. Prefrontal cortex (PFC) serves a top-down role to inhibit those bottom-up impulses, and PFC dysfunction impairs a person's ability to recognize social cues and increases the risk of impulsive aggressive responses by a person failing to make appropriate risk/reward assessments for inhibiting responses. Added sensory deficits in hearing, vision or pain together with sensory processing and appraisal deficits in cognition combine to foster behavioral disturbances of agitation, aggression and impulsive acts [1]. Of the PFC, specifically the ventromedial PFC and its connections to lower structures, such as the amygdala, serve this top-down inhibitory function [1, 2]. PFC-amygdala circuit connectivity is disrupted by dysfunction in associated serotonin and dopamine systems in several mental conditions. Enhancing serotonergic and dopaminergic signaling in and around this circuit provides a theoretical approach to pharmacologic agent selection for many of these behavioral disturbances. Severe mental and neurocognitive disorders, including traumatic brain injury (TBI), often show pathology in the brain regions associated with top-down and bottom-up structures, as described above [3].

A Traumatic Brain Injury Treatment of Behavioral Disturbances Traumatic Brain Injury occurs in 50 million persons globally and 3.5 million in the US [4]. Behavioral disturbances of concern in post-acute TBI include agitation, irritability, impulsive violence and aggression [2, 4]. There are few studies providing strong support for particular pharmacologic interventions in TBI. Systematic reviews reveal limited evidence of efficacy for individual agents. Nevertheless, there are data to suggest that certain medications can be used in a manner consistent with good clinical practice [2, 5].

Systematic reviews highlight trials of amantadine, propranolol and valproic acid as most supported for efficacy in TBI behavioral disturbances. Support from systematic reviews also exists for methylphenidate and carbamazepine, though the evidence for methylphenidate is not as strong as for the weak dopamine agonist amantadine, and use of carbamazepine has many disadvantages, including the need for slow titration to minimize ataxia, risk of hyponatremia, and potent induction of both cyp 450 3A4 and the efflux transporter P-glycoprotein. Asian patients should be screened for the HLA-B*1502 allele due to its association with carbamazepine-induced Stevens-Johnson Syndrome [2, 6–8, 9]. Antidepressants, in particular selective serotonin reuptake inhibitors (SSRIs), do show efficacy for depressive symptoms in TBI patients but not for aggression and agitation [2, 10]. Medication classes associated with only negative outcomes or side effects across multiple publications include benzodiazepines, phenytoin and opiates [4].

Importantly, while antipsychotics have frequently been used to target agitation in TBI patients, a 2019 systematic review found "while the class may reduce agitation, it is advisable to consider if other classes, such as beta-blockers or anti-epileptics, might provide a similar effect" with greater literature support and lesser risks of cognitive decrements [4].

Ⓑ Dementia/Neurocognitive Disorders Major Neurocognitive Disorders (Dementias) consist of a heterogeneous group of disorders, however the majority of studies have focused on the most common cause, Alzheimer's disease (AD), and to a lesser extent on vascular dementia.

Behavioral disturbances of most concern are similar to those found in TBI patients, though psychosocial interventions for dementias have the greatest literature support, are more likely to show effect in dementia patients, and, therefore, should be considered before the addition of pharmacologic interventions.

Psychosocial interventions including correcting visual and hearing impairments, ensuring adequate lighting, alleviation of pain, empiric routine use of nonopioid analgesics when patients' verbal abilities are limited, bright light therapy and orienting strategies have modest efficacy data [2].

Acetylcholinesterase inhibitors (AChEIs) have the strongest evidence of the pharmacologic options supporting their use for behavioral disturbances associated with mild to moderate AD by delaying the progression of the underlying illness [2, 11]. Memantine has also shown low to moderate quality evidence of efficacy in AD both as monotherapy and combined with AChEIs [2, 12].

Selective serotonin reuptake inhibitor antidepressants have a significant efficacy for aggressive dementia patients such that a 2011 Cochrane review concluded SSRIs and trazodone seemed to be reasonably well tolerated compared to placebo and antipsychotics. Of the SSRIs, citalopram and escitalopram are most studied but have QTc warnings, whereas sertraline does not and may be considered desirable from a drug-drug interaction risk, as well [2, 13].

A large, naturalistic study from the US Veterans Health Administration (VHA) provided mortality risk estimates for various agents in a population of 46,008 veterans with dementia. The study clarified the risk:benefit landscape when treating behavioral disturbances in patients with dementia. The number needed to harm (NNH), with harm defined as mortality over six months, ranged for antipsychotics from eight for haloperidol to 31 for quetiapine. Antidepressant use, on the other hand, was associated with a decreased risk of mortality. Takeaways from this study include that antipsychotics should not be considered as first-line agents in patients with dementia, and, if used, low doses of atypical antipsychotics, such as risperidone 0.25 mg/d or quetiapine 25 mg bid, should be considered [2, 14]. Nevertheless, antipsychotics may be considered in certain situations, such as continued agitation despite non-pharmacologic interventions, or when behavioral agitation or aggression are dangerous to the patient or others [15]. Atypical antipsychotics, including aripiprazole, should be considered due to greater tolerability. Once used for four months, antipsychotics may be tapered and discontinued often without worsening of behavioral disturbances [15, 16], with the possible exception of patients with significant psychosis [15, 17].

Evidence for use of anticonvulsants in dementia patients with behavioral disturbances is largely negative. In the VAH study, valproate was found to have a NNH of 20. Data with carbamazepine use are conflicting, and both tolerability and kinetic concerns limit its use. Low-dose lamotrigine (mean dose at study endpoint 46.3 ± 24.2 mg/d, range 25–100 mg/d) showed modest benefit in a 16-week trial with 40 inpatients to the extent that the doses of concomitant antipsychotics could be lowered [14, 18, 19].

Finally, although benzodiazepines are occasionally used on an emergent basis for acute agitation, there is no evidence to support their efficacy for persistent aggression, with significant concerns about tolerability [20].

Table 13.1 Medications for Behavioral Disturbances [2, 4, 5, 14, 15, 21, 22]

Medication	Indications	Comments
AChEIs	Mild-moderate Alzheimer Dz No TBI indication	• Differential response among agents, so try another if first one fails • Not for acute agitation
Amantadine	No dementia indication Behavioral disturbance in TBI	
Anticonvulsants	Behavioral disturbance in dementia Behavioral disturbance in TBI	• Scarce support of efficacy • Increased mortality risk with dementia • If used, consider: Valproate 40–60 mcg/ml Lamotrigine 25–100 mg/d • Positive findings supporting use • Carbamazepine has pharmacokinetic risks, ataxia, sedation, Stevens-Johnson risk in Asians make it less desirable • Phenytoin also has pharmacokinetic risks, side effects make it less desirable • Valproate has the most evidence support • Valproate 1000–1800 mg/d
Antidepressants	Behavioral disturbance in dementia Behavioral disturbance in TBI	• Modest efficacy • SSRIs are the most studied for behavioral disturbance in dementia • Not effective for affective symptoms • Citalopram and escitalopram QT risks • Citalopram/escitalopram 10–20 mg/d Sertraline 25–100 mg/d Trazadone 12.5–200 mg/d (multiple daily dosing) • Positive findings of weak quality • Have been helpful for depressive symptoms in TBI
Atypical Antipsychotics	Behavioral disturbance in dementia Behavioral disturbance in TBI	• Increased mortality risk with dementia • Modest benefit for behavioral disturbances • More effective if psychosis present • Less effective if severe dementia • Try to taper after four months of use • Aripiprazole 2–10 mg/d • Olanzapine 5–10 mg/d • Risperidone 0.5–2.0 mg/d • Quetiapine 25–300 mg/d • No evidence of efficacy for routine use for behavioral disturbance in TBI • If used, only consider quick treatment of a few doses for severe agitation • Consider second-line to amantadine, propranolol, valproate

Medication	Indications	Comments
(Typical) Antipsychotics	Avoid in either dementia or TBI	• Risks too high with dementia • No supporting evidence for TBI
Benzodiazepines	Behavioral disturbance in dementia Behavioral disturbance in TBI	• Known risks, no substantial benefits – avoid • Mostly negative findings for efficacy • May use only short-term for acute agitation
Buspirone	Behavioral disturbance in dementia Behavioral disturbance in TBI	• No supporting evidence • Low level of evidence, may be considered second-line
Dopamine Agonists	Behavioral disturbance in dementia Behavioral disturbance in TBI	• No supporting evidence • Amantadine has strongest evidence of efficacy of possible agents for behavioral disturbance in TBI • Initiate >4 weeks post-TBI • Amantadine 100–300 mg/d • Methylphenidate only mixed efficacy data for anger, inferior to amantadine
Lithium	Behavioral disturbance in dementia Behavioral disturbance in TBI	• No supporting evidence • Insufficient evidence to recommend
Propranolol	Behavioral disturbance in dementia Behavioral disturbance in TBI	• No supporting evidence • Positive findings support for behavioral disturbance in TBI • Titrate to 40–80 mg/d

Ⓒ Summary Points
• Behavioral disturbances cause increased risk for patients and caregivers.
• For dementia, psychosocial treatments have stronger evidence supporting efficacy than pharmacological interventions.
• For patients with behavioral disturbance, few pharmacological interventions have strong evidence to support their use.
• All pharmacological interventions with evidence of efficacy for behavioral disturbance have adverse risks associated that must be taken into account when considering a patient's risk:benefit analysis for a particular medication.

References

1. Siever, L. J. (2008). Neurobiology of aggression and violence. *Am J Psychiatry*, 165, 429–442.
2. Meyer, J. M., Cummings, M. A., Proctor, G., et al. (2016). Psychopharmacology of persistent violence and aggression. *Psychiatr Clin North Am*, 39, 541–556.
3. Rosenbloom, M. H., Schmahmann, J. D., Price, B. H. (2012). The functional neuroanatomy of decision-making. *J Neuropsychiatry Clin Neurosci*, 24, 266–277.
4. Nash, R. P., Weinberg, M. S., Laughon, S. L., et al. (2019). Acute pharmacological management of behavioral and emotional dysregulation following a traumatic brain injury: a systematic review of the literature. *Psychosomatics*, 60, 139–152.
5. Hicks, A. J., Clay, F. J., Hopwood, M., et al. (2019). The efficacy and harms of pharmacological interventions for aggression after traumatic brain injury: a systematic review. *Front Neurol*, 10, 1169.
6. Tangamornsuksan, W., Chaiyakunapruk, N., Somkrua, R., et al. (2013). Relationship between the HLA-B*1502 allele and carbamazepine-induced Stevens-Johnson syndrome and toxic epidermal necrolysis: a systematic review and meta-analysis. *JAMA Dermatol*, 149, 1025–1032.
7. Hammond, F. M., Bickett, A. K., Norton, J. H., et al. (2014). Effectiveness of amantadine hydrochloride in the reduction of chronic traumatic brain injury irritability and aggression. *J Head Trauma Rehabil*, 29, 391–399.
8. Sami, M. B., Faruqui, R. (2015). The effectiveness of dopamine agonists for treatment of neuropsychiatric symptoms post brain injury and stroke. *Acta Neuropsychiatr*, 27, 317–326.
9. Hammond, F. M., Malec, J. F., Zafonte, R. D., et al. (2017). Potential impact of amantadine on aggression in chronic traumatic brain injury. *J Head Trauma Rehabil*, 32, 308–318.
10. Hammond, F. M., Sherer, M., Malec, J. F., et al. (2015). Amantadine effect on perceptions of irritability after traumatic brain injury: results of the amantadine irritability multisite study. *J Neurotrauma*, 32, 1230–1238.
11. Cummings, J., Lai, T. J., Hemrungrojn, S., et al. (2016). Role of donepezil in the management of neuropsychiatric symptoms in Alzheimer's disease and dementia with Lewy bodies. *CNS Neurosci Ther*, 22, 159–166.
12. Gareri, P., Putignano, D., Castagna, A., et al. (2014). Retrospective study on the benefits of combined Memantine and cholinEsterase inhibitor treatMent in AGEd Patients affected with Alzheimer's disease: the MEMAGE study. *J Alzheimers Dis*, 41, 633–640.
13. Seitz, D. P., Adunuri, N., Gill, S. S., et al. (2011). Antidepressants for agitation and psychosis in dementia. *Cochrane Database Syst Rev*, 2011, CD008191.
14. Maust, D. T., Kim, H. M., Seyfried, L. S., et al. (2015). Antipsychotics, other psychotropics, and the risk of death in patients with dementia: number needed to harm. *JAMA Psychiatry*, 72, 438–445.
15. Deardorff, W. J., Grossberg, G. T. (2019). Behavioral and psychological symptoms in Alzheimer's dementia and vascular dementia. *Handb Clin Neurol*, 165, 5–32.
16. Reus, V. I., Fochtmann, L. J., Eyler, A. E., et al. (2016). The American Psychiatric Association practice guideline on the use of antipsychotics to treat agitation or psychosis in patients with dementia. *Am J Psychiatry*, 173, 543–546.
17. Devanand, D. P., Mintzer, J., Schultz, S., et al. (2012). The antipsychotic discontinuation in Alzheimer disease trial: clinical rationale and study design. *Am J Geriatr Psychiatry*, 20, 362–373.
18. Gallagher, D., Herrmann, N. (2014). Antiepileptic drugs for the treatment of agitation and aggression in dementia: do they have a place in therapy? *Drugs*, 74, 1747–1755.
19. Suzuki, H., Gen, K. (2015). Clinical efficacy of lamotrigine and changes in the dosages of concomitantly used psychotropic drugs in Alzheimer's disease with behavioural and psychological symptoms of dementia: a preliminary open-label trial. *Psychogeriatrics*, 15, 32–37.
20. Tampi, R. R., Tampi, D. J. (2014). Efficacy and tolerability of benzodiazepines for the treatment of behavioral and psychological symptoms of dementia: a systematic review of randomized controlled trials. *Am J Alzheimers Dis Other Demen*, 29, 565–574.
21. Plantier, D., Luaute, J., Group, S. (2016). Drugs for behavior disorders after traumatic brain injury: systematic review and expert consensus leading to French recommendations for good practice. *Ann Phys Rehabil Med*, 59, 42–57.
22. Keszycki, R. M., Fisher, D. W., Dong, H. (2019). The hyperactivity-impulsivity-irritability-disinhibition-aggression-agitation domain in Alzheimer's disease: current management and future directions. *Front Pharmacol*, 10, 1109.

Part II
Medication Reference Tables

First-Generation (Typical) Antipsychotics
2.01 Chlorpromazine

QUICK CHECK

A. BASIC INFORMATION [1]

Principle Trade Names
• Thorazine®
• Largactil® (outside the US)

Legal Status
• Prescription only
• Not controlled

Classifications
• Monoamine antagonist
• Typical or first-generation antipsychotic (FGA)

Generics Available
• Yes

Formulations
• Tablets: 10 mg; 25 mg; 50 mg; 100 mg; 200 mg
• Capsules: 30 mg; 75 mg; 150 mg
• Oral solution or syrup: 10 mg/5 ml; 25 mg/ 5 ml; 100 mg/5 ml; 40 mg/ml

• Injectable: 25 mg/ml
• Suppositories: 25 mg; 100 mg

FDA Indications
• Schizophrenia
• Mania
• Severe behavioral problems in children (1–12 years of age) marked by combativeness and/or explosive hyperexcitable behavior
• Nausea and vomiting
• Intractable hiccups
• Restlessness and apprehension before surgery
• Acute intermittent porphyria
• Adjunctively for the treatment of tetanus

Other Data-Supported Indications
• Agitation/aggression (severe, acute) associated with psychiatric disorders (e.g. bipolar disorder, schizophrenia), delirium, substance intoxication

Dopamine
• Antagonism at D_2 receptors may decrease positive psychotic symptoms, contribute to antimanic effects, decrease aggression and have antiemetic effects

Serotonin
• Antagonism at $5HT_{2A}$ receptors in the nigrostriatal tract diminishes risk for neurological motor symptoms

Epinephrine/norepinephrine
• Antagonism at α_1- and α_2-adrenergic receptors causes orthostatic hypotension

C. PLASMA CONCENTRATIONS AND TREATMENT RESPONSE [2, 3]

Initial Target Range
• Optimal initial target range is 3–72 ng/ml

Range for Treatment Resistance
• May consider levels up to 100 ng/ml

Typical Time to Response
• In responders to a given dose, some therapeutic improvement can be seen in two weeks

Time-Course of Improvement
• If no response after two weeks of a given dose, verify adherence and plasma level. Consider dose increase if no adverse effects and plasma level is < 72 ng/ml
• If no response after four weeks at maximum tolerated plasma concentration, withdraw treatment

D. TYPICAL TREATMENT RESPONSE [1]

Usual Target Symptoms
• Psychosis – positive symptoms
• Mania
• Violence and aggression

Common Short-Term Adverse Effects
• Somnolence
• Orthostatic hypotension, lightheadedness or syncope
• Dry mouth
• Constipation
• Gastroesophageal reflux, dyspepsia
• Blurred vision
• Urinary retention (males)
• Tachycardia
• Parkinsonism (higher doses)
• Akathisia (higher doses)

Rare Adverse Effects
• Prolonged QTc interval
• Seizure
• Neuroleptic malignant syndrome
• Increased risk of death or cerebrovascular events in elderly patients with dementia-related psychosis
• Elevated liver enzymes
• Hyperprolactinemia

Long-Term Effects
• Metabolic changes, including weight gain, hyperglycemia, dyslipidemia
• Tardive dyskinesia

E. PRE-TREATMENT WORKUP AND INITIAL LABORATORY TESTING [1]

History
• Obtain personal and family histories of diabetes, obesity, dyslipidemia

Physical
• General physical examination
• Vital signs and weight (for BMI)

Neurological
• AIMS
• Neurology consultation if personal history of active, poorly controlled seizure disorder

Blood Tests
• Within 90 days: liver function tests, fasting glucose and/or Hgb A1C lipid panel
• Metabolic monitoring every six months

Cardiac Tests
• ECG at higher dosages or if used with cyp 2D6 inhibitors

Urine Tests
• Not necessary

Pregnancy Test
• Pregnancy test (premenopausal females)
• Classified as risk not ruled out

Metabolic Syndrome Parameters
• Elevated waist circumference:
  ◦ Men – greater than 40 inches (102 cm)
  ◦ Women – greater than 35 inches (88 cm)
• Elevated triglycerides: equal to or greater than 150 mg/dl (1.7 mmol/l)
• Reduced HDL ("good") cholesterol:
  ◦ Men – less than 40 mg/dl (1.03 mmol/l)
  ◦ Women – less than 50 mg/dl (1.29 mmol/l)
• Elevated blood pressure: ≥130/80 mm Hg or use of medication for hypertension
• Elevated fasting glucose: equal to or greater than 100 mg/dl (5.6 mmol/l) or use of medication for hyperglycemia

Monthly
• Weight/BMI (or at each outpatient visit)

Semi-Annually (twice per year)
• Hgb A1C or fasting glucose
• Fasting lipid panel

Annually
• AIMS
• Prolactin if complaining of related adverse effects

Initial Dosing
Oral Equivalence with Other FGAs

Haloperidol	2 mg
Fluphenazine	2 mg
Thiothixene	5 mg
Trifluoperazine	5 mg
Perphenazine	8–10 mg
Loxapine	12.5 mg
Chlorpromazine	100 mg

• Initial oral doses for adult psychosis/ agitation 100–200 mg/day in divided doses to minimize orthostasis risk
• Initial IM doses must be 1/3 that of oral doses

Titration
• Based on tolerance of sedation, orthostasis, may proceed by 100 mg every 2–7 days until 200–300 mg qhs reached. Should be consolidated to qhs dosing once stable
• Expected range for response in adult schizophrenia is 200–800 mg/day (equivalent to 4–16 mg/day haloperidol) but higher doses may be required based on plasma levels

Half-Life
• Oral: 11.1 hrs
• IM: 11.1 hrs

Bioavailability
• Oral bioavailability by dose:

Mean (SD) Max
25 mg 8.07% (3.52) 14.7%
100 mg 18.4% (8.11) 34.2%
• IM doses are 1/3 that of usual oral doses

Adjustment for Hepatic Dysfunction (by Child-Pugh Criteria)
• Child-Pugh category A or B (mild-moderate hepatic impairment): no dosage adjustment necessary
• Child-Pugh category C (severe hepatic impairment): contraindicated

Adjustment for Renal Dysfunction
• No dosage adjustment necessary per the package insert
• However, dose reductions may be necessary in the presence of significant renal impairment

 Precautions with metabolic inducers (may require higher doses)
• Carbamazepine lowers plasma levels on average 61% (range 28–84%) [12]
• Phenobarbital lowers plasma levels 36–60% [13, 14]
• Limited data on phenytoin. Assume interaction is similar in scope to carbamazepine
• Cigarette or cannabis smoking increases clearance 38–50%

 Precautions with metabolic inhibitors (may require lower doses)
• Strong cyp 1A2 and cyp 2D6 inhibitors will increase exposure as much as 38% and 70% respectively

 Precautions with other protein-bound drugs
• May increase exposure to warfarin and digoxin

2.01 Chlorpromazine (Continued)

- Chlorpromazine has lower rates of acute adverse neurological effects than other FGAs, and its sedative effects may prove useful at times.

- Disadvantages of chlorpromazine include higher rates of orthostasis than most antipsychotics, significant weight gain, anticholinergic and sedative effects.

References

1. Meyer, J. M. (2018). Pharmacotherapy of psychosis and mania. In Brunton, L. L., Hilal-Dandan, R. and Knollmann, B. C. (eds.). *Goodman & Gilman's The Pharmacological Basis of Therapeutics*, 13th ed. Chicago, IL: McGraw-Hill, pp. 279–302.
2. Dahl, S. G. (1986). Plasma level monitoring of antipsychotic drugs. Clinical utility. *Clin Pharmacokinet*, 11, 36–61.
3. Van Putten, T., Marder, S. R., Wirshing, W. C., et al. (1991). Neuroleptic plasma levels. *Schizophr Bull*, 17, 197–216.
4. Yeung, P. K., Hubbard, J. W., Korchinski, E. D., et al. (1993). Pharmacokinetics of chlorpromazine and key metabolites. *Eur J Clin Pharmacol*, 45, 563–569.
5. Otagiri, M., Maruyama, T., Imai, T., et al. (1987). A comparative study of the interaction of warfarin with human alpha 1-acid glycoprotein and human albumin. *J Pharm Pharmacol*, 39, 416–420.
6. Castaneda-Hernandez, G., Bravo, G., Godfraind, T. (1991). Chlorpromazine treatment increases circulating digoxin like immunoreactivity in the rat. *Proc West Pharmacol Soc*, 34, 501–503.
7. Chetty, M., Miller, R., Moodley, S. V. (1994). Smoking and body weight influence the clearance of chlorpromazine. *Eur J Clin Pharmacol*, 46, 523–526.
8. Yoshii, K., Kobayashi, K., Tsumuji, M., et al. (2000). Identification of human cytochrome P450 isoforms involved in the 7-hydroxylation of chlorpromazine by human liver microsomes. *Life Sci*, 67, 175–184.
9. Sunwoo, Y., Ryu, J., Jung, C., et al. (2004). Disposition of chlorpromazine in Korean healthy subjects with CYP2D6*10B mutation. *Clin Pharmacol Ther*, 75, P90.
10. Gardiner, S. J., Begg, E. J. (2006). Pharmacogenetics, drug-metabolizing enzymes, and clinical practice. *Pharmacol Rev*, 58, 521–590.
11. Wojcikowski, J., Boksa, J., Daniel, W. A. (2010). Main contribution of the cytochrome P450 isoenzyme 1A2 (CYP1A2) to N-demethylation and 5-sulfoxidation of the phenothiazine neuroleptic chlorpromazine in human liver – a comparison with other phenothiazines. *Biochem Pharmacol*, 80, 1252–1259.
12. Raitasuo, V., Lehtovaara, R., Huttunen, M. O. (1994). Effect of switching carbamazepine to oxcarbazepine on the plasma levels of neuroleptics. A case report. *Psychopharmacology (Berl)*, 116, 115–116.
13. Curry, S. H., Davis, J. M., Janowsky, D. S., et al. (1970). Factors affecting chlorpromazine plasma levels in psychiatric patients. *Arch Gen Psychiatry*, 22, 209–215.
14. Loga, S., Curry, S., Lader, M. (1975). Interactions of orphenadrine and phenobarbitone with chlorpromazine: plasma concentrations and effects in man. *Br J Clin Pharmacol*, 2, 197–208.

2.02 Fluphenazine

A. BASIC INFORMATION [1]

Principle Trade Names
- Prolixin®
- Prolixin Decanoate®

Legal Status
- Prescription only
- Not controlled

Classifications
- Monoamine antagonist
- Typical or first-generation antipsychotic (FGA)

Generics Available
- Yes

Formulations
- Tablets: 1 mg; 2.5 mg; 5 mg; 10 mg
- Oral elixir or concentrate: 2.5 mg/5 ml, 5 mg/5 ml
- Injectable: 2.5 mg/ml
- Long-acting injectable (LAI): 25 mg/ml

FDA Indications
- Psychotic disorders

Other Data-Supported Indications
- Agitation/aggression (severe, acute) associated with psychiatric disorders (e.g. bipolar disorder, schizophrenia), delirium, substance intoxication

Dopamine
- Antagonism at D_2 receptors may decrease positive psychotic symptoms, contribute to antimanic effects and decrease aggression

C. PLASMA CONCENTRATIONS AND TREATMENT RESPONSE [2, 3]

Initial Target Range
• Optimal initial target range is 0.8–2.0 ng/ml

Range for Treatment Resistance
• May consider levels up to 4.0 ng/ml if tolerated

Typical Time to Response
• In responders to a given dose, some therapeutic improvement can be seen in two weeks

Time-Course of Improvement
• If no response after two weeks of a given dose, verify adherence and plasma level. Consider dose increase if no EPS and plasma level is < 0.8 ng/ml
• If no response after four weeks at maximum tolerated plasma concentration, withdraw treatment

D. TYPICAL TREATMENT RESPONSE [1]

Usual Target Symptoms
• Psychosis – positive symptoms
• Mania
• Violence and aggression

Common Short-Term Adverse Effects
• Parkinsonism
• Akathisia
• Acute or subacute dystonic reaction

Rare Adverse Effects
• Prolonged QTc interval
• Seizure
• Neuroleptic malignant syndrome
• Increased risk of death or cerebrovascular events in elderly patients with dementia-related psychosis
• Hyperprolactinemia

Long-Term Effects
• Tardive dyskinesia

E. PRE-TREATMENT WORKUP AND INITIAL LABORATORY TESTING [1]

History
• Obtain personal and family histories of diabetes, obesity, dyslipidemia

Physical
• General physical examination
• Vital signs and weight (for BMI)

Neurological
• AIMS
• Neurology consultation if personal history of active, poorly controlled seizure disorder

Blood Tests
• Within 90 days: liver function tests, fasting glucose and/or Hgb A1C lipid panel
• Metabolic monitoring every six months

Cardiac Tests
• None required

Urine Tests
• None required

Pregnancy Test
• Pregnancy test (premenopausal females)
• Classified as risk not ruled out

Metabolic Syndrome Parameters
• Elevated waist circumference:
  ○ Men – greater than 40 inches (102 cm)
  ○ Women – greater than 35 inches (88 cm)
• Elevated triglycerides: equal to or greater than 150 mg/dl (1.7 mmol/l)
• Reduced HDL ("good") cholesterol:
  ○ Men – less than 40 mg/dl (1.03 mmol/l)
  ○ Women – less than 50 mg/dl (1.29 mmol/l)
• Elevated blood pressure: ≥130/80 mm Hg or use of medication for hypertension
• Elevated fasting glucose: equal to or greater than 100 mg/dl (5.6 mmol/l) or use of medication for hyperglycemia

F. MONITORING

Monthly
• Weight/BMI (or at each outpatient visit)

Semi-Annually (twice per year)
• Hgb A1C or fasting glucose
• Fasting lipid panel

• With LAI fluphenazine, a plasma level every three months during the first six months is helpful until steady state is reached

Annually
• AIMS
• Plasma fluphenazine level
• Prolactin if complaining of related adverse effects

Initial Dosing
Oral Equivalence with Other FGAs

Haloperidol	2 mg
Fluphenazine	2 mg
Thiothixene	5 mg
Trifluoperazine	5 mg
Perphenazine	8–10 mg
Loxapine	12.5 mg
Chlorpromazine	100 mg

• Initial oral doses for adult psychosis/agitation 2.5–10 mg/day
• Initial IM doses must be 1/3 that of oral doses
• LAI: the T_{Max} for fluphenazine decanoate is 20–24 hours, and a 25 mg injection will yield a peak level of 1.2 ng/ml with a rapid decline over 72 hours [4]. Three-weekly loading injections of 50 mg will yield a plasma level of 1.09 ng/ml 17.5 days after the first injection [5]

Titration
• Based on tolerance of dopamine blockade and absence of EPS, may proceed by 5 mg every 2–7 days until 10–30 mg qhs reached if necessary
• Expected range for response in adult schizophrenia is 2.5–15 mg qhs (equivalent to 2.5–15 mg qhs haloperidol) but higher doses may be needed based on plasma levels

• LAI: maintenance doses of 25 mg every two weeks should result in a mean stable plasma level of 1.2 ng/ml [7]. The maximum injection volume is 3 ml, so doses >75 mg must be divided (e.g. a dose of 100 mg every two weeks should be given as 50 mg weekly). Doses can be increased every four weeks as needed to control positive psychotic symptoms

Half-Life
• Oral: 13 hours
• LAI: 14 days (chronic dosing)

Bioavailability
• Oral bioavailability low (3% in some studies)
• Acute IM bioavailability is 100%, so doses are 1/3 of usual oral doses

Adjustment for Hepatic Dysfunction (by Child-Pugh Criteria)
• Not studied. Use plasma levels to guide treatment, with extreme caution when treating Child-Pugh C patients

Adjustment for Renal Dysfunction
• Dose reductions may be necessary in the presence of significant renal impairment. Use plasma levels to guide treatment

H. MEDICATIONS TO AVOID IN COMBINATION/WARNINGS [9–11]

Precautions with metabolic inducers (may require higher doses)

- Carbamazepine lowers plasma levels on average 49%
- Cigarette smoking increases clearance 62%

Precautions with metabolic inhibitors (may require lower doses)

- Strong cyp 2D6 inhibitors will increase exposure 65%. Impact of strong 1A2 inhibitors not studied – recommend rechecking plasma fluphenazine levels if on the inhibitor for more than 14 days

Precautions with other protein-bound drugs

- None known

ART OF PSYCHOPHARMACOLOGY: TAKE-HOME PEARLS

- Fluphenazine has significantly less risk for orthostasis, anticholinergic effects and sedation than lower potency FGAs and provides potent dopamine D_2 antagonism.
- Fluphenazine has low risk for metabolic adverse effects.
- There are also oral concentrate, acute intramuscular and long-acting injectable formulations.
- Fluphenazine has markedly higher rates of adverse neurological effects than low potency FGAs and SGAs.

References

1. Meyer, J. M. (2018). Pharmacotherapy of psychosis and mania. In Brunton, L. L., Hilal-Dandan, R. and Knollmann, B. C. (eds.). *Goodman & Gilman's The Pharmacological Basis of Therapeutics*, 13th ed. Chicago, IL: McGraw-Hill, pp. 279–302.
2. Midha, K. K., Hubbard, J. W., Marder, S. R., et al. (1994). Impact of clinical pharmacokinetics on neuroleptic therapy in patients with schizophrenia. *J Psychiatry Neurosci*, 19, 254–264.
3. Meyer, J. M. (2014). A rational approach to employing high plasma levels of antipsychotics for violence associated with schizophrenia: case vignettes. *CNS Spectr*, 19, 432–438.
4. Ereshefsky, L., Saklad, S. R., Jann, M. W., et al. (1984). Future of depot neuroleptic therapy: pharmacokinetic and pharmacodynamic approaches. *J Clin Psychiatry*, 45, 50–59.
5. Jann, M. W., Ereshefsky, L., Saklad, S. R. (1985). Clinical pharmacokinetics of the depot antipsychotics. *Clin Pharmacokinet*, 10, 315–333.
6. Midha, K. K., Hawes, E. M., Hubbard, J. W., et al. (1988). Variation in the single dose pharmacokinetics of fluphenazine in psychiatric patients. *Psychopharmacology (Berl)*, 96, 206–211.
7. Marder, S. R., Midha, K. K., Van Putten, T., et al. (1991). Plasma levels of fluphenazine in patients receiving fluphenazine decanoate. Relationship to clinical response. *Br J Psychiatry*, 158, 658–665.
8. Koytchev, R., Alken, R. G., McKay, G., et al. (1996). Absolute bioavailability of oral immediate and slow release fluphenazine in healthy volunteers. *Eur J Clin Pharmacol*, 51, 183–187.
9. Ereshefsky, L., Jann, M. W., Saklad, S. R., et al. (1985). Effects of smoking on fluphenazine clearance in psychiatric inpatients. *Biol Psychiatry*, 20, 329–332.
10. Jann, M. W., Fidone, G. S., Hernandez, J. M., et al. (1989). Clinical implications of increased antipsychotic plasma concentrations upon anticonvulsant cessation. *Psychiatry Res*, 28, 153–159.
11. Goff, D. C., Midha, K. K., Sarid-Segal, O., et al. (1995). A placebo-controlled trial of fluoxetine added to neuroleptic in patients with schizophrenia. *Psychopharmacology (Berl)*, 117, 417–423.

2.03 Haloperidol

A. BASIC INFORMATION [1]

Principle Trade Names
- Haldol®
- Haldol Decanoate®

Legal Status
- Prescription only
- Not controlled

Classifications
- Monoamine antagonist
- Typical or first-generation antipsychotic (FGA)

Generics Available
- Yes

Formulations
- Tablets: 0.5 mg; 1 mg; 2 mg; 5 mg; 10 mg; 20 mg
- Oral concentrate (haloperidol lactate): 2 mg/5 ml
- Injectable: 5 mg/ml
- Long-acting injectable (LAI): 50 mg/ml; 100 mg/ml

FDA Indications
- Psychotic disorders
- Control of tics and vocal utterances of Tourette's Disorder in children and adults

Other Data-Supported Indications
- Agitation/aggression (severe, acute) associated with psychiatric disorders (e.g. bipolar disorder, schizophrenia), delirium, substance intoxication

Dopamine
- Antagonism at D_2 receptors may decrease positive psychotic symptoms, contribute to antimanic effects and decrease aggression

Initial Target Range
- Optimal initial target range is 2.0–12.0 ng/ml

Range for Treatment Resistance
- May consider levels up to 18 ng/ml if tolerated

Typical Time to Response
- In responders to a given dose, some therapeutic improvement can be seen in two weeks

Time-Course of Improvement
- If no response after two weeks of a given dose, verify adherence and plasma level. Consider dose increase if no EPS and plasma level is <2.0 ng/ml
- If no response after four weeks at maximum tolerated plasma concentration, withdraw treatment

Usual Target Symptoms
- Psychosis – positive symptoms
- Mania
- Violence and aggression

Common Short-Term Adverse Effects
- Parkinsonism
- Akathisia
- Acute or subacute dystonic reaction

Rare Adverse Effects
- Prolonged QTc interval
- Seizure
- Neuroleptic malignant syndrome
- Increased risk of death or cerebrovascular events in elderly patients with dementia-related psychosis
- Hyperprolactinemia

Long-Term Effects
- Tardive dyskinesia

History
- Obtain personal and family histories of diabetes, obesity, dyslipidemia

Physical
- General physical examination
- Vital signs and weight (for BMI)

Neurological
- AIMS
- Neurology consultation if personal history of active, poorly controlled seizure disorder

Blood Tests
- Within 90 days: liver function tests, fasting glucose and/or Hgb A1C lipid panel
- Metabolic monitoring every six months

Cardiac Tests
- None required, but may be considered in those with a history of cardiovascular disorders or on multiple agents that prolong the QT interval

Urine Tests
- None required

Pregnancy Test
- Pregnancy test (premenopausal females)
- Classified as risk not ruled out

Metabolic Syndrome Parameters
- Elevated waist circumference:
  - Men – greater than 40 inches (102 cm)
  - Women – greater than 35 inches (88 cm)
- Elevated triglycerides: equal to or greater than 150 mg/dl (1.7 mmol/l)
- Reduced HDL ("good") cholesterol:
  - Men – less than 40 mg/dl (1.03 mmol/l)
  - Women – less than 50 mg/dl (1.29 mmol/l)
- Elevated blood pressure: ≥130/80 mm Hg or use of medication for hypertension
- Elevated fasting glucose: equal to or greater than 100 mg/dl (5.6 mmol/l) or use of medication for hyperglycemia

Monthly
• Weight/BMI (or at each outpatient visit)

Semi-Annually (twice per year)
• Hgb A1C or fasting glucose
• Fasting lipid panel
• If on LAI haloperidol, a plasma level every three months during the first six months is helpful until steady state is reached

Annually
• AIMS
• Plasma haloperidol level
• Prolactin if complaining of related adverse effects

Initial Dosing
Oral Equivalence with Other FGAs

Haloperidol	2 mg
Fluphenazine	2 mg
Thiothixene	5 mg
Trifluoperazine	5 mg
Perphenazine	8–10 mg
Loxapine	12.5 mg
Chlorpromazine	100 mg

• Initial oral doses for adult psychosis/agitation 2.5–10 mg/day
• Initial IM doses must be 60% of oral doses
• LAI: the T_{Max} for haloperidol decanoate is 5–7 days. Three-weekly loading injections of 100 mg will yield a plasma level equivalent of 10 mg qhs of oral haloperidol [7]. Monthly maintenance dose will be two times the loading dose and should commence two weeks after the third loading injection [7]

Titration
• Based on tolerance of dopamine blockade and absence of EPS, may proceed by 5 mg every 2–7 days until 10–30 mg qhs reached if necessary
• Expected range for response in adult schizophrenia is 2.5–15 mg qhs (equivalent to 2.5–15 mg qhs fluphenazine) but higher doses may be needed based on plasma levels

• LAI: monthly maintenance dose is 20 times the oral dose. The maximum injection volume is 3 ml, so doses > 300 mg/month must be divided and half of the monthly dose administered every two weeks. Doses can be increased every four weeks as needed to control positive psychotic symptoms

Half-Life
• Oral: 24 hours (half-life prolonged in cyp 2D6 poor or slow metabolizers)
• LAI: 21 days (chronic dosing)

Bioavailability
• Oral bioavailability 60%
• Acute IM bioavailability is 100%, so doses are 60% of usual oral doses

Adjustment for Hepatic Dysfunction (by Child-Pugh Criteria)
• Not studied. Use plasma levels to guide treatment, with extreme caution when treating Child-Pugh C patients

Adjustment for Renal Dysfunction
• Not studied. Use plasma levels to guide treatment

Precautions with metabolic inducers (may require higher doses)

- Carbamazepine, phenobarbital or phenytoin decrease mean plasma levels by 40–72%
- Rifampin decreased plasma haloperidol levels by a mean of 70% [10]

Precautions with metabolic inhibitors (may require lower doses)

- Strong cyp 2D6 inhibitors will increase exposure approximately 25–50% [9]

- Individuals with only one functional 2D6 gene experience two-fold greater trough serum levels, those with no functioning alleles three- to four-fold higher [11, 12]
- Strong cyp 1A2 inhibitors increase exposure on average 62.5% (range 48–79%) [9]

Precautions with other protein-bound drugs

- None known

- Haloperidol has significantly less risk for orthostasis, anticholinergic effects and sedation than lower potency FGAs and provides potent dopamine D_2 antagonism.
- Haloperidol has low risk for metabolic adverse effects.
- There are also oral concentrate, acute IM and LAI formulations.
- Haloperidol has markedly higher rates of neurological adverse effects than low potency FGAs and SGAs.

References

1. Meyer, J. M. (2018). Pharmacotherapy of psychosis and mania. In Brunton, L. L., Hilal-Dandan, R. and Knollmann, B. C. (eds.). *Goodman & Gilman's The Pharmacological Basis of Therapeutics*, 13th ed. Chicago, IL: McGraw-Hill, pp. 279–302.
2. Van Putten, T., Marder, S. R., Wirshing, W. C., et al. (1991). Neuroleptic plasma levels. *Schizophr Bull*, 17, 197–216.
3. Wei, F. C., Jann, M. W., Lin, H. N., et al. (1996). A practical loading dose method for converting schizophrenic patients from oral to depot haloperidol therapy. *J Clin Psychiatry*, 57, 298–302.
4. Kapur, S., Zipursky, R., Roy, P., et al. (1997). The relationship between D2 receptor occupancy and plasma levels on low dose oral haloperidol: a PET study. *Psychopharmacology (Berl)*, 131, 148–152.
5. Meyer, J. M. (2014). A rational approach to employing high plasma levels of antipsychotics for violence associated with schizophrenia: case vignettes. *CNS Spectr*, 19, 432–438.
6. Chang, W. H., Juang, D. J., Lin, S. K., et al. (1995). Disposition of haloperidol and reduced haloperidol plasma levels after single dose haloperidol decanoate administration. *Human Psychopharmacol*, 10, 47–51.
7. Wei, F. C., Jann, M. W., Lin, H. N., et al. (1996). A practical loading dose method for converting schizophrenic patients from oral to depot haloperidol therapy. *J Clin Psychiatry*, 57, 298–302.
8. Meyer, J. M. (2019). Monitoring and improving antipsychotic adherence in outpatient forensic diversion programs. *CNS Spectr*, doi: 10.1017/S1092852919000865
9. Kudo, S., Ishizaki, T. (1999). Pharmacokinetics of haloperidol: an update. *Clin Pharmacokinet*, 37, 435–456.
10. Mylan Institutional LLC (2019). *Haloperidol Package Insert*. Rockford, Illinois.
11. Suzuki, A., Otani, K., Mihara, K., et al. (1997). Effects of the CYP2D6 genotype on the steady-state plasma concentrations of haloperidol and reduced haloperidol in Japanese schizophrenic patients. *Pharmacogenetics*, 7, 415–418.
12. Panagiotidis, G., Arthur, H. W., Lindh, J. D., et al. (2007). Depot haloperidol treatment in outpatients with schizophrenia on monotherapy: impact of CYP2D6 polymorphism on pharmacokinetics and treatment outcome. *Ther Drug Monit*, 29, 417–422.

2.04 Loxapine

A. BASIC INFORMATION [1]

Principle Trade Names
- Loxitane®
- Adasuve®

Legal Status
- Prescription only
- Not controlled

Classifications
- Monoamine antagonist
- Typical or first-generation antipsychotic (FGA)

Generics Available
- Yes

Formulations
- Tablets or capsules: 5 mg; 10 mg; 25 mg; 50 mg
- Inhalation powder: 10 mg in a single-use inhaler

FDA Indications
- Schizophrenia
- Acute treatment of agitation associated with schizophrenia or bipolar I disorder in adults (inhaled form)

Other Data-Supported Indications
- Agitation/aggression (severe, acute) associated with psychiatric disorders (e.g. bipolar disorder, schizophrenia), delirium, substance intoxication

Dopamine
- Antagonism at D_2 receptors may decrease positive psychotic symptoms, contribute to antimanic effects and decrease aggression

C. PLASMA CONCENTRATIONS AND TREATMENT RESPONSE [2–4]

Initial Target Range
• Optimal initial target range is 3.0–7.5 ng/ml

Range for Treatment Resistance
• May consider levels up to 18 ng/ml if tolerated

Typical Time to Response
• In responders to a given dose, some therapeutic improvement can be seen in two weeks

Time-Course of Improvement
• If no response after two weeks of a given dose, verify adherence and plasma level. Consider dose increase if no EPS and plasma level is <3.0 ng/ml
• If no response after four weeks at maximum tolerated plasma concentration, withdraw treatment

D. TYPICAL TREATMENT RESPONSE [1]

Usual Target Symptoms
• Psychosis – positive symptoms
• Mania
• Violence and aggression

Common Short-Term Adverse Effects
• Parkinsonism
• Akathisia
• Acute or subacute dystonic reaction

Rare Adverse Effects
• Seizure
• Neuroleptic malignant syndrome
• Increased risk of death or cerebrovascular events in elderly patients with dementia-related psychosis
• Hyperprolactinemia

Long-Term Effects
• Tardive dyskinesia

E. PRE-TREATMENT WORKUP AND INITIAL LABORATORY TESTING [1]

History
• Obtain personal and family histories of diabetes, obesity, dyslipidemia

Physical
• General physical examination
• Vital signs and weight (for BMI)

Neurological
• AIMS
• Neurology consultation if personal history of active, poorly controlled seizure disorder

Blood Tests
• Within 90 days: liver function tests, fasting glucose and/or Hgb A1C lipid panel
• Metabolic monitoring every six months

Cardiac Tests
• None required, but may be considered in those with a history of cardiovascular disorders or on multiple agents that prolong the QT interval

Urine Tests
• None required

Pregnancy Test
• Pregnancy test (premenopausal females)
• Classified as risk not ruled out

Metabolic Syndrome Parameters
• Elevated waist circumference:
  ◦ Men – greater than 40 inches (102 cm)
  ◦ Women – greater than 35 inches (88 cm)
• Elevated triglycerides: equal to or greater than 150 mg/dl (1.7 mmol/l)
• Reduced HDL ("good") cholesterol:
  ◦ Men – less than 40 mg/dl (1.03 mmol/l)
  ◦ Women – less than 50 mg/dl (1.29 mmol/l)
• Elevated blood pressure: ≥130/80 mm Hg or use of medication for hypertension
• Elevated fasting glucose: equal to or greater than 100 mg/dl (5.6 mmol/l) or use of medication for hyperglycemia

Monthly
• Weight/BMI (or at each outpatient visit)

Semi-Annually (twice per year)
• Hgb A1C or fasting glucose
• Fasting lipid panel

Annually
• AIMS
• Plasma loxapine level
• Prolactin if complaining of related adverse effects

Initial Dosing
Oral Equivalence with Other FGAs

Haloperidol	2 mg
Fluphenazine	2 mg
Thiothixene	5 mg
Trifluoperazine	5 mg
Perphenazine	8–10 mg
Loxapine	12.5 mg
Chlorpromazine	100 mg

• Initial oral doses for adult psychosis/ agitation 20–50 mg/day
• For acute agitation, inhalation dose is 10 mg per 24-hour period

Titration
• Based on tolerance of dopamine blockade and absence of EPS, may proceed by 25 mg every 2–7 days until 60–100 mg qhs reached if necessary
• Expected range for response in adult schizophrenia is 25–100 mg qhs (equivalent to 4–16 mg qhs haloperidol) but higher doses may be needed based on plasma levels. Maximum recommended dose is 250 mg qhs

Half-Life
• Oral: 4–7 hours (active metabolites have longer half-lives)
• Inhaled: 7.6 hours

Bioavailability
• Oral bioavailability 33%
• Inhaled bioavailability 100%

Adjustment for Hepatic Dysfunction (by Child-Pugh Criteria)
• Not studied. Use plasma levels to guide treatment, with extreme caution when treating Child-Pugh C patients

Adjustment for Renal Dysfunction
• Not studied. Use plasma levels to guide treatment

 Precautions with metabolic inducers (may require higher doses)
• No impact of smoking, but no data on use with inducers of other cyp enzymes. Consider monitoring of plasma levels, but due to multiple cyp isoforms involved, likelihood of clinically significant kinetic interactions is minimal

 Precautions with metabolic inhibitors (may require lower doses)
• Multiple cyp isoforms are involved in loxapine metabolism, so likelihood of clinically significant kinetic interactions is minimal

 Precautions with other protein-bound drugs
• None known

2.04 Loxapine (Continued)

- Loxapine has significantly less risk for orthostasis, anticholinergic effects and sedation than lower potency FGAs and provides potent dopamine D_2 antagonism.
- Loxapine has low risk for metabolic adverse effects.

- There is also an inhaled formulation for acute agitation.
- Loxapine has lower rates of acute neurological adverse effects than higher potency FGAs, but it is an FGA with neurological adverse effects rates that are higher than SGAs.

References

1. Meyer, J. M. (2018). Pharmacotherapy of psychosis and mania. In Brunton, L. L., Hilal-Dandan, R. and Knollmann, B. C. (eds.). *Goodman & Gilman's The Pharmacological Basis of Therapeutics*, 13th ed. Chicago, IL: McGraw-Hill, pp. 279–302.
2. Simpson, G. M., Cooper, T. B., Lee, J. H., et al. (1978). Clinical and plasma level characteristics of intramuscular and oral loxapine. *Psychopharmacology (Berl)*, 56, 225–232.
3. Kapur, S., Zipursky, R. B., Jones, C., et al. (1996). The D_2 receptor occupancy profile of loxapine determined using PET. *Neuropsychopharmacol*, 15, 562–566.
4. Kapur, S., Zipursky, R., Remington, G., et al. (1997). PET evidence that loxapine is an equipotent blocker of 5-HT2 and D_2 receptors: implications for the therapeutics of schizophrenia. *Am J Psychiatry*, 154, 1525–1529.
5. Alexza Pharmaceuticals Inc. (2011). Adasuve (loxapine) inhalation powder NDA 022549 – Psychopharmacologic Drug Advisory Committee briefing document, December 12, 2011. Food and Drug Administration.
6. Luo, J. P., Vashishtha, S. C., Hawes, E. M., et al. (2011). In vitro identification of the human cytochrome p450 enzymes involved in the oxidative metabolism of loxapine. *Biopharm Drug Dispos*, 32, 398–407.
7. Galen US Inc. (2019). *Adasuve Package Insert*. Souderton, Pennsylvania.

A. BASIC INFORMATION [1]

Principle Trade Names
• Trilafon®

Legal Status
• Prescription only
• Not controlled

Classifications
• Monoamine antagonist
• Typical or first-generation antipsychotic (FGA)

Generics Available
• Yes

Formulations
• Tablets: 2 mg; 4 mg; 8 mg; 16 mg

• A combination of low-dose amitriptyline and perphenazine is available, but has no use in modern psychiatry
• Long-acting injectable (LAI): perphenazine enanthate or decanoate – not available in the US, limited availability in the EU

FDA Indications
• Schizophrenia
• Emesis

Other Data-Supported Indications
• Agitation/aggression (severe, acute) associated with psychiatric disorders (e.g. bipolar disorder, schizophrenia), delirium, substance intoxication

Dopamine
• Antagonism at D_2 receptors may decrease positive psychotic symptoms, contribute to antimanic effects and decrease aggression. It also provides antiemetic effects

C. PLASMA CONCENTRATIONS AND TREATMENT RESPONSE [2, 3]

Initial Target Range
- Optimal initial target range is 0.81–2.4 ng/ml

Range for Treatment Resistance
- May consider levels up to 5.0 ng/ml if tolerated

Typical Time to Response
- In responders to a given dose, some therapeutic improvement can be seen in two weeks

Time-Course of Improvement
- If no response after two weeks of a given dose, verify adherence and plasma level. Consider dose increase if no adverse neurological effects and plasma level is <0.81 ng/ml
- If no response after four weeks at maximum tolerated plasma concentration, withdraw treatment

D. TYPICAL TREATMENT RESPONSE [1]

Usual Target Symptoms
- Psychosis – positive symptoms
- Mania
- Violence and aggression

Common Short-Term Adverse Effects
- Parkinsonism
- Akathisia
- Acute or subacute dystonic reaction

Rare Adverse Effects
- Seizure
- Neuroleptic malignant syndrome
- Increased risk of death or cerebrovascular events in elderly patients with dementia-related psychosis
- Hyperprolactinemia

Long-Term Effects
- Tardive dyskinesia

E. PRE-TREATMENT WORKUP AND INITIAL LABORATORY TESTING [1]

History
- Obtain personal and family histories of diabetes, obesity, dyslipidemia

Physical
- General physical examination
- Vital signs and weight (for BMI)

Neurological
- AIMS
- Neurology consultation if personal history of active, poorly controlled seizure disorder

Blood Tests
- Within 90 days: liver function tests, fasting glucose and/or Hgb A1C lipid panel
- Metabolic monitoring every six months

Cardiac Tests
- None required, but may be considered in those with a history of cardiovascular disorders or on multiple agents that prolong the QT interval

Urine Tests
- None required

Pregnancy Test
- Pregnancy test (premenopausal females)
- Classified as risk not ruled out

Metabolic Syndrome Parameters
- Elevated waist circumference:
  - Men – greater than 40 inches (102 cm)
  - Women – greater than 35 inches (88 cm)
- Elevated triglycerides: equal to or greater than 150 mg/dl (1.7 mmol/l)
- Reduced HDL ("good") cholesterol:
  - Men – less than 40 mg/dl (1.03 mmol/l)
  - Women – less than 50 mg/dl (1.29 mmol/l)
- Elevated blood pressure: ≥130/80 mm Hg or use of medication for hypertension
- Elevated fasting glucose: equal to or greater than 100 mg/dl (5.6 mmol/l) or use of medication for hyperglycemia

F. MONITORING

Monthly
• Weight/BMI (or at each outpatient visit)

Semi-Annually (twice per year)
• Hgb A1C or fasting glucose
• Fasting lipid panel

Annually
• AIMS
• Plasma perphenazine level
• Prolactin if complaining of related adverse effects

Initial Dosing
Oral Equivalence with Other FGAs

Haloperidol   2 mg
Fluphenazine   2 mg
Thiothixene   5 mg
Trifluoperazine   5 mg
Perphenazine   8–10 mg
Loxapine   12.5 mg
Chlorpromazine   100 mg

• Initial oral doses for adult psychosis/agitation 20–50 mg/day
• For acute agitation, inhalation dose is 10 mg per 24-hour period

Titration
• Based on tolerance of dopamine blockade and absence of adverse neurological effects, may proceed by 8–16 mg every 2–7 days until 16–32 mg qhs reached if necessary
• Expected range for response in adult schizophrenia is 16–48 mg qhs (equivalent to 4–12 mg qhs haloperidol) but higher doses may be needed based on plasma levels. Maximum recommended dose is 64 mg qhs

Half-Life
• Oral: 9–12 hours

Bioavailability
• Oral bioavailability 60%

Adjustment for Hepatic Dysfunction (by Child-Pugh Criteria)
• Not studied. Use plasma levels to guide treatment, with extreme caution when treating Child-Pugh C patients

Adjustment for Renal Dysfunction
• Not studied. Use plasma levels to guide treatment

H. MEDICATIONS TO AVOID IN COMBINATION/WARNINGS [4]

 Precautions with metabolic inducers (may require higher doses)
• Poorly documented in the literature. Suggest plasma level monitoring with use of strong inducers for more than 14 days (e.g. phenytoin, carbamazepine, rifampin)

 Precautions with metabolic inhibitors (may require lower doses)
• Strong 2D6 inhibitors will increase perphenazine levels two-fold to 13-fold. Plasma levels must be monitored and doses decreased by at least 50% initially

 Precautions with other protein-bound drugs
• None known

ART OF PSYCHOPHARMACOLOGY: TAKE-HOME PEARLS

- Perphenazine has significantly less risk for orthostasis, anticholinergic effects and sedation than lower potency FGAs and provides potent dopamine D_2 antagonism.

- Perphenazine has low risk for metabolic adverse effects.
- Perphenazine has lower rates of acute adverse neurological effects than higher potency FGAs, but it is an FGA with adverse neurological effect rates higher than SGAs.

References

1. Meyer, J. M. (2018). Pharmacotherapy of psychosis and mania. In Brunton, L. L., Hilal-Dandan, R. and Knollmann, B. C. (eds.). *Goodman & Gilman's The Pharmacological Basis of Therapeutics*, 13th ed. Chicago, IL: McGraw-Hill, pp. 279–302.
2. Van Putten, T., Marder, S. R., Wirshing, W. C., et al. (1991). Neuroleptic plasma levels. *Schizophr Bull*, 17, 197–216.
3. Patteet, L., Morrens, M., Maudens, K. E., et al. (2012). Therapeutic drug monitoring of common antipsychotics. *Ther Drug Monit*, 34, 629–651.
4. Ozdemir, V., Naranjo, C. A., Herrmann, N., et al. (1997). Paroxetine potentiates the central nervous system side effects of perphenazine: contribution of cytochrome P4502D6 inhibition in vivo. *Clin Pharmacol Ther*, 62, 334–347.

A. BASIC INFORMATION [1]

Principle Trade Names
• Navane®

Legal Status
• Prescription only
• Not controlled

Classifications
• Monoamine antagonist
• Typical or first-generation antipsychotic (FGA)

Generics Available
• Yes

Formulations
• Capsules: 1 mg; 2 mg; 5 mg; 10 mg

FDA Indications
• Schizophrenia

Other Data-Supported Indications
• Agitation/aggression (severe, acute) associated with psychiatric disorders (e.g. bipolar disorder, schizophrenia), delirium, substance intoxication

Dopamine
• Antagonism at D_2 receptors may decrease positive psychotic symptoms, contribute to antimanic effects and decrease aggression. It also provides antiemetic effects

Initial Target Range
• Optimal initial target range is 1.0–10.0 ng/ml

Range for Treatment Resistance
• May consider levels up to 12 ng/ml if tolerated

Typical Time to Response
• In responders to a given dose, some therapeutic improvement can be seen in two weeks

Time-Course of Improvement
• If no response after two weeks of a given dose, verify adherence and plasma level. Consider dose increase if no adverse neurological effects and plasma level is <1.0 ng/ml
• If no response after four weeks at maximum tolerated plasma concentration, withdraw treatment

Usual Target Symptoms
• Psychosis – positive symptoms
• Mania
• Violence and aggression

Common Short-Term Adverse Effects
• Parkinsonism
• Akathisia
• Acute or subacute dystonic reaction

Rare Adverse Effects
• Seizure
• Neuroleptic malignant syndrome
• Increased risk of death or cerebrovascular events in elderly patients with dementia-related psychosis
• Hyperprolactinemia

Long-Term Effects
• Tardive dyskinesia

History
• Obtain personal and family histories of diabetes, obesity, dyslipidemia

Physical
• General physical examination
• Vital signs and weight (for BMI)

Neurological
• AIMS
• Neurology consultation if personal history of active, poorly controlled seizure disorder

Blood Tests
• Within 90 days: liver function tests, fasting glucose and/or Hgb A1C lipid panel
• Metabolic monitoring every six months

Cardiac Tests
• None required, but may be considered in those with a history of cardiovascular disorders or on multiple agents that prolong the QT interval

Urine Tests
• None required

Pregnancy Test
• Pregnancy test (premenopausal females)
• Classified as risk not ruled out

Metabolic Syndrome Parameters
• Elevated waist circumference:
  ○ Men – greater than 40 inches (102 cm)
  ○ Women – greater than 35 inches (88 cm)
• Elevated triglycerides: equal to or greater than 150 mg/dl (1.7 mmol/L)
• Reduced HDL ("good") cholesterol:
  ○ Men – less than 40 mg/dl (1.03 mmol/l)
  ○ Women – less than 50 mg/dl (1.29 mmol/l)
• Elevated blood pressure: ≥130/80 mm Hg or use of medication for hypertension
• Elevated fasting glucose: equal to or greater than 100 mg/dl (5.6 mmol/l) or use of medication for hyperglycemia

Monthly
• Weight/BMI (or at each outpatient visit)

Semi-Annually (twice per year)
• Hgb A1C or fasting glucose
• Fasting lipid panel

Annually
• AIMS
• Plasma thiothixene level
• Prolactin if complaining of related adverse effects

Initial Dosing
Oral Equivalence with Other FGAs

Haloperidol	2 mg
Fluphenazine	2 mg
Thiothixene	5 mg
Trifluoperazine	5 mg
Perphenazine	8–10 mg
Loxapine	12.5 mg
Chlorpromazine	100 mg

• Initial oral doses for adult psychosis/ agitation 10–20 mg/day

Titration
• Based on tolerance of dopamine blockade and absence of adverse neurological effects, may proceed by 5 mg every 2–7 days until 15–20 mg qhs reached if necessary
• Expected range for response in adult schizophrenia is 20–30 mg qhs (equivalent to 8–12 mg qhs haloperidol) but higher doses may be needed based on plasma levels. Maximum recommended dose is 60 mg qhs

Half-Life
• Oral: 16.4 hours

Bioavailability
• Oral bioavailability "well absorbed"

Adjustment for Hepatic Dysfunction (by Child-Pugh Criteria)
• Not studied. Use plasma levels to guide treatment, with extreme caution when treating Child-Pugh C patients

Adjustment for Renal Dysfunction
• Not studied. Use plasma levels to guide treatment

 Precautions with metabolic inducers (may require higher doses)
• Strong inducers lower plasma levels over 70%. Suggest monitoring of plasma levels when strong inducers (e.g. phenytoin, carbamazepine, rifampin) are used for more than 14 days. Smokers require 45% higher dosages to achieve comparable plasma levels to nonsmokers

 Precautions with metabolic inhibitors (may require lower doses)
• Strong 2D6 inhibitors do not increase thiothixene levels. No data on use with strong cyp 1A2 inhibitors, but cimetidine, a weak/moderate inhibitor of cyp 1A2, 2C19, 2D6 and 3A4, was associated with > three-fold increase in plasma levels. Monitoring of plasma levels suggested when used with inhibitors of cyp 1A2 or 3A4, and possibly also 2C19 (omeprazole, esomeprazole)

 Precautions with other protein-bound drugs
• None known

2.06 Thiothixene (Continued)

- Thiothixene has significantly less risk for orthostasis, anticholinergic effects and sedation than lower potency FGAs and provides potent dopamine D_2 antagonism.
- Thiothixene has low risk for metabolic adverse effects.

- Thiothixene has lower rates of acute adverse neurological effects than higher potency FGAs, but it is an FGA with adverse neurological effect rates higher than SGAs.

References

1. Meyer, J. M. (2018). Pharmacotherapy of psychosis and mania. In Brunton, L. L., Hilal-Dandan, R. and Knollmann, B. C. (eds.). *Goodman & Gilman's The Pharmacological Basis of Therapeutics*, 13th ed. Chicago, IL: McGraw-Hill, pp. 279–302.
2. Kim, D. Y., Hollister, L. E. (1984). Drug-refractory chronic schizophrenics: doses and plasma concentrations of thiothixene. *J Clin Psychopharmacol*, 4, 32–35.
3. Mavroidis, M. L., Kanter, D. R., Hirschowitz, J., et al. (1984). Clinical relevance of thiothixene plasma levels. *J Clin Psychopharmacol*, 4, 155–157.
4. Guthrie, S. K., Hariharan, M., Kumar, A. A., et al. (1997). The effect of paroxetine on thiothixene pharmacokinetics. *J Clin Pharm Ther*, 22, 221–226.
5. Ereshefsky, L., Saklad, S. R., Watanabe, M. D., et al. (1991). Thiothixene pharmacokinetic interactions: a study of hepatic enzyme inducers, clearance inhibitors, and demographic variables. *J Clin Psychopharmacol*, 11, 296–301.

A. BASIC INFORMATION [1]

Principle Trade Names
• Stelazine®

Legal Status
• Prescription only
• Not controlled

Classifications
• Monoamine antagonist
• Typical or first-generation antipsychotic (FGA)

Generics Available
• Yes

Formulations
• Tablets: 1 mg; 2 mg; 5 mg; 10 mg

FDA Indications
• Schizophrenia
• Generalized nonpsychotic anxiety (no longer used for this purpose)

Other Data-Supported Indications
• Agitation/aggression (severe, acute) associated with psychiatric disorders (e.g. bipolar disorder, schizophrenia), delirium, substance intoxication

Dopamine
• Antagonism at D_2 receptors may decrease positive psychotic symptoms, contribute to antimanic effects and decrease aggression. It also provides antiemetic effects

Initial Target Range
- Optimal initial target range is 1.0–2.3 ng/ml

Range for Treatment Resistance
- May consider levels up to 3.5 ng/ml if tolerated

Typical Time to Response
- In responders to a given dose, some therapeutic improvement can be seen in two weeks

Time-Course of Improvement
- If no response after two weeks of a given dose, verify adherence and plasma level. Consider dose increase if no adverse neurological effects and plasma level is <1.0 ng/ml
- If no response after four weeks at maximum tolerated plasma concentration, withdraw treatment

Usual Target Symptoms
- Psychosis – positive symptoms
- Mania
- Violence and aggression

Common Short-Term Adverse Effects
- Parkinsonism
- Akathisia
- Acute or subacute dystonic reaction

Rare Adverse Effects
- Seizure
- Neuroleptic malignant syndrome
- Increased risk of death or cerebrovascular events in elderly patients with dementia-related psychosis
- Hyperprolactinemia

Long-Term Effects
- Tardive dyskinesia

History
- Obtain personal and family histories of diabetes, obesity, dyslipidemia

Physical
- General physical examination
- Vital signs and weight (for BMI)

Neurological
- AIMS
- Neurology consultation if personal history of active, poorly controlled seizure disorder

Blood Tests
- Within 90 days: liver function tests, fasting glucose and/or Hgb A1C lipid panel
- Metabolic monitoring every six months

Cardiac Tests
- None required, but may be considered in those with a history of cardiovascular disorders or on multiple agents that prolong the QT interval

Urine Tests
- None required

Pregnancy Test
- Pregnancy test (premenopausal females)
- Classified as risk not ruled out

Metabolic Syndrome Parameters
- Elevated waist circumference:
  - Men – greater than 40 inches (102 cm)
  - Women – greater than 35 inches (88 cm)
- Elevated triglycerides: equal to or greater than 150 mg/dl (1.7 mmol/l)
- Reduced HDL ("good") cholesterol:
  - Men – less than 40 mg/dl (1.03 mmol/l)
  - Women – less than 50 mg/dl (1.29 mmol/l)
- Elevated blood pressure: ≥130/80 mm Hg or use of medication for hypertension
- Elevated fasting glucose: equal to or greater than 100 mg/dl (5.6 mmol/l) or use of medication for hyperglycemia

Monthly
- Weight/BMI (or at each outpatient visit)

Semi-Annually (twice per year)
- Hgb A1C or fasting glucose
- Fasting lipid panel

Annually
- AIMS
- Plasma trifluoperazine level
- Prolactin if complaining of related adverse effects

Initial Dosing

Oral Equivalence with Other FGAs

Haloperidol	2 mg
Fluphenazine	2 mg
Thiothixene	5 mg
Trifluoperazine	5 mg
Perphenazine	8–10 mg
Loxapine	12.5 mg
Chlorpromazine	100 mg

- Initial oral doses for adult psychosis/agitation 10–20 mg/day

Titration
- Based on tolerance of dopamine blockade and absence of adverse neurological effects, may proceed by 5 mg every 2–7 days until 15–20 mg qhs reached if necessary
- Expected range for response in adult schizophrenia is 15–20 mg qhs (equivalent to 6–8 mg qhs haloperidol) but higher doses may be needed based on plasma levels. Maximum recommended dose is 40 mg qhs

Half-Life
- Oral: 12.5–15.7 hours

Bioavailability
- Oral bioavailability not determined

Adjustment for Hepatic Dysfunction (by Child-Pugh Criteria)
- Not studied. Use plasma levels to guide treatment, with extreme caution when treating Child-Pugh C patients

Adjustment for Renal Dysfunction
- Not studied. Use plasma levels to guide treatment

 Precautions with metabolic inducers (may require higher doses)
- Limited data. Use plasma levels to guide treatment when strong inducers added (carbamazepine, phenytoin, phenobarbital). No impact of smoking

 Precautions with metabolic inhibitors (may require lower doses)
- Limited data, but one case report of severe neurological side effects upon addition of paroxetine, a strong cyp 2D6 inhibitor. Use dose reduction and plasma levels to guide treatment when moderate or strong cyp 2D6 inhibitors added

 Precautions with other protein-bound drugs
- None known

ART OF PSYCHOPHARMACOLOGY: TAKE-HOME PEARLS

- Trifluoperazine has significantly less risk for orthostasis, anticholinergic effects and sedation than lower potency FGAs and provides potent dopamine D_2 antagonism.
- Trifluoperazine has low risk for metabolic adverse effects.

- Trifluoperazine has lower rates of acute adverse neurological effects than higher potency FGAs, but it is an FGA with adverse neurological effect rates higher than SGAs.

References

1. Meyer, J. M. (2018). Pharmacotherapy of psychosis and mania. In Brunton, L. L., Hilal-Dandan, R. and Knollmann, B. C. (eds.). *Goodman & Gilman's The Pharmacological Basis of Therapeutics*, 13th ed. Chicago, IL: McGraw-Hill, pp. 279–302.
2. Janicak, P. G., Javaid, J. I., Sharma, R. P., et al. (1989). Trifluoperazine plasma levels and clinical response. *J Clin Psychopharmacol*, 9, 340–346.
3. Midha, K. K., Korchinski, E. D., Verbeeck, R. K., et al. (1983). Kinetics of oral trifluoperazine disposition in man. *Br J Clin Pharmacol*, 15, 380–382.
4. Midha, K. K., Hawes, E. M., Hubbard, J. W., et al. (1988). A pharmacokinetic study of trifluoperazine in two ethnic populations. *Psychopharmacology (Berl)*, 95, 333–338.
5. Nicholson, S. D. (1992). Extra pyramidal side effects associated with paroxetine. *West Engl Med J*, 107, 90–91.

Second-Generation (Atypical) Antipsychotics
2.08 Asenapine

A. BASIC INFORMATION [1, 2]

Principle Trade Names
- Saphris®
- Secuado®

Legal Status
- Prescription only
- Not controlled

Classifications
- Monoamine antagonist
- Atypical antipsychotic
- Second-generation antipsychotic (SGA)
- Mood stabilizer

Generics Available
- No

Formulations
- Tablet, sublingual: 2.5 mg; 5 mg; 10 mg
- Patch 24-hour, transdermal: 3.8 mg/24 hours; 5.7 mg/24 hours; 7.6 mg/24 hours

FDA Indications
- Schizophrenia
- Schizoaffective disorder
- Other psychotic disorder
- Bipolar mood disorder – acute manic or mixed episodes and maintenance after achieving responder status for two weeks
- Adjunct to lithium and/or valproate

Other Data-Supported Indications
- Severe persistent assaultive behavior
- Severe persistent self-injurious behavior
- Agitation/aggression (severe, acute) associated with psychiatric disorders (e.g. bipolar disorder, schizophrenia), substance intoxication, or other organic causes
- Psychosis/agitation associated with dementia
- Behavioral disturbances in children and adolescents
- Disorders associated with problems with impulse control

Dopamine

- Antagonism at D_2 receptors may decrease positive psychotic symptoms and contribute to mood stabilization

Serotonin

- Robust antagonism at 5HT receptors (1A/B, 2A/B/C, 5–7) enhances dopamine release in the mesocortical, nigrostriatal, and tuberoinfundibular tracts and likely improves frontal lobe functioning, diminishing neurological motor symptoms, and avoiding prolactin elevation, respectively
- Antagonism at $5HT_{2C}$ and $5HT_7$ may contribute to antidepressant actions

Epinephrine/norepinephrine

- Antagonism at α_1- and α_2-adrenergic receptors causes orthostatic hypotension
- Antagonism at α_2-adrenergic receptors may contribute to antidepressant actions

C. PLASMA CONCENTRATIONS AND TREATMENT RESPONSE [2, 3, 4]

Initial Target Range

- No established plasma therapeutic range

Range for Treatment Resistance

- No established plasma therapeutic range

Typical Time to Response

- Therapeutic improvement can be seen for 1–12 weeks.

Time-Course of Improvement

- If no response by four weeks at maximum tolerated dose, taper and withdraw therapy

D. TYPICAL TREATMENT RESPONSE [2, 4, 5]

Usual Target Symptoms

- Psychosis – positive and negative symptoms
- Cognitive symptoms
- Affective symptoms
- Suicidal behavior
- Violence and aggression

Common Short-Term Adverse Effects

- Somnolence
- Nausea
- Orthostatic hypotension
- Tachycardia
- Lightheadedness or syncope
- Dyspepsia

Rare Adverse Effects

- Prolonged QTc interval
- Obtundation and/or confusion
- Seizure
- Cerebrovascular events in demented elderly
- Extrapyramidal side effects

- Neuroleptic malignant syndrome
- Hyperglycemia with ketoacidosis
- Oral hypoesthesia
- Type 1 hypersensitivity reactions (anaphylaxis, angioedema, hypotension, tachycardia, swollen tongue, difficulty breathing, wheezing, rash)
- Increased risk of death or cerebrovascular events in elderly patients with dementia-related psychosis
- Neuroleptic malignant syndrome (much reduced risk compared to conventional antipsychotics)

Long-Term Effects

- Constipation
- Dry mouth
- Akathisia
- Elevated liver enzymes
- Hyperprolactinemia
- Metabolic changes, including weight gain, hyperglycemia, dyslipidemia

History
- Obtain personal and family histories of diabetes
- Personal history of:
  - high BMI
  - dyslipidemia (elevated TGs or cholesterol)

Physical
- General physical examination
- Vital signs
- BMI
- Waist circumference

Neurological
- Check for myoclonus or myoclonic jerks
- AIMS
- Neurology consultation if personal history of active, poorly controlled seizure disorder

Blood Tests
Within 30 days:
- Complete metabolic panel
- Fasting blood sugar and/or Hgb A1c
- Lipid panel

Cardiac Tests
- ECG

Urine Tests
- Urinalysis

Pregnancy Test
- Pregnancy test (premenopausal females)
- Classified as risk not ruled out

Metabolic Syndrome Parameters
- Elevated waist circumference:
  - Men – greater than 40 inches (102 cm)
  - Women – greater than 35 inches (88 cm)
- Elevated triglycerides: equal to or greater than 150 mg/dl (1.7 mmol/l)
- Reduced HDL ("good") cholesterol:
  - Men – less than 40 mg/dl (1.03 mmol/l)
  - Women – less than 50 mg/dl (1.29 mmol/l)
- Elevated blood pressure: ≥ 130/80 mm Hg or use of medication for hypertension
- Elevated fasting glucose: equal to or greater than 100 mg/dl (5.6 mmol/l) or use of medication for hyperglycemia

Monthly
- Weight
- BMI

Semi-Annually (twice per year)
- Hgb A1c or fasting glucose
- Fasting lipid panel
- BMI
- ECG (if on other medications that may prolong QTc as per the package insert)

Annually
- ECG
- AIMS

- Waist circumference
- Hgb A1c or fasting glucose
- Nutritional consultation if
  - waist circumference increases from <35 inches to >35 inches in females OR increases from <40 inches to >40 inches in males
  - weight increases 5% in one month, 7.5% in three months, or 10% in six months
  - BMI increases from normal to overweight (<25 to >25) OR from overweight to obese (25–29.9 to 30 or higher)
- Prolactin level
- Breast exam (both males/females)

Initial Dosing
- Administer initial dose of 5–10 mg BID
- If treating manic state, initiate at 10 mg BID

Titration
- If tolerated and clinically indicated, titrate to a maximum of 20 mg daily

Half-Life
- Sublingual: ~24 hours
- Transdermal: ~30 hours

Bioavailability
- 95% protein-bound
- Sublingual: 35%
- If swallowed: <2%

- Decreased if administered with food or liquid

Adjustment for Hepatic Dysfunction (by Child-Pugh Criteria)
- Child-Pugh category A or B (mild-moderate hepatic impairment): no dosage adjustment necessary
- Child-Pugh category C (severe hepatic impairment): contraindicated

Adjustment for Renal Dysfunction
- No dosage adjustment necessary per the package insert
- However, dose reductions may be necessary in the presence of significant renal impairment

H. MEDICATIONS TO AVOID IN COMBINATION/WARNINGS [2]

 Precautions with metabolic inducers – 3A4

(may require higher doses)
- Carbamazepine
- Phenytoin
- Omeprazole
- Phenobarbital
- Rifampin
- Cigarette use

 Precautions with metabolic inhibitors – 1A2, 2D6, 3A4

(may require lower doses)
- Fluvoxamine
- Ciprofloxacin

- Cimetidine
- Paroxetine
- Fluoxetine
- High-dose caffeine

 Precautions with other protein-bound drugs
- Asenapine is 95% protein-bound and may displace other protein-bound drugs (e.g. warfarin and digoxin)

ART OF PSYCHOPHARMACOLOGY: TAKE-HOME PEARLS

- Asenapine can be used as rapid-acting PRN for agitation or transient worsening of psychosis or mania due to rapid onset of action.
- A limitation is that asenapine does not result in full remission of psychotic symptoms

(only reduces symptoms by approximately 30%) in schizophrenia.
- Asenapine should not be recommended in patients who are nonadherent.

References

1. Organon Inc. LLC. (2013). *Saphris Package Insert*. Roseland, New Jersey.
2. California Department of State Hospitals. (2019). *DSH Psychotropic Medication Policy: Asenapine Protocol*. Sacramento, California.
3. Bishara, D., Taylor, D. (2008). Upcoming agents for the treatment of schizophrenia: mechanism of action, efficacy and tolerability. *Drugs*, 68, 2269–2292.
4. Vieta, E., Sanchez-Moreno, J. (2008). Acute and long-term treatment of mania. *Dialogues Clin Neurosci*, 10, 165–179.
5. Friberg, L. E., de Greef, R., Kerbusch, T., et al. (2009). Modeling and simulation of the time course of asenapine exposure response and dropout patterns in acute schizophrenia. *Clin Pharmacol Ther*, 86, 84–91.

2.09 Clozapine

A. BASIC INFORMATION [1–4]

Principle Trade Names
- Clozaril®
- FazaClo® (ODT)
- Leponex®
- Versacloz® (oral suspension)

Legal Status
- Prescription only
- Not controlled

Classifications
- Monoamine antagonist
- Atypical antipsychotic
- Second-generation antipsychotic (SGA)
- Mood stabilizer

Generics Available
- Yes, for tablets and ODT

Formulations
- Tablets: 25 mg; 100 mg
- Orally dissolving tablets (ODT): 25 mg; 100 mg
- Liquid: 50 mg/ml
- Injectable immediate-release: 25 mg/ml (not approved in the US)

FDA Indications
- Treatment-resistant schizophrenia and schizoaffective disorder
- Recurrent suicidality in schizophrenia or schizoaffective disorder

Other Data-Supported Indications
- Treatment-resistant bipolar mood disorder
- Aggressive/violent patients not responsive to other treatments
- Dopamine antagonist-intolerant psychosis (e.g. Parkinson's disease psychosis)
- Psychogenic polydipsia

Dopamine
- Modest antagonist at D_2 and D_3 receptors
- May modestly decrease positive psychotic symptoms and contribute to mood stabilization
- Clinical effects of robust binding at D_4 receptors is unknown

Serotonin
- Robust antagonism at $5HT_{2A}$ receptors increases dopamine release in the mesocortical, nigrostriatal, and tuberoinfundibular tracts and likely improves frontal lobe functioning, diminishing neurological motor symptoms, and avoiding prolactin elevation, respectively
- Antagonism at $5HT_{2C}$ receptors likely increases carbohydrate craving
- Clinical effects of binding at $5HT_{1A}$ receptors are unknown

Acetylcholine
- Central agonism at M_4 receptors may exert antipsychotic effects
- Antagonism at other muscarinic receptors produces anticholinergic effects including blurred near vision, decreased gastrointestinal motility and urinary retention

Glutamate
- Allosteric modulation (increase) in glutamate signal transduction is likely a major factor in treating psychosis and improving frontal lobe functions including cognition, reduction in negative symptoms, and improving executive functions

Histamine
- Inverse agonism at H_1 receptors produces sedation

Epinephrine/norepinephrine
- Antagonism at α-adrenergic receptors causes orthostatic hypotension

Enkephalin
- Antagonism at σ-opioid cytoplasmic receptors may decrease gastrointestinal motility

Initial Target Range
- 350–600 ng/ml

Range for Treatment Resistance
- 600–1000 ng/ml (more resistant patients)

Typical Time to Response
- Median time to response is three weeks after achieving a minimum of 350 ng/ml at trough
- If no response, recheck plasma concentration and continue titration

Time-Course of Improvement
- Some patients show ongoing improvements for up to 24 months at a therapeutic concentration

D. TYPICAL TREATMENT RESPONSE [1, 2–4, 7, 6]

Usual Target Symptoms
- Psychosis – positive and negative symptoms
- Cognitive symptoms
- Affective symptoms
- Suicidal behavior
- Violence and aggression

Common Short-Term Adverse Effects
- Sedation
- Orthostasis
- Tachycardia
- Benign fever (~20%)

Rare Adverse Effects
- Myocarditis (within first six weeks of treatment)
- Dilated cardiomyopathy (long-term risk)
- Venous thromboembolism

- Hyperglycemia with ketoacidosis
- Seizures (with high dosages)
- Severe neutropenia
- Tardive dyskinesia
- Paralytic ileus
- Increased risk of death or cerebrovascular events in elderly patients with dementia-related psychosis
- Neuroleptic malignant syndrome (in conjunction with other antipsychotics)

Long-Term Effects
- Constipation
- Enuresis
- Sialorrhea
- Metabolic syndrome, including weight gain, central adiposity, hypertension, hyperglycemia, dyslipidemia

E. PRE-TREATMENT WORKUP AND INITIAL LABORATORY TESTING [1, 2–4, 6, 8, 9]

History
Obtain personal and family histories of:
- cardiac disease
- obesity
- dyslipidemia
- hypertension
- diabetes mellitus
- epilepsy
- gastrointestinal disease or injury
- prostatic hypertrophy

Physical
Obtain a general physical examination with emphasis on:
- cardiovascular examination (including blood pressure with orthostatic measurements, pulse rate, respiratory rate and temperature)
- gastrointestinal examination
- BMI
- waist circumference

Neurological
- Check for myoclonus or myoclonic jerks
- AIMS

Blood Tests
- ANC (within one week prior to clozapine start)
- Complete metabolic panel
- Fasting blood sugar and/or Hgb A1c

- Lipid panel
- KUB (if clinically indicated)

Cardiac Tests
- ECG
- Vital signs
- Orthostatic BP measurements twice (separated by at least one hour)

Urine Tests
- Urinalysis

Pregnancy Test
- Pregnancy test (premenopausal females)
- Classified as no increased risk in human pregnancies

Metabolic Syndrome Parameters
- Elevated waist circumference:
  - Men – greater than 40 inches (102 cm)
  - Women – greater than 35 inches (88 cm)
- Elevated triglycerides: equal to or greater than 150 mg/dl (1.7 mmol/l)
- Reduced HDL ("good") cholesterol:
  - Men – less than 40 mg/dl (1.03 mmol/l)
  - Women – less than 50 mg/dl (1.29 mmol/l)
- Elevated blood pressure: ≥130/80 mm Hg or use of medication for hypertension
- Elevated fasting glucose: equal to or greater than 100 mg/dl (5.6 mmol/l) or use of medication for hyperglycemia

F. MONITORING [3, 6, 10, 11]

First Two Weeks of Treatment
• Daily VS + orthostatic measurements

Monthly
• Fasting blood sugar (for first three months only)
• BMI (monthly for three months, then quarterly)

Quarterly
• Hgb A1c
• Fasting lipid panel
• BMI
• KUB (if ↑ risk)
• AIMS [if (+), until (-) twice]

Biannually (twice per year)
• ECG (if on other medications that may prolong QTc as per the package insert)

Annually
• ECG
• AIMS
• Prolactin level

Other
• Initial plasma clozapine concentration range = 350–600 ng/ml
• For more ill patients, plasma clozapine concentration range = 600–1000 ng/ml

G. DOSING AND KINETICS [1, 2, 4, 6 – 12]

Initial Dosing
• Administer initial dose of 12.5–25 mg PO qhs
• For elderly or those sensitive to orthostasis, initiate at 6.25–12.5 mg PO qhs

Titration
• If tolerated, increase dose the following day to 25 mg BID and titrate by 12.5 to 25–50 mg twice per week (target dose by end of second week = 200 mg daily; obtain trough plasma level at this dose for fine tuning dosage)
• For elderly or those sensitive to orthostasis and if tolerated, increase dose the following day to 12.5 mg BID and titrate by 12.5–25 mg twice per week (target dose by end of first week = 100 mg daily; obtain trough plasma level at this dose for fine tuning dosage)

Half-Life
• 6 to 26 hours with a mean of 14.2 hours
• ~ 80% of clozapine is excreted in a metabolized state
• After titration, clozapine can often be consolidated to a single bedtime dose

Bioavailability
• 60–70%

Adjustment for Hepatic Dysfunction (by Child-Pugh Criteria)
• No dosage adjustments per the package insert
• However, dose reductions may be necessary in the presence of significant hepatic impairment

Adjustment for Renal Dysfunction
• No dosage adjustments per the package insert
• However, dose reductions may be necessary in the presence of severe impairment (Child-Pugh category C) or renal impairment

H. MEDICATIONS TO AVOID IN COMBINATION/WARNINGS [1, 2–4, 6]

 Precautions with medications that suppress bone marrow function and cause neutropenia

- Antineoplastic drugs
- Antiretroviral medications
- Carbamazepine
- Propylthiouracil

 Precautions with type 1 C antiarrhythmic medications

- Propafenone
- Flecainide
- Ecainide
- Quinidine

 Precautions with hypersensitivity

- Loxapine
- Amoxapine

 Precautions with CNS depressants

- Benzodiazepines (avoid concurrent use during first week of titration)
- Barbiturates

 Precautions with anticholinergic agents

- Benztropine
- Trihexyphenidyl
- Olanzapine

- Quetiapine
- Chlorpromazine
- Oxybutynin
- Other antimuscarinics

 Precautions with strong cyp 1A2 inhibitors

- Fluvoxamine
- Ciprofloxacin
- Use 1/3 the dose of clozapine

 Precautions with strong cyp 1A2 inducers

- Cigarette smoke
- Phenytoin

 Precautions with strong cyp 2D6 inhibitors

- Bupropion
- Duloxetine
- Paroxetine
- Fluoxetine

 Precautions with strong cyp 3A4 inhibitors

- Ketoconazole

 Precautions with highly protein-bound drugs

- Digoxin
- Warfarin

 I. MEDICAL PRECAUTIONS AND CONTRAINDICATIONS [1, 2–4, 6, 13, 14]

Use precautions in patients with

- Pregnancy (classified as no increased risk)
- Current serious medical illness/debilitated medical status
- Personal/family history of morbid obesity, severe diabetes mellitus or dyslipidemia
- History of seizure disorder
- Serious hepatic/renal/cardiopulmonary disease
- Enlarged prostate

 ## Do NOT Use in patients with

- Prior clozapine-induced severe neutropenia unless benefits clearly outweigh risk
- Present, severe CNS depression or coma
- Pre-treatment ANC <1500 cells/mm³ or (<1000 cells/mm³ in benign ethnic neutropenia/BEN)
- Nonadherence to required lab monitoring

- Uncontrolled seizure disorder
- Medically unstable status which could be complicated by clozapine treatment
- Acute narrow-angle glaucoma
- Bowel obstruction
- Paralytic ileus
- Unstable hypotension
- Unstable tachyarrhythmias
- Unstable febrile illness
- <6 years of age
- Hypersensitivity

May rechallenge if benefits clearly outweigh risks

- Continual, ongoing treatment with filgrastim 300 mcg once to three times weekly has been shown to stimulate the bone marrow at a rate faster than antibodies can destroy them

2.09 Clozapine (Continued)

 J. RECOMMENDED ABSOLUTE NEUTROPHIL COUNT MONITORING FOR GENERAL POPULATION [3; 6; 13; 14; 15]

ANC level	Treatment Recommendations	ANC Monitoring
≥1500/mm³	• Initiate treatment • If treatment interrupted for <30 days, continue monitoring as before • If treatment interrupted for ≥30 days, monitor as if new patient	• Weekly for months 1–6 • Q-2 weeks for months 7–12 • Q-4 weeks after 1 year
(Mild neutropenia) 1000–1499/mm³	• Continue treatment	• Weekly x 3 weeks until ANC ≥1500/mm³ • Once ANC ≥1500/mm³, return to patient's last "Normal Range" ANC monitoring interval

(Moderate neutropenia) 500–999/mm³	• Interrupt treatment for suspected clozapine-induced neutropenia
	• Infection workup (CXR, cultures (throat, blood, urine))
	• Appropriate antibiotics
	• Treat:
	    Lithium 300–900 mg qhs
	    OR
	    Filgrastim 300mcg SQ
	• May rechallenge clozapine
		• Daily ANC until ≥1000 mm³
		
		THEN
		
		• Weekly x 3 weeks until ANC ≥1500/mm³
		• Once ANC ≥1500/mm³, check ANC weekly x 4 weeks, then return to patient's last "Usual Range" ANC monitoring interval

(Severe neutropenia) <500/mm³	• STOP clozapine! • Diphenhydramine or benztropine taper • STAT filgrastim 480 mcg SQ (prior to transfer) • Immediate transfer to reverse-isolation room in acute care hospital • Filgrastim QD • Infection workup (CXR, cultures (throat, blood, urine)) • Appropriate antibiotics • Do not rechallenge unless benefits clearly outweigh risk	• Daily ANC check until ANC ≥1500/mm³ THEN • Weekly x 4 weeks until ANC ≥1500/mm³ • Report to Clozapine REMS

K. RECOMMENDED ABSOLUTE NEUTROPHIL COUNT MONITORING FOR BEN POPULATION [3, 6, 13, 14, 15]

ANC level	Treatment Recommendations	ANC Monitoring
(Established baseline) $\geq$**1000/mm³**	• Obtain at least two baseline ANC levels before initiating treatment • If treatment interrupted for <30 days, continue monitoring as before • If treatment interrupted for $\geq$30 days, monitor as if new patient	• Weekly for months 1–6 • Q-2 weeks for months 7–12 • Q-4 weeks after 1 year
(BEN neutropenia) **500–999/mm³**	• Continue treatment • Note that some BEN patients exhibit a stable ANC <1000 cells per cubic mm and this section would not apply to them unless their ANC declines below their characteristic baseline	• Weekly x 3 weeks until ANC $\geq$1000/mm³ or known baseline • Once ANC $\geq$1000/mm³, return to patient's last "Normal BEN Range" ANC monitoring interval**
(BEN severe neutropenia) **<500/mm³**	• STOP clozapine! • Diphenhydramine or benztropine taper • STAT filgrastim 480 mcg SQ (prior to transfer) • Immediate transfer to reverse-isolation room in acute care hospital • Filgrastim QD • Infection workup (CXR, cultures (throat, blood, urine)) • Appropriate antibiotics • Hematology consultation • Do NOT rechallenge unless benefits clearly outweigh risk	• Daily ANC check until ANC $\geq$1000/mm³ (or known baseline) THEN • Weekly x 3 weeks until ANC $\geq$1500/mm³ or known baseline) • Report to Clozapine REMS

2.09 Clozapine (Continued)

ART OF PSYCHOPHARMACOLOGY: TAKE-HOME PEARLS

- Clozapine is more effective for treatment-resistant schizophrenia, producing a response in up to 60% of such patients.
- Clozapine is effective for violent, aggressive patients.
- Clozapine is effective for patients with tardive dyskinesia without risk of worsening their movement disorder.
- Clozapine reduces risk in patients with suicidal ideation or behavior.
- Conversely, clozapine carries greater risks for patients with diabetes, obesity and/or dyslipidemia.

- Similarly, clozapine is more problematic for patients with intolerable sialorrhea or orthostasis.
- Clozapine is not used first-line due to side effects and monitoring burden.
- However, some studies have shown that clozapine is associated with the lowest risk of mortality among all antipsychotics; hence, use of clozapine may not be reserved only for treatment-resistant cases.
- If benefits clearly outweigh the risks, clozapine can be rechallenged successfully using concomitant filgrastim in about 70% of cases.

References

1. Jazz Pharmaceuticals Inc. *Fazaclo Package Insert*. Palo Alto, California.
2. HLS Therapeutics (U.S.) Inc. (2019). *Clozaril Package Insert*. Rosemont, Pennsylvania.
3. Meyer, J. M. (2019). *The Clozapine Handbook: Stahl's Handbooks*. New York: Cambridge University Press.
4. TruPharma LLC. (2020). *Versacloz Package Insert*. Tampa, Florida.
5. Remington, G., Agid, O., Foussias, G., et al. (2013). Clozapine and therapeutic drug monitoring: is there sufficient evidence for an upper threshold? *Psychopharmacology (Berl)*, 225, 505–518.
6. California Department of State Hospitals. (2019). *DSH Psychotropic Medication Policy: Clozapine Protocol*. Sacramento, California.
7. De Berardis, D., Rapini, G., Olivieri, L., et al. (2018). Safety of antipsychotics for the treatment of schizophrenia: a focus on the adverse effects of clozapine. *Ther Adv Drug Saf*, 9, 237–256.
8. Maguire, G. A. (2002). Comprehensive understanding of schizophrenia and its treatment. *Am J Health Syst Pharm*, 59, S4–11.
9. Solmi, M., Murru, A., Pacchiarotti, I., et al. (2017). Safety, tolerability, and risks associated with first- and second-generation antipsychotics: a state-of-the-art clinical review. *Ther Clin Risk Manag*, 13, 757–777.
10. Jin, H., Meyer, J. M., Jeste, D. V. (2002). Phenomenology of and risk factors for new-onset diabetes mellitus and diabetic ketoacidosis associated with atypical antipsychotics: an analysis of 45 published cases. *Ann Clin Psychiatry*, 14, 59–64.
11. American Diabetes Association, American Psychiatric Association, American Association of Clinical Endocrinologists, et al. (2004). Consensus development conference on antipsychotic drugs and obesity and diabetes. *Obes Res*, 12, 362–368.
12. Howland, R. H. (2010). Potential adverse effects of discontinuing psychotropic drugs. *J Psychosoc Nurs Ment Health Serv*, 48, 11–14.
13. Lally, J., Malik, S., Krivoy, A., et al. (2017). The use of granulocyte colony-stimulating factor in clozapine rechallenge: a systematic review. *J Clin Psychopharmacol*, 37, 600–604.
14. Lally, J., Malik, S., Whiskey, E., et al. (2017). Clozapine-associated agranulocytosis treatment with granulocyte colony-stimulating factor/granulocyte-macrophage colony-stimulating factor: a systematic review. *J Clin Psychopharmacol*, 37, 441–446.
15. Andres, E., Zimmer, J., Mecili, M., et al. (2011). Clinical presentation and management of drug-induced agranulocytosis. *Expert Rev Hematol*, 4, 143–151.

2.10 Iloperidone

A. BASIC INFORMATION [1, 2]

Principle Trade Names
- Fanapt®
- Fanapt® Titration Pack

Legal Status
- Prescription only
- Not controlled

Classifications
- Monoamine antagonist
- Atypical antipsychotic
- Second-generation antipsychotic (SGA)
- Mood stabilizer

Generics Available
- No

Formulations
- Tablet: 1 mg; 2 mg; 4 mg; 6 mg; 8 mg; 10 mg; 12 mg

FDA Indications
- Schizophrenia
- Schizophrenia maintenance

Other Data-Supported Indications
- Other psychotic disorders
- Bipolar mood disorder – manic or mixed episodes
- Major depressive episode with psychotic features (also as adjunct for mood)
- Severe persistent assaultive behavior
- Severe persistent self-injurious behavior
- Severe, persistent stereotypic or impulsive behaviors

B. MECHANISMS OF ACTION [1, 2, 3]

Dopamine

- Antagonism at D_2 receptors may decrease positive psychotic symptoms and contribute to mood stabilization, as well as cause motor side effects and hyperprolactinemia

Serotonin

- Robust antagonism at $5HT_{2A}$ receptors enhances dopamine release in the mesocortical, nigrostriatal, and tuberoinfundibular tracts and likely improves frontal lobe functioning, diminishing neurological motor symptoms, and decreases risk for hyperprolactinemia

Epinephrine/norepinephrine

- Antagonism at α_1-adrenergic receptors causes orthostatic hypotension, sedation and dizziness
- It is the most potent α-adrenergic antagonist of the SGA medications, requiring gradual titration

C. PLASMA CONCENTRATIONS AND TREATMENT RESPONSE [2, 3, 5]

Initial Target Range

- No established plasma therapeutic range

Range for Treatment Resistance

- No established plasma therapeutic range

Typical Time to Response

- Therapeutic improvement can be seen for 1–20 weeks

Time-Course of Improvement

- If no response by four weeks at maximum tolerated dose, taper and withdraw therapy

D. TYPICAL TREATMENT RESPONSE [1, 2, 3, 4]

Usual Target Symptoms

- Psychosis – positive and negative symptoms
- Cognitive symptoms
- Affective symptoms

Common Short-Term Adverse Effects

- Cephalgia
- Sedation
- Insomnia
- Agitation
- Anxiety
- Orthostatic hypotension
- Tachycardia
- Lightheadedness or syncope
- Dyspepsia and other upper gastrointestinal (GI) symptoms

Rare Adverse Effects

- Prolonged QTc interval
- Cerebrovascular events in demented elderly
- Hyperglycemia with ketoacidosis
- Type 1 hypersensitivity reactions (anaphylaxis, angioedema, hypotension, tachycardia, swollen tongue, difficulty breathing, wheezing, rash)
- Neuroleptic malignant syndrome (reduced risk compared to conventional antipsychotics)

Long-Term Effects

- Hyperprolactinemia
- Extrapyramidal side effects (reversible)
- Metabolic changes (weight gain, hyperglycemia, dyslipidemia)
- Tardive dyskinesia (demented elderly)

E. PRE-TREATMENT WORKUP AND INITIAL LABORATORY TESTING[2, 6, 7]

History
- Obtain personal/family histories of diabetes
- Personal history of: high BMI; dyslipidemia (elevated TGs or cholesterol)

Physical
- General physical examination
- Vital signs
- BMI
- Waist circumference

Neurological
- Check for myoclonus or myoclonic jerks
- AIMS
- Neurology consultation if personal history of active, poorly controlled seizure disorder

Blood Tests
Within 30 days:
- Complete metabolic panel
- Fasting blood sugar or Hgb A1c
- Lipid panel

Cardiac Tests
- ECG

Urine Tests
- Urinalysis

Pregnancy Test
- Pregnancy test (premenopausal females)
- Classified as risk not ruled out

Metabolic Syndrome Parameters
- Elevated waist circumference:
  ∘ Men – greater than 40 inches (102 cm)
  ∘ Women – greater than 35 inches (88 cm)
- Elevated triglycerides: equal to or greater than 150 mg/dl (1.7 mmol/l)
- Reduced HDL ("good") cholesterol:
  ∘ Men – less than 40 mg/dl (1.03 mmol/l)
  ∘ Women – less than 50 mg/dl (1.29 mmol/l)
- Elevated blood pressure: ≥130/80 mm Hg or use of medication for hypertension
- Elevated fasting glucose: equal to or greater than 100 mg/dl (5.6 mmol/l) or use of medication for hyperglycemia

F. MONITORING [6, 8]

Monthly
- Weight
- BMI

Semi-Annually (twice per year)
- Hgb A1c or fasting glucose
- Fasting lipid panel
- ECG (if on other medications that may prolong QTc as per the package insert)

Annually
- ECG
- AIMS
- Waist circumference

- Hgb A1c or fasting glucose
- Nutritional consultation if
  ∘ waist circumference increases from <35 inches to >35 inches in females OR increases from <40 inches to >40 inches in males
  ∘ weight increases 5% in one month, 7.5% in three months, or 10% in six months
  ∘ BMI increases from normal to overweight (<25 to >25) OR from overweight to obese (25–29.9 to 30 or higher)
- Prolactin level
- Breast exam (both males/females)

Initial Dosing
• Administer initial dose of 1–2 mg BID

Titration
• If tolerated and clinically indicated, titrate slowly to a maximum of 24 mg daily

Half-Life
• 18–33 hours

Bioavailability
• >95% protein-bound

Adjustment for Hepatic Dysfunction (by Child-Pugh Criteria)
• Child-Pugh category A or B (mild-moderate hepatic impairment): no dosage adjustment necessary
• Child-Pugh category C (severe hepatic impairment): contraindicated

Adjustment for Renal Dysfunction
• No dosage adjustment necessary per the package insert
• However, dose reductions may be necessary in the presence of significant renal impairment

H. MEDICATIONS TO AVOID IN COMBINATION/WARNINGS [1, 2, 3, 4]

Precautions with metabolic inducers – 3A4 (may require two-fold higher doses)
• Carbamazepine
• Phenytoin
• Omeprazole
• Phenobarbital
• Rifampin
• Oxcarbazepine

Precautions with metabolic inhibitors – 2D6, 3A4 (may require lower doses)
• Fluvoxamine
• Paroxetine

• Fluoxetine
• Bupropion
• Sertraline
• Ketoconazole
• Erythromycin
• Clarithromycin
• Diltiazem

Avoid with
• Cimetidine
• Grapefruit juice
• Protease inhibitors

I. MEDICAL PRECAUTIONS AND CONTRAINDICATIONS [1, 2]

Use precautions in patients with
• Cardiac arrhythmias
• Family history of sudden death
• Significant risk of electrolyte imbalances (e.g. diarrhea, diuretic treatment)
• Concomitant use of drugs with demonstrated propensity to prolong QT interval (e.g. mefloquine, pimozide)

Do NOT Use in patients if
• Hypersensitivity
• >65 years or older (Beers Criteria)

- Iloperidone can be used in some patients with treatment-refractory psychosis or bipolar disorder.
- Iloperidone does not result in full remission of psychotic symptoms (only reduces symptoms by approximately 30%) in schizophrenia patients.

- Iloperidone is not recommended in patients with treatment nonadherence, unstable mood or aggression.
- Iloperidone is not helpful for cognitive deficits.
- Iloperidone typically produces few to no neurological side effects.
- A four-week depot preparation is in development.

References

1. Vanda Pharmaceuticals Inc. (2009). *Fanapt Package Insert.* Washington, D.C.
2. California Department of State Hospitals. (2019). *DSH Psychotropic Medication Policy: Iloperidone Protocol.* Sacramento, California.
3. Stahl, S. M. (2002). *Antipsychotic Agents,* 2nd ed. New York: Cambridge University Press.
4. Remington, G. J. (2003). *Antipsychotics,* 13th ed. Toronto: Hogrefe and Huber Co.
5. Kane, J. M., Lauriello, J., Laska, E., et al. (2008). Long-term efficacy and safety of iloperidone: results from 3 clinical trials for the treatment of schizophrenia. *J Clin Psychopharmacol,* 28, S29–35.
6. Meyer, J. M. (2001). Effects of atypical antipsychotics on weight and serum lipid levels. *J Clin Psychiatry,* 62 Suppl. 27, 27–34; discussion 40–41.
7. American Diabetes Association, American Psychiatric Association, American Association of Clinical Endocrinologists, et al. (2004). Consensus development conference on antipsychotic drugs and obesity and diabetes. *Obes Res,* 12, 362–368.
8. California Department of State Hospitals. (2019). *DSH Psychotropic Medication Policy: Asenapine Protocol.* Sacramento, California.

2.11 Lumateperone

A. BASIC INFORMATION [1]

Principle Trade Names
• Caplyta®

Legal Status
• Prescription only (first available 2020)
• Not controlled

Classifications
• Monoamine antagonist
• Atypical antipsychotic
• Second-generation antipsychotic (SGA)

Generics Available
• No

Formulations
• Capsule: 42 mg

FDA Indications
• Schizophrenia

Other Data-Supported Indications
• None

B. MECHANISMS OF ACTION [1, 2]

Dopamine
• Antagonism at D_2 receptors may decrease positive psychotic symptoms and contribute to mood stabilization, as well as cause motor side effects and hyperprolactinemia
• Dopamine antagonism, however, is relatively weak.

Serotonin
• Robust antagonism at $5HT_{2A}$ receptors enhances dopamine release in the mesocortical, nigrostriatal, and tuberoinfundibular tracts and likely improves frontal lobe functioning, diminishing neurological motor symptoms, and decreases risk for hyperprolactinemia

Epinephrine/norepinephrine
• Antagonism at α_1-adrenergic receptors causes drowsiness and dizziness

C. PLASMA CONCENTRATIONS AND TREATMENT RESPONSE [1]

Initial Target Range
• No established plasma therapeutic range

Range for Treatment Resistance
• No established plasma therapeutic range

Typical Time to Response
• Therapeutic improvement may be seen for 1–20 weeks

Time-Course of Improvement
• If no response by four weeks at maximum tolerated dose, taper and withdraw therapy

D. TYPICAL TREATMENT RESPONSE [1]

Usual Target Symptoms
• Psychosis – positive and negative symptoms

Common Short-Term Adverse Effects
• Sedation
• Somnolence
• Orthostatic hypotension
• Syncope
• Cognitive impairment
• Motor impairment

Rare Adverse Effects
• Cerebrovascular events in demented elderly
• Dysphagia
• Hyperglycemia with ketoacidosis
• Leukopenia

• Neutropenia
• Type 1 hypersensitivity reactions (anaphylaxis, angioedema, hypotension, tachycardia, swollen tongue, difficulty breathing, wheezing, rash)
• Increased creatine phosphokinase
• Increased hepatic transaminases
• Neuroleptic malignant syndrome (reduced risk compared to conventional antipsychotics)

Long-Term Effects
• Dry mouth
• Body temperature dysregulation
• Metabolic changes (weight gain, hyperglycemia, dyslipidemia)
• Decreased appetite

E. PRE-TREATMENT WORKUP AND INITIAL LABORATORY TESTING [3, 4]

History
• Obtain personal/family histories of diabetes
• Personal history of: high BMI; dyslipidemia (elevated TGs or cholesterol)

Physical
• General physical examination
• Vital signs
• BMI
• Waist circumference

Neurological
• Check for myoclonus or myoclonic jerks
• AIMS
• Neurology consultation if personal history of active, poorly controlled seizure disorder

Blood Tests
Within 30 days:
• Complete metabolic panel
• Fasting blood sugar or Hgb A1c
• Lipid panel

Cardiac Tests
• ECG

Urine Tests
• Urinalysis

Pregnancy Test
• Pregnancy test (premenopausal females)
• Classified as risk not ruled out

Metabolic Syndrome Parameters
• Elevated waist circumference:
  ◦ Men – greater than 40 inches (102 cm)
  ◦ Women – greater than 35 inches (88 cm)
• Elevated triglycerides: equal to or greater than 150 mg/dl (1.7 mmol/l)
• Reduced HDL ("good") cholesterol:
  ◦ Men – less than 40 mg/dl (1.03 mmol/l)
  ◦ Women – less than 50 mg/dl (1.29 mmol/l)
• Elevated blood pressure: ≥130/80 mm Hg or use of medication for hypertension
• Elevated fasting glucose: equal to or greater than 100 mg/dl (5.6 mmol/l) or use of medication for hyperglycemia

2.11 Lumateperone (Continued)

F. MONITORING [4]

Monthly
- Weight
- BMI

Semi-Annually (twice per year)
- Hgb A1c or fasting glucose
- Fasting lipid panel
- ECG (if on other medications that may prolong QTc as per the package insert)

Annually
- ECG
- AIMS

- Waist circumference
- Hgb A1c or fasting glucose
- Nutritional consultation if:
  - waist circumference increases from <35 inches to >35 inches in females OR increases from <40 inches to >40 inches in males
  - weight increases 5% in one month, 7.5% in three months, or 10% in six months
  - BMI increases from normal to overweight (<25 to >25) OR from overweight to obese (25–29.9 to 30 or higher)
- Prolactin level
- Breast exam (both males/females)

G. DOSING AND KINETICS [1, 2]

Initial Dosing
- Administer initial dose of 42 mg once daily with food

Titration
- No titration needed

Half-Life
- 18 hours

Bioavailability
- 4.4% bioavailable (>97% protein-bound)

Adjustment for Hepatic Dysfunction (by Child-Pugh Criteria)
- Child-Pugh category A (mild hepatic impairment): no dosage adjustment necessary
- Child-Pugh category B or C (moderate-severe hepatic impairment): contraindicated

Adjustment for Renal Dysfunction
- No dosage adjustment necessary per the package insert
- However, dose reductions may be necessary in the presence of significant renal impairment

H. MEDICATIONS TO AVOID IN COMBINATION/WARNINGS [1]

Avoid with metabolic inducers – 3A4
- Carbamazepine
- Phenytoin
- Omeprazole
- Phenobarbital
- Rifampin
- Oxcarbazepine

Avoid with metabolic inhibitors – 3A4
- Fluvoxamine
- Fluconazole
- Itraconazole
- Voriconazole

- Nefazodone
- Cyclosporine
- Erythromycin
- Clarithromycin
- Diltiazem
- Verapamil
- Ritonavir
- Nelfinavir
- Grapefruit juice

Avoid with UGT inhibitors
- Valproic acid
- Probenecid

I. MEDICAL PRECAUTIONS AND CONTRAINDICATIONS [1]

⚠ Do NOT Use in patients if
- Hypersensitivity
- Elderly patients with dementia-related psychosis

ART OF PSYCHOPHARMACOLOGY: TAKE-HOME PEARLS

- Lumateperone can be used in some patients with treatment-refractory psychosis or bipolar disorder.
- Lumateperone does not result in full remission of psychotic symptoms (only reduces symptoms by approximately 30%) in schizophrenia patients.

- Lumateperone is not recommended in patients with treatment nonadherence, unstable mood or aggression.
- Lumateperone is not helpful for affective or cognitive symptoms.
- Lumateperone produces few to no neurological side effects.
- No long-acting formulation of lumateperone is available

References

1. Intra-cellular Therapies, I. (2019). *Caplyta (Lumateperone) Package Insert*. Towson, Maryland.
2. Lexicomp. Lumateperone: Drug Information. Available from: https://www.accessdata.fda.gov/drugsatfda_docs/label/2019/209500s000lbl.pdf
3. American Diabetes Association, American Psychiatric Association, American Association of Clinical Endocrinologists, et al. (2004). Consensus development conference on antipsychotic drugs and obesity and diabetes. *Obes Res*, 12, 362–368.
4. Marder, S. R., Essock, S. M., Miller, A. L., et al. (2004). Physical health monitoring of patients with schizophrenia. *Am J Psychiatry*, 161, 1334–1349.

2.12 Lurasidone

☰ A. BASIC INFORMATION [1]

Principle Trade Names
• Latuda®

Legal Status
• Prescription only
• Not controlled

Classifications
• Monoamine antagonist
• Atypical antipsychotic
• Second-generation antipsychotic (SGA)
• Mood stabilizer

Generics Available
• No

Formulations
• Tablet: 20 mg; 40 mg; 60 mg; 80 mg; 120 mg

FDA Indications
• Schizophrenia
• Bipolar depression

Other Data-Supported Indications
• Other psychotic disorders
• Bipolar mood disorder – acute manic or mixed episodes and maintenance after achieving responder status for two weeks
• Major depressive disorder with current psychotic features
• Severe persistent self-injurious behavior
• Agitation/aggression (severe, acute) associated with psychiatric disorders (e.g. bipolar disorder, schizophrenia), substance intoxication, or other organic causes
• Psychosis/agitation associated with dementia
• Behavioral disturbances in children and adolescents
• Disorders associated with problems with impulse control

B. MECHANISM OF ACTION [1, 2]

Dopamine
- Antagonism at D_2 receptors may decrease positive psychotic symptoms and contribute to mood stabilization

Serotonin
- Robust antagonism at $5HT_{2A}$ receptors enhances dopamine release in the mesocortical, nigrostriatal, and tuberoinfundibular tracts and likely improves frontal lobe functioning, diminishing neurological motor symptoms, and avoiding prolactin elevation, respectively

- Antagonism at $5HT_7$ may contribute to antidepressant actions

Epinephrine/norepinephrine
- Antagonism at α_2-adrenergic receptors causes orthostatic hypotension
- Antagonism at α_2-adrenergic receptors may contribute to antidepressant actions

C. PLASMA CONCENTRATIONS AND TREATMENT RESPONSE [3]

Initial Target Range
- No established plasma therapeutic range

Range for Treatment Resistance
- No established plasma therapeutic range

Typical Time to Response
- Therapeutic improvement can be seen for 1–20 weeks

Time-Course of Improvement
- If no response by four weeks at maximum tolerated dose, taper and withdraw therapy

D. TYPICAL TREATMENT RESPONSE [1, 2, 3–5]

Usual Target Symptoms
- Psychosis – positive and negative symptoms
- Cognitive symptoms
- Affective symptoms
- Suicidal behavior
- Violence and aggression

Common Short-Term Adverse Effects
- Akathisia (diminished by evening dosing)
- Cephalgia
- Sedation (dose-dependent)
- Agitation and anxiety
- Orthostatic hypotension
- Dyspepsia and other upper GI symptoms

Rare Adverse Effects
- Tachycardia, first-degree AV block
- Hyperglycemic ketoacidosis
- Type 1 hypersensitivity reactions (anaphylaxis, angioedema, hypotension, tachycardia, swollen tongue, difficulty breathing, wheezing, rash)

- Increased risk of death or cerebrovascular events in elderly patients with dementia-related psychosis
- Neuroleptic malignant syndrome (much reduced risk compared to conventional antipsychotics)

Long-Term Effects
- Constipation
- Dry mouth
- Akathisia
- Hyperprolactinemia
- Metabolic changes, including weight gain, hyperglycemia, dyslipidemia (very rare, if at all)

History
- Obtain personal and family histories of diabetes
- Personal history of:
  - high BMI
  - dyslipidemia (elevated TGs or cholesterol)

Physical
- General physical examination
- Vital signs
- BMI
- Waist circumference

Neurological
- Check for myoclonus or myoclonic jerks
- AIMS
- Neurology consultation if personal history of active, poorly controlled seizure disorder

Blood Tests
Within 30 days:
- Complete metabolic panel
- Fasting blood sugar and Hgb A1c
- Lipid panel

Cardiac Tests
- ECG

Urine Tests
- Urinalysis

Pregnancy Test
- Pregnancy test (premenopausal females)
- Classified as risk not ruled out
- No increased risk in animal studies

Metabolic Syndrome Parameters
- Elevated waist circumference:
  - Men – greater than 40 inches (102 cm)
  - Women – greater than 35 inches (88 cm)
- Elevated triglycerides: equal to or greater than 150 mg/dl (1.7 mmol/l)
- Reduced HDL ("good") cholesterol:
  - Men – less than 40 mg/dl (1.03 mmol/l)
  - Women – less than 50 mg/dl (1.29 mmol/l)
- Elevated blood pressure: ≥130/80 mm Hg or use of medication for hypertension
- Elevated fasting glucose: equal to or greater than 100 mg/dl (5.6 mmol/l) or use of medication for hyperglycemia

Monthly
- Weight
- BMI

Semi-Annually (twice per year)
- Hgb A1c or fasting glucose
- Fasting lipid panel
- BMI

Annually
- ECG
- AIMS
- Waist circumference

- Hgb A1c or fasting glucose
- Nutritional consultation if:
  - waist circumference increases from <35 inches to >35 inches in females OR increases from <40 inches to >40 inches in males
  - weight increases 5% in one month, 7.5% in three months, or 10% in six months
  - BMI increases from normal to overweight (<25 to >25) OR from overweight to obese (25–29.9 to 30 or higher)
- Prolactin level
- Breast exam (both males/females)

Initial Dosing

- Administer initial dose of 40–80 mg QD 30 minutes after evening meal
- If mild-moderate hepatic/renal disease/impairment, initiate at 20 mg QD 30 minutes after evening meal

Titration

- If tolerated and clinically indicated, titrate to a maximum of 160 mg daily
- If mild-moderate hepatic/renal disease/impairment, titrate to a maximum of 80 mg daily

Half-Life

- 7.5–10 hours

Bioavailability

- ~99% protein-bound
- 9–19% bioavailable in fed state

Adjustment for Hepatic Dysfunction (by Child-Pugh Criteria)

- Child-Pugh category A (mild hepatic impairment): no dosage adjustment necessary
- Child-Pugh category B or C (moderate-severe hepatic impairment): initiate at 20 mg daily with maximum dosage of 80 mg daily

Adjustment for Renal Dysfunction

- eGFR ≥50 ml/min: no dosage adjustment necessary per the package insert
- eGFR <50 ml/min: initiate at 20 mg daily with maximum dosage of 80 mg daily

Precautions with weak-moderate inducers – 3A4

(may require higher doses)
- Oxcarbazepine

Avoid with strong 3A4 inducers

- Carbamazepine
- Phenytoin
- Phenobarbital
- Rifampin

Precautions with weak-moderate inhibitors – 3A4

(may require lower doses)
- Diltiazem

Avoid with strong 3A4 inhibitors

- Fluvoxamine
- Ciprofloxacin
- Cimetidine
- Paroxetine
- Fluoxetine
- Ketoconazole

Use precautions in patients with

- Cerebrovascular disease
- Conditions that predispose to hypotension (e.g. dehydration, hypovolemia, concomitant antihypertensive medications)
- Serious hepatic/renal/cardiopulmonary disease (maximum dose of 80 mg daily)
- Active/poorly controlled seizure disorder
- Current/historical tardive dyskinesia
- Pregnancy

- History of prolactin-sensitive/dependent tumors or other concomitant conditions/drugs known to elevate prolactin
- Parkinson's disease
- Elderly demented patients with psychosis
- History of leukopenia or neutropenia

⚠ Do NOT Use in patients with

- Hypersensitivity
- Severe hepatic/renal disease/impairment
- Concurrent treatment with strong CYP3A4 inducers

- Lurasidone is metabolically neutral.
- Lurasidone is very efficacious in bipolar depression.
- Lurasidone does not cause QTc prolongation.
- Lurasidone does not result in full remission of positive psychotic symptoms (only reduces symptoms by approximately 30%) in schizophrenia patients.
- Lurasidone must be taken with food (350 kcal) for effective absorption.
- Lurasidone is not recommended in patients who are treatment nonadherent.

References

1. Sunovion Pharmaceuticals Inc. *Latuda (Lurasidone) Package Insert*. Fort Lee, New Jersey.
2. California Department of State Hospitals. (2019). *DSH Psychotropic Medication Policy: Lurasidone Protocol*. Sacramento, California.
3. Nakamura, M., Ogasa, M., Guarino, J., et al. (2009). Lurasidone in the treatment of acute schizophrenia: a double-blind, placebo-controlled trial. *J Clin Psychiatry*, 70, 829–836.
4. Cucchiaro J., P. A., et al. (2010). Safety of lurasidone: pooled analysis of five placebo-controlled trials in patients with schizophrenia. New Orleans, LA: American Psychiatric Association.
5. Solmi, M., Murru, A., Pacchiarotti, I., et al. (2017). Safety, tolerability, and risks associated with first- and second-generation antipsychotics: a state-of-the-art clinical review. *Ther Clin Risk Manag*, 13, 757–777.
6. American Diabetes Association, American Psychiatric Association, American Association of Clinical Endocrinologists, et al. (2004). Consensus development conference on antipsychotic drugs and obesity and diabetes. *Obes Res*, 12, 362–368.
7. Marder, S. R., Essock, S. M., Miller, A. L., et al. (2004). Physical health monitoring of patients with schizophrenia. *Am J Psychiatry*, 161, 1334–1349.

2.13 Olanzapine

A. BASIC INFORMATION [1–5]

Principle Trade Names
- Zyprexa®
- Zyprexa Zydis® (ODT)
- Zyprexa Relprevv®

Legal Status
- Prescription
- Not controlled

Classifications
- Monoamine antagonist
- Atypical antipsychotic
- Second-generation antipsychotic (SGA)
- Mood stabilizer

Generics Available
- Yes, for tablets and ODT

Formulations
- Tablets: 2.5 mg; 5 mg; 7.5 mg; 10 mg; 15 mg; 20 mg
- Orally dissolving tablets (ODT): 5 mg; 10 mg; 15 mg; 20 mg
- Injectable, immediate-release: 10 mg
- Suspension (LAI): 210 mg; 300 mg; 405 mg

FDA Indications
- Schizophrenia
- Bipolar disorder – acute manic or mixed episodes, and maintenance
- Acute agitation/aggression associated with schizophrenia and bipolar I mania
- Treatment-resistant depression (in combination with fluoxetine, Symbyax®)

Other Data-Supported Indications
- Other psychotic disorders
- Severe persistent assaultive behavior
- Severe persistent self-injurious behavior
- Agitation/aggression (severe, acute) associated with psychiatric disorders (e.g. bipolar disorder, schizophrenia), substance intoxication, or other organic causes
- Psychosis/agitation associated with dementia
- Behavioral disturbances in children and adolescents
- Disorders associated with problems with impulse control
- Anorexia nervosa
- Major depression with psychotic features

Dopamine
- Robust antagonism at D_2 and D_3 receptors decreases positive psychotic symptoms and contributes to mood stabilization
- Clinical effects of robust binding at D_4 receptors is unknown

Serotonin
- Robust antagonism at $5HT_{2A}$ receptors increases dopamine release in the mesocortical, nigrostriatal, and tuberoinfundibular tracts and likely improves frontal lobe functioning, diminishing neurological motor symptoms, and avoiding prolactin elevation, respectively
- Antagonism at $5HT_{2C}$ receptors likely increases carbohydrate craving and may contribute to improved cognitive and affective symptoms

Acetylcholine
- Antagonism at $M1_{1-5}$ receptors produces anticholinergic effects including blurred near vision, dry mouth, decreased gastrointestinal motility, and urinary retention

Glutamate
- At high plasma concentrations (120–200 ng/ml), allosteric modulation (increase) in glutamate signal transduction may be a major factor in treating psychosis and improving frontal lobe functions including cognition, reduction in negative symptoms, and improving executive functions

Histamine
- Inverse agonism at H_1 receptors produces sedation and weight gain

Epinephrine/norepinephrine
- Antagonism at α_1-adrenergic receptors causes orthostatic hypotension

Initial Target Range
- 40–120 ng/ml

Range for Treatment Resistance
- 120–150 ng/ml (more resistant patients)

Typical Time to Response
- Therapeutic improvement can be seen within one to two weeks for aggression, agitation, insomnia
- Therapeutic improvement can be seen within three to six weeks for control of mania and positive psychotic symptoms
- Therapeutic improvement can be seen between one to six weeks

Time-Course of Improvement
- If no response by four weeks at maximum tolerated dose or in upper therapeutic plasma concentration range (120–200 ng/ml), taper and withdraw therapy or cross-titrate with clozapine

D. TYPICAL TREATMENT RESPONSE [1–5]

Usual Target Symptoms
- Psychosis – positive and negative symptoms
- Cognitive symptoms
- Affective symptoms
- Suicidal behavior
- Violence and aggression

Common Short-Term Adverse Effects
- Dry mouth
- Sedation
- Dizziness
- Orthostasis
- Tachycardia

Rare Adverse Effects
- Drug Reaction with Eosinophilia and Systemic Symptoms (DRESS)
- Transaminitis/pancreatitis

- Hyperglycemia with ketoacidosis
- Seizures (rare)
- Increased risk of death or cerebrovascular events in elderly patients with dementia-related psychosis
- Neuroleptic malignant syndrome (in conjunction with other antipsychotics)

Long-Term Effects
- Constipation
- Urinary retention
- Enuresis
- Peripheral edema
- Pain – joint, back, chest, extremity
- Abnormal gait
- Ecchymosis
- Metabolic syndrome, including weight gain, central adiposity, hypertension, hyperglycemia, dyslipidemia

E. PRE-TREATMENT WORKUP AND INITIAL LABORATORY TESTING [5, 6]

History
- Obtain personal and family histories of diabetes
- Personal history of high BMI and/or dyslipidemia (elevated TGs or cholesterol)

Physical
- General physical examination
- Vital signs
- BMI
- Waist circumference

Neurological
- Check for myoclonus or myoclonic jerks
- AIMS
- Neurology consultation if personal history of active, poorly controlled seizure disorder

Blood Tests
Within 30 days:
- Complete metabolic panel
- Fasting blood sugar and/or Hgb A1c
- Lipid panel

Cardiac Tests
- ECG

Urine Tests
- Urinalysis

Pregnancy Test
- Pregnancy test (premenopausal females)
- Classified as no increased risk

Metabolic Syndrome Parameters
- Elevated waist circumference:
  ○ Men – greater than 40 inches (102 cm)
  ○ Women – greater than 35 inches (88 cm)
- Elevated triglycerides: equal to or greater than 150 mg/dl (1.7 mmol/l)
- Reduced HDL ("good") cholesterol:
  ○ Men – less than 40 mg/dl (1.03 mmol/l)
  ○ Women – less than 50 mg/dl (1.29 mmol/l)
- Elevated blood pressure: ≥130/80 mm Hg or use of medication for hypertension
- Elevated fasting glucose: equal to or greater than 100 mg/dl (5.6 mmol/l) or use of medication for hyperglycemia

Monthly
- Fasting blood sugar (for first three months)
- BMI
- Weight

Quarterly
- Fasting glucose and/or Hgb A1c
- Fasting lipid panel

Biannually (twice per year)
- ECG (if on other medications that may prolong QTc as per the package insert)

Annually
- ECG
- AIMS [if (+), until (-) twice]
- Prolactin level

- Nutritional consultation if:
  - waist circumference increases from <35 inches to >35 inches in females OR increases from <40 inches to >40 inches in males
  - weight increases 5% in one month, 7.5% in three months, or 10% in six months
  - BMI increases from normal to overweight (<25 to >25) OR from overweight to obese (25–29.9 to 30 or higher)
- Prolactin level
- Breast exam (both males/females)

Other
- Initial plasma olanzapine concentration range = 40–120 ng/ml
- For more ill patients, plasma olanzapine concentration range = 120–200 ng/ml

Initial Dosing
- Tablets or ODT:
  - Administer initial dose of 10–20 mg PO qhs
  - In acute agitated states, initiate at 40 mg qhs and taper as agitation decreases
- Suspension/(LAI):
  - available doses are 150 mg, 210 mg, 300 mg, and 405 mg
  - lower two doses may be given Q2–4 weeks
  - depot designed for Q4-weeks dosing interval

Titration
- Tablets or ODT: if tolerated, titrate to a maximum of 60 mg daily
- Suspension/(LAI): no oral cross-over or loading needed

Half-Life
- Oral and short-acting IM: 21–54 hours with a mean of 37 hours; approximately 1.5 times greater in elderly
- Extended-release injection: ~30 days
- ~40% of olanzapine is removed via first-pass metabolism
- After titration, olanzapine can often be consolidated to a single bedtime dose

Bioavailability
- Well absorbed (not affected by food)
- Tablets and ODT are bioequivalent

Adjustment for Hepatic Dysfunction (by Child-Pugh Criteria)
- No dosage adjustments per the package insert
- However, dose reductions may be necessary in the presence of significant hepatic impairment
- In combination with fluoxetine, initial olanzapine dose should be limited to 2.5–5 mg daily

Adjustment for Renal Dysfunction
- No dosage adjustments per the package insert
- Not removed by dialysis

H. MEDICATIONS TO AVOID IN COMBINATION/WARNINGS [3–5]

Precautions with anticholinergic agents

- Benztropine
- Trihexyphenidyl
- Clozapine
- Quetiapine
- Chlorpromazine
- Oxybutynin
- Other antimuscarinics

Precautions with antihypertensive agents

- May increase effect of antihypertensive medications

Precautions with dopamine agonists

- May antagonize levodopa and other dopamine agonists

Precautions with strong cyp 1A2 inhibitors (may require lower doses)

- Fluvoxamine
- Ciprofloxacin
- Cimetidine
- High-dose caffeine

Precautions with strong cyp 1A2 inducers (may require higher doses)

- Phenytoin
- Carbamazepine
- Omeprazole
- Phenobarbital
- Rifampin
- Cigarette smoke

I. MEDICAL PRECAUTIONS AND CONTRAINDICATIONS [3–5]

Precautions with depot olanzapine

- 0.1–0.2% risk of rapid drug/vehicle dissociation leading to delirium, obtundation and coma
- Overall risk ~2%

Required for each depot injection

- Direct nursing observation for a minimum of three hours
- If delirium, obtundation or coma occur, transfer to an acute care facility should be strongly considered
- Rare post-injection deaths have been reported

Risk for Drug Reaction with Eosinophilia and Systemic Symptoms (DRESS)

- May begin as a rash but could progress to other body parts
- Can include fever, swollen lymph nodes, swollen face, organ inflammation and increased WBC count (eosinophilia)
- May be fatal

Use precautions in patients with

- Conditions that predispose to hypotension (dehydration, overheating)
- Prostatic hypertrophy
- Constipation
- Elevated risk for aspiration pneumonia

⚠ Do NOT Use in patients with

- Unstable medical conditions:
  - acute myocardial infarction
  - unstable angina
  - severe hypotension and/or bradycardia
  - sick sinus syndrome
  - recent heart surgery
- History of acute narrow-angle glaucoma
- Bowel obstruction
- Paralytic ileus
- Hypersensitivity

2.13 Olanzapine (Continued)

- Olanzapine can be used in some patients with treatment-resistant psychosis or bipolar disorder.
- Olanzapine is a preferred augmenting agent in bipolar depression or treatment-resistant unipolar depression.

- The immediate-release olanzapine injection is useful when rapid onset of anti-agitation action without drug titration is needed.
- Alternative antipsychotics should be considered for patients who have personal or family history of diabetes mellitus, obesity and/or dyslipidemia.

References

1. Janowsky, D. S., Barnhill, L. J.. Davis, J. M. (2003). Olanzapine for self-injurious, aggressive, and disruptive behaviors in intellectually disabled adults: a retrospective, open-label, naturalistic trial. *J Clin Psychiatry*, 64, 1258–1265.
2. Keck, P. E., Jr. (2005). The role of second-generation antipsychotic monotherapy in the rapid control of acute bipolar mania. *J Clin Psychiatry*, 66 Suppl. 3, 5–11.
3. California Department of State Hospitals. (2019). *DSH Psychotropic Medication Policy: Olanzapine Protocol*. Sacramento, California.
4. Eli Lilly and Company. (2019). *Zyprexa Package Insert*. Available from: https://www.accessdata.fda.gov/drugsatfda_docs/label/2009/020592s051,021086s030,021253s036lbl.pdf (last accessed November 7, 2020).
5. Eli Lilly and Company. (2019). *Zyprexa Relprevv Package Insert*. Indianapolis, Indiana.
6. Meyer, J. M. (2001). Effects of atypical antipsychotics on weight and serum lipid levels. *J Clin Psychiatry*, 62 Suppl. 27, 27–34; discussion 40–41.
7. American Diabetes Association, American Psychiatric Association, American Association of Clinical Endocrinologists, et al. (2004). Consensus development conference on antipsychotic drugs and obesity and diabetes. *Obes Res*, 12, 362–368.
8. Callaghan, J. T., Bergstrom, R. F., Ptak, L. R., et al. (1999). Olanzapine. Pharmacokinetic and pharmacodynamic profile. *Clin Pharmacokinet*, 37, 177–193.
9. Baker, R. W., Kinon, B. J., Maguire, G. A., et al. (2003). Effectiveness of rapid initial dose escalation of up to forty milligrams per day of oral olanzapine in acute agitation. *J Clin Psychopharmacol*, 23, 342–348.
10. Botts, S., Littrell, R., de Leon, J. (2004). Variables associated with high olanzapine dosing in a state hospital. *J Clin Psychiatry*, 65, 1138–1143.

2.14 Paliperidone

A. BASIC INFORMATION [1–3]

Principle Trade Names
- Invega®
- Invega Sustenna®
- Invega Trinza®

Legal Status
- Prescription only
- Not controlled

Classifications
- Monoamine antagonist
- Atypical antipsychotic
- Second-generation antipsychotic (SGA)
- Mood stabilizer

Generics Available
- Yes, for extended-release tablets

Formulations
- Extended-release tablet: 1.5 mg; 3 mg; 6 mg; 9 mg
- Suspension, intramuscular:
- Invega Sustenna®: 39 mg; 78 mg; 117 mg; 156 mg; 234 mg
- Invega Trinza®: 273 mg; 410 mg; 546 mg; 819 mg

FDA Indications
- Schizophrenia
- Schizoaffective disorder

Other Data-Supported Indications
- Other psychotic disorders
- Bipolar mood disorder – acute manic or mixed episodes and maintenance after achieving responder status for two weeks
- Major depressive disorder with current psychotic features
- Severe persistent self-injurious behavior
- Agitation/aggression (severe, acute) associated with psychiatric disorders (e.g. bipolar disorder, schizophrenia), substance intoxication, or other organic causes
- Psychosis/agitation associated with dementia
- Behavioral disturbances in children and adolescents
- Disorders associated with problems with impulse control

B. MECHANISMS OF ACTION [1–3]

Dopamine
- Antagonism at D_2 receptors may decrease positive psychotic symptoms and contribute to mood stabilization

Serotonin
- Robust antagonism at $5HT_{2A}$ receptors enhances dopamine release in the mesocortical, nigrostriatal, and tuberoinfundibular tracts and likely improves frontal lobe functioning, diminishing neurological motor symptoms, and avoiding prolactin elevation, respectively

- Antagonism at $5HT_7$ may contribute to antidepressant actions

Epinephrine/norepinephrine
- Antagonism at α_1-adrenergic receptors may cause orthostatic hypotension
- Antagonism at α_2-adrenergic receptors may contribute to antidepressant actions

C. PLASMA CONCENTRATIONS AND TREATMENT RESPONSE [1–3, 4–7]

Initial Target Range
- 28–112 ng/ml

Range for Treatment Resistance
- 28–112 ng/ml
- Probably should be in the upper half of the therapeutic range

Typical Time to Response
- Therapeutic improvement can be seen for 1–20 weeks

Time-Course of Improvement
- If no response to tablets by four weeks at maximum tolerated dose, taper and withdraw therapy
- Do not use depot formulation if no response to tablet

D. TYPICAL TREATMENT RESPONSE [1, 2, 4–6, 8]

Usual Target Symptoms
- Psychosis – positive and negative symptoms
- Cognitive symptoms
- Affective symptoms
- Suicidal behavior
- Violence and aggression

Common Short-Term Adverse Effects
- Akathisia (diminished by evening dosing)
- Cephalgia
- Sedation (dose-dependent)
- Agitation and anxiety
- Orthostatic hypotension
- Dyspepsia and other upper GI symptoms

Rare Adverse Effects
- QT interval prolongation
- Hyperglycemic ketoacidosis

- Type 1 hypersensitivity reactions (anaphylaxis, angioedema, hypotension, tachycardia, swollen tongue, difficulty breathing, wheezing, rash)
- Increased risk of death or cerebrovascular events in elderly patients with dementia-related psychosis
- Neuroleptic malignant syndrome (much reduced risk compared to conventional antipsychotics)

Long-Term Effects
- Constipation
- Dry mouth
- Akathisia
- Hyperprolactinemia
- Metabolic changes, including weight gain, hyperglycemia, dyslipidemia (very rare, if at all)

History
• Obtain personal and family histories of diabetes
• Personal history of:
  ○ high BMI
  ○ dyslipidemia (elevated TGs or cholesterol)

Physical
• General physical examination
• Vital signs
• BMI
• Waist circumference

Neurological
• Check for myoclonus or myoclonic jerks
• AIMS
• Neurology consultation if personal history of active, poorly controlled seizure disorder

Blood Tests
Within 30 days:
• Complete metabolic panel
• Fasting blood sugar & Hgb A1c
• Lipid panel

Cardiac Tests
• ECG

Urine Tests
• Urinalysis

Pregnancy Test
• Pregnancy test (premenopausal females)
• Classified as risk not ruled out

Metabolic Syndrome Parameters
• Elevated waist circumference:
  ○ Men – greater than 40 inches (102 cm)
  ○ Women – greater than 35 inches (88 cm)
• Elevated triglycerides: equal to or greater than 150 mg/dl (1.7 mmol/l)
• Reduced HDL ("good") cholesterol:
  ○ Men – less than 40 mg/dl (1.03 mmol/l)
  ○ Women – less than 50 mg/dl (1.29 mmol/l)
• Elevated blood pressure: ≥130/80 mm Hg or use of medication for hypertension
• Elevated fasting glucose: equal to or greater than 100 mg/dl (5.6 mmol/l) or use of medication for hyperglycemia

Monthly
• Weight
• BMI

Semi-Annually (twice per year)
• Hgb A1c or fasting glucose
• Fasting lipid panel
• BMI

Annually
• ECG
• AIMS
• Waist circumference

• Hgb A1c or fasting glucose
• Nutritional consultation if:
  ○ waist circumference increases from <35 inches to >35 inches in females OR increases from <40 inches to >40 inches in males
  ○ weight increases 5% in one month, 7.5% in three months, or 10% in six months
  ○ BMI increases from normal to overweight (<25 to >25) OR from overweight to obese (25–29.9 to 30 or higher)
• Prolactin level
• Breast exam (both males/females)

Initial Dosing
- Tablets:
  - administer initial dose of 3–6 mg QD
  - in elderly or those with moderate-severe renal impairment, begin with 1.5 mg QD
- Suspension/depot in deltoid muscle:
  - administer initial injection of 234 mg
  - in elderly or those with hepatic/renal impairment, begin with 156 mg

Titration
- Tablets:
  - if tolerated and clinically indicated, titrate to a maximum of 12 mg daily
  - in mild renal impairment, titrate to a maximum of 6 mg daily
  - in moderate-severe renal impairment, titrate to a maximum of 3 mg daily
- Suspension/depot:
  - give second injection of 156 mg one week after initial injection; maintenance doses (39 mg, 78 mg, 117 mg, 156 mg, and 234 mg – depending on clinical response with 117 mg as the modal maintenance dose) are given every four weeks in deltoid or gluteal muscle
  - in elderly or those with hepatic/renal disease/impairment, give second injection of 117 mg one week after initial injection; maintenance doses (39 mg, 78 mg, 117 mg, and 156 mg – depending on clinical response) are given every four weeks in deltoid or gluteal muscle

Half-life
- Tablet: 23 hours (24–51 hours with renal impairment)
- Suspension/depot (monthly): 25–49 days
- Suspension/depot (three-month IM):
  - deltoid injection range: 84–95 days
  - gluteal injection range: 118–139 days

Bioavailability
- 74% protein-bound
- 28% bioavailable (oral)

Adjustment for Hepatic Dysfunction (by Child-Pugh Criteria)
- Child-Pugh category A or B (mild-moderate hepatic impairment): no dosage adjustment necessary
- Child-Pugh category C (severe hepatic impairment): no dosage adjustments in manufacturer's labeling (not studied)

Adjustment for Renal Dysfunction
- eGFR 50–79 ml/min: dose range from 3 mg to maximum of 6 mg daily
- eGFR 10–49 ml/min: dose range from 1.5 mg to maximum of 3 mg daily
- eGFR <10 mg/min: use not recommended

H. MEDICATIONS TO AVOID IN COMBINATION/WARNINGS [1–3, 7]

Precautions with cyp 3A4 inducers (may require higher doses)
- Carbamazepine
- Oxcarbazepine
- Phenytoin
- Rifampin

Precautions with cyp 2D6 inhibitors (may require lower doses)
- Bupropion
- Duloxetine
- Paroxetine
- Fluoxetine

Precautions with cyp 3A4 inhibitors (may require lower doses)
- Fluvoxamine
- Ciprofloxacin
- Cimetidine
- Paroxetine
- Fluoxetine
- Ketoconazole

Use precautions in patients with

- Cerebrovascular disease
- Conditions that predispose to hypotension (e.g. dehydration, hypovolemia, concomitant antihypertensive medications)
- Diabetes mellitus
- Dyslipidemia
- Concomitant use of medications known to cause elevated blood glucose (e.g. steroids, niacin, thiazide diuretics, atypical antipsychotics)
- Severe cardiovascular disease
- Hepatic disease (less important for paliperidone than risperidone due to limited hepatic metabolism)
- Renal impairment
- Active/poorly controlled seizure disorder
- Current/historical tardive dyskinesia
- Pregnancy or breastfeeding
- History of prolactin-sensitive/dependent tumors or other concomitant conditions/drugs known to elevate prolactin
- Parkinson's disease
- Elderly demented patients with psychosis
- History of leukopenia or neutropenia

 Do NOT Use in patients with

- Hypersensitivity
- Severe renal disease/impairment

- Paliperidone may cause less weight gain than some antipsychotics, e.g. clozapine and olanzapine, but more than others.
- Some patients respond to paliperidone better than the parent drug, risperidone.
- Paliperidone may cause more motor side effects than other atypical antipsychotics, especially when administered to patients with Parkinson's disease or Lewy body dementia.
- Paliperidone does not result in full remission of positive psychotic symptoms (only reduces symptoms by approximately 30%) in schizophrenia patients.
- Depot paliperidone is not recommended in those who do not show good clinical response to oral formulation.
- Depot paliperidone does not require simultaneous oral medication.
- Depot paliperidone is absorbed more slowly from the gluteal muscle than the deltoid.

References

1. Janssen Pharmaceuticals Inc. (2019). *Invega Package Insert*. Titusville, New Jersey.
2. Janssen Pharmaceuticals Inc. (2019). *Invega Sustenna Package Insert*. Titusville, New Jersey.
3. Janssen Pharmaceuticals Inc. (2019). *Invega Trinza Package Insert*. Titusville, New Jersey.
4. Kane, J., Canas, F., Kramer, M., et al. (2007). Treatment of schizophrenia with paliperidone extended-release tablets: a 6-week placebo-controlled trial. *Schizophr Res*, 90, 147–161.
5. Kramer, M., Simpson, G., Maciulis, V., et al. (2007). Paliperidone extended-release tablets for prevention of symptom recurrence in patients with schizophrenia: a randomized, double-blind, placebo-controlled study. *J Clin Psychopharmacol*, 27, 6–14.
6. Meltzer, H. Y., Bobo, W. V., Nuamah, I. F., et al. (2008). Efficacy and tolerability of oral paliperidone extended-release tablets in the treatment of acute schizophrenia: pooled data from three 6-week, placebo-controlled studies. *J Clin Psychiatry*, 69, 817–829.
7. California Department of State Hospitals. (2019). *DSH Psychotropic Medication Policy: Paliperidone Protocol*. Sacramento, California.
8. Nasrallah, H. A. (2008). Atypical antipsychotic-induced metabolic side effects: insights from receptor-binding profiles. *Mol Psychiatry*, 13, 27–35.
9. Meyer, J. M. (2001). Effects of atypical antipsychotics on weight and serum lipid levels. *J Clin Psychiatry*, 62 Suppl. 27, 27–34; discussion 40–41.
10. American Diabetes Association, American Psychiatric Association, American Association of Clinical Endocrinologists, et al. (2004). Consensus development conference on antipsychotic drugs and obesity and diabetes. *Diabetes Care*, 27, 596–601.

2.15 Quetiapine

A. BASIC INFORMATION [1, 2]

Principle Trade Names
• Seroquel®
• Seroquel XR®

Legal Status
• Prescription only
• Not controlled

Classifications
• Monoamine antagonist
• Atypical antipsychotic
• Second-generation antipsychotic (SGA)
• Mood stabilizer

Generics Available
• Yes, for tablet and extended-release tablets

Formulations
• Tablet: 25 mg; 50 mg; 100 mg; 200 mg; 300 mg; 400 mg
• Tablet, extended release: 25 mg; 50 mg; 100 mg; 200 mg; 300 mg; 400 mg

FDA Indications
• Schizophrenia
• Schizoaffective disorder
• Other psychotic disorder
• Bipolar mood disorder – acute manic or mixed episodes and maintenance after achieving responder status for two weeks
• Adjunct to lithium and/or valproate
• Bipolar depression
• Depression

Other Data-Supported Indications
• Severe persistent assaultive behavior
• Severe persistent self-injurious behavior
• Agitation/aggression (severe, acute) associated with psychiatric disorders (e.g. bipolar disorder, schizophrenia), substance intoxication, or other organic causes
• Psychosis/agitation associated with dementia
• Behavioral disturbances in children and adolescents
• Disorders associated with problems with impulse control
• Severe treatment-resistant anxiety

Dopamine

- Antagonism at D_2 receptors decreases positive psychotic symptoms and contributes to mood stabilization
- Rapid dissociation from D_2 receptors limits antipsychotic efficacy but also decreases adverse neurological effects, e.g. dystonias, akathisia and parkinsonism

Serotonin

- Robust antagonism at 5HT receptors (1A/B, 2A/B/C, 5–7) enhances dopamine release in the mesocortical, nigrostriatal, and tuberoinfundibular tracts and likely improves frontal lobe functioning, diminishing neurological motor symptoms, and avoiding prolactin elevation, respectively

Epinephrine and Norepinephrine

- Antagonism at α_1-adrenergic receptors may cause orthostatic hypotension
- Norquetiapine acts as an inhibitor of the norepinephrine reuptake transporter (likely responsible for antidepressant properties)

Acetylcholine

- Muscarinic antagonism may cause a variety of anticholinergic adverse effects, e.g. decreased recall, blurred near vision, xerostomia, decreased gastrointestinal motility and urinary retention (males)

Histamine

- Antagonism at H_1 receptors may cause anxiolytic effects and sedation

Initial Target Range

- No established plasma therapeutic range

Range for Treatment Resistance

- No established plasma therapeutic range

Typical Time to Response

- Therapeutic improvement can be seen for 1–12 weeks

Time-Course of Improvement

- If no response by four weeks at maximum tolerated dose, taper and withdraw therapy

Usual Target Symptoms

- Psychosis – positive and negative symptoms
- Cognitive symptoms of psychosis
- Affective symptoms
- Suicidal behavior
- Violence and aggression

Common Short-Term Adverse Effects

- Somnolence
- Incoordination
- Orthostatic hypotension
- Lightheadedness or syncope

Rare Adverse Effects

- Prolonged QTc interval
- Hyperglycemia with ketoacidosis
- Type 1 hypersensitivity reactions (anaphylaxis, angioedema, hypotension, tachycardia, swollen tongue, difficulty breathing, wheezing, rash)

- Increased risk of death or cerebrovascular events in elderly patients with dementia-related psychosis
- Neuroleptic malignant syndrome (much reduced risk compared to conventional antipsychotics)
- Pulmonary edema

Long-Term Effects

- Hyperprolactinemia
- Renal impairment
- Metabolic changes, including weight gain, hyperglycemia, dyslipidemia

History
- Obtain personal and family histories of diabetes
- Personal history of:
  - high BMI
  - dyslipidemia (elevated TGs or cholesterol)

Physical
- General physical examination
- Vital signs
- BMI
- Waist circumference

Neurological
- Check for myoclonus or myoclonic jerks
- AIMS
- Neurology consultation if personal history of active, poorly controlled seizure disorder

Blood Tests
Within 30 days:
- Complete metabolic panel
- Fasting blood sugar and/or Hgb A1c
- Lipid panel

Cardiac Tests
- ECG

Urine Tests
- Urinalysis

Pregnancy Test
- Pregnancy test (premenopausal females)
- Classified as risk not ruled out

Metabolic Syndrome Parameters
- Elevated waist circumference:
  - Men – greater than 40 inches (102 cm)
  - Women – greater than 35 inches (88 cm)
- Elevated triglycerides: equal to or greater than 150 mg/dl (1.7 mmol/l)
- Reduced HDL ("good") cholesterol:
  - Men – less than 40 mg/dl (1.03 mmol/l)
  - Women – less than 50 mg/dl (1.29 mmol/l)
- Elevated blood pressure: ≥130/80 mm Hg or use of medication for hypertension
- Elevated fasting glucose: equal to or greater than 100 mg/dl (5.6 mmol/l) or use of medication for hyperglycemia

Monthly
- Weight
- BMI

Semi-Annually (twice per year)
- Hgb A1c or fasting glucose
- Fasting lipid panel
- BMI
- ECG (if on other medications that may prolong QTc as per the package insert)

Annually
- ECG
- AIMS
- Waist circumference
- Hgb A1c or fasting glucose
- Nutritional consultation if:
  - waist circumference increases from <35 inches to >35 inches in females OR increases from <40 inches to >40 inches in males
  - weight increases 5% in one month, 7.5% in three months, or 10% in six months
  - BMI increases from normal to overweight (<25 to >25) OR from overweight to obese (25–29.9 to 30 or higher)
- Prolactin level
- Breast exam (both males/females)

G. DOSING AND KINETICS [1, 2, 4]

Initial Dosing
• Administer initial dose of 25–50 mg BID
• For acute mania, initiate at 50 mg BID
• For extended-release formulation, initiate at 200 mg qhs

Titration
• If tolerated and clinically indicated, titrate by 25–50 mg BID or TID per day, or as clinically indicated to a maximum dose of 1200 mg daily
• For extended-release formulation, titrate by 200–400 mg weekly

Half-Life
• Tablet: ~6hrs
• Tablet, extended release: ~7hrs

Bioavailability
• 100%

Adjustment for Hepatic Dysfunction (by Child-Pugh Criteria)
• Child-Pugh category A or B (mild-moderate hepatic impairment): dosage adjustment suggested with lower clearance in hepatic impairment (30% lower)

Adjustment for Renal Dysfunction
• No dosage adjustment necessary per the package insert

H. MEDICAL PRECAUTIONS AND CONTRAINDICATIONS [1, 2, 3]

Use precautions in patients with
• Personal/family history of diabetes mellitus
• Glucose intolerance/hyperglycemia
• History of high BMI
• HTN
• Obesity
• Exposure to alpha/beta blockers
• Concomitant use of medications known to cause elevated blood glucose (e.g. steroids, niacin, thiazide diuretics, atypical antipsychotics)
• Past or current dyslipidemia
• Cerebrovascular disease/conditions predisposing to hypotension (e.g. dehydration, hypovolemia, and treatment with antihypertensive medications)
• Severe cardiovascular disease, history of myocardial infarction/ischemia or heart failure
• Past or current liver disease or treatment with potentially hepatotoxic drugs
• Active or poorly controlled seizure disorder requiring anticonvulsant treatment
• Past or current tardive dyskinesia
• Elderly demented with psychosis
• Pregnancy or breastfeeding
• History of leukopenia or agranulocytosis

⚠ Do NOT Use in patients with
• Hypersensitivity

ART OF PSYCHOPHARMACOLOGY: TAKE-HOME PEARLS

- Quetiapine may be the preferred antipsychotic for psychosis in Parkinson's disease and Lewy body dementia.
- A limitation is that quetiapine does not result in full remission of psychotic symptoms (only reduces symptoms by approximately 30%) in schizophrenia.

- Quetiapine is approved for bipolar depression.
- Quetiapine has essentially only rare adverse motor effects or prolactin elevation.

References

1. AstraZeneca Pharmaceuticals LP. (2020). *Seroquel Package Insert*. Wilmington, Delaware.
2. AstraZeneca Pharmaceuticals LP. (2020). *Seroquel XR Package Insert*. Wilmington, Delaware.
3. California Department of State Hospitals. (2019). *DSH Psychotropic Medication Policy: Quetiapine Protocol*. Sacramento, California.
4. DeVane, C. L., Nemeroff, C. B. (2001). Clinical pharmacokinetics of quetiapine: an atypical antipsychotic. *Clin Pharmacokinet*, 40, 509–522.
5. Meyer, J. M. (2001). Effects of atypical antipsychotics on weight and serum lipid levels. *J Clin Psychiatry*, 62 Suppl. 27, 27–34; discussion 40–41.
6. American Diabetes Association, American Psychiatric Association, American Association of Clinical Endocrinologists, et al. (2004). Consensus development conference on antipsychotic drugs and obesity and diabetes. *Diabetes Care*, 27, 596–601.
7. Citrome, L. (2017). Activating and sedating adverse effects of second-generation antipsychotics in the treatment of schizophrenia and major depressive disorder: absolute risk increase and number needed to harm. *J Clin Psychopharmacol*, 37, 138–147.

2.16 Risperidone

A. BASIC INFORMATION [1–4]

Principle Trade Names
• Risperdal®
• Risperdal M-tab® (oral disintegrating tablet)
• Risperdal Consta®
• Perseris®

Legal Status
• Prescription only
• Not controlled

Classifications
• Monoamine antagonist
• Atypical antipsychotic
• Second-generation antipsychotic (SGA)
• Mood stabilizer

Generics Available
• Yes, for tablet, ODT, oral solution

Formulations
• Tablet: 0.25 mg; 0.5 mg; 1 mg; 2 mg; 3 mg; 4 mg
• Oral disintegrating tablet: 0.5 mg; 1 mg; 2 mg; 3 mg; 4 mg
• Oral solution: 1 mg/ml
• Suspension, intramuscular ER: 12.5 mg; 25 mg; 37.5 mg; 50 mg
• Subcutaneous: 90 mg; 120 mg

FDA Indications
• Schizophrenia
• Other psychotic disorders
• Bipolar mood disorder – acute manic or mixed episodes or maintenance (as monotherapy or adjunct to lithium/valproate)
• Autism-related irritability in children aged 5–16 years

Other Data-Supported Indications
• Major depressive disorder with current psychotic features
• Severe persistent self-injurious behavior
• Agitation/aggression (severe, acute) associated with psychiatric disorders (e.g. bipolar disorder, schizophrenia), substance intoxication, or other organic causes
• Behavioral disturbances in children and adolescents
• Disorders associated with problems with impulse control

Dopamine

- Antagonism at D_2 receptors may decrease positive psychotic symptoms and contribute to mood stabilization

Serotonin

- Robust antagonism at $5HT_{2A}$ receptors enhances dopamine release in the mesocortical, nigrostriatal, and tuberoinfundibular tracts and likely improves frontal lobe functioning, diminishing neurological motor symptoms, and avoiding prolactin elevation, respectively

Epinephrine/norepinephrine

- Antagonism at α_2-adrenergic receptors may cause orthostatic hypotension
- Antagonism at α_2-adrenergic receptors may contribute to antidepressant actions

C. PLASMA CONCENTRATIONS AND TREATMENT RESPONSE [1-4, 5]

Initial Target Range

- 28–112 ng/ml

Range for Treatment Resistance

- 28–112 ng/ml
- Probably should be in the upper half of the therapeutic range

Typical Time to Response

- Therapeutic improvement can be seen for 1–20 weeks

Time-Course of Improvement

- If no response to tablets by four weeks at maximum tolerated dose, taper and withdraw therapy
- Do not use depot formulation if no response to tablet

D. TYPICAL TREATMENT RESPONSE [1-4, 5, 6-8]

Usual Target Symptoms

- Psychosis – positive and negative symptoms
- Cognitive symptoms
- Affective symptoms
- Suicidal behavior
- Violence and aggression

Common Short-Term Adverse Effects

- Akathisia (diminished by evening dosing)
- Cephalgia
- Sedation (dose-dependent)
- Agitation and anxiety
- Orthostatic hypotension
- Dyspepsia and other upper gastrointestinal (GI) symptoms

Rare Adverse Effects

- QT interval prolongation
- Hyperglycemic ketoacidosis

- Type 1 hypersensitivity reactions (anaphylaxis, angioedema, hypotension, tachycardia, swollen tongue, difficulty breathing, wheezing, rash)
- Increased risk of death or cerebrovascular events in elderly patients with dementia-related psychosis
- Neuroleptic malignant syndrome (much reduced risk compared to conventional antipsychotics)

Long-Term Effects

- Constipation
- Dry mouth
- Akathisia
- Hyperprolactinemia
- Metabolic changes, including weight gain, hyperglycemia, dyslipidemia (very rare, if at all)

History
- Obtain personal and family histories of diabetes
- Personal history of:
  - high BMI
  - dyslipidemia (elevated TGs or cholesterol)

Physical
- General physical examination
- Vital signs
- BMI
- Waist circumference

Neurological
- Check for myoclonus or myoclonic jerks
- AIMS
- Neurology consultation if personal history of active, poorly controlled seizure disorder

Blood Tests
Within 30 days:
- Complete metabolic panel
- Fasting blood sugar and Hgb A1c
- Lipid panel

Cardiac Tests
- ECG

Urine Tests
- Urinalysis

Pregnancy Test
- Pregnancy test (premenopausal females)
- Classified as risk not ruled out

Metabolic Syndrome Parameters
- Elevated waist circumference:
  - Men – greater than 40 inches (102 cm)
  - Women – greater than 35 inches (88 cm)
- Elevated triglycerides: equal to or greater than 150 mg/dl (1.7 mmol/l)
- Reduced HDL ("good") cholesterol:
  - Men – less than 40 mg/dl (1.03 mmol/l)
  - Women – less than 50 mg/dl (1.29 mmol/l)
- Elevated blood pressure: ≥130/80 mm Hg or use of medication for hypertension
- Elevated fasting glucose: equal to or greater than 100 mg/dl (5.6 mmol/l) or use of medication for hyperglycemia

Monthly
- Weight
- BMI

Semi-Annually (twice per year)
- Hgb A1c or fasting glucose
- Fasting lipid panel
- BMI

Annually
- ECG
- AIMS
- Waist circumference
- Hgb A1c or fasting glucose
- Nutritional consultation if:
  - waist circumference increases from <35 inches to >35 inches in females OR increases from <40 inches to >40 inches in males
  - weight increases 5% in one month, 7.5% in three months, or 10% in six months
  - BMI increases from normal to overweight (<25 to >25) OR from overweight to obese (25–29.9 to 30 or higher)
- Prolactin level
- Breast exam (both males/females)

Initial Dosing

- Tablets/oral solution:
  - Administer initial dose of 0.5 mg–1 mg BID
  - In elderly or those with hepatic/renal impairment, begin with 0.25–0.5 mg BID
- IM depot: administer initial injection of 25–37.5 mg
- For IM depot in those with hepatic/renal impairment:
  - Initiate with 0.5 mg BID for one week, then 1 mg BID or 2 mg QD for the second week
  - If tolerated, begin 12.5–25 mg IM every two weeks and continue PO dosing for three weeks after the first IM injection
- For SubQ depot in those with hepatic/renal impairment: (use with caution; has not been studied)
  - Initiate with PO dosing and titrate up to 3 mg QD
- If tolerated and effective, initiate 90 mg SQ monthly

Titration

- Tablets/oral solution:
  - If tolerated and clinically indicated, titrate to a maximum of 4–8 mg daily
  - In elderly or those with hepatic/renal impairment, titration should progress slowly by no more than 0.5 mg BID weekly with increases to dosages >1.5 mg BID occurring at intervals of ≥1 week
- IM depot: if inadequate response, increase by 12.5 mg increments every four weeks to a maximum dose of 50 mg every two weeks

Half-Life

- Tablet/oral solution: 20 hours (prolonged in elderly patients, renal impairment)
- IM depot (biweekly): three to six days
- SubQ (monthly): nine to 11 days

Bioavailability

- 70% bioavailable

Adjustment for Hepatic Dysfunction (by Child-Pugh Criteria)

- Child-Pugh category A or B (mild-moderate hepatic impairment): no dosage adjustment necessary in manufacturer's labeling, but dose reduction may be appropriate
- Child-Pugh category C (severe hepatic impairment): titrate by no more than 0.5 mg BID with increases to dosages >1.5 mg BID occurring at intervals ≥1 week

Adjustment for Renal Dysfunction

- eGFR ≥30 ml/min: no dosage adjustments in manufacturer's labeling, but reduction in dosage may be appropriate
- eGFR <30 mg/min: titrate by no more than 0.5 mg BID with increases to dosages >1.5 mg BID occurring at intervals ≥1 week

H. MEDICATIONS TO AVOID IN COMBINATION/WARNINGS [1–4, 5]

Precautions with cyp 3A4 inducers (may require higher doses)

- Carbamazepine
- Oxcarbazepine
- Phenytoin
- Rifampin

Precautions with cyp 2D6 inhibitors (may require lower doses)

- Bupropion
- Duloxetine
- Paroxetine
- Fluoxetine

Precautions with cyp 3A4 inhibitors (may require lower doses)

- Fluvoxamine
- Ciprofloxacin
- Cimetidine
- Paroxetine
- Fluoxetine
- Ketoconazole

I. MEDICAL PRECAUTIONS AND CONTRAINDICATIONS [1–4, 5]

Use precautions in patients with
- Cerebrovascular disease
- Conditions that predispose to hypotension (e.g. dehydration, hypovolemia, concomitant antihypertensive medications)
- Diabetes mellitus
- Dyslipidemia
- Concomitant use of medications known to cause elevated blood glucose (e.g. steroids, niacin, thiazide diuretics, atypical antipsychotics)
- Severe cardiovascular disease
- Hepatic disease (less important for paliperidone than risperidone due to limited hepatic metabolism)
- Renal impairment
- Active/poorly controlled seizure disorder
- Current/historical tardive dyskinesia
- Pregnancy or breastfeeding
- History of prolactin-sensitive/dependent tumors or other concomitant conditions/ drugs known to elevate prolactin
- Parkinson's disease
- Elderly demented patients with psychosis
- History of leukopenia or neutropenia

⚠ Do NOT Use in patients with
- Hypersensitivity
- Comorbid phenylketonuria (M-tabs contain aspartate)

ART OF PSYCHOPHARMACOLOGY: TAKE-HOME PEARLS

- Risperidone is a well-accepted agent for dementia with aggressive features.
- Risperidone is a well-accepted agent for children with behavioral disturbances but with greater sedation and weight gain than in adult populations.
- Like paliperidone, risperidone may cause more motor side effects than other atypical antipsychotics, especially when administered to patients with Parkinson's disease or Lewy body dementia.
- Like paliperidone, risperidone does not result in full remission of positive psychotic symptoms (only reduces symptoms by approximately 30%) in schizophrenia patients.
- Depot risperidone is not recommended in those who do not show good clinical response to oral formulation.
- Depot risperidone requires simultaneous oral medication for three weeks.

References

1. Indivior Inc. (2019). *Perseris Package Insert*. North Chesterfield, Virginia.
2. Janssen Pharmaceuticals Inc. (2020). *Risperdal Package Insert*. Titusville, New Jersey.
3. Janssen Pharmaceuticals Inc. (2020). *Risperdal M-tab Package Insert*. Titusville, New Jersey.
4. Janssen Pharmaceuticals Inc. (2020). *Risperdal Consta Package Insert*. Titusville, New Jersey.
5. California Department of State Hospitals. (2019). *DSH Psychotropic Medication Policy: Risperidone Protocol*. Sacramento, California.
6. Meyer, J. M. (2001). Effects of atypical antipsychotics on weight and serum lipid levels. *J Clin Psychiatry*, 62 Suppl. 27, 27–34; discussion 40–41.
7. Haddad, P. M., Anderson, I. M. (2002). Antipsychotic-related QTc prolongation, torsade de pointes and sudden death. *Drugs*, 62, 1649–1671.
8. American Diabetes Association, American Psychiatric Association, American Association of Clinical Endocrinologists, et al. (2004). Consensus development conference on antipsychotic drugs and obesity and diabetes. *Obes Res*, 12, 362–368.
9. Jin, H., Meyer, J. M., Jeste, D. V. (2002). Phenomenology of and risk factors for new-onset diabetes mellitus and diabetic ketoacidosis associated with atypical antipsychotics: an analysis of 45 published cases. *Ann Clin Psychiatry*, 14, 59–64.
10. Marder, S. R., Essock, S. M., Miller, A. L., et al. (2004). Physical health monitoring of patients with schizophrenia. *Am J Psychiatry*, 161, 1334–1349.
11. Meyer, J. M. (2017). Converting oral to long-acting injectable antipsychotics: a guide for the perplexed. *CNS Spectr*, 22, 14–28.
12. Meyer, J. M. (2018). Converting oral to long-acting injectable antipsychotics: a guide for the perplexed – CORRIGENDUM. *CNS Spectr*, 23, 186.

2.17 Ziprasidone

A. BASIC INFORMATION [1]

Principle Trade Names
• Geodon®

Legal Status
• Prescription only
• Not controlled

Classifications
• Monoamine antagonist
• Atypical antipsychotic
• Second-generation antipsychotic (SGA)
• Mood stabilizer

Generics Available
• Yes

Formulations
• Capsule: 20 mg; 40 mg; 60 mg; 80 mg
• Solution (IM): 20 mg

FDA Indications
• Schizophrenia
• Bipolar mood disorder

Other Data-Supported Indications
• Other psychotic disorders
• Bipolar mood disorder – acute manic or mixed episodes and maintenance after achieving responder status for two weeks
• Major depressive disorder with current psychotic features
• Severe persistent self-injurious behavior
• Agitation/aggression (severe, acute) associated with psychiatric disorders (e.g. bipolar disorder, schizophrenia), substance intoxication, or other organic causes
• Psychosis/agitation associated with dementia
• Behavioral disturbances in children and adolescents
• Disorders associated with problems with impulse control

B. MECHANISMS OF ACTION [1]

Dopamine
• Antagonism at D_2 receptors may decrease positive psychotic symptoms and contribute to mood stabilization

Serotonin
• Weak activity at serotonin transporter

Epinephrine/norepinephrine
• Weak norepinephrine activity

Initial Target Range
- No established plasma therapeutic range

Range for Treatment Resistance
- No established plasma therapeutic range

Typical Time to Response
- Therapeutic improvement can be seen for 1–20 weeks

Time-Course of Improvement
- If no response by four weeks at maximum tolerated dose, taper and withdraw therapy

Usual Target Symptoms
- Psychosis – positive and negative symptoms
- Cognitive symptoms
- Affective symptoms
- Suicidal behavior
- Violence and aggression

Common Short-Term Adverse Effects
- Akathisia
- Sedation
- Orthostatic hypotension

Rare Adverse Effects
- QT interval prolongation
- Arrhythmia
- Hyperglycemic ketoacidosis
- Priapism

- Type 1 hypersensitivity reactions (anaphylaxis, angioedema, hypotension, tachycardia, swollen tongue, difficulty breathing, wheezing, rash)
- Increased risk of death or cerebrovascular events in elderly patients with dementia-related psychosis
- Neuroleptic malignant syndrome (much reduced risk compared to conventional antipsychotics)

Long-Term Effects
- Akathisia
- Hyperprolactinemia
- Metabolic changes, including weight gain, hyperglycemia, dyslipidemia (very rare, if at all)
- Neurological signs

PRE-TREATMENT WORKUP AND INITIAL LABORATORY TESTING [1, 2, 5, 6]

History
- Obtain personal and family histories of diabetes
- Personal history of:
  - high BMI
  - dyslipidemia (elevated TGs or cholesterol)

Physical
- General physical examination
- Vital signs
- BMI
- Waist circumference

Neurological
- Check for myoclonus or myoclonic jerks
- AIMS
- Neurology consultation if personal history of active, poorly controlled seizure disorder

Blood Tests
Within 30 days:
- Complete metabolic panel
- Fasting blood sugar and Hgb A1c
- Lipid panel

Cardiac Tests
- ECG

Urine Tests
- Urinalysis

Pregnancy Test
- Pregnancy test (premenopausal females)
- Classified as risk not ruled out
- No increased risk in animal studies, except failure to thrive in rat pups

Metabolic Syndrome Parameters
- Elevated waist circumference:
  - Men – greater than 40 inches (102 cm)
  - Women – greater than 35 inches (88 cm)
- Elevated triglycerides: equal to or greater than 150 mg/dl (1.7 mmol/l)
- Reduced HDL ("good") cholesterol:
  - Men – less than 40 mg/dl (1.03 mmol/l)
  - Women – less than 50 mg/dl (1.29 mmol/l)
- Elevated blood pressure: ≥130/80 mm Hg or use of medication for hypertension
- Elevated fasting glucose: equal to or greater than 100 mg/dl (5.6 mmol/l) or use of medication for hyperglycemia

 F. MONITORING [5–9]

Monthly
- Weight
- BMI

Semi-Annually (twice per year)
- Hgb A1c or fasting glucose
- Fasting lipid panel
- BMI

Annually
- ECG
- AIMS
- Waist circumference
- Hgb A1c or fasting glucose
- Nutritional consultation if:
  - waist circumference increases from <35 inches to >35 inches in females OR increases from <40 inches to >40 inches in males
  - weight increases 5% in one month, 7.5% in three months, or 10% in six months
  - BMI increases from normal to overweight (<25 to >25) OR from overweight to obese (25–29.9 to 30 or higher)
- Prolactin level
- Breast exam (both males/females)

G. DOSING AND KINETICS [1, 2, 4]

Initial Dosing

- Administer initial dose of 40–60 mg BID 30 minutes after morning and evening meals

Titration

- If tolerated and clinically indicated, titrate by 20–40 mg daily to a maximum of 240 mg daily

Half-Life

- Adults: 7 hours
- Children: 3.3–4.1 hours

Bioavailability

- Oral: 60% with food
- IM: 100%

Adjustment for Hepatic Dysfunction (by Child-Pugh Criteria)

- No dosage adjustment is recommended
- However, drug undergoes extensive hepatic metabolism and systemic exposure may be increased; use with caution

Adjustment for Renal Dysfunction

- For oral, no dosage adjustment necessary
- For IM, an excipient in the formulation is cleared by renal filtration, so use with caution

H. MEDICATIONS TO AVOID IN COMBINATION/WARNINGS [1, 2]

 Precautions with drugs which have demonstrated QT prolongation

- Dofetilide
- Chlorpromazine
- Haloperidol
- Thioridazine
- Droperidol
- Pimozide

- Sparfloxacin
- Gatifloxacin
- Halofantrine
- Meflozuine
- Pentamidine
- Arsenic trioxide
- Levomethadyl acetate
- Dolasetron mesylate
- Probucol
- Tacrolimus

I. MEDICAL PRECAUTIONS AND CONTRAINDICATIONS [1, 2]

Use precautions in patients with

- Cerebrovascular disease
- Conditions that predispose to hypotension (e.g. dehydration, hypovolemia, concomitant antihypertensive medications)
- Concomitant use of drugs which have demonstrated QT prolongation
- Significant hepatic impairment
- Current/historical tardive dyskinesia
- Historical NMS
- Pregnancy
- History of prolactin-sensitive/dependent tumors or other concomitant conditions/ drugs known to elevate prolactin
- Parkinson's disease
- Significant risk of electrolyte imbalances, especially hypokalemia (e.g. diarrhea, diuretic treatment)
- History of leukopenia or severe neutropenia
- Elderly demented patients with psychosis

⚠ Do NOT Use in patients with

- Hypersensitivity
- Pre-existing prolonged QT prolongation (with persistent findings of QTc interval >450 ms in males or >470 ms in females)
- Recent history of cardiac arrhythmia
- Recent myocardial infarction
- Uncompensated heart failure

ART OF PSYCHOPHARMACOLOGY: TAKE-HOME PEARLS

- Ziprasidone is usually metabolically neutral.
- Ziprasidone rarely, but may, causes QTc prolongation.
- Ziprasidone does not result in full remission of positive psychotic symptoms (only reduces symptoms by approximately 30%) in schizophrenia patients.

- Ziprasidone must be taken with food (500 kcal) for effective absorption.
- Ziprasidone is not recommended in patients who are treatment nonadherent.

References

1. Pfizer Inc. (2020). *Geodon Package Insert.* New York, New York.
2. California Department of State Hospitals. (2019). *DSH Psychotropic Medication Policy: Paliperidone Protocol.* Sacramento, California.
3. Huhn, M., Nikolakopoulou, A., Schneider-Thoma, J., et al. (2019). Comparative efficacy and tolerability of 32 oral antipsychotics for the acute treatment of adults with multi-episode schizophrenia: a systematic review and network meta-analysis. *Lancet*, 394, 939–951.
4. Leucht, S., Crippa, A., Siafis, S., et al. (2020). Dose-response meta-analysis of antipsychotic drugs for acute schizophrenia. *Am J Psychiatry*, 177, 342–353.
5. Meyer, J. M. (2001). Effects of atypical antipsychotics on weight and serum lipid levels. *J Clin Psychiatry*, 62 Suppl. 27, 27–34; discussion 40–41.
6. American Diabetes Association, American Psychiatric Association, American Association of Clinical Endocrinologists, et al. (2004). Consensus development conference on antipsychotic drugs and obesity and diabetes. *Diabetes Care*, 27, 596–601.
7. Aronow, W. S., Shamliyan, T. A. (2018). Effects of atypical antipsychotic drugs on QT interval in patients with mental disorders. *Ann Transl Med*, 6, 147.
8. Beach, S. R., Celano, C. M., Sugrue, A. M., et al. (2018). QT prolongation, Torsades de Pointes, and psychotropic medications: a 5-year update. *Psychosomatics*, 59, 105–122.
9. Pillinger, T., McCutcheon, R. A., Vano, L., et al. (2020). Comparative effects of 18 antipsychotics on metabolic function in patients with schizophrenia, predictors of metabolic dysregulation, and association with psychopathology: a systematic review and network meta-analysis. *Lancet Psychiatry*, 7, 64–77.

Dopamine Partial Agonist Antipsychotics
2.18 Aripiprazole

A. BASIC INFORMATION [1–4]

Principle Trade Names
- Abilify®
- Abilify Maintena®
- Abilify MyCite®
- Aristada®

Legal Status
- Prescription only
- Not controlled

Classifications
- Monoamine partial agonist
- Atypical antipsychotic
- Third-generation antipsychotic (TGA)
- Mood stabilizer

Generics Available
- Yes, excluding depot formulations

Formulations
- Tablet: 2 mg; 5 mg; 10 mg; 15 mg; 20 mg; 30 mg
- Disintegrating tablet: 10 mg; 15 mg
- Solution (IM): 1 mg/ml (150 ml)
- Depot (Abilify Maintena®): 300 mg; 400 mg
- Depot (Aristada®): 441 mg; 662 mg; 882 mg; 1064 mg
- Depot nanocrystals (Aristada Initio®): 675 mg

FDA Indications
- Schizophrenia
- Bipolar mood disorder
- Depression (adjunct)
- Autism-related irritability in children (6–17 years)
- Tourette's disorder in children (6–18 years)

Other Data-Supported Indications
- Other psychotic disorders
- Bipolar depression
- Severe persistent self-injurious behavior
- Agitation/aggression (severe, acute) associated with psychiatric disorders (e.g. bipolar disorder, schizophrenia), substance intoxication, or other organic causes
- Psychosis/agitation associated with dementia
- Behavioral disturbances in children and adolescents
- Disorders associated with problems with impulse control

Dopamine
- Partial agonism at D_2 receptors may decrease positive psychotic symptoms and contribute to mood stabilization
- Partial agonism at D_2 receptors also may cause motor side effects (akathisia), nausea/vomiting and activation

Serotonin
- Partial agonism at $5HT_{1A}$ receptors may reduce impulsivity
- Antagonism at $5HT_{2A}$ receptors may reduce depression

Epinephrine/norepinephrine
- α_1-adrenergic antagonism may cause dizziness, sedation and hypotension

C. PLASMA CONCENTRATIONS AND TREATMENT RESPONSE [6–8]

Initial Target Range
- No established plasma therapeutic range

Range for Treatment Resistance
- No established plasma therapeutic range

Typical Time to Response
- Therapeutic improvement can be seen for 1–20 weeks

Time-Course of Improvement
- If no response by four weeks at maximum tolerated dose, taper and withdraw therapy

D. TYPICAL TREATMENT RESPONSE [1, 2–4, 5]

Usual Target Symptoms
- Psychosis – positive and negative symptoms
- Cognitive symptoms
- Affective symptoms
- Suicidal behavior
- Violence and aggression

Common Short-Term Adverse Effects
- Agitation
- Anorexia
- Blurred vision
- Dyspepsia
- Esophageal dysmotility
- Nausea/vomiting
- Headache
- Insomnia
- Sedation
- Orthostatic hypotension/dizziness

Rare Adverse Effects
- Rare impulse control problems
- Rare seizures

- Type 1 hypersensitivity reactions (anaphylaxis, angioedema, hypotension, tachycardia, swollen tongue, difficulty breathing, wheezing, rash)
- Increased risk of death or cerebrovascular events in elderly patients with dementia-related psychosis
- Neuroleptic malignant syndrome (much reduced risk compared to conventional antipsychotics)
- Rare tardive dyskinesia

Long-Term Effects
- Akathisia
- Constipation
- Hyperprolactinemia
- Metabolic changes, including weight gain, hyperglycemia, dyslipidemia (very rare, if at all)
- Neurological signs

History
- Obtain personal and family histories of diabetes
- Personal history of:
  - high BMI
  - dyslipidemia (elevated TGs or cholesterol)

Physical
- General physical examination
- Vital signs
- BMI
- Waist circumference

Neurological
- Check for myoclonus or myoclonic jerks
- AIMS
- Neurology consultation if personal history of active, poorly controlled seizure disorder

Blood Tests
- Within 30 days:
  - Complete metabolic panel
  - Fasting blood sugar and Hgb A1c
  - Lipid panel

Cardiac Tests
- ECG

Urine Tests
- Urinalysis

Pregnancy Test
- Pregnancy test (premenopausal females)
- Classified as risk not ruled out
- No increased risk in animal studies

Metabolic Syndrome Parameters
- Elevated waist circumference:
  - Men – greater than 40 inches (102 cm)
  - Women – greater than 35 inches (88 cm)
- Elevated triglycerides: equal to or greater than 150 mg/dl (1.7 mmol/l)
- Reduced HDL ("good") cholesterol:
  - Men – less than 40 mg/dl (1.03 mmol/l)
  - Women – less than 50 mg/dl (1.29 mmol/l)
- Elevated blood pressure: ≥130/80 mm Hg or use of medication for hypertension
- Elevated fasting glucose: equal to or greater than 100 mg/dl (5.6 mmol/l) or use of medication for hyperglycemia

Monthly
- Weight
- BMI

Semi-Annually (twice per year)
- Hgb A1c or fasting glucose
- Fasting lipid panel
- BMI

Annually
- ECG
- AIMS
- Waist circumference
- Hgb A1c or fasting glucose

- Nutritional consultation if:
  - waist circumference increases from <35 inches to >35 inches in females OR increases from <40 inches to >40 inches in males
  - weight increases 5% in one month, 7.5% in three months, or 10% in six months
  - BMI increases from normal to overweight (<25 to >25) OR from overweight to obese (25–29.9 to 30 or higher)
- Prolactin level
- Breast exam (both males/females)

Initial Dosing
- Oral: administer initial dose of 5–30 mg daily
- Depot (Maintena®): initial dose of 400 mg IM (gluteal or deltoid) Q-28 days with continued PO aripiprazole 10–20 mg QD for the first 14 days after first injection
- Depot (Aristada®): initial dose of 441 mg (deltoid ok), 662 mg, 882 mg, or 1064 mg (three higher doses via gluteal only) with continued PO aripiprazole for the first 21 days or concurrent dose of Aristada Initio® 675 mg with initial injection

Titration
- Oral: if tolerated and clinically indicated, titrate by 15–30 mg daily to a maximum of 45 mg daily
- Depot:
  - Maintena® – continue 400 mg IM Q-28 days

- Depot:
  - Aristada® 441 mg IM continued Q-28 days
  - Aristada® 662 mg IM continued Q-28 days
  - Aristada® 882 mg IM continued Q-42 days
  - Aristada® 1064 mg IM continued Q-56 days

Half-Life
- Tablet: 75 hours
- Maintena®: 46.5 days
- Aristada®: ~30–47 days

Bioavailability
- Oral: 87%
- IM: 100%

Adjustment for Hepatic Dysfunction (by Child-Pugh Criteria)
- No dosage adjustment is recommended

Adjustment for Renal Dysfunction
- No dosage adjustment necessary

 H. MEDICATIONS TO AVOID IN COMBINATION/WARNINGS [1, 2–4, 7]

 Precautions with strong cyp 3A4 inducers – may require dose increases
- Carbamazepine
- Oxcarbazepine
- Phenytoin
- Phenobarbital
- Primidone
- Some glucocorticoids

 Precautions with strong cyp 3A4 inhibitors – may require dose decreases
- Ketoconazole

 Precautions with strong cyp 2D6 inhibitors – may require dose decreases
- Bupropion
- Paroxetine

- Erythromycin
- Cimetidine
- Fluvoxamine
- Fluoxetine – lowest possible dose if concomitantly prescribed

 Do NOT use depot formulations with strong cyp 3A4 or 2D6 inhibitors
- Ketoconazole
- Bupropion
- Paroxetine
- Erythromycin
- Cimetidine
- Fluvoxamine
- Fluoxetine

I. MEDICAL PRECAUTIONS AND CONTRAINDICATIONS [1, 2–4, 7]

Use precautions in patients with
- Pregnancy
- Historical or current tardive dyskinesia
- History of leukopenia or severe neutropenia
- Elderly demented patients with psychosis

⚠ Do NOT Use in patients with
- Hypersensitivity
- PKU individual taking wafer (contains phenylalanine)
- Dementia and advanced age

 ART OF PSYCHOPHARMACOLOGY: TAKE-HOME PEARLS

- Aripiprazole is usually metabolically neutral.
- Aripiprazole is less sedating than most other antipsychotics.
- Aripiprazole does not result in full remission of positive psychotic symptoms (only reduces symptoms by approximately 30%) in schizophrenia patients.
- Aripiprazole is approved as adjunctive treatment for depression in combination with SSRIs or SNRIs.
- Aripiprazole can be used to reverse hyperprolactinemia/galactorrhea induced by other antipsychotics by reversing the dopamine 2 actions of other antipsychotics.

 ## References

1. Otsuka USA Pharmaceutical Inc. (2017). *Abilify Maintena Package Insert*. Rockville, Maryland.
2. Alkermes Inc. (2020). *Aristada Package Insert*. Wilmington, Ohio.
3. Otsuka USA Pharmaceutical Inc. (2020). *Abilify MyCite Package Insert*. Rockville, Maryland.
4. Otsuka USA Pharmaceutical Inc. (2020). *Abilify Package Insert*. Rockville, Maryland.
5. de la Iglesia-Larrad, J. I., Barral, C., Casado-Espada, N. M., et al. (2019). Benzodiazepine abuse, misuse, dependence, and withdrawal among schizophrenic patients: a review of the literature. *Psychiatry Res*, 284, 112660.
6. Romeo, B., Blecha, L., Locatelli, K., et al. (2018). Meta-analysis and review of dopamine agonists in acute episodes of mood disorder: efficacy and safety. *J Psychopharmacol*, 32, 385–396.
7. California Department of State Hospitals. (2019). *DSH Psychotropic Medication Policy: Aripiprazole Protocol*. Sacramento, California.
8. Leucht, S., Crippa, A., Siafis, S., et al. (2020). Dose-response meta-analysis of antipsychotic drugs for acute schizophrenia. *Am J Psychiatry*, 177, 342–353.
9. Meyer, J. M. (2001). Effects of atypical antipsychotics on weight and serum lipid levels. *J Clin Psychiatry*, 62 Suppl. 27, 27–34; discussion 40–41.
10. American Diabetes Association, American Psychiatric Association, American Association of Clinical Endocrinologists, et al. (2004). Consensus development conference on antipsychotic drugs and obesity and diabetes. *Diabetes Care*, 27, 596–601.
11. Marder, S. R., Essock, S. M., Miller, A. L., et al. (2004). Physical health monitoring of patients with schizophrenia. *Am J Psychiatry*, 161, 1334–1349.

2.19 Brexpiprazole

Principle Trade Names
• Rexulti®

Legal Status
• Prescription only
• Not controlled

Classifications
• Monoamine partial agonist
• Atypical antipsychotic
• Third-generation antipsychotic (TGA)
• Mood stabilizer

Generics Available
• Yes

Formulations
• Tablet: 0.25 mg; 0.5 mg; 1 mg; 2 mg; 3 mg; 4 mg

FDA Indications
• Schizophrenia
• Treatment-resistant depression (adjunct)

Other Data-Supported Indications
• Other psychotic disorders
• Acute mania/mixed mania
• Bipolar maintenance
• Bipolar depression
• Severe persistent self-injurious behavior
• Agitation/aggression (severe, acute) associated with psychiatric disorders (e.g. bipolar disorder, schizophrenia), substance intoxication, or other organic causes
• Psychosis/agitation associated with dementia
• Behavioral disturbances in children and adolescents
• Disorders associated with problems with impulse control

B. MECHANISMS OF ACTION [1]

Dopamine
• Partial agonism at D_2 receptors may decrease positive psychotic symptoms and contribute to mood stabilization
• Partial agonism at D_2 receptors also may cause motor side effects (akathisia), nausea/vomiting and activation

Serotonin
• Partial agonism at $5HT_{1A}$ receptors may reduce impulsivity
• Antagonism at $5HT_{2A}$ and $5HT_7$ receptors may improve mood and cognition

Epinephrine/norepinephrine
• α_1-adrenergic antagonism may cause dizziness, sedation and hypotension

Initial Target Range
• No established plasma therapeutic range

Range for Treatment Resistance
• No established plasma therapeutic range

Typical Time to Response
• Therapeutic improvement can be seen for 1–20 weeks

Time-Course of Improvement
• If no response by four weeks at maximum tolerated dose, taper and withdraw therapy

Usual Target Symptoms
• Psychosis – positive and negative symptoms
• Cognitive symptoms
• Affective symptoms
• Suicidal behavior
• Violence and aggression

Common Short-Term Adverse Effects
• Agitation
• Anorexia
• Anxiety
• Blurred vision
• Dyspepsia
• Esophageal dysmotility
• Nausea/vomiting
• Headache
• Sedation
• Orthostatic hypotension/dizziness

Rare Adverse Effects
• Rare impulse control problems
• Rare seizures

• Type 1 hypersensitivity reactions (anaphylaxis, angioedema, hypotension, tachycardia, swollen tongue, difficulty breathing, wheezing, rash)
• Increased risk of death or cerebrovascular events in elderly patients with dementia-related psychosis
• Neuroleptic malignant syndrome (much reduced risk compared to conventional antipsychotics)
• Rare tardive dyskinesia

Long-Term Effects
• Akathisia
• Constipation
• Hyperprolactinemia
• Metabolic changes, including weight gain, hyperglycemia, dyslipidemia (very rare, if at all)
• Neurological signs

History
- Obtain personal and family histories of diabetes
- Personal history of:
  - high BMI
  - dyslipidemia (elevated TGs or cholesterol)

Physical
- General physical examination
- Vital signs
- BMI
- Waist circumference

Neurological
- Check for myoclonus or myoclonic jerks
- AIMS
- Neurology consultation if personal history of active, poorly controlled seizure disorder

Blood Tests
Within 30 days:
- Complete metabolic panel
- Fasting blood sugar and Hgb A1c
- Lipid panel

Cardiac Tests
- ECG

Urine Tests
- Urinalysis

Pregnancy Test
- Pregnancy test (premenopausal females)
- Classified as risk not ruled out
- No increased risk in animal studies

Metabolic Syndrome Parameters
- Elevated waist circumference:
  - Men – greater than 40 inches (102 cm)
  - Women – greater than 35 inches (88 cm)
- Elevated triglycerides: equal to or greater than 150 mg/dl (1.7 mmol/l)
- Reduced HDL ("good") cholesterol:
  - Men – less than 40 mg/dl (1.03 mmol/l)
  - Women – less than 50 mg/dl (1.29 mmol/l)
- Elevated blood pressure: ≥130/80 mm Hg or use of medication for hypertension
- Elevated fasting glucose: equal to or greater than 100 mg/dl (5.6 mmol/l) or use of medication for hyperglycemia

Monthly
- Weight
- BMI

Semi-Annually (twice per year)
- Hgb A1c or fasting glucose
- Fasting lipid panel
- BMI

Annually
- ECG
- AIMS
- Waist circumference
- Hgb A1c or fasting glucose

- Nutritional consultation if:
  - waist circumference increases from <35 inches to >35 inches in females OR increases from <40 inches to >40 inches in males
  - weight increases 5% in one month, 7.5% in three months, or 10% in six months
  - BMI increases from normal to overweight (<25 to >25) OR from overweight to obese (25–29.9 to 30 or higher)
- Prolactin level
- Breast exam (both males/females)

G. DOSING AND KINETICS [1, 2]

Initial Dosing
- Administer initial dose of 1–2 mg daily

Titration
- If tolerated and clinically indicated, titrate up to 3 mg daily for adjunctive treatment of depression
- If tolerated and clinically indicated, titrate up to 4 mg daily for psychosis

Half-Life
- 91 hours

Bioavailability
- 95%

Adjustment for Hepatic Dysfunction (by Child-Pugh Criteria)
- Child-Pugh category A: no dosage adjustments
- Child-Pugh category B or C, maximum:
  - Major depressive disorder: 2 mg once daily
  - Schizophrenia: 3 mg daily

Adjustment for Renal Dysfunction
- CrCl ≥60 ml/min: no dose adjustment necessary
- CrCl <60 ml/min, maximum:
  - Major depressive disorder: 2 mg once daily
  - Schizophrenia: 3 mg daily

 H. MEDICATIONS TO AVOID IN COMBINATION/WARNINGS [1, 2]

 ### Precautions with strong cyp 3A4 inducers – may require dose increases
- Carbamazepine
- Oxcarbazepine
- Phenytoin
- Phenobarbital
- Primidone
- Some glucocorticoids

 ### Precautions with strong cyp 3A4 inhibitors – may require dose decreases
- Ketoconazole

 ### Precautions with strong cyp 2D6 inhibitors – may require dose decreases
- Bupropion
- Paroxetine
- Erythromycin
- Cimetidine
- Fluvoxamine
- Fluoxetine – lowest possible dose if concomitantly prescribed

 I. MEDICAL PRECAUTIONS AND CONTRAINDICATIONS [1, 2]

Use precautions in patients with
- Pregnancy
- Historical or current tardive dyskinesia
- History of leukopenia or severe neutropenia
- Elderly demented patients with psychosis

 ART OF PSYCHOPHARMACOLOGY: TAKE-HOME PEARLS

- Brexpiprazole is usually metabolically neutral.
- Brexpiprazole is less sedating than most other antipsychotics.
- Brexpiprazole does not result in full remission of positive psychotic symptoms (only reduces symptoms by approximately 30%) in schizophrenia patients.
- Brexpiprazole is approved as adjunctive treatment for depression in combination with SSRIs or SNRIs.

2.19 Brexpiprazole (Continued)

 References

1. Otsuka USA Pharmaceutical Inc. (2020). *Rexulti Package Insert.* Deerfield, Illinois.
2. California Department of State Hospitals. (2019). *DSH Psychotropic Medication Policy: Brexpiprazole Protocol.* Sacramento, California.
3. Meyer, J. M. (2001). Effects of atypical antipsychotics on weight and serum lipid levels. *J Clin Psychiatry*, 62 Suppl. 27, 27–34; discussion 40–41.
4. American Diabetes Association, American Psychiatric Association, American Association of Clinical Endocrinologists, et al. (2004). Consensus development conference on antipsychotic drugs and obesity and diabetes. *Diabetes Care*, 27, 596–601.
5. Marder, S. R., Essock, S. M., Miller, A. L., et al. (2004). Physical health monitoring of patients with schizophrenia. *Am J Psychiatry*, 161, 1334–1349.

2.20 Cariprazine

A. BASIC INFORMATION [1]

Principle Trade Names
- Vraylar®

Legal Status
- Prescription only
- Not controlled

Classifications
- Monoamine partial agonist
- Atypical antipsychotic
- Third-generation antipsychotic (TGA)
- Mood stabilizer

Generics Available
- Yes

Formulations
- Capsule: 1.5 mg; 3 mg; 4.5 mg; 6 mg

FDA Indications
- Schizophrenia
- Acute mania/mixed mania

Other Data-Supported Indications
- Other psychotic disorders
- Bipolar maintenance
- Bipolar depression
- Treatment-resistant depression
- Severe persistent self-injurious behavior
- Agitation/aggression (severe, acute) associated with psychiatric disorders (e.g. bipolar disorder, schizophrenia), substance intoxication, or other organic causes
- Psychosis/agitation associated with dementia
- Behavioral disturbances in children and adolescents
- Disorders associated with problems with impulse control

Dopamine

- Partial agonism at D_2 receptors may decrease positive psychotic symptoms and contribute to mood stabilization
- Partial agonism at D_2 receptors also may cause motor side effects (akathisia), nausea/vomiting and activation

Serotonin

- Partial agonism at $5HT_{1A}$ receptors may reduce impulsivity
- Antagonism at $5HT_{2A}$ and $5HT_7$ receptors may improve mood and cognition

Epinephrine/norepinephrine

- α_1-adrenergic antagonism may cause dizziness, sedation and hypotension

Initial Target Range

- No established plasma therapeutic range

Range for Treatment Resistance

- No established plasma therapeutic range

Typical Time to Response

- Therapeutic improvement can be seen for 1–20 weeks

Time-Course of Improvement

- If no response by four weeks at maximum tolerated dose, taper and withdraw therapy

Usual Target Symptoms

- Psychosis – positive and negative symptoms
- Cognitive symptoms
- Affective symptoms
- Suicidal behavior
- Violence and aggression

Common Short-Term Adverse Effects

- Agitation
- Anorexia
- Anxiety
- Blurred vision
- Dyspepsia
- Esophageal dysmotility
- Nausea/vomiting
- Headache
- Sedation
- Orthostatic hypotension/dizziness

Rare Adverse Effects

- Rare impulse control problems
- Rare seizures

- Type 1 hypersensitivity reactions (anaphylaxis, angioedema, hypotension, tachycardia, swollen tongue, difficulty breathing, wheezing, rash)
- Increased risk of death or cerebrovascular events in elderly patients with dementia-related psychosis
- Neuroleptic malignant syndrome (much reduced risk compared to conventional antipsychotics)
- Rare tardive dyskinesia

Long-Term Effects

- Akathisia
- Constipation
- Hyperprolactinemia
- Metabolic changes, including weight gain, hyperglycemia, dyslipidemia (very rare, if at all)
- Neurological signs

History
• Obtain personal and family histories of diabetes
• Personal history of:
  ○ high BMI
  ○ dyslipidemia (elevated TGs or cholesterol)

Physical
• General physical examination
• Vital signs
• BMI
• Waist circumference

Neurological
• Check for myoclonus or myoclonic jerks
• AIMS
• Neurology consultation if personal history of active, poorly controlled seizure disorder

Blood Tests
Within 30 days:
• Complete metabolic panel
• Fasting blood sugar and Hgb A1c
• Lipid panel

Cardiac Tests
• ECG

Urine Tests
• Urinalysis

Pregnancy Test
• Pregnancy test (premenopausal females)
• Classified as risk not ruled out
• No increased risk in animal studies

Metabolic Syndrome Parameters
• Elevated waist circumference:
  ○ Men – greater than 40 inches (102 cm)
  ○ Women – greater than 35 inches (88 cm)
• Elevated triglycerides: equal to or greater than 150 mg/dl (1.7 mmol/l)
• Reduced HDL ("good") cholesterol:
  ○ Men – less than 40 mg/dl (1.03 mmol/l)
  ○ Women – less than 50 mg/dl (1.29 mmol/l)
• Elevated blood pressure: ≥130/80 mm Hg or use of medication for hypertension
• Elevated fasting glucose: equal to or greater than 100 mg/dl (5.6 mmol/l) or use of medication for hyperglycemia

Monthly
• Weight
• BMI

Semi-Annually (twice per year)
• Hgb A1c or fasting glucose
• Fasting lipid panel
• BMI

Annually
• ECG
• AIMS
• Waist circumference
• Hgb A1c or fasting glucose

• Nutritional consultation if:
  ○ waist circumference increases from <35 inches to >35 inches in females OR increases from <40 inches to >40 inches in males
  ○ weight increases 5% in one month, 7.5% in three months, or 10% in six months
  ○ BMI increases from normal to overweight (<25 to >25) OR from overweight to obese (25–29.9 to 30 or higher)
• Prolactin level
• Breast exam (both males/females)

Initial Dosing
• Administer initial dose of 1.5–3 mg daily

Titration
• If tolerated and clinically indicated, titrate up to 6 mg daily

Half-Life
• Two to five days (parent drug)
• Circa 18 days (active metabolite)

Bioavailability
• High oral bioavailability

Adjustment for Hepatic Dysfunction (by Child-Pugh Criteria)
• Child-Pugh category A: no dosage adjustments
• Child-Pugh category B or C: use not recommended

Adjustment for Renal Dysfunction
• CrCl ≥60 ml/min: no dose adjustment necessary
• CrCl <60 ml/min: use not recommended

H. MEDICATIONS TO AVOID IN COMBINATION/WARNINGS [1, 2]

 Precautions with strong cyp 3A4 inducers – may require dose increases
• Carbamazepine
• Oxcarbazepine
• Phenytoin
• Phenobarbital
• Primidone
• Some glucocorticoids

 Precautions with strong cyp 3A4 inhibitors – may require dose decreases
• Ketoconazole

 Precautions with strong cyp 2D6 inhibitors – may require dose decreases
• Bupropion
• Paroxetine
• Erythromycin
• Cimetidine
• Fluvoxamine
• Fluoxetine – lowest possible dose if concomitantly prescribed

I. MEDICAL PRECAUTIONS AND CONTRAINDICATIONS [1, 2]

Use precautions in patients with
• Pregnancy
• Historical or current tardive dyskinesia
• History of leukopenia or severe neutropenia
• Elderly demented patients with psychosis

ART OF PSYCHOPHARMACOLOGY: TAKE-HOME PEARLS

• Cariprazine is usually metabolically neutral.
• Cariprazine is less sedating than most other antipsychotics.

• Cariprazine does not result in full remission of positive psychotic symptoms (only reduces symptoms by approximately 30%) in schizophrenia patients.

References

1. Allergan USA Inc. (2019). *Vraylar Package Insert*. Madison, New Jersey.
2. California Department of State Hospitals. (2019). *DSH Psychotropic Medication Policy: Ziprasidone Protocol*. Sacramento, California.
3. Leucht, S., Crippa, A., Siafis, S., et al. (2020). Dose-response meta-analysis of antipsychotic drugs for acute schizophrenia. *Am J Psychiatry*, 177, 342–353.
4. Cutler, A. J., Durgam, S., Wang, Y., et al. (2018). Evaluation of the long-term safety and tolerability of cariprazine in patients with schizophrenia: results from a 1-year open-label study. *CNS Spectr*, 23, 39–50.
5. Azorin, J. M., Simon, N. (2019). Dopamine receptor partial agonists for the treatment of bipolar disorder. *Drugs*, 79, 1657–1677.
6. Earley, W., Burgess, M. V., Rekeda, L., et al. (2019). Cariprazine treatment of bipolar depression: a randomized double-blind placebo-controlled phase 3 study. *Am J Psychiatry*, 176, 439–448.
7. Chakrabarty, T., Keramatian, K., Yatham, L. N. (2020). Treatment of mixed features in bipolar disorder: an updated view. *Curr Psychiatry Rep*, 22, 15.
8. Meyer, J. M. (2001). Effects of atypical antipsychotics on weight and serum lipid levels. *J Clin Psychiatry*, 62 Suppl. 27, 27–34; discussion 40–41.
9. American Diabetes Association, American Psychiatric Association, American Association of Clinical Endocrinologists, et al. (2004). Consensus development conference on antipsychotic drugs and obesity and diabetes. *Diabetes Care*, 27, 596–601.
10. Marder, S. R., Essock, S. M., Miller, A. L., et al. (2004). Physical health monitoring of patients with schizophrenia. *Am J Psychiatry*, 161, 1334–1349.

Medications for Motor/Neurologic Adverse Effects

2.21 Amantadine

A. BASIC INFORMATION [1–8]

Principle Trade Names
- Gocovri®
- Osmolex®
- Symadine®
- Symmetrel®

Legal Status
- Prescription only
- Not controlled

Classifications
- Antiviral
- Anti-Parkinsonian (dyskinesia)

Generics Available
- Yes, for immediate-release tablets and syrup

Formulations
- Tablets (oral immediate-release): 100 mg
- Capsules (oral osmotic capsule): 129 mg; 193 mg; 258 mg
- Capsule (extended-release): 68.5 mg; 137 mg
- Syrup (oral): 50 mg/5 ml

FDA Indications
- Antiviral for influenza, type A (no longer recommended)
- Parkinsonism (dyskinesia)

Other Data-Supported Indications
- Antipsychotic-induced dystonia or parkinsonism
- Tardive dyskinesia
- Other tardive motor syndromes (sparse data)
- Mitigation of antipsychotic-induced weight gain
- Multiple sclerosis-associated fatigue

Antiviral
- Antagonism of influenza virus A M_2 proton channel, inhibiting viral replication
- 100% of tested influenza A strains has become resistant to this mechanism of action
- Ineffective against influenza B

Acetylcholine
- Antagonist at nicotinic α_7 receptors
- Modest antagonist at muscarinic receptors

Dopamine
- Modestly increases dopamine release
- Moderately blocks dopamine reuptake

- These mechanisms likely account for beneficial motor effects

Enkephalin
- Agonist at σ opioid receptors
- Likely promotes dopamine release

Epinephrine and norepinephrine
- Moderately increases release

Glutamate
- Noncompetitive antagonist at NMDA receptors
- Decreases calcium influx at the NMDA calcium channel, dampening cell excitation
- Mechanism is similar to that of memantine

C. PLASMA CONCENTRATIONS AND TREATMENT RESPONSE [8, 12, 13, 14]

Initial Target Range
- No established therapeutic plasma concentration range

Range for Treatment Resistance
- No established therapeutic plasma concentration range

Typical Time to Response
- Acute Parkinsonian, dyskinetic and dystonic symptoms typically show improvement over two to seven days

- Dyskinetic movements in tardive dyskinesia may begin to improve more slowly but may continue to improve over several weeks

Time-Course of Improvement
- If no improvement is seen after two to four weeks at maximum dosing, then withdraw the treatment
- In tardive dyskinesia, biweekly (every two weeks) AIMS examinations across the first six to twelve weeks of treatment may be beneficial in judging treatment efficacy. In research trials, the average reduction in AIMS scores was 15%

D. TYPICAL TREATMENT RESPONSE [1, 8, 13, 15]

Usual Target Symptoms
- Muscle rigidity
- Dyskinetic movements
- Dystonic tremor
- Bradykinesia
- Fatigue in multiple sclerosis

Common Short-Term Adverse Effects
- Dry mouth
- Dysphoria and anxiety
- Headache
- Increased pulse and blood pressure transient during titration
- Dizziness
- Post-dose nausea
- Constipation
- Diarrhea
- Drowsiness
- Anxiety dreams

Rare Adverse Effects
- Hallucinosis
- Compulsive behaviors, including gambling and sexual behaviors
- Suicidal ideation
- Déjà vu, especially when combined with other dopaminergic agents
- Dependent edema
- Stevens-Johnson Syndrome
- Livedo reticularis (very rare)
- Anticholinergic delirium in overdose
- Death in overdoses > one gram (very rare)

Long-Term Effects
- Generally well tolerated in long-term treatment
- May accumulate in the context of progressive renal disease

History
- Personal history of renal disease
- Familial history of renal disease

Physical
- Current findings suggestive of urinary tract disease (e.g. fever associated with lower back pain, urinary frequency or dysuria)
- Prostatic enlargement
- Gross hematuria
- Cloudy urine

Neurological
- Single or polyfocal tics
- Unstable seizure disorder

Blood Tests
- Electrolytes
- BUN, creatinine and eGFR

Cardiac Tests
- ECG if evidence of unstable cardiovascular disease

Urine Tests
- Urinalysis
- Renal ultrasound if kidney disease (e.g. polycystic disease suspected)

Pregnancy Test
- Pregnancy test (premenopausal females)
- Classified as risk not ruled out

During titration or after dose adjustments
- Check status of target symptoms after one to two weeks
- For tardive dyskinesia, monitor periodic AIMS scores to track efficacy
- Check for common adverse effects as clinically indicated or after dose adjustment

Maintenance
- Recheck target symptoms as clinically indicated but at least annually
- Recheck BUN, creatinine and EGFR every six to twelve months or more frequently if the initial EGFR was <70 ml/min
- Recheck for emergence of adverse effects at least annually

Initial Dosing
- For immediate-release formulations, the typical initial dose is 100 mg QAM
- For extended-release formulations:
  ◦ Gocovri®): initially give 137 mg q bedtime
  ◦ (Osmolex®): initially give 129 mg q bedtime

Titration
- Increase immediate-release by 100 mg per week to as much as 100 mg TID or 200 mg BID
- Increase ER formulations weekly as needed to as much as 274 mg (Gocovri®) or 193 mg or 258 mg (Osmolex®) q bedtime

Half-Life
- 10–31 hours

Bioavailability
- 86–90%
- 67% protein-bound

Adjustment for Hepatic Dysfunction (by Child-Pugh Criteria)
- Minimal hepatic metabolism (mostly acetylation)
- No adjustment required

Adjustment for Renal Dysfunction
- Depends entirely on renal clearance
- Contraindicated in end-stage renal disease

H. MEDICATIONS TO AVOID IN COMBINATION/WARNINGS [11, 19]

 Dopaminergic stimulants

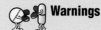 **Warnings**

- Use with caution, as the combination may promote déjà vu, hallucinosis, loss of appetite or worsening of a primary psychotic disorder

- Contraindicated in end-stage renal disease, as amantadine depends entirely on renal clearance

 ART OF PSYCHOPHARMACOLOGY: TAKE-HOME PEARLS

- Amantadine can provide an effective treatment of antipsychotic-induced neurologic symptoms without increasing anticholinergic burden.

- Amantadine can modestly reduce dyskinetic movements in tardive dyskinesia.
- Amantadine may mitigate against antipsychotic-induced weight gain.

References

1. Blanchet, P. J., Metman, L. V., Chase, T. N. (2003). Renaissance of amantadine in the treatment of Parkinson's disease. *Adv Neurol*, 91, 251–257.
2. da Silva-Junior, F. P., Braga-Neto, P., Sueli Monte, F., et al. (2005). Amantadine reduces the duration of levodopa-induced dyskinesia: a randomized, double-blind, placebo-controlled study. *Parkinsonism Relat Disord*, 11, 449–452.
3. Citrome, L. (2016). Emerging pharmacological therapies in schizophrenia: what's new, what's different, what's next? *CNS Spectr*, 21, 1–12.
4. Duwe, S. (2017). Influenza viruses – antiviral therapy and resistance. *GMS Infect Dis*, 5, Doc04.
5. Yang, T. T., Wang, L., Deng, X. Y., et al. (2017). Pharmacological treatments for fatigue in patients with multiple sclerosis: a systematic review and meta-analysis. *J Neurol Sci*, 380, 256–261.
6. Zheng, W., Wang, S., Ungvari, G. S., et al. (2017). Amantadine for antipsychotic-related weight gain: meta-analysis of randomized placebo-controlled trials. *J Clin Psychopharmacol*, 37, 341–346.
7. Elkurd, M. T., Bahroo, L. B., Pahwa, R. (2018). The role of extended-release amantadine for the treatment of dyskinesia in Parkinson's disease patients. *Neurodegener Dis Manag*, 8, 73–80.
8. Hirjak, D., Kubera, K. M., Bienentreu, S., et al. (2019). Antipsychotic-induced motor symptoms in schizophrenic psychoses – Part 1: dystonia, akathisia and parkinsonism. *Nervenarzt*, 90, 1–11.
9. Deleu, D., Northway, M. G., Hanssens, Y. (2002). Clinical pharmacokinetic and pharmacodynamic properties of drugs used in the treatment of Parkinson's disease. *Clin Pharmacokinet*, 41, 261–309.
10. Musharrafieh, R., Ma, C., Wang, J. (2020). Discovery of M2 channel blockers targeting the drug-resistant double mutants M2-S31 N/L26I and M2-S31 N/V27A from the influenza A viruses. *Eur J Pharm Sci*, 141, 105124.
11. PubChem. (2020). Amantadine, CID = 2130. Available from: https://pubchem.ncbi.nlm.nih.gov/compound/amantadine (last accessed November 27, 2020).
12. Paik, J., Keam, S. J. (2018). Amantadine extended-release (GOCOVRI): a review in levodopa-induced dyskinesia in Parkinson's disease. *CNS Drugs*, 32, 797–806.
13. Mazzucchi, S., Frosini, D., Bonuccelli, U., et al. (2015). Current treatment and future prospects of dopa-induced dyskinesias. *Drugs Today (Barc)*, 51, 315–329.
14. Lin, C. C., Ondo, W. G. (2018). Non-VMAT2 inhibitor treatments for the treatment of tardive dyskinesia. *J Neurol Sci*, 389, 48–54.
15. Pahwa, R., Tanner, C. M., Hauser, R. A., et al. (2015). Amantadine extended release for levodopa-induced dyskinesia in Parkinson's disease (EASED Study). *Mov Disord*, 30, 788–795.
16. Faulkner, M. A. (2014). Safety overview of FDA-approved medications for the treatment of the motor symptoms of Parkinson's disease. *Expert Opin Drug Saf*, 13, 1055–1069.
17. Dubaz, O. M., Wu, S., Cubillos, F., et al. (2019). Changes in prescribing practices of dopaminergic medications in individuals with Parkinson's disease by expert care centers from 2010 to 2017: The Parkinson's Foundation Quality Improvement Initiative. *Mov Disord Clin Pract*, 6, 687–692.
18. Aoki, F. Y., Sitar, D. S. (1988). Clinical pharmacokinetics of amantadine hydrochloride. *Clin Pharmacokinet*, 14, 35–51.
19. Perez-Lloret, S., Rascol, O. (2018). Efficacy and safety of amantadine for the treatment of L-DOPA-induced dyskinesia. *J Neural Transm (Vienna)*, 125, 1237–1250.

2.22 Benztropine

A. BASIC INFORMATION [1–6]

Principle Trade Names
• Cogentin®

Legal Status
• Prescription only
• Not controlled

Classifications
• Anticholinergic
• Anti-Parkinsonian (second-line)

Generics Available
• Yes

Formulations
• Oral Tablets: 0.5 mg; 1 mg; 2 mg
• Injectable: 1 mg/ml

FDA Indications
• Parkinsonism

Other Data-Supported Indications
• Acute dystonia
• Dystonic tremor
• Rabbit syndrome (a tardive dystonic tremor)
• Prevention of cholinergic rebound
• Sialorrhea

B. MECHANISMS OF ACTION [6, 7–9]

Acetylcholine
• Antagonist at muscarinic receptors, especially M_1 and M_3

Dopamine
• Indirectly decreases dopamine reuptake

Histamine
• Modest antagonist at histamine H_1 receptors

Myelin
• May stimulate oligodendrogliocytes to produce more myelin (e.g. in multiple sclerosis)

C. PLASMA CONCENTRATIONS AND TREATMENT RESPONSE [10, 11]

Initial Target Range
• No established therapeutic range

Range for Treatment Resistance
• No established therapeutic range

Typical Time to Response
• Less than 60 minutes with oral administration
• Less than 30 minutes with intramuscular administration
• Less than 10 minutes with intravenous administration

D. TYPICAL TREATMENT RESPONSE [6, 10, 11, 12–14]

Usual Target Symptoms
- Parkinsonism, including bradykinesia, rigidity, tremor, hypophonia and festinating gait
- Acute medication-induced dystonia
- Dystonic tremor
- Sialorrhea

Common Short-Term Adverse Effects
- Decreased memory consolidation
- Decreased concentration
- Drowsiness
- Blurred near vision (loss of accommodation)
- Dry mouth
- Constipation

Rare Adverse Effects
- Altered sense of time
- Acute angle closure glaucoma
- Anticholinergic delirium
- Paralytic ileus/bowel obstruction
- Urinary retention (aggravated by BPH)
- Anhidrosis
- Hyperthermia (aggravated by hot weather)

Long-Term Effects
- Increased dental caries with prolonged xerostomia
- Questionable acceleration of neurocognitive disorders

E. PRE-TREATMENT WORKUP AND INITIAL LABORATORY TESTING [2, 3, 8, 15]

History
- Narrow-angle or angle closure glaucoma
- Present xerostomia
- Constipation/ileus/bowel obstruction
- BPH or urinary retention
- Anhidrosis or hyperthermia
- Delirium or neurocognitive disorder (dementia)

Physical
- Vitals, especially pulse rate and temperature
- Check for dry mucous membranes, flushed face, dilated pupils
- Check for physical signs of constipation/fecal impaction/bowel obstruction
- Check for bladder distention

Neurological
- Delirium, as reflected by fluctuating level of consciousness, confusion, disorientation, and possible hallucinosis
- Neurocognitive disorder, as reflected by memory impairments, cognitive impairments, language impairments, deficits in executive functions, disorientation, and possible behavioral disturbances or psychosis

Blood Tests
- Liver function tests if hepatic impairment suspected

Cardiac Tests
- ECG if significant tachycardia present or known cardiac disease is present

Urine Tests
- Measurement of residual urine if retention suspected

Pregnancy Test
- Pregnancy test (premenopausal females)
- Classified as risk not ruled out

Other Tests (ECG, etc.)
- KUB if fecal impaction/paralytic ileus/bowel obstruction suspected
- ECG if significant tachycardia or known cardiovascular disease

F. MONITORING [16–18]

Titration or After Dose Adjustment
- Check for common adverse effects, as most are dose-dependent
- Check pulse rate and temperature

Maintenance
- Recheck periodically for common adverse effects

- Periodically monitor bowel function
- In circa 70% of cases where anticholinergic medications were initiated to treat medication-induced neurological symptoms, the anticholinergic can be tapered and discontinued after three months without recurrence of neurological adverse effects

G. DOSING AND KINETICS [6, 19]

Titration
- If well tolerated, increase dose by 0.5–1.0 mg BID or TID
- Maximum recommended dose is 2.0 mg TID
- For PRN use: 0.5–2.0 mg PO, IM or IV (slow push)
- For routine use: 0.5–2.0 mg PO or IM BID

Half-Life
- 12–24 hours

Bioavailability
- Oral: undetermined (low), but incompletely absorbed with multiple metabolites
- Injectable: 100%

Adjustment for Hepatic Dysfunction (by Child-Pugh Criteria)
- No dose adjustment for categories A or B
- Contraindicated for category C

Adjustment for Renal Dysfunction
- None per the PI but may require dose reduction in end-stage renal disease

H. MEDICATIONS TO AVOID IN COMBINATION/WARNINGS [14, 20–22, 23]

 Antipsychotics

- Use with caution in combination with highly anticholinergic antipsychotics, e.g. chlorpromazine, clozapine, olanzapine, quetiapine, etc.

 Antidepressants

- Use with caution in combination with highly anticholinergic antidepressants, e.g. tricyclic antidepressants

 Muscarinic Antagonists

- Avoid combining multiple muscarinic receptor antagonists, as anticholinergic effects are additive

 Sympathomimetics

- Avoid combined use in cases where angle closure glaucoma, significant tachycardia or hyperthermia are risks

 Opioids

- Combined use substantially increases risks of constipation, fecal impaction, paralytic ileus and bowel obstruction

 Warnings

- May induce acute narrow-angle glaucoma
- Do not use in delirium, except in cholinergic rebound delirium, e.g. after abrupt clozapine discontinuation
- Do not use in neurocognitive disorders

ART OF PSYCHOPHARMACOLOGY: TAKE-HOME POINTS

- Anticholinergic medications, like benztropine, are excellent rescue medications for acute dystonia or parkinsonism; however, long-term use should be avoided. If long-term treatment for dystonia is needed, consider a trial of amantadine.
- Anticholinergic medications typically worsen tardive movement disorders (e.g. tardive dyskinesia), except for "rabbit syndrome"

which is a vertical 5 Hz dystonic tremor of the nose and upper lip.
- Give a tapering dose after abrupt discontinuation of clozapine to avert cholinergic rebound. A typical taper would be 2 mg BID then decreased by 0.5 mg per week to discontinuation.
- Benztropine is prone to diversion and abuse in forensic settings.

References

1. Szafranski, T., Gmurkowski, K. (1999). Clozapine withdrawal. A review. *Psychiatr Pol*, 33, 51–67.
2. Faulkner, M. A. (2014). Safety overview of FDA-approved medications for the treatment of the motor symptoms of Parkinson's disease. *Expert Opin Drug Saf*, 13, 1055–1069.
3. Thenganatt, M. A., Jankovic, J. (2014). Treatment of dystonia. *Neurotherapeutics*, 11, 139–152.
4. Sridharan, K., Sivaramakrishnan, G. (2018). Pharmacological interventions for treating sialorrhea associated with neurological disorders: a mixed treatment network meta-analysis of randomized controlled trials. *J Clin Neurosci*, 51, 12–17.
5. Orayj, K., Lane, E. (2019). Patterns and determinants of prescribing for Parkinson's disease: a systematic literature review. *Parkinsons Dis*, 2019, 9237181.
6. PubChem. (2020). Benztropine, CID = 238053. Retrieved April 21, 2020.
7. Modell, J. G., Tandon, R., Beresford, T. P. (1989). Dopaminergic activity of the antimuscarinic antiparkinsonian agents. *J Clin Psychopharmacol*, 9, 347–351.
8. Deleu, D., Northway, M. G., Hanssens, Y. (2002). Clinical pharmacokinetic and pharmacodynamic properties of drugs used in the treatment of Parkinson's disease. *Clin Pharmacokinet*, 41, 261–309.
9. Green, A. J. (2014). The best basic science paper in MS in 2013: antimuscarinic therapies in remyelination. *Mult Scler*, 20, 1814–1816.
10. Robottom, B. J., Weiner, W. J., Factor, S. A. (2011). Movement disorders emergencies. Part 1: Hypokinetic disorders. *Arch Neurol*, 68, 567–572.
11. Rajan, S., Kaas, B., Moukheiber, E. (2019). Movement disorders emergencies. *Semin Neurol*, 39, 125–136.
12. Mazzucchi, S., Frosini, D., Bonuccelli, U., et al. (2015). Current treatment and future prospects of dopa-induced dyskinesias. *Drugs Today (Barc)*, 51, 315–329.
13. Barbe, A. G. (2018). Medication-induced xerostomia and hyposalivation in the elderly: culprits, complications, and management. *Drugs Aging*, 35, 877–885.
14. Andre, L., Gallini, A., Montastruc, F., et al. (2019). Association between anticholinergic (atropinic) drug exposure and cognitive function in longitudinal studies among individuals over 50 years old: a systematic review. *Eur J Clin Pharmacol*, 75, 1631–1644.
15. Ogino, S., Miyamoto, S., Miyake, N., et al. (2014). Benefits and limits of anticholinergic use in schizophrenia: focusing on its effect on cognitive function. *Psychiatry Clin Neurosci*, 68, 37–49.
16. Kopala, L. C. (1996). Spontaneous and drug-induced movement disorders in schizophrenia. *Acta Psychiatr Scand Suppl*, 389, 12–17.
17. Gao, K., Kemp, D. E., Ganocy, S. J., et al. (2008). Antipsychotic-induced extrapyramidal side effects in bipolar disorder and schizophrenia: a systematic review. *J Clin Psychopharmacol*, 28, 203–209.
18. Lupu, A. M., Clinebell, K., Gannon, J. M., et al. (2017). Reducing anticholinergic medication burden in patients with psychotic or bipolar disorders. *J Clin Psychiatry*, 78, e1270–e1275.
19. Close, S. P., Elliott, P. J., Hayes, A. G., et al. (1990). Effects of classical and novel agents in a MPTP-induced reversible model of Parkinson's disease. *Psychopharmacology (Berl)*, 102, 295–300.
20. Meyer, S., Meyer, O., Kressig, R. W. (2010). Drug-induced delirium. *Ther Umsch*, 67, 79–83.
21. Onder, G., Liperoti, R., Foebel, A., et al. (2013). Polypharmacy and mortality among nursing home residents with advanced cognitive impairment: results from the SHELTER study. *J Am Med Dir Assoc*, 14, 450 e7–12.
22. Robles Bayon, A., Gude Sampedro, F. (2014). Inappropriate treatments for patients with cognitive decline. *Neurologia*, 29, 523–532.
23. Ueki, T., Nakashima, M. (2019). Relationship between constipation and medication. *J UOEH*, 41, 145–151.

2.23 Diphenhydramine

A. BASIC INFORMATION [1–7]

Principle Trade Names
- Benadryl®
- Unisom®
- Sominex®

Legal Status
- OTC
- Not controlled

Classifications
- Antihistamine
- Sedative
- Anticholinergic
- Local anesthetic
- Anti-nausea agent

Generics Available
- Yes

Formulations
- Oral tablets/capsules: 25 mg; 50 mg
- Oral solution: 12.5 mg/5 ml
- Injectable: 50 mg/ml

- Suppository: 12.5 mg; 25 mg
- Topical: 1%; 2%
- Also available in an array of combination products

FDA Indications
- Allergy
- Occasional insomnia
- Parkinsonism
- Motion sickness

Other Data-Supported Indications
- Acute dystonia
- Dystonic tremor
- Rabbit syndrome (a tardive dystonic tremor)
- Anxiety
- Pruritis
- Pain (topical anesthetic)

B. MECHANISMS OF ACTION [6, 8–10]

Acetylcholine
- Antagonist at muscarinic receptors M_{1-5}, accounting for benefits with respect to antipsychotic-induced adverse motor effects

Histamine
- Inverse agonist at H_1 histamine receptors, accounting for anti-allergy and sedating/anxiolytic effects

Serotonin
- Modest inhibitor of the serotonin reuptake transporter

Sodium
- Inhibitor of intracellular sodium channels, likely accounting for topical anesthetic effects

Potassium
- Inhibitor of the HERG potassium rectifier channel, accounting for QT interval prolongation at high concentrations or in overdose

C. PLASMA CONCENTRATIONS AND TREATMENT RESPONSE [11, 12]

Initial Target Range
- No established therapeutic range

Range for Treatment Resistance
- No established therapeutic range

Typical Time to Response
- Oral: <60 minutes
- Intramuscular: <30 minutes
- Intravenous: < 10 minutes
- Rectal: <60 minutes
- Topical: < 30 minutes
- Peak effect in two to three hours after oral dose
- May require several weeks to achieve maximum benefit in chronic conditions

D. TYPICAL TREATMENT RESPONSE [6, 11, 12, 13–15]

Usual Target Symptoms
- Parkinsonism, including bradykinesia, rigidity, tremor, hypophonia and festinating gait
- Acute medication-induced dystonia
- Dystonic tremor
- Allergic reactions
- Anxiety/insomnia
- Pain (topical)
- Nausea/motion sickness

Common Short-Term Adverse Effects
- Decreased memory consolidation
- Decreased concentration
- Sedation
- Euphoria/dysphoria
- Nausea/vomiting at high doses
- Mydriasis
- Dry mouth
- Constipation

Rare Adverse Effects
- Hallucinosis
- Hives
- Seizure
- Acute angle closure glaucoma
- Tachycardia/palpitations/QT prolongation
- Torsades de Pointes (very rare, most cases associated with overdose)
- Paradoxical excitement (more likely in young children and the elderly)
- Ataxia/incoordination
- Anticholinergic delirium
- Paralytic ileus/bowel obstruction
- Urinary retention (aggravated by BPH)
- Anhidrosis
- Hyperthermia (aggravated by hot weather)

Long-Term Effects
- Increased dental caries with prolonged xerostomia
- Questionable acceleration of neurocognitive disorders

History
- Narrow-angle or angle closure glaucoma
- Present xerostomia
- Constipation/ileus/bowel obstruction
- BPH or urinary retention
- Anhidrosis or hyperthermia
- Delirium or neurocognitive disorder (dementia)

Physical
- Vitals, especially pulse rate and temperature
- Check for dry mucous membranes, flushed face, dilated pupils
- Check for physical signs of constipation/fecal impaction/bowel obstruction
- Check for bladder distention

Neurological
- Delirium, as reflected by fluctuating levels of consciousness, confusion, disorientation, and possible hallucinosis
- Neurocognitive disorder, as reflected by memory impairments, cognitive impairments, language impairments, deficits in executive functions, disorientation, and possible behavioral disturbances or psychosis
- Excessive sedation or ataxia/incoordination

Blood Tests
- None

Cardiac Tests
- ECG if significant tachycardia/palpitations present or known cardiac disease, especially involving QT prolongation

Urine Tests
- Measurement of residual urine if retention suspected

Pregnancy Test
- Pregnancy test (premenopausal females)
- Classified as no increased risk

Other Tests (ECG, etc.)
- KUB if fecal impaction/paralytic ileus/bowel obstruction suspected
- ECG if significant tachycardia/palpitations or known cardiovascular disease, especially if QT prolongation has been present

Titration or After Dose Adjustment
- Check for common adverse effects, as most are dose-dependent
- Check pulse rate and temperature

Maintenance
- Recheck periodically for common adverse effects

- Periodically monitor bowel function
- In circa 70% of cases where anticholinergic medications were initiated to treat medication-induced neurological symptoms, the anticholinergic can be tapered and discontinued after three months without recurrence of neurological adverse effects

Titration
- If well tolerated, increase dose to as much as 50 mg TID as needed
- Maximum recommended dose is 50 mg TID
- For PRN use: 12.5–50 mg PO, IM or per rectum. Intravenous dosing is more variable but should not exceed 150 mg per 24 hours
- For routine use: 12.5–50 mg PO, IM or per rectum TID. Intravenous diphenhydramine should be given via drip not to exceed 150 mg per day. Topical diphenhydramine may be applied to optimal clinical effectiveness

Half-Life
- 2.4–13.5 hours, with a mean of 4.3 hours

Adjustment for Hepatic Dysfunction (by Child-Pugh Criteria)
- No adjustment for categories A or B
- 80–90% reduction for category C
- Topical dosing unaffected

Adjustment for Renal Dysfunction
- Dose reduction may be needed in end-stage renal disease

H. MEDICATIONS TO AVOID IN COMBINATION/WARNINGS [6, 15, 22–24, 25]

 Antipsychotics

• Use with caution in combination with highly antihistaminic/anticholinergic antipsychotics, e.g. chlorpromazine, clozapine, olanzapine, quetiapine, etc.

 Antidepressants

• Use with caution in combination with highly antihistaminic/anticholinergic antidepressants, e.g. tricyclic antidepressants

 Antihistamines

• Avoid combining with medications that are centrally acting H_1 histamine receptor inverse agonists or antagonists, as effects are additive

 Muscarinic Antagonists

• Avoid combining multiple muscarinic receptor antagonists, as anticholinergic effects are additive

 Sympathomimetics

• Avoid combined use in cases where angle closure glaucoma, significant tachycardia or hyperthermia are risks

 Opioids

• Combined use substantially increases risks of constipation, fecal impaction, paralytic ileus and bowel obstruction. Diphenhydramine also may interfere with the analgesic effects of morphine and related opioids, but not endogenous enkephalins

 Warnings

• May induce acute narrow-angle glaucoma
• Use with caution in hyperthyroidism or hypertension
• Do not use in delirium, except in cholinergic rebound delirium, e.g. after abrupt clozapine discontinuation (less well supported than benztropine for this use given potential excessive sedation or paradoxical excitation)
• Avoid use if history indicates allergy to diphenhydramine
• Avoid use if risk of QT interval prolongation is present
• Do not use in bronchial asthma
• Do not use in pyloric or duodenal obstruction or bladder neck obstruction
• Contraindicated in breastfeeding
• Contraindicated in neonates or premature infants
• Do not use in neurocognitive disorders

ART OF PSYCHOPHARMACOLOGY: TAKE-HOME POINTS

• Anticholinergic medications, like diphenhydramine, are excellent rescue medications for acute dystonia or parkinsonism; however, long-term use should be avoided. If long-term treatment for dystonia is needed, consider a trial of amantadine.
• Anticholinergic medications typically worsen tardive movement disorders (e.g. tardive dyskinesia), except for "rabbit syndrome" which is a vertical 5 Hz dystonic tremor of the nose and upper lip.

• Diphenhydramine is effective in some cases of anxiety or insomnia but adds to overall anticholinergic burden. In contrast, hydroxyzine is a potent, centrally acting, sedating antihistamine that lacks affinity for muscarinic receptors.

References

1. Szafranski, T., Gmurkowski, K. (1999). Clozapine withdrawal. A review. *Psychiatr Pol*, 33, 51–67.
2. Faulkner, M. A. (2014). Safety overview of FDA-approved medications for the treatment of the motor symptoms of Parkinson's disease. *Expert Opin Drug Saf*, 13, 1055–1069.
3. Thenganatt, M. A., Jankovic, J. (2014). Treatment of dystonia. *Neurotherapeutics*, 11, 139–152.
4. Stahl, S. M. (2017). Diphenhydramine. In *Stahl's Essential Psychopharmacology Prescriber's Guide* (eds.). Cambridge: Cambridge University Press, pp. 217–219.
5. Orayj, K., Lane, E. (2019). Patterns and determinants of prescribing for Parkinson's disease: a systematic literature review. *Parkinsons Dis*, 2019, 9237181.
6. PubChem. (2020). Trihexyphenidyl, CID = 5572. Retrieved April 21, 2020.
7. Shirley, D. W., Sterrett, J., Haga, N., et al. (2020). The therapeutic versatility of antihistamines: a comprehensive review. *Nurse Pract*, 45, 8–21.
8. Modell, J. G., Tandon, R., Beresford, T. P. (1989). Dopaminergic activity of the antimuscarinic antiparkinsonian agents. *J Clin Psychopharmacol*, 9, 347–351.
9. Deleu, D., Northway, M. G., Hanssens, Y. (2002). Clinical pharmacokinetic and pharmacodynamic properties of drugs used in the treatment of Parkinson's disease. *Clin Pharmacokinet*, 41, 261–309.
10. Fresnius-Kabi USA. (2019). *Diphenhydramine Package Insert*. Lake Zurich, Illinois.
11. Robottom, B. J., Weiner, W. J., Factor, S. A. (2011). Movement disorders emergencies. Part 1: hypokinetic disorders. *Arch Neurol*, 68, 567–572.
12. Rajan, S., Kaas, B., Moukheiber, E. (2019). Movement disorders emergencies. *Semin Neurol*, 39, 125–136.
13. Mazzucchi, S., Frosini, D., Bonuccelli, U., et al. (2015). Current treatment and future prospects of dopa-induced dyskinesias. *Drugs Today (Barc)*, 51, 315–329.
14. Barbe, A. G. (2018). Medication-induced xerostomia and hyposalivation in the elderly: culprits, complications, and management. *Drugs Aging*, 35, 877–885.
15. Andre, L., Gallini, A., Montastruc, F., et al. (2019). Association between anticholinergic (atropinic) drug exposure and cognitive function in longitudinal studies among individuals over 50 years old: a systematic review. *Eur J Clin Pharmacol*, 75, 1631–1644.
16. Ogino, S., Miyamoto, S., Miyake, N., et al. (2014). Benefits and limits of anticholinergic use in schizophrenia: focusing on its effect on cognitive function. *Psychiatry Clin Neurosci*, 68, 37–49.
17. Kopala, L. C. (1996). Spontaneous and drug-induced movement disorders in schizophrenia. *Acta Psychiatr Scand Suppl*, 389, 12–17.
18. Gao, K., Kemp, D. E., Ganocy, S. J., et al. (2008). Antipsychotic-induced extrapyramidal side effects in bipolar disorder and schizophrenia: a systematic review. *J Clin Psychopharmacol*, 28, 203–209.
19. Lupu, A. M., Clinebell, K., Gannon, J. M., et al. (2017). Reducing anticholinergic medication burden in patients with psychotic or bipolar disorders. *J Clin Psychiatry*, 78, e1270–e1275.
20. Paton, D. M., Webster, D. R. (1985). Clinical pharmacokinetics of H1-receptor antagonists (the antihistamines). *Clin Pharmacokinet*, 10, 477–497.
21. Close, S. P., Elliott, P. J., Hayes, A. G., et al. (1990). Effects of classical and novel agents in a MPTP-induced reversible model of Parkinson's disease. *Psychopharmacology (Berl)*, 102, 295–300.
22. Meyer, S., Meyer, O., Kressig, R. W. (2010). Drug-induced delirium. *Ther Umsch*, 67, 79–83.
23. Onder, G., Liperoti, R., Foebel, A., et al. (2013). Polypharmacy and mortality among nursing home residents with advanced cognitive impairment: results from the SHELTER study. *J Am Med Dir Assoc*, 14(6), 450 e7–12.
24. Robles Bayon, A., Gude Sampedro, F. (2014). Inappropriate treatments for patients with cognitive decline. *Neurologia*, 29, 523–532.
25. Ueki, T., Nakashima, M. (2019). Relationship between constipation and medication. *J UOEH*, 41, 145–151.

A. BASIC INFORMATION [1–5]

Principle Trade Names
• Artane®
• Parkin®
• Pacitan®
• Hexymer®

Legal Status
• Prescription only
• Not controlled

Classifications
• Anticholinergic
• Anti-Parkinsonian (second-line)

Generics Available
• Yes

Formulations
• Oral tablets: 2 mg; 5 mg
• Oral elixir: 2 mg/5 ml

FDA Indications
• Parkinsonism

Other Data-Supported Indications
• Acute dystonia
• Dystonic tremor
• Rabbit syndrome (a tardive dystonic tremor)
• Spasticity

B. MECHANISMS OF ACTION [6, 7]

Acetylcholine
• Antagonist at muscarinic receptors, especially M_1

Dopamine
• Indirectly decreases dopamine reuptake and may allosterically bind to dopamine receptors

C. PLASMA CONCENTRATIONS AND TREATMENT RESPONSE [8, 9]

Initial Target Range
• No established therapeutic range

Range for Treatment Resistance
• No established therapeutic range

Typical Time to Response
• Less than 60 minutes
• Peak effect in two to three hours

2.24 Trihexyphenidyl (Continued)

D. TYPICAL TREATMENT RESPONSE [5, 8, 9, 10–12]

Usual Target Symptoms
- Parkinsonism, including bradykinesia, rigidity, tremor, hypophonia and festinating gait
- Acute medication-induced dystonia
- Dystonic tremor
- Muscle spasticity

Common Short-Term Adverse Effects
- Decreased memory consolidation
- Decreased concentration
- Sedation
- Euphoria
- Anxiety at high doses
- Mydriasis
- Headache
- Dry mouth
- Constipation

Rare Adverse Effects
- Hallucinosis
- Acute angle closure glaucoma
- Tachycardia/palpitations
- Anticholinergic delirium
- Paralytic ileus/bowel obstruction
- Urinary retention (aggravated by BPH)
- Anhidrosis
- Hyperthermia (aggravated by hot weather)

Long-Term Effects
- Increased dental caries with prolonged xerostomia
- Questionable acceleration of neurocognitive disorders

E. PRE-TREATMENT WORKUP AND INITIAL LABORATORY TESTING [2, 3, 7, 13]

History
- Narrow-angle or angle closure glaucoma
- Present xerostomia
- Constipation/ileus/bowel obstruction
- BPH or urinary retention
- Anhidrosis or hyperthermia
- Delirium or neurocognitive disorder (dementia)

Physical
- Vitals, especially pulse rate and temperature
- Check for dry mucous membranes, flushed face, dilated pupils
- Check for physical signs of constipation/fecal impaction/bowel obstruction
- Check for bladder distention

Neurological
- Delirium, as reflected by fluctuating level of consciousness, confusion, disorientation, and possible hallucinosis
- Neurocognitive disorder, as reflected by memory impairments, cognitive impairments, language impairments, deficits in executive functions, disorientation, and possible behavioral disturbances or psychosis

Blood Tests
- None

Cardiac Tests
- ECG if significant tachycardia/palpitations present or known cardiac disease is present

Urine Tests
- Measurement of residual urine if retention suspected

Pregnancy Test
- Pregnancy test (premenopausal females)
- Classified as risk not ruled out

Other Tests (ECG, etc.)
- KUB if fecal impaction/paralytic ileus/bowel obstruction suspected
- ECG if significant tachycardia/palpitations or known cardiovascular disease

Titration or After Dose Adjustment
- Check for common adverse effects, as most are dose-dependent
- Check pulse rate and temperature

Maintenance
- Recheck periodically for common adverse effects

- Periodically monitor bowel function
- In circa 70% of cases where anticholinergic medications were initiated to treat medication-induced neurological symptoms, the anticholinergic can be tapered and discontinued after three months without recurrence of neurological adverse effects

Titration
- If well tolerated, increase dose to 5 mg TID as needed
- Maximum recommended dose is 5 mg TID
- For PRN use: 2–5 mg PO
- For routine use: 2–5 mg PO TID

Half-Life
- 3.3–4.1 hours

Bioavailability
- 100%

Adjustment for Hepatic Dysfunction (by Child-Pugh Criteria)
- None

Adjustment for Renal Dysfunction
- Excreted mostly unchanged in urine, requiring dose reduction in renal impairment (EGFR <50 ml/min)

Antipsychotics
- Use with caution in combination with highly anticholinergic antipsychotics, e.g. chlorpromazine, clozapine, olanzapine, quetiapine, etc.

Antidepressants
- Use with caution in combination with highly anticholinergic antidepressants, e.g. tricyclic antidepressants

Muscarinic Antagonists
- Avoid combining multiple muscarinic receptor antagonists, as anticholinergic effects are additive

Sympathomimetics
- Avoid combined use in cases where angle closure glaucoma, significant tachycardia or hyperthermia are risks

Opioids
- Combined use substantially increases risks of constipation, fecal impaction, paralytic ileus and bowel obstruction

Warnings
- May induce acute narrow-angle glaucoma
- Do not use in delirium, except in cholinergic rebound delirium, e.g. after abrupt clozapine discontinuation (less well supported than benztropine for this use)
- Do not use in neurocognitive disorders

2.24 Trihexyphenidyl (Continued)

ART OF PSYCHOPHARMACOLOGY: TAKE-HOME PEARLS

- Anticholinergic medications, like trihexyphenidyl, are excellent rescue medications for acute dystonia or parkinsonism; however, long-term use should be avoided. If long-term treatment for dystonia is needed, consider a trial of amantadine.

- Anticholinergic medications typically worsen tardive movement disorders (e.g. tardive dyskinesia), except for "rabbit syndrome" which is a vertical 5 Hz dystonic tremor of the nose and upper lip.
- Trihexyphenidyl is very prone to diversion and abuse in forensic settings due to its short half-life, rapid onset of action and euphoric effects.

 References

1. Szafranski, T., Gmurkowski, K. (1999). Clozapine withdrawal. A review. *Psychiatr Pol*, 33, 51–67.
2. Faulkner, M. A. (2014). Safety overview of FDA-approved medications for the treatment of the motor symptoms of Parkinson's disease. *Expert Opin Drug Saf*, 13, 1055–1069.
3. Thenganatt, M. A., Jankovic, J. (2014). Treatment of dystonia. *Neurotherapeutics*, 11, 139–152.
4. Orayj, K., Lane, E. (2019). Patterns and determinants of prescribing for Parkinson's disease: a systematic literature review. *Parkinsons Dis*, 2019, 9237181.
5. PubChem. (2020). Trihexyphenidyl, CID = 5572. Retrieved April 21, 2020.
6. Modell, J. G., Tandon, R., Beresford, T. P. (1989). Dopaminergic activity of the antimuscarinic antiparkinsonian agents. *J Clin Psychopharmacol*, 9, 347–351.
7. Deleu, D., Northway, M. G., Hanssens, Y. (2002). Clinical pharmacokinetic and pharmacodynamic properties of drugs used in the treatment of Parkinson's disease. *Clin Pharmacokinet*, 41, 261–309.
8. Robottom, B. J., Weiner, W. J., Factor, S. A. (2011). Movement disorders emergencies. Part 1: hypokinetic disorders. *Arch Neurol*, 68, 567–572.
9. Rajan, S., Kaas, B., Moukheiber, E. (2019). Movement disorders emergencies. *Semin Neurol*, 39, 125–136.
10. Mazzucchi, S., Frosini, D., Bonuccelli, U., et al. (2015). Current treatment and future prospects of dopa-induced dyskinesias. *Drugs Today (Barc)*, 51, 315–329.
11. Barbe, A. G. (2018). Medication-induced xerostomia and hyposalivation in the elderly: culprits, complications, and management. *Drugs Aging*, 35, 877–885.
12. Andre, L., Gallini, A., Montastruc, F., et al. (2019). Association between anticholinergic (atropinic) drug exposure and cognitive function in longitudinal studies among individuals over 50 years old: a systematic review. *Eur J Clin Pharmacol*, 75, 1631–1644.
13. Ogino, S., Miyamoto, S., Miyake, N., et al. (2014). Benefits and limits of anticholinergic use in schizophrenia: focusing on its effect on cognitive function. *Psychiatry Clin Neurosci*, 68, 37–49.
14. Kopala, L. C. (1996). Spontaneous and drug-induced movement disorders in schizophrenia. *Acta Psychiatr Scand Suppl*, 389, 12–17.
15. Gao, K., Kemp, D. E., Ganocy, S. J., et al. (2008). Antipsychotic-induced extrapyramidal side effects in bipolar disorder and schizophrenia: a systematic review. *J Clin Psychopharmacol*, 28, 203–209.
16. Lupu, A. M., Clinebell, K., Gannon, J. M., et al. (2017). Reducing anticholinergic medication burden in patients with psychotic or bipolar disorders. *J Clin Psychiatry*, 78, e1270–e1275.
17. Close, S. P., Elliott, P. J., Hayes, A. G., et al. (1990). Effects of classical and novel agents in a MPTP-induced reversible model of Parkinson's disease. *Psychopharmacology (Berl)*, 102, 295–300.
18. Meyer, S., Meyer, O., Kressig, R. W. (2010). Drug-induced delirium. *Ther Umsch*, 67, 79–83.
19. Onder, G., Liperoti, R., Foebel, A., et al. (2013). Polypharmacy and mortality among nursing home residents with advanced cognitive impairment: results from the SHELTER study. *J Am Med Dir Assoc*, 14(6), 450 e7–12.
20. Robles Bayon, A., Gude Sampedro, F. (2014). Inappropriate treatments for patients with cognitive decline. *Neurologia*, 29, 523–532.
21. Ueki, T., Nakashima, M. (2019). Relationship between constipation and medication. *J UOEH*, 41, 145–151.

A. BASIC INFORMATION [1–5]

Principle Trade Names
- Tegretol®
- Tegretol-XR®
- Carbatrol®
- Epitol®
- Equetro®

Legal Status
- Prescription only
- Not controlled

Classifications
- Glutamate, voltage-gated sodium and calcium channel blocker
- Voltage-sensitive sodium and calcium channel antagonist
- Anticonvulsant
- Antineuralgic
- Mood stabilizer

Generics Available
- Yes

Formulations
- Capsule extended-release: 100 mg; 200 mg; 300 mg
- Suspension, oral: 100 mg/5 ml
- Tablet: 200 mg
- Tablet, chewable: 100 mg
- Tablet extended-release: 100 mg; 200 mg; 400 mg

FDA Indications
- Partial seizures with complex symptomatology
- Generalized tonic-clonic (grand mal) seizures
- Mixed seizure patterns
- Pain associated with trigeminal neuralgia
- Acute mania/mixed mania

Other Data-Supported Indications
- Glossopharyngeal neuralgia
- Bipolar mood disorder, including rapid cycling and mixed mood states
- Bipolar depression
- Post-traumatic stress disorder
- Psychosis, schizophrenia (adjunctive)

Glutamate
- Inhibition of glutamate release may depress activity in the nucleus ventralis of the thalamus

Voltage-Sensitive Sodium Channels
- Antagonism at these sodium channels in the thalamus may decrease temporal stimulation leading to neural discharge by limiting influx of sodium ions across the cell membrane
- Sodium channel antagonism may stimulate the release of antidiuretic hormone

Initial Target Range
- Epilepsy: 4–12 mcg/ml
- Bipolar: 4–8 mcg/ml

Range for Treatment Resistance
- Bipolar: 8–12 mcg/ml

Typical Time to Response
- Seizures should be reduced by two weeks
- Therapeutic improvement of mood instability may be seen between 4–20 weeks

Time-Course of Improvement
- If no response by four weeks at maximum tolerated dose, taper and withdraw therapy

Usual Target Symptoms
- Seizure activity
- Chronic pain
- Alcohol and benzodiazepine withdrawal symptoms
- Positive psychotic symptoms
- Psychomotor agitation
- Mood lability
- Impulsivity
- Irritability

Common Short-Term Adverse Effects
- Nausea
- Vomiting
- Diarrhea
- Constipation
- Ataxia
- Nystagmus
- Sedation
- Headache
- Confusion
- Visual hallucinations
- Rash

Rare Adverse Effects
- Aplastic anemia
- Leukopenia and severe neutropenia
- Thrombocytopenia
- Drug Reaction with Eosinophilia and Systemic Symptoms (DRESS)
- Toxic epidermal necrolysis (TEN)
- Stevens-Johnson Syndrome (SJS)
- Syndrome of inappropriate antidiuretic hormone secretion (SIADH)
- Delayed cardiac conduction, which may be associated with CHF, syncope and bradycardia
- Increased frequency of generalized convulsions in patients with absence seizures
- Increased intraocular pressure
- Altered thyroid function
- Suicidality

Long-Term Effects
- Genitourinary dysfunction, increased BUN, and oliguria
- Cholestatic jaundice
- Decreased diabetic control

History
• Current pregnancy
• Planned pregnancy
• Planned breastfeeding

Physical
• General physical examination
• Vital signs

Blood Tests
• Within 30 days:
  ◦ CBC with differential including platelets
  ◦ Complete metabolic panel
  ◦ Serum amylase
  ◦ Liver function tests

Cardiac Tests
• ECG

Urine Tests
• Urinalysis

Pregnancy Test
• Pregnancy test (premenopausal females)
• Classified as evidence of risk present

Weekly (first 4 weeks)
• Plasma carbamazepine concentration (auto-induces metabolism)
• Electrolytes
• CBC with differential including platelets

Biweekly (every two weeks for months two and three)
• Plasma carbamazepine concentration
• Electrolytes
• CBC with differential including platelets

Monthly (months four through six)
• Electrolytes
• CBC with differential including platelets

Semi-Annually (twice per year after first six months)
• CBC with differential including platelets
• Complete metabolic panel
• Serum amylase
• Liver function tests

Annually
• ECG

Initial Dosing
• Administer initial dose of 200 mg BID to TID
• Elderly/medically fragile: initiate at 100 mg BID

Titration
• If tolerated and clinically indicated, titrate by 200 mg daily
• Elderly/medically fragile: if tolerated and clinically indicated, titrate by 200 mg every three to four days

Half-Life
• Capsule/tablet: 25–65 hours
• Extended-release: 35–40 hours

Bioavailability
• 75–85%
• Extended-release: 89%

Adjustment for Hepatic Dysfunction (by Child-Pugh Criteria)
• No dosage adjustments provided in the manufacturer's labeling
• Use with caution and consider dose reduction

Adjustment for Renal Dysfunction
• No dosage adjustments necessary
• Subsequent dose adjustments should be based on patient response, tolerability and serum concentrations
• Hemodialysis/peritoneal dialysis:
  ◦ No dosage adjustment necessary
  ◦ Subsequent dose adjustments should be based on patient response, tolerability and serum concentrations

Precautions with strong cyp 3A4 inducers – may require dose increases

- Carbamazepine
- Oxcarbazepine
- Phenytoin
- Phenobarbital
- Primidone
- Some glucocorticoids

Precautions with strong cyp 2D6 inhibitors – may require dose decreases

- Paroxetine
- Erythromycin
- Cimetidine
- Fluvoxamine
- Fluoxetine

Precautions with medications which carry significant risks of blood dyscrasias

- Clozapine
- Antineoplastic drugs
- Antiviral medications

Do NOT use with

- Monoamine oxidase inhibitors (MAOIs)
  - May induce potential hypertensive crisis
  - May use 14 days after discontinuation of MAOI

Other precautions

- Doxycycline: half-life decreased
- Warfarin: decreased blood level and half-life decreased
- Oral contraceptives: breakthrough bleeding or pregnancy may occur due to lower contraceptive serum levels

Use precautions in patients with

- Cardiovascular disease, especially affecting cardiac conduction
- Anemia, thrombocytopenia or leukopenia
- Acute intermittent porphyria
- Known hepatic or pancreatic disease
- Diabetes
- Renal disease
- Glaucoma
- Pregnancy

Contraindicated

- Hypersensitivity to carbamazepine, tricyclic compounds, or any components of the prescribed preparation
- History of blood dyscrasia due to carbamazepine
- History of carbamazepine-induced SIADH
- Presence of absence seizures (may induce status epilepticus)
- Breastfeeding
- Persons of Asian descent with HLA-B*1502 allele (may cause toxic epidermal necrolysis or Stevens-Johnson Syndrome)

Discontinuation indicated if

- SIADH results in decline of plasma sodium to <125 mg/dl
- Platelets decline to 100,000 cells/mm^3
- WBC declines to <3500 cells/mm^3
- ANC declines to <1500 cells/mm^3
- RBC declines to <4,000,000 cells/mm^3
- Reticulocytes decline to <0.3%
- Serum iron declines to <150 g/dl
- Persisting or worsening skin rash
- Signs and symptoms of hepatotoxicity (e.g. nausea, vomiting, jaundice or RUQ tenderness)
- Persisting sore throat
- Persisting infection
- Increased bruising/bleeding

- Carbamazepine is efficacious for seizures and pain.
- Although it is formally approved for acute mania and mixed mood states, carbamazepine does not result in full remission of mood instability.
- The extended-release formulation has improved efficacy and tolerability in bipolar disorder compared to immediate-release carbamazepine.
- The risk for serious side effects is greatest during the first few months of carbamazepine treatment.

- Because it is a strong cyp 3A4 inducer, carbamazepine can significantly lower the plasma levels of many drugs including anticonvulsants, some antibiotics, blood thinners and oral contraceptives, as well as its own (autoinduction) plasma concentration.
- Carbamazepine can increase potential for bone marrow depression if used concomitantly with clozapine or other medications which could suppress bone marrow function and cause neutropenia.
- Carbamazepine has many drug-drug interactions, which make it difficult to use in patients who are prescribed concomitant medications.

 References

1. Novartis Pharmaceutical Corporation. (2007). *Tegretol-XR Package Insert*. East Hanover, New Jersey.
2. Validus Pharmaceuticals LLC. (2007). *Equetro Package Insert*. Parsippany, New Jersey.
3. Teva Pharmaceuticals USA Inc. (2018). *Epitol Package Insert*. North Wales, Pennsylvania.
4. Novartis Pharmaceutical Corporation. (2020). *Tegretol Package Insert*. East Hanover, New Jersey.
5. Shire US Inc. (2020). *Carbatrol Package Insert*. Lexington, Massachusetts.
6. California Department of State Hospitals. (2019). *DSH Psychotropic Medication Policy: Carbamazepine Protocol*. Sacramento, California.
7. Capule, F., Tragulpiankit, P., Mahasirimongkol, S., et al. (2020). Association of carbamazepine-induced Stevens-Johnson syndrome/toxic epidermal necrolysis with the HLA-B75 serotype or HLA-B*15:21 allele in Filipino patients. *Pharmacogenomics J*, 20, 533–541.
8. Soria, A., Bernier, C., Veyrac, G., et al. (2020). Drug reaction with eosinophilia and systemic symptoms may occur within 2 weeks of drug exposure: a retrospective study. *J Am Acad Dermatol*, 82, 606–611.
9. Birnbaum, A. K., Meador, K. J., Karanam, A., et al. (2020). Antiepileptic drug exposure in infants of breastfeeding mothers with epilepsy. *JAMA Neurol*, 77, 441–450.

2.26 Lamotrigine

A. BASIC INFORMATION [1–3]

Principle Trade Names
- Lamictal®
- Lamictal ODT®
- Lamictal XR®
- Subvenite®

Legal Status
- Prescription only
- Not controlled

Classifications
- Glutamate, voltage-gated sodium channel blocker
- Voltage-sensitive sodium channel antagonist
- Anticonvulsant
- Mood stabilizer

Generics Available
- Yes

Formulations
- Tablet: 25 mg; 100 mg; 150 mg 200 mg
- Tablet, chewable: 5 mg; 25 mg
- Tablet, oral disintegrating: 25 mg; 50 mg; 100 mg; 200 mg
- Tablet extended-release: 25 mg; 50 mg; 100 mg; 200 mg; 250 mg; 300 mg

FDA Indications
- Partial seizures (adjunctive)
- Generalized tonic-clonic seizures (adjunctive)
- Conversion to monotherapy in adults with partial seizures who are receiving treatment with carbamazepine, phenytoin, phenobarbital, primidone or valproate
- Bipolar I disorder

Other Data-Supported Indications
- Other seizure disorders
- Epilepsy
- Neuropathic pain/chronic pain
- Bipolar depression
- Psychosis, schizophrenia (adjunctive)

Glutamate
• Inhibition of glutamate release may depress activity in the thalamus

Voltage-Sensitive Sodium Channels
• Antagonism at these sodium channels may stabilize neuronal membranes and cause decrease stimulation leading to neural discharge by limiting influx of sodium ions across the cell membrane

Serotonin
• Weak inhibitory effect on $5HT_3$ receptor in vitro inhibits dihydrofolate reductase

Initial Target Range
• Epilepsy: 3–15 mcg/ml
• Bipolar: 1–6 mcg/ml

Range for Treatment Resistance
• Same as above

Typical Time to Response
• Seizures may be reduced by two weeks but may take longer
• Therapeutic improvement of mood instability may be seen between 4–20 weeks

Time-Course of Improvement
• If no response by four weeks at maximum tolerated dose, taper and withdraw therapy

Usual Target Symptoms
• Seizure activity
• Depressed mood
• Chronic pain
• Positive psychotic symptoms (adjunctive)
• Psychomotor agitation
• Mood lability
• Impulsivity
• Irritability

Common Short-Term Adverse Effects
• Nausea
• Vomiting
• Dyspepsia
• Sedation
• Insomnia
• Headache
• Diplopia
• Blurred vision
• Tremor
• Ataxia
• Benign rash (~10%)
• Rhinitis

Rare Adverse Effects
• Blood dyscrasias
• Aseptic meningitis
• Drug Reaction with Eosinophilia and Systemic Symptoms (DRESS)
• Toxic epidermal necrolysis (TEN)
• Stevens-Johnson Syndrome (SJS)
• Photosensitivity
• Withdrawal seizures with abrupt discontinuation
• Sudden death during epileptic episode
• Suicidality

Long-Term Effects
• Safe – no significant long-term effects
• Recommend ophthalmological checks, as lamotrigine binds to tissue that contains melanin

History
• General history, including concomitant medications

Physical
• General physical examination, especially skin examination
• Vital signs

Neurological
• Neurology consultation if personal history of active, poorly controlled seizure disorder

Blood Tests
• Within 30 days:
  ○ CBC with differential
  ○ Complete metabolic panel
  ○ Liver function tests

Cardiac Tests
• ECG

Urine Tests
• Urinalysis

Pregnancy Test
• Pregnancy test (premenopausal females)
• Classified as evidence of risk present

Weekly (for three months beginning at titration completion)
• Inquiry and/or inspection of individual for skin rash

Quarterly or Semi-Annually
• CBC with differential including platelets
• Complete metabolic panel
• Liver function tests

Annually
• ECG

When valproate or enzyme-inducing drugs dosages are changed
• Inquiry and/or inspection of individual for skin rash weekly for three months after this type of medication change

Initial Dosing
• Seizure treatment with concomitant valproate: initiate with 25 mg QOD for weeks one and two
• Seizure treatment with concomitant enzyme-inducing antiepileptics and NOT on valproate: initiate with 50 mg QD for weeks one and two
• Psychiatric treatment with concomitant valproate: initiate with 25 mg QOD for weeks one and two
• Psychiatric treatment with concomitant enzyme-inducing antiepileptics and NOT on valproate: initiate with 50 mg QD for weeks one and two

Titration
• Seizure with concomitant valproate:
  ○ If tolerated and clinically indicated, titrate to 25 mg daily for weeks three and four
  ○ If tolerated and clinically indicated, titrate further by 25–50 mg per day every for one to two weeks to reach maintenance level (usual maintenance dosage 100–400 mg daily in two divided doses)
• Seizure treatment with concomitant enzyme-inducing antiepileptics and NOT on valproate:
  ○ If tolerated and clinically indicated, titrate to 50 mg BID for weeks three and four
  ○ If tolerated and clinically indicated, titrate further by 100 mg per day every one to two weeks to reach maintenance level (usual maintenance dosage 300–500 mg daily in two divided doses)
• Psychiatric treatment with concomitant valproate:
  ○ If tolerated and clinically indicated, titrate to 25 mg daily for weeks three and four
  ○ If tolerated and clinically indicated, titrate to 50 mg daily for week five

○ If tolerated and clinically indicated, titrate to 100 mg daily for weeks six and seven (usual maintenance dosage 200–400 mg daily)
• Psychiatric treatment with concomitant enzyme-inducing antiepileptics and NOT on valproate:
○ If tolerated and clinically indicated, titrate to 50 mg BID for weeks three and four
○ If tolerated and clinically indicated, titrate to 100 mg BID for week five
○ If tolerated and clinically indicated, titrate to 150 mg BID for week six
○ If tolerated and clinically indicated, titrate to 200 mg BID for week seven onward (usual maintenance dosage 400 mg daily)

Half-Life
• Immediate-release and extended-release: 25–33 hours; 25–43 hours in elderly
• Concomitant VPA: 48–70 hours
• Concomitant phenytoin, phenobarbital, primidone or carbamazepine: 13–14 hours
• Hemodialysis: 13 hours during dialysis; 57 hours between dialysis
• Child-Pugh category A: 46 ± 20 hours
• Child-Pugh category B: 72 ± 44 hours
• Child-Pugh category C without ascites: 67 ± 11 hours
• Child-Pugh category C with ascites: 100 ± 48 hours

Bioavailability
• Immediate-release and extended-release: 98%
• With concomitant Antiepileptic Drugs (AED) (phenytoin, phenobarbital, primidone or carbamazepine): 21–70% lower

Adjustment for Hepatic Dysfunction (by Child-Pugh Criteria)
• Child-Pugh category A: No dosage adjustments necessary
• Child-Pugh category B and C without ascites: Decrease initial, titration and maintenance doses by ~25%; adjust according to clinical response and tolerance
• Child-Pugh category B and C with ascites: Decrease initial, titration and maintenance doses by ~50%; adjust according to clinical response and tolerance

Adjustment for Renal Dysfunction
• No dosage adjustments necessary provided in manufacturer's labeling
• Decreased maintenance dosage may be effective in patients with significant renal impairment; has not been adequately studied; use with caution

Adjustment with discontinuation of valproate
• Lamotrigine dosage may need to be increased (valproic acid inhibits lamotrigine metabolism) by 50 mg in the first week and by another 50 mg in the second week

Adjustment with discontinuation of enzyme-inducing antiepileptics
• Lamotrigine dosage may need to be decreased (valproic acid inhibits lamotrigine metabolism) by 100 mg in the second week after discontinuation of AED and by another 100 mg in the third week

Adjustment with other drugs
• Lamotrigine dosage accounts for possible increase in lamotrigine metabolism when lamotrigine is added to oral contraceptives with estrogens (particularly ethinylestradiol), rifampin or oxcarbazepine

Adjustments due to autoinduction
• If an individual previously responding to lamotrigine loses his/her response, a blood level may be obtained to consider: a) lack of adherence, and b) the possibility of lamotrigine's induction of its own metabolism, particularly in individuals NOT taking enzyme-inducing antiepileptic drugs (e.g. after a few weeks, up to six weeks, of a stable dose, levels spontaneously decrease by one-third to one-quarter)

Discontinuation due to adverse event
• Dose is discontinued at the first sign of rash (unless rash is clearly not drug related, with documentation) and medical consultation and CBC with differential and liver function tests are obtained

Tapered discontinuation
• If discontinued due to reasons other than safety, dose is decreased by 50% per week over at least two weeks

H. MEDICATIONS TO AVOID IN COMBINATION/WARNINGS [1–3]

 Valproate

- Increases plasma concentration and half-life of lamotrigine
- Requires lowering dosage of lamotrigine by ~50%
- Increased risk of serious rash when used concomitantly with lamotrigine

 Enzyme-inducing antiepileptic drugs (e.g. carbamazepine, phenytoin, phenobarbital, primidone)

- May increase clearance of lamotrigine and lower its plasma concentration

 Precautions with medications which carry significant risks of blood dyscrasias

- Clozapine
- Antineoplastic drugs
- Antiviral medications

 Oral contraceptives

- May decrease plasma levels of lamotrigine

I. MEDICAL PRECAUTIONS AND CONTRAINDICATIONS [1, 2, 3, 5]

Use precautions in patients with
- Hepatic impairment
- Renal impairment
- Pregnancy
- Breastfeeding

Contraindicated
- Hypersensitivity to lamotrigine
- History of serious rash with systemic symptoms associated with prior lamotrigine treatment

Discontinuation indicated if
- Serious rash develops

ART OF PSYCHOPHARMACOLOGY: TAKE-HOME PEARLS

- Lamotrigine is efficacious for seizures and pain.
- Although it is formally approved for acute mania and mixed mood states, lamotrigine does not result in full remission of mood instability and may promote mood elevation in some patients. It is most effective for bipolar depression.
- The risk for developing serious rash is increased with higher doses of lamotrigine, faster dose titrations, concomitant use of valproate, and in children under 12 years of age.
- Lamotrigine may cause serious, potentially fatal rash.
- Lamotrigine may increase suicidality.
- Lamotrigine has many drug-drug interactions, which make it difficult to use in patients who are prescribed concomitant medications.

 References

1. GlaxoSmithKline LLC. (2009). *Lamictal Package Insert*. Research Triangle Park, North Carolina.
2. GlaxoSmithKline LLC. (2019). *Lamictal XR Package Insert*. Research Triangle Park, North Carolina.
3. OWP Pharmaceuticals Inc. (2020). *Subvenite Package Insert*. North Paerville, Illinois.
4. Sills, G. J., Rogawski, M. A. (2020). Mechanisms of action of currently used antiseizure drugs. *Neuropharmacology*, 168, 107966.
5. California Department of State Hospitals. (2019). *DSH Psychotropic Medication Policy: Lamotrigine Protocol*. Sacramento, California.

6. Li, Y., Zhang, F., Xu, Y., et al. (2018). Pharmacokinetics, safety, and tolerability of lamotrigine chewable/dispersible tablet following repeat-dose administration in healthy Chinese volunteers. *Clin Pharmacol Drug Dev*, 7, 627–633.
7. Nevitt, S. J., Tudur Smith, C., Weston, J., et al. (2018). Lamotrigine versus carbamazepine monotherapy for epilepsy: an individual participant data review. *Cochrane Database Syst Rev*, 6, CD001031.
8. Tawhari, I., Tawhari, F., Aljuaid, M. (2018). Lamotrigine-induced drug reaction with eosinophilia and systemic symptoms (DRESS) during primary Epstein-Barr virus (EBV) infection. *BMJ Case Rep*, 2018, 2018, brc2017222416.
9. Vazquez, M., Maldonado, C., Guevara, N., et al. (2018). Lamotrigine-valproic acid interaction leading to Stevens-Johnson syndrome. *Case Rep Med*, 2018, 5371854.
10. Oya, K., Sakuma, K., Esumi, S., et al. (2019). Efficacy and safety of lithium and lamotrigine for the maintenance treatment of clinically stable patients with bipolar disorder: a systematic review and meta-analysis of double-blind, randomized, placebo-controlled trials with an enrichment design. *Neuropsychopharmacol Rep*, 39, 241–246.
11. Panebianco, M., Bresnahan, R., Ramaratnam, S., et al. (2020). Lamotrigine add-on therapy for drug-resistant focal epilepsy. *Cochrane Database Syst Rev*, 3, CD001909.
12. Pensel, M. C., Nass, R. D., Tauboll, E., et al. (2020). Prevention of sudden unexpected death in epilepsy: current status and future perspectives. *Expert Rev Neurother*, 20, 497–508.
13. Stephen, L. J., Brodie, M. J. (2020). Pharmacological management of the genetic generalised epilepsies in adolescents and adults. *CNS Drugs*, 34, 147–161.

2.27 Lithium

A. BASIC INFORMATION [1–5]

Principle Trade Names
- Lithium Carbonate®
- Lithium Citrate®
- Lithobid®
- Lithostat®

Legal Status
- Prescription only
- Not controlled

Classifications
- Glutamate, voltage-gated sodium channel blocker
- Voltage-sensitive sodium channel antagonist
- Anticonvulsant
- Mood stabilizer

Generics Available
- Yes

Formulations
- Tablet: 150 mg; 300 mg; 600 mg
- Tablet, extended-release: 300 mg; 450 mg
- Solution: 8 meq/5 ml

FDA Indications
- Bipolar I disorder – mania
- Bipolar I disorder – maintenance
- Suicidality

Other Data-Supported Indications
- Bipolar depression
- Schizoaffective disorder
- Major depressive disorder (adjunctive)
- Vascular headache
- Neutropenia
- Psychomotor agitation or assaultiveness

Sodium transporter
• Unknown action in nerve and muscle cells

Serotonin
• Possible alteration in metabolism of serotonin with unknown effects

Catecholamines
• Possible alteration in metabolism of catecholamines with unknown effects

Second Messenger Systems
• Possible alteration of intracellular signaling
  ○ Inhibition of inositol monophosphatase may affect neurotransmission via phosphatidyl inositol second messenger system
  ○ Reduction of protein kinase C activity may affect genomic expression associated with neurotransmission
  ○ Increase in cytoprotective proteins may activate signaling cascade used by endogenous growth factors and increase gray matter content possibly by activation of neurogenesis and neurotrophic actions

C. PLASMA CONCENTRATIONS AND TREATMENT RESPONSE [1, 4, 5, 6–9, 10, 11]

Initial Target Range
• Major depression: 0.6–0.8 meq/l
• Bipolar: 0.8–1.0 meq/l
• Acute/severe mania: 1.0–1.4 meq/l

Range for Treatment Resistance
• Same as above

Typical Time to Response
• Therapeutic improvement of mood instability may be seen between one to three weeks
• Neutropenia resolution may be seen within three to four weeks

Time-Course of Improvement
• If no response by four weeks at maximum tolerated dose, taper and withdraw therapy

D. TYPICAL TREATMENT RESPONSE [1, 4, 5, 6–9, 10, 11]

Usual Target Symptoms
• Mania
• Depression
• Psychomotor agitation
• Mood lability
• Impulsivity
• Irritability
• Suicidality

Common Short-Term Adverse Effects
• Dyspepsia
• Diarrhea
• Tremor
• Polyuria/polydipsia
• Hypothyroidism
• Exacerbation of dermatitis, acne, psoriasis
• Weight gain

Warning Signs of Toxicity
• T-wave inversion
• Vomiting
• Dysarthria
• Ataxia
• Vertigo
• Confusion
• Lethargy
• Hyperreflexia
• Coarse hand tremor

Factors Promoting toxicity
• Too little sodium (e.g. due to low-salt diet, fad diet or salt substitute)
• Dehydration (due to diuretics, excessive sweating, fever, or poor fluid intake secondary to physical/mental illness)
• Drug interactions (e.g. thiazide diuretics, ACE inhibitors, and NSAIDS except for sulindac)

E. PRE-TREATMENT WORKUP AND INITIAL LABORATORY TESTING [1, 4, 5, 6–9, 10, 11]

History
• General history, especially history of thyroid disease, renal disease, cardiac disease and potential pregnancy

Physical
• General physical examination, especially thyroid gland
• Vital signs

Blood Tests
• Within 30 days:
  ○ CBC with differential
  ○ Complete metabolic panel
  ○ Thyroid function tests, including thyroid stimulating hormone (TSH)

Cardiac Tests
• ECG

Urine Tests
• Urinalysis

Pregnancy Test
• Pregnancy test (premenopausal females)
• Classified as evidence of risk present

F. MONITORING [1, 4, 5, 7]

Weekly (first four weeks)
• Plasma lithium concentration

Monthly (months two and three)
• Plasma lithium concentration

Semi-Annually (first year of lithium treatment)
• CBC with differential including platelets
• Complete metabolic panel
• TSH
• Plasma lithium concentration

Annually
• ECG
• CBC with differential including platelets
• Complete metabolic panel
• TSH
• Plasma lithium concentration

After any dose increase
• Plasma lithium concentration five to seven days after dose increase

Initial Dosing

- Mania/mood instability: initiate with immediate-release formulation 600–900 mg qhs
- Acute severe mania: if eGFR is >60 ml/min, load with Lithobid (extended-release formulation – to help decrease gastrointestinal (GI) side effects of nausea and diarrhea) at 30 mg/kg (adjusted to the nearest 300 mg dosage increment) in three divided doses over a six-hour time span on the first day at 4 pm, 6 pm and 8 pm (Note: the total daily dose should not exceed 3000 mg.)
- Neutropenia: initiate with 300 mg qhs

Titration

- Mania/mood instability: if tolerated and clinically indicated, titrate by 300 mg qhs until plasma lithium measurement falls in the therapeutic range (0.8–1.2 meq/l) when checked five to seven days after dose adjustment
- Acute severe mania: a 12-hour trough plasma level should be obtained the morning after loading to help guide subsequent dosing (target = 1.2–1.4 meq/l for acute severe mania)
  ○ If plasma concentration the next morning is <1.0 meq/l, give immediate-release lithium 1200 mg qhs with a follow-up lithium level to be rechecked five to seven days later for finer adjustment of the dose

○ If plasma concentration the next morning is >1.0 meq/l, give immediate-release lithium 900 mg qhs
- Neutropenia: if tolerated and clinically indicated, titrate by 300 mg qhs until plasma lithium measurement falls between 0.6–1.0 meq/l when checked five to seven days after dose adjustment

Half-Life

- Immediate-release and extended-release: 18–36 hours; 28.5 hours in elderly

Bioavailability

- 80–100%

Adjustment for Hepatic Dysfunction (by Child-Pugh Criteria)

- No dosage adjustments necessary

Adjustment for Renal Dysfunction

- CrCl 50–89 ml/min: initiate therapy with low dose; titrate slowly with frequent monitoring
- CrCl <50 ml/min: avoid use

Precautions with antidepressants

- Antidepressants can destabilize mood in patients with a bipolar diathesis
- May induce rapid cycling
- May induce suicidality

Avoid use with

- Thiazide diuretics
- ACE inhibitors
- NSAIDs (except for sulindac)

I. MEDICAL PRECAUTIONS AND CONTRAINDICATIONS [1, 4, 5, 7]

Use precautions in patients with
- Hypothyroidism
- History of current cystic acne
- Bradycardia or cardiomyopathy associated with bradycardia
- Pregnancy (increased risk for Epstein's anomaly during use in first trimester or breastfeeding)
- Concurrent thiazide diuretics, ACE inhibitors, or NSAIDs (except sulindac)
- Dehydration
- Renal transplant
- Peritoneal dialysis
- Hemodialysis

Contraindicated
- Hypersensitivity
- Acute or unstable renal failure
- Psoriasis
- Sick sinus syndrome
- Brugada syndrome
- Sodium depletion

ART OF PSYCHOPHARMACOLOGY: TAKE-HOME PEARLS

- Lithium is efficacious for mania and as an adjunct for treatment-resistant depression.
- Lithium is effective in decreasing impulsivity and persistent/chronic suicidality.
- Lithium is first-line treatment for mood stabilization and may be the best agent for euphoric mania.
- Lithium can help resolve mild neutropenia.
- Historically, it was thought that lithium may not be the best option for rapid cycling and mixed states of bipolar illness; however, recent data suggest that lithium and valproate are equally effective in these contexts.
- Lithium yields good results in combination with atypical antipsychotics and/or mood-stabilizing anticonvulsants, such as valproate.
- Lithium requires monitoring of plasma concentration (narrow therapeutic window), renal function and thyroid function.
- Elderly patients will require lower doses of lithium to achieve therapeutic serum levels and may be more sensitive to adverse effects.

References

1. ANI Pharmaceuticals Inc. *Lithobid Package Insert*. Baudette, Minnesota.
2. Calabrese, J. R., Shelton, M. D., Rapport, D. J., et al. (2005). A 20-month, double-blind, maintenance trial of lithium versus divalproex in rapid-cycling bipolar disorder. *Am J Psychiatry*, 162, 2152–2161.
3. Kemp, D. E., Gao, K., Ganocy, S. J., et al. (2009). A 6-month, double-blind, maintenance trial of lithium monotherapy versus the combination of lithium and divalproex for rapid-cycling bipolar disorder and co-occurring substance abuse or dependence. *J Clin Psychiatry*, 70, 113–121.
4. Mission Pharmacal. (2015). *Lithostat Package Insert*. San Antonio, Texas.
5. West-Ward Pharmaceuticals Corp. (2019). *Lithium Carbonate Package Insert*. Eatontown, New Jersey.
6. Smith, K. A., Cipriani, A. (2017). Lithium and suicide in mood disorders: updated meta-review of the scientific literature. *Bipolar Disord*, 19, 575–586.
7. California Department of State Hospitals. (2019). *DSH Psychotropic Medication Policy: Lithium Protocol*. Sacramento, California.
8. Oya, K., Sakuma, K., Esumi, S., et al. (2019). Efficacy and safety of lithium and lamotrigine for the maintenance treatment of clinically stable patients with bipolar disorder: a systematic review and meta-analysis of double-blind, randomized, placebo-controlled trials with an enrichment design. *Neuropsychopharmacol Rep*, 39, 241–246.
9. Undurraga, J., Sim, K., Tondo, L., et al. (2019). Lithium treatment for unipolar major depressive disorder: systematic review. *J Psychopharmacol*, 33, 167–176.
10. Bahji, A., Ermacora, D., Stephenson, C., et al. (2020). Comparative efficacy and tolerability of pharmacological treatments for the treatment of acute bipolar depression: a systematic review and network meta-analysis. *J Affect Disord*, 269, 154–184.
11. Silva, E., Higgins, M., Hammer, B., et al. (2020). Clozapine rechallenge and initiation despite neutropenia – a practical, step-by-step guide. *BMC Psychiatry*, 20, 279.

2.28 Valproic Acid

A. BASIC INFORMATION [1–4]

Principle Trade Names
- Depakote®
- Depakote Sprinkles®
- Depakote ER®
- Depakene®
- Divalproex®
- Depakon®

Legal Status
- Prescription only
- Not controlled

Classifications
- Voltage-gated sodium channel blocker
- Anticonvulsant
- Mood stabilizer
- Migraine prophylactic
- Histone D-acetylase inhibitor
- Chemotherapy agent

Generics Available
- Yes

Formulations
- Tablet/capsule: 125 mg; 250 mg; 500 mg
- Tablet, extended-release: 250 mg; 500 mg
- Solution, oral: 250 mg/5 ml
- Solution, IV: 100 mg/ml (limited to emergent seizure treatment)

FDA Indications
- Bipolar I disorder – mania, mixed episodes
- Seizures – complex partial, simple absence, complex absence
- Migraine prophylaxis

Other Data-Supported Indications
- Bipolar disorder maintenance
- Bipolar depression (limited benefit)
- Schizoaffective disorder
- Psychosis/schizophrenia (adjunctive)
- Persistent or recurring self-injurious behaviors
- Aggressive/violent patients not responsive to other treatments
- Selected solid tumors (adjunctive)

Sodium transporter
- Blocks voltage-dependent sodium channels by unknown mechanism to suppress high-frequency repetitive neuronal firing

Gamma-aminobutyric acid (GABA)
- Increases availability of GABA to brain neurons by unknown mechanism but likely increased synthesis and release
- May enhance action of GABA at postsynaptic receptor sites
- May mimic GABAergic action at postsynaptic receptor sites

Histone D-acetylase
- Inhibits acetylation of DNA, slowing DNA copying

C. PLASMA CONCENTRATIONS AND TREATMENT RESPONSE [1–4, 5]

Initial Target Range
- Acute/severe mania: 100–120 mcg/ml
- Maintenance: 80–120 mcg/ml

Range for Treatment Resistance
- Same as for acute/severe mania

Typical Time to Response
- Therapeutic improvement of mood instability may be seen within a few days

- Optimization of mood stabilization may be seen within three to four weeks
- Seizures and migraines may improve within three to four weeks

Time-Course of Improvement
- If no response by four weeks at maximum tolerated dose, taper and withdraw therapy

D. TYPICAL TREATMENT RESPONSE [1–3, 4, 5, 6–15, 16, 17]

Usual Target Symptoms
- Mania
- Psychomotor agitation
- Mood lability
- Impulsivity
- Irritability
- Seizures
- Migraine headache
- Solid tumor growth

Common Short-Term Adverse Effects
- Gastrointestinal (GI) symptoms (nausea, vomiting, dyspepsia, abdominal pain, diarrhea, anorexia and constipation)
- Somnolence
- Tremor
- Dizziness
- Diplopia
- Amblyopia/blurred vision
- Nystagmus
- Emotional lability

- Amnesia
- Respiratory symptoms (flu-like syndrome, infection, bronchitis, rhinitis)

Rare Adverse Effects
- Hepatotoxicity (usually within first six months of treatment; symptoms include lethargy, malaise, anorexia, jaundice and weakness)
- Hyperammonemic encephalopathy
- Pancreatitis
- Thrombocytopenia
- Suicidal ideation

Long-Term Effects
- Teratogenic effects
- Alopecia
- Nail pigmentation
- Edema
- Weight loss/gain
- Possible association with polycystic ovary syndrome
- Possible impairment in bone metabolism

E. PRE-TREATMENT WORKUP AND INITIAL LABORATORY TESTING [1–4, 5]

History
- General history, especially history of hyperammonemia, hyperammonemic encephalopathy, potential pregnancy and planned breastfeeding

Physical
- General physical examination
- Vital signs

Blood Tests
- Within 30 days:
  ○ CBC with differential, including platelet count

  ○ Complete metabolic panel
  ○ Liver function tests

Cardiac Tests
- ECG

Urine Tests
- Urinalysis

Pregnancy Test
- Pregnancy test (premenopausal females)
- Classified as evidence of risk present
- Fetal exposure decreases IQ by circa ten points
- Roughly doubles risk of autism

F. MONITORING [1–4, 5]

Monthly (first six months)
- CBC with differential including platelets
- Complete metabolic panel
- Liver function tests

Semi-Annually/Annually
- CBC with differential including platelets
- Complete metabolic panel
- Liver function tests

Five to seven days after any dosage increase
- Serum trough VPA level

After any evidence of:
Encephalopathy
Coma
Mental retardation
Cyclical vomiting with lethargy
Episodic extreme irritability
Ataxia
Low BUN
Protein avoidance
- Check ammonia and glutamine levels

Initial Dosing
- Seizure disorders:
  - Initiate at 10–15 mg/kg/day in two to three divided doses (once daily if extended-release formulation)
  - For elderly, use a lower starting dose due to decrease in unbound clearance of valproate and possible increase in sensitivity to somnolence
- Mania/mood instability: initiate with 750–1000 mg in divided doses (once daily with extended release formulation)
- Acute severe mania or mixed states: load with 20–30 mg/kg/day

Titration
- Seizure disorders:
  - If tolerated and clinically indicated, titrate by 5–10 mg/kg/week to achieve optimal clinical response
  - For elderly, titrate more slowly and with regular monitoring to achieve optimal clinical response if tolerated and clinically indicated
- Mania/mood instability: if tolerated and clinically indicated, titrate up or down to achieve therapeutic plasma concentration (80–100 mcg/ml) when checked five to seven days after dose adjustment
- Acute severe mania: if tolerated and clinically indicated, titrate up or down to achieve therapeutic plasma concentration (100–120 mcg/ml) when checked five to seven days after dose adjustment

Half-Life
- 9–19 hours

Bioavailability
- ~90 %
- 70–95% protein-bound

Adjustment for Hepatic Dysfunction (by Child-Pugh Criteria)
- Child-Pugh category A or B: use not recommended
- Child-Pugh category C: contraindicated

Adjustment for Renal Dysfunction
- Mild to severe impairment: no dosage adjustment required (including hemodialysis)
- Monitoring only total serum VPA may be misleading, as protein binding is reduced in patients with renal impairment

H. MEDICATIONS TO AVOID IN COMBINATION/WARNINGS [1–4, 5]

 Precautions with strong inducers – may require dose increases
- Carbamazepine
- Phenytoin
- Phenobarbital
- Primidone
- Ethosuximide
- Rifampin
- Lamotrigine (milder effects)
- Oxcarbazepine (milder effects)

 Precautions with strong inhibitors – may require dose decreases
- Aspirin/salicylates
- Cimetidine
- Fluoxetine

 Precautions with AIDS medications
- Some AIDS medications may be hepatic inducers; monitor VPA level and adjust dosage as necessary
- Some AIDS medications may be hepatic inhibitors; monitor VPA level and adjust dosage as necessary

 Precautions with drugs which undergo glucuronidation or metabolism via cyp 2C9
- Adding/discontinuing valproate may increase levels of phenobarbital, phenytoin, carbamazepine, oxcarbazepine and ethosuximide
- If valproate is discontinued, lamotrigine dosage may need to be increased (valproic acid inhibits lamotrigine metabolism) by 50% in the first week with further inhibition in the second week of exposure

 Precautions with benzodiazepines
- Valproate may increase levels of several benzodiazepines (e.g. diazepam)
- Combined clonazepam-valproate may result in absence seizures or status epilepticus

 Precautions with tricyclic antidepressants
- TCA levels increase by 50–60% after addition of valproate

 Precautions with other highly protein-bound medications
- Careful monitoring of INR is required, as valproate can displace warfarin from protein binding

I. MEDICAL PRECAUTIONS AND CONTRAINDICATIONS [1–4, 5]

Use precautions in patients with
- Pregnancy (increased risk for neural tube defects, autism and decreased intelligence)
- Breastfeeding (delays in cognitive development/performance; doubles risk for autism spectrum disorder)
- Significant baseline abnormalities in blood counts
- Concurrent treatment with myelotoxic agents
- History of adverse hematological reaction to any drug
- Renal disease/impairment
- Congenital metabolic disorders and/or organic brain disease
- Elderly with excessive somnolence and/or with decreased food/fluid intake

Contraindicated
- Hypersensitivity
- Pre-existing unstable hepatic disease
- Significant hepatic dysfunction
- Known urea cycle disorders (e.g. hyperammonemic encephalopathy, persistent hyperammonemia)
- Pre-existing thrombocytopenia with platelets <100 K cells/mm^3
- Pre-existing clinical presentation consistent with active pancreatitis

ART OF PSYCHOPHARMACOLOGY: TAKE-HOME PEARLS

- Valproic acid, like lithium, is a first-line treatment option for mixed states and rapid cycling in bipolar disorder.
- Valproic acid is efficacious for mania but less so for the depressed phase of bipolar disorder.
- Valproic acid does not result in full remission of symptoms (only reduces symptoms by approximately 30%); hence, patients may need combination therapy.
- Valproic acid yields good results in combination with lithium and/or atypical antipsychotics.
- Valproic acid requires monitoring of plasma concentrations (highly protein-bound) and liver function.
- Elderly patients will require lower doses of valproic to achieve therapeutic serum levels and may be more sensitive to adverse effects.

References

1. AbbVie Inc. (2020). *Depakote Package Insert*. North Chicago, Illinois.
2. AbbVie Inc. (2020). *Depakote Sprinkles Package Insert*. North Chicago, Illinois.
3. AbbVie Inc. (2020). *Depakote ER Package Insert*. North Chicago, Illinois.
4. Zydus Pharmaceuticals (USA) Inc. (2020). *Divalproex Package Insert*. Pennington, New Jersey.
5. California Department of State Hospitals. (2019). *DSH Psychotropic Medication Policy: Valproic Acid/Divalproex Protocol*. Sacramento, California.
6. Lonergan, E. T., Cameron, M., Luxenberg, J. (2004). Valproic acid for agitation in dementia. *Cochrane Database Syst Rev*, CD003945.
7. Sykes, L., Wood, E., Kwan, J. (2014). Antiepileptic drugs for the primary and secondary prevention of seizures after stroke. *Cochrane Database Syst Rev*, CD005398.
8. Trinka, E., Hofler, J., Zerbs, A., et al. (2014). Efficacy and safety of intravenous valproate for status epilepticus: a systematic review. *CNS Drugs*, 28, 623–639.
9. Hayes, J. F., Marston, L., Walters, K., et al. (2016). Adverse renal, endocrine, hepatic, and metabolic events during maintenance mood stabilizer treatment for bipolar disorder: a population-based cohort study. *PLoS Med*, 13, e1002058.
10. Nevitt, S. J., Sudell, M., Weston, J., et al. (2017). Antiepileptic drug monotherapy for epilepsy: a network meta-analysis of individual participant data. *Cochrane Database Syst Rev*, 12, CD011412.
11. Thomson, S. R., Mamulpet, V., Adiga, S. (2017). Sodium valproate induced alopecia: a case series. *J Clin Diagn Res*, 11, FR01–FR02.
12. Baillon, S. F., Narayana, U., Luxenberg, J. S., et al. (2018). Valproate preparations for agitation in dementia. *Cochrane Database Syst Rev*, 10, CD003945.
13. Graham, R. K., Tavella, G., Parker, G. B. (2018). Is there consensus across international evidence-based guidelines for the psychotropic drug management of bipolar disorder during the perinatal period? *J Affect Disord*, 228, 216–221.
14. Baudou, E., Benevent, J., Montastruc, J. L., et al. (2019). Adverse effects of treatment with valproic acid during the neonatal period. *Neuropediatrics*, 50, 31–40.
15. Baumgartner, J., Hoeflich, A., Hinterbuchinger, B., et al. (2019). Fulminant onset of valproate-associated hyperammonemic encephalopathy. *Am J Psychiatry*, 176, 900–903.
16. Jochim, J., Rifkin-Zybutz, R. P., Geddes, J., et al. (2019). Valproate for acute mania. *Cochrane Database Syst Rev*, 10, CD004052.
17. Chakrabarty, T., Keramatian, K., Yatham, L. N. (2020). Treatment of mixed features in bipolar disorder: an updated view. *Curr Psychiatry Rep*, 22, 15.

Selective Serotonin Reuptake Inhibitor Antidepressants
2.29 Citalopram

A. BASIC INFORMATION [1, 2]

Principle Trade Names
• Celexa®

Legal Status
• Prescription only
• Not controlled

Classifications
• Selective serotonin reuptake inhibitor (SSRI)
• Antidepressant

Generics Available
• Yes

Formulations
• Tablet: 10 mg; 20 mg; 40 mg
• Oral solution: 10 mg/5 ml

FDA Indications
• Major depressive disorder

Other Data-Supported Indications
• Agitation in Alzheimer's disease
• Anxiety associated with major depressive disorder
• Generalized anxiety disorder
• Obsessive-compulsive disorder
• Panic disorder
• Post-traumatic stress disorder
• Social anxiety disorder

B. MECHANISMS OF ACTION [3, 4]

Serotonin
• Binds directly to 5HT transporter, potently and selectively inhibits 5HT reuptake
• Downregulates and desensitizes the $5HT_{1A}$ receptor with the downstream effect of increasing 5HT levels in the cortex

Other
• May overcome mood-related changes in synaptic plasticity and neurogenesis by increasing brain derived neurotrophic factor (BDNF) and inducing signaling through certain BDNF receptors

C. PLASMA CONCENTRATIONS AND TREATMENT RESPONSE [5]

Initial Target Range
• No established plasma therapeutic range

Range for Treatment Resistance
• No established plasma therapeutic range

Typical Time to Response
• At least four weeks to attain response with six weeks needed to attain remission. Remission can take up to 12 weeks

Time-Course of Improvement
• If no response by six to eight weeks following titration to maximum tolerated dose, switch to an alternate antidepressant or augment with a second medication, e.g. lithium, triiodothyronin, second-generation antipsychotic, etc.

D. TYPICAL TREATMENT RESPONSE [1, 2, 6]

Usual Target Symptoms
• Affective symptoms
• Anxiety
• Mood-related cognitive symptoms
• Suicidality and suicidal behavior

Common Short-Term Adverse Effects
• Diarrhea
• Dry mouth
• Nausea
• Sweating
• Somnolence or insomnia
• Tremor

Rare Adverse Effects
• Acute angle closure glaucoma
• Agitation
• Akathisia
• Dose-dependent QT interval prolongation
• Hyponatremia

• Treatment-emergent suicidal ideation and suicide in young patients
• Increased risk of upper gastrointestinal (GI) bleed
• May trigger switch to hypomania or mania in bipolar disorder
• Serotonin syndrome
• Type 1 hypersensitivity reactions (anaphylaxis, angioedema, hypotension, tachycardia, swollen tongue, difficulty breathing, wheezing, rash)
• Associated with neonatal withdrawal syndrome
• Associated with rare neonatal pulmonary hypertension

Long-Term Effects
• Discontinuation syndrome
• Sexual dysfunction with anorgasmia being the most common dose-dependent sexual side effect, but also may impair libido, arousal and erectile function

E. PRE-TREATMENT WORKUP AND INITIAL LABORATORY TESTING [1, 2]

History
• General history
• Personal history of:
  ○ heart disease, e.g. congenital long QT syndrome, bradycardia, recent acute myocardial infarction or uncompensated heart failure
  ○ predisposition to hypokalemia, hypomagnesemia
  ○ GI bleed
• Medication history including drugs that prolong the QT interval

Physical
• General physical examination
• Vital signs

Blood Tests
• Basic metabolic panel
• Serum magnesium (if at risk for electrolyte disturbance)
• Liver function panel

Cardiac Tests
• ECG

Pregnancy Test
• Pregnancy test (premenopausal females)
• Classified as risk not ruled out

MONITORING [1]

Quarterly to Annually
- In patients at risk for QT prolongation:
  - Serum potassium and magnesium
  - ECG

 DOSING AND KINETICS [1]

Initial Dosing
- Administer an initial dose of 20 mg daily
- Decrease the initial dose to 10 mg daily in special populations:
  - In patients ≥60 years of age
  - Patients with severe hepatic impairment
  - cyp 2C19 poor metabolizers or those taking a cyp 2C19 inhibitor

Titration
- If tolerated and clinically indicated, titrate to a maximum of 40 mg daily
- In the special population groups listed above, the maximum dose is 20 mg daily

Half-Life
- 35 hours

Bioavailability
- 80%
- Bioavailability is not affected by food

Adjustment for Hepatic Dysfunction (by Child-Pugh Criteria)
- Child-Pugh category A or B (mild-moderate hepatic impairment): no dosage adjustment necessary
- Child-Pugh category C (severe hepatic impairment): use with caution and monitor QT interval

Adjustment for Renal Dysfunction
- No dosage adjustment necessary per the package insert
- However, dose reductions may be necessary in the presence of significant renal impairment

 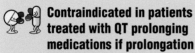 H. MEDICATIONS TO AVOID IN COMBINATION/WARNINGS [1]

 Precautions with cyp 2C19 inhibitors (requires lower dose due to risk of QT interval prolongation)
- Cimetidine
- Clopidogrel
- Efavirenz
- Fluvoxamine
- Fluoxetine
- Isoniazid

Contraindicated in patients treated with QT prolonging medications if prolongation is present
- Class IA antiarrhythmics
- Class III antiarrhythmics
- Antipsychotic medications
- Certain antibiotics, e.g. moxifloxacin
- Other medications known to prolong the QT interval, e.g. methadone

 Contraindicated in patients treated with monoamine oxidase inhibitors (MAOIs) due to risk of serotonin syndrome (either concomitant treatment or treatment within 14 days of stopping an MAOI)
- MAOIs, including linezolid or intravenous methylene blue

- Citalopram is the most selective SSRI and is a racemic mixture with essentially all of its 5HT reuptake inhibition due to the S(+)-enantiomer (escitalopram).
- Citalopram is generally well tolerated with few side effects.

- QT interval prolongation is an infrequently reported adverse effect of citalopram; nevertheless, attention to factors including age, cardiovascular health, dose, concomitant QT-prolonging medications, and medications that may increase the citalopram plasma level is warranted.

References

1. Aurobindo Pharma Limited. (2019). *Citalopram Package Insert*. East Windsor, New Jersey.
2. California Department of State Hospitals. (2019). *DSH Psychotropic Medication Policy: SSRI Protocol*. Sacramento, California.
3. Gray, N. A., Milak, M. S., DeLorenzo, C., et al. (2013). Antidepressant treatment reduces serotonin-1A autoreceptor binding in major depressive disorder. *Biol Psychiatry*, 74, 26–31.
4. Kraus, C., Castren, E., Kasper, S., et al. (2017). Serotonin and neuroplasticity – links between molecular, functional and structural pathophysiology in depression. *Neurosci Biobehav Rev*, 77, 317–326.
5. Gaynes, B. N., Rush, A. J., Trivedi, M. H., et al. (2008). The STAR*D study: treating depression in the real world. *Clevel Clin J Med*, 75, 57–66.
6. Ferguson, J. M. (2001). SSRI antidepressant medications: adverse effects and tolerability. *Prim Care Companion J Clin Psychiatry*, 3, 22.

2.30 Escitalopram

A. BASIC INFORMATION [1, 2]

Principle Trade Names
• Lexapro®

Legal Status
• Prescription only
• Not controlled

Classifications
• Selective serotonin reuptake inhibitor (SSRI)
• Antidepressant

Generics Available
• Yes

Formulations
• Tablet: 5 mg; 10 mg; 20 mg
• Oral solution: 1 mg/ml

FDA Indications
• Major depressive disorder in adults and adolescents
• Generalized anxiety disorder

Other Data-Supported Indications
• Agitation in Alzheimer's disease
• Obsessive-compulsive disorder
• Panic disorder
• Post-traumatic stress disorder
• Premenstrual dysphoric disorder
• Social anxiety disorder

B. MECHANISMS OF ACTION [3, 4]

Serotonin
• Binds directly to 5HT transporter, potently and selectively inhibits 5HT reuptake
• Downregulates and desensitizes the $5HT_{1A}$ receptor with the downstream effect of increasing 5HT levels in the cortex
• Competitively and reversibly antagonizes $5HT_{2C}$ receptors resulting in an increase in DA and NE activity in the prefrontal cortex

Other
• May overcome mood-related changes in synaptic plasticity and neurogenesis by increasing brain derived neurotrophic factor (BDNF) and inducing signaling through certain BDNF receptors

Initial Target Range
- No established plasma therapeutic range

Range for Treatment Resistance
- No established plasma therapeutic range

Typical Time to Response
- Faster onset of action than citalopram with improvements seen by week one or two
- At least four weeks to attain response with six weeks needed to attain remission. Remission can take up to 12 weeks

Time-Course of Improvement
- If no response by six to eight weeks at maximum tolerated dose, switch to an alternate antidepressant or augment with a second medication, e.g. lithium, triiodothyronine, second-generation antipsychotic, etc.

Usual Target Symptoms
- Affective symptoms
- Anxiety
- Mood-related cognitive symptoms
- Suicidality and suicidal behavior

Common Short-Term Adverse Effects
- Insomnia
- Fatigue
- Nausea
- Sweating
- Somnolence

Rare Adverse Effects
- Acute angle closure glaucoma
- Agitation
- Akathisia
- Hyponatremia (mostly in elderly patients and reversible with drug discontinuation)
- Treatment-emergent suicidal ideation and suicide in young patients

- Increased risk of upper gastrointestinal (GI) bleed
- May trigger switch to hypomania or mania in bipolar disorder
- Seizures
- Serotonin syndrome
- Type 1 hypersensitivity reactions (anaphylaxis, angioedema, hypotension, tachycardia, swollen tongue, difficulty breathing, wheezing, rash)
- Associated with neonatal withdrawal syndrome
- Associated with rare neonatal pulmonary hypertension

Long-Term Effects
- Discontinuation syndrome
- Sexual dysfunction

History
- General history
- Personal history of GI bleed

Physical
- Vital signs
- General physical examination

Blood Tests
- Basic metabolic panel
- Liver function panel

Pregnancy Test
- Pregnancy test (premenopausal females)
- Classified as risk not ruled out

Healthy patients
• None

Initial Dosing
• Administer an initial dose of 10 mg daily

Titration
• If tolerated and clinically indicated, titrate to a maximum of 20 mg daily
• In most elderly patients, adolescents, and patients with hepatic impairment, the maximum dose is 10 mg daily

Half-Life
• 27–32 hours

Bioavailability
• 80%
• 56% protein-bound
• Bioavailability is not affected by food

Adjustment for Hepatic Dysfunction (by Child-Pugh Criteria)
• Child-Pugh category A or B (mild-moderate hepatic impairment): no dosage adjustment necessary
• Child-Pugh category C (severe hepatic impairment): maximum dose is 10 mg daily

Adjustment for Renal Dysfunction
• No dosage adjustment necessary per the package insert
• However, dose reductions may be necessary in the presence of significant renal impairment

 Contraindicated in patients treated with monoamine oxidase inhibitors (MAOIs) due to risk of serotonin syndrome (either with concomitant treatment or treatment within 14 days of stopping an MAOI)

Do not start an MAOI for at least five to seven days after discontinuing escitalopram
• MAOIs, including linezolid and intravenous methylene blue

 Possible increased risk of bleeding when combined with drugs that interfere with hemostasis
• Aspirin
• NSAIDs
• Warfarin

• Escitalopram may be one of the best tolerated antidepressants with few side effects and no appreciable effect on the major cytochrome P450 isoforms.

• As the S(+)-enantiomer of citalopram, escitalopram exerts essentially all the 5HT reuptake inhibition. There is evidence that escitalopram is more potent and demonstrates better efficacy than citalopram.

References

1. California Department of State Hospitals. (2019). *DSH Psychotropic Medication Policy: SSRI Protocol.* Sacramento, California.
2. Jubilant Cadista Pharmaceuticals Inc. (2019). *Escitalopram Package Insert. Salisbury,* Maryland.
3. Gray, N. A., Milak, M. S., DeLorenzo, C., et al. (2013). Antidepressant treatment reduces serotonin-1A autoreceptor binding in major depressive disorder. *Biol Psychiatry,* 74, 26–31.
4. Kraus, C., Castren, E., Kasper, S., et al. (2017). Serotonin and neuroplasticity – links between molecular, functional and structural pathophysiology in depression. *Neurosci Biobehav Rev,* 77, 317–326.
5. Sánchez, C., Bøgesø, K. P., Ebert, B., et al. (2004). Escitalopram versus citalopram: the surprising role of the R-enantiomer. *Psychopharmacology,* 174, 163–176.
6. Gaynes, B. N., Rush, A. J., Trivedi, M. H., et al. (2008). The STAR*D study: treating depression in the real world. *Clevel Clin J Med,* 75, 57–66.
7. Ferguson, J. M. (2001). SSRI antidepressant medications: adverse effects and tolerability. *Prim Care Companion J Clin Psychiatry,* 3, 22.

2.31 Fluoxetine

A. BASIC INFORMATION [1, 2]

Principle Trade Names
- Prozac®
- Sarafem®
- Symbyax® (fluoxetine olanzapine combination)

Legal Status
- Prescription only
- Not controlled

Classifications
- Selective serotonin reuptake inhibitor (SSRI)
- Antidepressant

Generics Available
- Yes

Formulations
- Tablet: 10 mg; 20 mg; 40 mg
- Capsule: 10 mg; 20 mg; 40 mg
- Delayed-release capsules: 90 mg
- Oral solution: 20 mg/5 ml

FDA Indications
- Major depressive disorder in patients eight years and older
- Obsessive-compulsive disorder (OCD) in patients seven years and older
- Panic disorder, with and without agoraphobia
- Bulimia nervosa
- Premenstrual dysphoric disorder
- Depressive episodes associated with bipolar I disorder (fluoxetine and olanzapine in combination, monotherapy contraindicated)
- Treatment-resistant depression (fluoxetine and olanzapine in combination)

Other Data-Supported Indications
- Agitation in Alzheimer's disease
- Anxiety associated with major depressive disorder
- Generalized anxiety disorder
- Post-traumatic stress disorder
- Social anxiety disorder

Serotonin

- Binds directly to 5HT transporter, potently and selectively inhibits 5HT reuptake
- Downregulates and desensitizes the 5HT$_{1A}$ receptor with the downstream effect of increasing 5HT levels in the cortex
- Antagonizes 5HT$_{2C}$ receptors, possibly increasing extracellular concentrations of norepinephrine and dopamine in the prefrontal cortex

Other

- May overcome mood-related changes in synaptic plasticity and neurogenesis by increasing brain derived neurotrophic factor (BDNF) and inducing signaling through certain BDNF receptors

Initial Target Range

- No established plasma therapeutic range

Range for Treatment Resistance

- No established plasma therapeutic range

Typical Time to Response

- At least four weeks to attain response with six weeks needed to attain remission. Remission can take up to 12 weeks

Time-Course of Improvement

- If no response by six to eight weeks to maximum tolerated dose, switch to an alternate antidepressant or augment with a second medication, e.g. lithium, triiodothyronine, second-generation antipsychotic, etc.

Usual Target Symptoms

- Affective symptoms
- Anxiety
- Mood-related cognitive symptoms
- Binge eating and purging
- Suicidality and suicidal behavior

Common Short-Term Adverse Effects

- Agitation, anxiety and activation
- Anorexia
- Diarrhea
- Dry mouth
- Dyspepsia
- Nausea
- Insomnia or somnolence
- Sweating
- Tremor

Rare Adverse Effects

- Acute angle closure glaucoma
- Akathisia
- Hyponatremia (mostly in elderly patients and reversible with drug discontinuation)
- Treatment-emergent suicidal ideation and suicide in young patients

- Increased risk of upper gastrointestinal (GI) bleed
- May trigger switch to hypomania or mania in bipolar disorder
- Serotonin syndrome
- Type 1 hypersensitivity reactions, e.g. anaphylaxis, angioedema, hypotension, tachycardia, swollen tongue, difficulty breathing, wheezing, rash
- Third trimester fetal exposure may result in lower birth weight and premature delivery
- Rare pulmonary hypertension or discontinuation syndrome in exposed neonates

Long-Term Effects

- Drug interactions, e.g. fluoxetine and norfluoxetine are inhibitors of multiple cytochrome P450 enzymes:
  - Potent inhibition of cyp 2D6 and cyp 2C19
  - Moderate inhibition of cyp 3A4 and cyp 2C9
- Sexual dysfunction
- Weight loss

History
- General history
- Current medications
- Personal history of GI bleed

Physical
- Vital signs
- General physical examination

Blood Tests
- Basic metabolic panel
- Liver function panel

Pregnancy Test
- Test premenopausal females
- Classified as risk not ruled out

In healthy patients
None

Initial Dosing
- Administer an initial dose of 20 mg each morning in patients with depression or OCD
- Administer an initial dose of 60 mg each morning to patients with bulimia
- Decrease the initial dose to 10 mg daily in special populations:
  - Children and adolescents
  - In patients ≥60 years of age
  - Patients with severe hepatic impairment

Titration
- If tolerated and clinically indicated, titrate to clinical effect. Maximum dose is 80 mg daily
- In the special population groups listed above, a lower maximum dose should be considered

Half-Life
- Fluoxetine: four to six days after chronic administration
- Norfluoxetine (active metabolite): four to 16 days after acute and chronic administration

Bioavailability
- 60–80%
- 94.5% protein-bound
- Bioavailability is not affected by food

Adjustment for Hepatic Dysfunction (by Child-Pugh Criteria)
- Child-Pugh category A or B (mild-moderate hepatic impairment): no dosage adjustment necessary
- Child-Pugh category C (severe hepatic impairment): lower the dose or give less frequently

Adjustment for Renal Dysfunction
- No dosage adjustment necessary per the package insert
- However, dose reductions may be necessary in the presence of significant renal impairment

H. MEDICATIONS TO AVOID IN COMBINATION/WARNINGS [1, 8]

 Contraindicated in patients taking certain dopamine receptor antagonists

- Pimozide
  - Pimozide can prolong the QT interval. Fluoxetine's inhibition of cyp 2D6 can increase the level of pimozide resulting in increased risk of QT prolongation
- Thioridazine
  - Thioridazine can prolong the QT interval. Fluoxetine's inhibition of cyp 2D6 can increase the level of thioridazine resulting in increased risk of QT prolongation
  - Do not start thioridazine within five weeks of stopping fluoxetine

 Contraindicated in patients treated with monoamine oxidase inhibitors (MAOIs) due to risk of serotonin syndrome (either concomitant treatment or treatment within 14 days of stopping an MAOI)

Do not start an MAOI for at least five weeks after discontinuing fluoxetine

- MAOIs, including linezolid and intravenous methylene blue

 Drugs metabolized by cyp 2D6 due to fluoxetine's potent inhibition of this enzyme

- Certain antidepressants, e.g. tricyclic antidepressants (TCAs) and others
- Certain antipsychotics, e.g. phenothiazides, risperidone, clozapine and others
- Antiarrhythmics, e.g. flecainide and others
- Codeine
- Certain beta blockers
- Atomoxetine
- Tamoxifen

 Drugs that are metabolized by cyp 3A4 due to fluoxetine's moderate inhibition of this enzyme

- Certain benzodiazepines, e.g. alprazolam, diazepam, triazolam
- Trazodone
- Certain cholesterol lowering medications, e.g. simvastatin
- Buspirone

 Possible increased risk of bleeding when combined with drugs that interfere with hemostasis

- Aspirin
- NSAIDs
- Warfarin

 Drugs tightly bound to plasma proteins as due to fluoxetine's tight binding, plasma concentrations of other protein-bound drugs may shift

- Warfarin
- Antibiotics, e.g. penicillins, sulfonamides, tetracyclines
- Antiepileptics, e.g. phenytoin, divalproex
- NSAIDs
- Sedatives, e.g. benzodiazepines, barbiturates

ART OF PSYCHOPHARMACOLOGY: TAKE-HOME PEARLS [8, 9]

- Activating qualities make fluoxetine a strong consideration for patients with atypical depression.
- While fluoxetine is generally well tolerated, some patients with anxiety or panic disorder may find it too activating.
- Fluoxetine's inhibition of multiple cyp 450 isoenzymes results in problematic drug-drug interactions.

References

1. Aurobindo Pharma Limited. (2019). *Fluoxetine Package Insert and Label.* East Windsor, New Jersey.
2. California Department of State Hospitals. (2019). *DSH Psychotropic Medication Policy: SSRI Protocol.* Sacramento, California.
3. Ni, Y., Miledi, R. (1997). Blockage of 5HT2C serotonin receptors by fluoxetine (Prozac). *Proc Natl Acad Sci,* 94, 2036–2040.
4. Gray, N. A., Milak, M. S., DeLorenzo, C., et al. (2013). Antidepressant treatment reduces serotonin-1A autoreceptor binding in major depressive disorder. *Biol Psychiatry,* 74, 26–31.
5. Kraus, C., Castren, E., Kasper, S., et al. (2017). Serotonin and neuroplasticity – links between molecular, functional and structural pathophysiology in depression. *Neurosci Biobehav Rev,* 77, 317–326.
6. Gaynes, B. N., Rush, A. J., Trivedi, M. H., et al. (2008). The STAR*D study: treating depression in the real world. *Clevel Clin J Med,* 75, 57–66.
7. Ferguson, J. M. (2001). SSRI antidepressant medications: adverse effects and tolerability. *Prim Care Companion J Clin Psychiatry,* 3, 22.
8. Sager, J. E., Lutz, J. D., Foti, R. S., et al. (2014). Fluoxetine- and norfluoxetine-mediated complex drug–drug interactions: in vitro to in vivo correlation of effects on CYP2D6, CYP2C19, and CYP3A4. *Clin Pharmacol Ther,* 95, 653–662.
9. Spina, E., de Leon, J. (2014). Clinically relevant interactions between newer antidepressants and second-generation antipsychotics. *Expert Opin Drug Metab Toxicol,* 10, 721–746.

2.32 Fluvoxamine

A. BASIC INFORMATION [1–3]

Principle Trade Names
• Luvox®
• Luvox CR®

Legal Status
• Prescription only
• Not controlled

Classifications
• Selective serotonin reuptake inhibitor (SSRI)
• Antidepressant

Generics Available
• Yes

Formulations
• Tablet: 25 mg; 50 mg; 100 mg
• Extended-release capsule: 100 mg; 200 mg

FDA Indications
• Obsessive-compulsive disorder in patients eight years and older (fluvoxamine) and in adults (fluvoxamine CR)
• Social anxiety disorder (fluvoxamine CR)

Other Data-Supported Indications
• Depression
• Generalized anxiety disorder
• Panic disorder
• Post-traumatic stress disorder

Serotonin
• Binds directly to 5HT transporter, potently and selectively inhibits 5HT reuptake
• Downregulates and desensitizes the $5HT_{1A}$ receptor with the downstream effect of increasing 5HT levels in the cortex
• Competitively and reversibly antagonizes $5HT_{2C}$ receptors resulting in an increase in DA and NE activity in the prefrontal cortex

Other
• Potent σ_1 receptor chaperone receptor agonist. σ_1 agonism may play a role in treatment of certain neuropsychiatric diseases
• May overcome mood-related changes in synaptic plasticity and neurogenesis by increasing brain derived neurotrophic factor (BDNF) and inducing signaling through certain BDNF receptors

C. PLASMA CONCENTRATIONS AND TREATMENT RESPONSE [7]

Initial Target Range
- No established plasma therapeutic range

Range for Treatment Resistance
- No established plasma therapeutic range

Typical Time to Response
- At least four weeks to attain response with six weeks needed to attain remission. Remission can take up to 12 weeks

Time-Course of Improvement
- If no response by six to eight weeks at maximum tolerated dose, switch to an alternate antidepressant or augment with a second medication, e.g. lithium, triiodothyronine, second-generation antipsychotic, etc.

D. TYPICAL TREATMENT RESPONSE [2, 3, 8]

Usual Target Symptoms
- Affective symptoms
- Anxiety
- Mood-related cognitive symptoms
- Obsessions and compulsions
- Suicidality and suicidal behavior

Common Short-Term Adverse Effects
- Nausea
- Somnolence
- Insomnia
- Nervousness
- Dyspepsia
- Vomiting
- Dizziness
- Sweating
- Tremor

Rare Adverse Effects
- Acute angle closure glaucoma
- Hyponatremia (mostly in elderly patients and reversible with drug discontinuation)
- Treatment-emergent suicidal ideation and suicide in young patients

- Increased risk of upper gastrointestinal (GI) bleed
- May trigger switch to hypomania or mania in bipolar disorder
- Serotonin syndrome
- Seizures
- Type 1 hypersensitivity reactions (anaphylaxis, angioedema, hypotension, tachycardia, swollen tongue, difficulty breathing, wheezing, rash)
- Third trimester fetal exposure may result in lower birth weight and premature delivery
- Rare pulmonary hypertension or discontinuation syndrome in exposed neonates

Long-Term Effects
- Drug interactions, e.g. fluvoxamine is a potent inhibitor of cyp 1A2 and a moderate inhibitor of cyp 2C19
- Discontinuation syndrome
- Sexual dysfunction

E. PRE-TREATMENT WORKUP AND INITIAL LABORATORY TESTING [2]

History
- General history
- Personal history of GI bleed

Physical
- Vital signs
- General physical examination

Blood Tests
- Basic metabolic panel
- Liver function panel

Pregnancy Test
- Pregnancy test (premenopausal females)
- Classified as risk not ruled out

Healthy patients
• None

Initial Dosing
• For immediate-release administer an initial dose of 50 mg at bedtime
• For controlled release begin with a dose of 100 mg at bedtime
• Decrease the initial dose in children, adolescents, the elderly, and medically frail patients

Titration
• If tolerated and clinically indicated, titrate to a dose range of 50–200 mg/day in patients under 18 years and 100–300 mg in adults
• Doses greater than 100 mg should be given in divided doses
• Modify the titration and maximal dose in elderly patients

Half-Life
• 15.6 hours

Bioavailability
• 44–62%
• Bioavailability is not affected by food

Adjustment for Hepatic Dysfunction (by Child-Pugh Criteria)
• Child-Pugh category A or B (mild-moderate hepatic impairment): no dosage adjustment necessary
• Child-Pugh category C (severe hepatic impairment): decrease starting and maximum dose

Adjustment for Renal Dysfunction
• No dosage adjustment necessary per the package insert
• However, dose reductions may be necessary in the presence of significant renal impairment

Tobacco Smokers
• 25% increase in fluvoxamine metabolism due to induction of cyp 1A2 by polycyclic aromatic hydrocarbons in smoke

H. MEDICATIONS TO AVOID IN COMBINATION/WARNINGS [1, 3, 10]

 Drugs metabolized by cyp 1A2 due to fluvoxamine's potent inhibition of this enzyme

- Alosetron
- Certain chemotherapeutic agents, e.g. bendamustine, erlotinib, pomalidomide
- Caffeine
- Clozapine
- Duloxetine
- Melatonin and related drugs, e.g. agomelatine, ramelteon, tasimelteon
- Olanzapine
- Pirfenidone
- Propranolol
- Tertiary-amine tricyclic antidepressants, e.g. imipramine, amitriptyline, clomipramine
- Theophylline and theophylline derivatives
- Tizanidine

 Drugs metabolized by cyp 3A4 due to fluvoxamine's weak inhibition of this enzyme

- Carbamazepine
- Lemborexant
- Lomitapide
- Methadone
- Certain benzodiazepines, e.g. alprazolam, diazepam, triazolam

 Drugs metabolized by cyp 2C19 due to fluvoxamine's weak inhibition of this enzyme

- Cilostazol
- Citalopram
- Warfarin

 Contraindicated in patients treated with monoamine oxidase inhibitors (MAOIs) due to risk of serotonin syndrome (either with concomitant treatment or treatment within 14 days of stopping an MAOI)

Do not start an MAOI for at least five to seven days after discontinuing fluvoxamine

- MAOIs, including linezolid and intravenous methylene blue

 Possible increased risk of bleeding when combined with drugs that interfere with hemostasis

- Aspirin
- NSAIDs
- Warfarin

 Contraindicated in patients taking certain dopamine receptor antagonists

- Pimozide
  - Pimozide can prolong the QT interval. Fluvoxamine's inhibition of cyp 1A2 and cyp 3A4 can increase the plasma level of pimozide resulting in increased risk of QT prolongation
- Thioridazine
  - Thioridazine can prolong the QT interval. Fluvoxamine's inhibition of cyp 1A2, cyp 2C19 and other enzymes can increase the plasma level of thioridizine resulting in increased risk of QT prolongation

 ART OF PSYCHOPHARMACOLOGY: TAKE-HOME PEARLS [10, 11]

- Fluvoxamine is not just an OCD drug. Moreover, it has no greater effect on OCD than the other SSRIs.
- Due to fluvoxamine's inhibition of multiple cyp 450 isoenzymes, drug interactions are common and include multiple drugs from different drug classes. Of particular importance in patients with treatment-resistant psychosis is fluvoxamine's inhibition of cyp isoenzymes involved in clozapine and olanzapine metabolism resulting in higher drug plasma levels.
- Although fluvoxamine has a relatively short half-life, antidepressant discontinuation syndrome is less common due to a longer brain half-life.

References

1. Actavis Pharma, I. (2017). *Fluvoxamine Extended Release Package Insert.* Parsippany, New Jersey.
2. California Department of State Hospitals. (2019). *DSH Psychotropic Medication Policy: SSRI Protocol.* Sacramento, California.
3. Apotex Corp. (2020). *Fluvoxamine Package Insert. Weston,* Florida.
4. Gray, N. A., Milak, M. S., DeLorenzo, C., et al. (2013). Antidepressant treatment reduces serotonin-1A autoreceptor binding in major depressive disorder. *Biol Psychiatry,* 74, 26–31.
5. Tsai, S. Y., Pokrass, M. J., Klauer, N. R., et al. (2014). Sigma-1 receptor chaperones in neurodegenerative and psychiatric disorders. *Expert Opin Ther Targets,* 18, 1461–1476.
6. Kraus, C., Castren, E., Kasper, S., et al. (2017). Serotonin and neuroplasticity – links between molecular, functional and structural pathophysiology in depression. *Neurosci Biobehav Rev,* 77, 317–326.
7. Gaynes, B. N., Rush, A. J., Trivedi, M. H., et al. (2008). The STAR*D study: treating depression in the real world. *Clevel Clin J Med,* 75, 57–66.
8. Ferguson, J. M. (2001). SSRI antidepressant medications: adverse effects and tolerability. *Prim Care Companion J Clin Psychiatry,* 3, 22.
9. Oliveira, P., Ribeiro, J., Donato, H., et al. (2017). Smoking and antidepressants pharmacokinetics: a systematic review. *Ann Gen Psychiatry,* 16, 17.
10. Spina, E., de Leon, J. (2014). Clinically relevant interactions between newer antidepressants and second-generation antipsychotics. *Expert Opin Drug Metab Toxicol,* 10, 721–746.
11. Strauss, W. L., Layton, M. E., Dager, S. R. (1998). Brain elimination half-life of fluvoxamine measured by 19 F magnetic resonance spectroscopy. *Am J Psychiatry,* 155, 380–384.

2.33 Paroxetine

A. BASIC INFORMATION [1–3]

Principle Trade Names
- Paxil®
- Paxil CR®
- Brisdelle®
- Pexeva®

Legal Status
- Prescription only
- Not controlled

Classifications
- Selective serotonin reuptake inhibitor (SSRI)
- Antidepressant

Generics Available
- Yes

Formulations
- Tablet: 10 mg; 20 mg; 30 mg; 40 mg
- Capsule: 7.5 mg
- Extended-release tablets: 12.5 mg; 25 mg; 37.5 mg

FDA Indications
- Major depressive disorder
- Generalized anxiety disorder
- Obsessive-compulsive disorder (OCD)
- Panic disorder, with and without agoraphobia
- Post-traumatic stress disorder
- Premenstrual dysphoric disorder
- Social anxiety disorder
- Vasomotor symptoms (Brisdelle®)

B. MECHANISMS OF ACTION [1–3, 4]

Serotonin
- Binds directly to 5HT transporter, selectively and potently inhibiting 5HT reuptake
- Downregulates and desensitizes the $5HT_{1A}$ receptor with the downstream effect of increasing 5HT levels in the cortex

Norepinephrine
- Shows moderate affinity for the NE transporter, inhibiting NE reuptake in a dose-dependent fashion

Acetylcholine
- Weakly antagonizes muscarinic (M_3) cholinergic receptors

Other
- May overcome mood-related changes in synaptic plasticity and neurogenesis by increasing brain derived neurotrophic factor (BDNF) and inducing signaling through certain BDNF receptors

Initial Target Range
- No established plasma therapeutic range

Range for Treatment Resistance
- No established plasma therapeutic range

Typical Time to Response
- At least four weeks to attain response with six weeks needed to attain remission. Remission can take up to 12 weeks

Time-Course of Improvement
- If no response by six to eight weeks at maximum tolerated dose, switch to an alternate antidepressant or augment with a second medication, e.g. lithium, triiodothyronine, second-generation antipsychotic, etc.

Usual Target Symptoms
- Affective symptoms
- Anxiety
- Mood-related cognitive symptoms
- Suicidality and suicidal behavior
- Vasomotor symptoms

Common Short-Term Adverse Effects
- Anorexia
- Diarrhea or constipation
- Dizziness
- Dry mouth
- Dyspepsia
- Headache
- Insomnia or somnolence
- Nausea
- Sedation
- Sweating
- Tremor

Rare Adverse Effects
- Acute angle closure glaucoma
- Akathisia
- Hyponatremia (mostly in elderly patients and reversible with drug discontinuation)
- Treatment-emergent suicidal ideation and suicide in young patients

- Increased risk of upper gastrointestinal (GI) bleed
- May trigger switch to hypomania or mania in bipolar disorder
- Serotonin syndrome
- Seizures
- Type 1 hypersensitivity reactions, e.g. anaphylaxis, angioedema, hypotension, tachycardia, swollen tongue, difficulty breathing, wheezing, rash
- Increased risk of cardiovascular malformations (atrial and ventricular septal defects) in infants when exposed to paroxetine during the first trimester
- Third trimester fetal exposure may result in lower birth weight and premature delivery
- Rare pulmonary hypertension or discontinuation syndrome in exposed neonates

Long-Term Effects
- Discontinuation syndrome is common, may be more severe than with other SSRIs
- Drug interactions, e.g. paroxetine is a potent inhibitor of cyp 2D6
- Sexual dysfunction
- Weight gain

History
- General history
- Current medications
- Personal history of GI bleed

Physical
- Vital signs
- General physical examination

Blood Tests
- Basic metabolic panel
- Liver function panel

Pregnancy Test
- Test premenopausal females
- Classified as risk not ruled out

F. MONITORING [1, 3]

In healthy patients
- None

G. DOSING AND KINETICS [1, 3, 5]

Initial Dosing
- Administer an initial dose of 20 mg each morning (25 mg controlled-released (CR)) in patients with depression, OCD, social anxiety disorder or generalized anxiety disorder
- Administer an initial dose of 10 mg each morning (12.5 mg CR) in patients with panic disorder
- Decrease the initial dose to 10 mg daily (12.5 mg CR) in special populations:
  - Children and adolescents
  - In patients ≥60 years of age
- Administer an initial dose of 7.5 mg at bedtime for treatment of vasomotor symptoms
- Paroxetine CR tablets must be swallowed whole. If crushed, chewed or dissolved, the controlled-release properties will be lost

Titration
- If tolerated and clinically indicated, titrate to clinical effect. Maximum dose is 60 mg daily
- Maximum dose for treating vasomotor symptoms is 7.5 mg nightly
- In the special population groups listed above, the maximum dose is 40 mg/day

Half-Life
- 21 hours

Bioavailability
- Extensively absorbed but also undergoes extensive first-pass metabolism
- 93–95% protein-bound
- When administered with food, the total drug exposure is not significantly changed although paroxetine reaches a greater peak plasma level more quickly

Adjustment for Hepatic Dysfunction (by Child-Pugh Criteria)
- Child-Pugh category A or B (mild-moderate hepatic impairment): no dosage adjustment necessary
- Child-Pugh category C (severe hepatic impairment): lower the starting dose to 10 mg/day, increase the interval between titrations, and titrate to a lower maximum dose, e.g. 40 mg/day

Adjustment for Renal Dysfunction
- Mean plasma concentration is four times greater in patients with creatinine clearance <30 ml/min
- Lower the starting dose to 10 mg/day, increase the interval between titrations, and titrate to a lower maximum dose, e.g. 40 mg/day

H. MEDICATIONS TO AVOID IN COMBINATION/ WARNINGS [6, 7]

 Contraindicated in patients taking certain dopamine receptor antagonists

- Pimozide
  - Pimozide can prolong the QT interval. Paroxetine's inhibition of cyp 2D6 can increase the level of pimozide resulting in increased risk of QT prolongation
- Thioridazine
  - Thioridazine can prolong the QT interval. Paroxetine's inhibition of cyp 2D6 can increase the level of thioridazine resulting in increased risk of QT prolongation

 Contraindicated in patients treated with monoamine oxidase inhibitors (MAOIs) due to risk of serotonin syndrome (either concomitant treatment or treatment within 14 days of stopping an MAOI)

Do not start an MAOI for at least 14 days after discontinuing paroxetine

- MAOIs, including linezolid and intravenous methylene blue

 Precautions in patients co-administered drugs metabolized by cyp 2D6 due to paroxetine's potent inhibition of this enzyme

- Certain antidepressants, e.g. TCAs and others
- Certain antipsychotics, e.g. phenothiazides, risperidone, clozapine and others
- Antiarrhythmics, e.g. flecainide and others
- Codeine
- Certain beta blockers
- Atomoxetine
- Tamoxifen

 Possible increased risk of bleeding when combined with drugs that interfere with hemostasis

- Aspirin
- NSAIDs
- Warfarin

ART OF PSYCHOPHARMACOLOGY: TAKE-HOME PEARLS [2, 4, 7]

- Of the SSRIs, paroxetine is the most potent inhibitor of the 5HT transporter and of the NE transporter. At doses of 40 mg daily, paroxetine may be functioning as a dual serotonin and norepinephrine reuptake inhibitor in many patients.
- Discontinuation syndrome has been reported more frequently and tends to be more severe with paroxetine than with other SSRIs. Symptoms can be reduced by either tapering slowly, switching to the liquid formulation for slower tapering, or switching to an SSRI with a longer half-life, e.g. fluoxetine.

- Developed to reduce GI side effects, the enteric coating on paroxetine CR delays drug release until the tablet has left the stomach. Due to the tablet's delayed-release properties, up to 20% does not enter systemic circulation. The dose of paroxetine CR is 1.25x the dose of paroxetine.
- Like fluoxetine, paroxetine's potent inhibition of cyp 2D6 results in problematic drug-drug interactions with many different classes of drugs. Paroxetine can also inhibit its own metabolism resulting in higher than expected drug plasma levels.

📖 References

1. California Department of State Hospitals. (2019). *DSH Psychotropic Medication Policy: SSRI Protocol*. Sacramento, California.
2. Rhodes Pharmaceuticals L.P. (2019). *Paroxetine Extended Release Package Insert*. Coventry, Rhode Island.
3. Solco Healthcare U.S. LLC. (2020). *Paroxetine Package Insert*. Somerset, New Jersey.
4. Gilmor, M. L., Owens, M. J., Nemeroff, C. B. (2002). Inhibition of norepinephrine uptake in patients with major depression treated with paroxetine. *Am J Psychiatry*, 159, 1702–1710.
5. Gaynes, B. N., Rush, A. J., Trivedi, M. H., et al. (2008). The STAR*D study: treating depression in the real world. *Clevel Clin J Med*, 75, 57–66.
6. Ferguson, J. M. (2001). SSRI antidepressant medications: adverse effects and tolerability. *Prim Care Companion J Clin Psychiatry*, 3, 22.
7. Spina, E., de Leon, J. (2014). Clinically relevant interactions between newer antidepressants and second-generation antipsychotics. *Expert Opin Drug Metab Toxicol*, 10, 721–746.

A. BASIC INFORMATION [1, 2]

Principle Trade Names
• Zoloft®

Legal Status
• Prescription only
• Not controlled

Classifications
• Selective serotonin reuptake inhibitor (SSRI)
• Antidepressant

Generics Available
• Yes

Formulations
• Tablet: 25 mg; 50 mg; 100 mg
• Oral solution: 20 mg/1 ml

FDA Indications
• Major depressive disorder
• Obsessive-compulsive disorder (OCD)
• Panic disorder
• Post-traumatic stress disorder (PTSD)
• Premenstrual dysphoric disorder (PMDD)
• Social anxiety disorder

Other Data-Supported Indications
• Agitation in Alzheimer's disease
• Generalized anxiety disorder

B. MECHANISMS OF ACTION [1-3, 6]

Serotonin
• Binds directly to 5HT transporter, potently and selectively inhibits 5HT reuptake
• Downregulates and desensitizes the $5HT_{1A}$ receptor with the downstream effect of increasing 5HT levels in the cortex

Dopamine
• Inhibits the dopamine transporter, increasing dopamine neurotransmission

Other
• High affinity for the σ_1 receptor, functioning as an inverse agonist
• May overcome mood-related changes in synaptic plasticity and neurogenesis by increasing brain derived neurotrophic factor (BDNF) and inducing signaling through certain BDNF receptors

C. PLASMA CONCENTRATIONS AND TREATMENT RESPONSE [7]

Initial Target Range
• No established plasma therapeutic range

Range for Treatment Resistance
• No established plasma therapeutic range

Typical Time to Response
• At least four weeks to attain response with six weeks needed to attain remission. Remission can take up to 12 weeks

Time-Course of Improvement
• If no response by six to eight weeks at maximum tolerated dose, switch to an alternate antidepressant or augment with a second medication, e.g. lithium, triiodothyronine, second-generation antipsychotic, etc.

D. TYPICAL TREATMENT RESPONSE [1, 8]

Usual Target Symptoms
• Affective symptoms
• Anxiety
• Mood-related cognitive symptoms
• Obsessions and compulsions
• Suicidality and suicidal behavior

Common Short-Term Adverse Effects
• Nausea
• Decreased appetite
• Diarrhea/loose stool
• Dyspepsia
• Sweating
• Tremor

Rare Adverse Effects
• Acute angle closure glaucoma
• Akathisia
• Hyponatremia (mostly in elderly patients and reversible with drug discontinuation)

• Treatment-emergent suicidal ideation and suicide in young patients
• Increased risk of upper gastrointestinal (GI) bleed
• May trigger switch to hypomania or mania in bipolar disorder
• Serotonin syndrome
• Seizures
• Type 1 hypersensitivity reactions, e.g. anaphylaxis, angioedema, hypotension, tachycardia, swollen tongue, difficulty breathing, wheezing, rash
• Third trimester fetal exposure may result in lower birth weight and premature delivery
• Rare pulmonary hypertension or discontinuation syndrome in exposed neonates

Long-Term Effects
• Drug interactions, e.g. sertraline is a weak-moderate inhibitor of cyp 2D6
• Sexual dysfunction

E. PRE-TREATMENT WORKUP AND INITIAL LABORATORY TESTING [2]

History
• General history
• Current medications
• Personal history of GI bleed

Physical
• Vital signs
• General physical examination

Blood Tests
• Basic metabolic panel
• Liver function panel

Pregnancy Test
• Test premenopausal females
• Classified as risk not ruled out

F. MONITORING [1]

In healthy patients
• None

Initial Dosing

- Administer an initial dose of 50 mg once daily in patients with depression, OCD or PMDD (intermittent dosing during luteal phase)
- Administer an initial dose of 25 mg daily in patients with PTSD, anxiety disorders or PMDD with continuous dosing

Titration

- If tolerated and clinically indicated, titrate by 25–50 mg increments weekly, to clinical effect. Maximum dose is 200 mg daily in healthy adults

Half-Life

- 26 hours

Bioavailability

- 44%

- 98% protein-bound
- Sertraline binds weakly to α_1-glycoproteins and doesn't displace highly protein-bound drugs such as warfarin
- When taken with food, sertraline reaches peak plasma concentration sooner

Adjustment for Hepatic Dysfunction (by Child-Pugh Criteria)

- Child-Pugh category A (mild hepatic impairment): decrease the dose to one-half of the recommended initial and maintenance dose. Maximum dose is 100 mg/day
- Child-Pugh category B or C (moderate or severe hepatic impairment): not recommended due to sertraline's extensive hepatic metabolism

Adjustment for Renal Dysfunction

- No dosage adjustment is necessary in mild, moderate or severe renal impairment

Contraindicated in patients taking pimozide

- Pimozide can prolong the QT interval. Sertraline's inhibition of cyp 2D6 can increase the level of pimozide resulting in increased risk of QT prolongation

Contraindicated in patients treated with monoamine oxidase inhibitors (MAOIs) due to risk of serotonin syndrome (either with concomitant treatment or treatment within 14 days of stopping an MAOI)

Do not start an MAOI for at least five to seven days after discontinuing sertraline

- MAOIs, including linezolid and intravenous methylene blue

Precautions with drugs metabolized by cyp 2D6 due to sertraline's dose-dependent, weak-moderate inhibition of this enzyme

- Certain antidepressants, e.g. TCAs and others
- Certain antipsychotics, e.g. phenothiazines, risperidone, clozapine and others
- Antiarrhythmics, e.g. flecainide and others
- Codeine
- Certain beta blockers
- Atomoxetine
- Tamoxifen

Possible increased risk of bleeding when combined with drugs that interfere with hemostasis

- Aspirin
- NSAIDs
- Warfarin

Possible false positive on urine drug screen

- Sertraline may result in a false positive for benzodiazepines on immunoassay urine drug screen. Consider confirmatory testing with gas chromatography/mass spectroscopy

- Sertraline is one of the most well-tolerated SSRIs with few side effects and modest effect on the major cyp isoenzymes.
- Safe in patients with mild-severe renal impairment.

- Similar to fluoxetine, sertraline tends to be activating early in treatment benefiting patients with lethargy and apathy. Activation may be due to sertraline's inhibition of dopamine reuptake.

References

1. Exelam Pharmaceuticals Inc. (2018). *Sertraline Package Insert*. Lawrenceville, Georgia.
2. California Department of State Hospitals. (2019). *DSH Psychotropic Medication Policy: SSRI Protocol*. Sacramento, California.
3. Nemeroff, C. B., Owens, M. J. (2004). Pharmacologic differences among the SSRIs: focus on monoamine transporters and the HPA axis. *CNS Spectr*, 9, 23–31.
4. Gray, N. A., Milak, M. S., DeLorenzo, C., et al. (2013). Antidepressant treatment reduces serotonin-1A autoreceptor binding in major depressive disorder. *Biol Psychiatry*, 74, 26–31.
5. Kraus, C., Castren, E., Kasper, S., et al. (2017). Serotonin and neuroplasticity – links between molecular, functional and structural pathophysiology in depression. *Neurosci Biobehav Rev*, 77, 317–326.
6. Matsushima, Y., Terada, K., Kamei, C., et al. (2019). Sertraline inhibits nerve growth factor-induced neurite outgrowth in PC12 cells via a mechanism involving the sigma-1 receptor. *Eur J Pharmacol*, 853, 129–135.
7. Gaynes, B. N., Rush, A. J., Trivedi, M. H., et al. (2008). The STAR*D study: treating depression in the real world. *Clevel Clin J Med*, 75, 57–66.
8. Ferguson, J. M. (2001). SSRI antidepressant medications: adverse effects and tolerability. *Prim Care Companion J Clin Psychiatry*, 3, 22.
9. Stahl, S. M. (2004). Selectivity of SSRIs: individualising patient care through rational treatment choices. *Int J Psychiatry Clin Pract*, 8, 3–10.

A. BASIC INFORMATION [1]

Principle Trade Names
• Viibryd®
• Viibryd Titration Pack®

Legal Status
• Prescription only
• Not controlled

Classifications
• Selective serotonin reuptake inhibitor (SSRI)
• 5HT$_{1A}$ receptor partial agonist
• Antidepressant

Generics Available
• Yes

Formulations
• Tablet: 10 mg; 20 mg; 40 mg

FDA Indications
• Major depressive disorder

Other Data-Supported Indications
• Generalized anxiety disorder
• Obsessive-compulsive disorder (OCD)

Serotonin
• Binds directly to 5HT transporter, potently and selectively inhibits 5HT reuptake
• 5HT elevation results in desensitizing 5HT$_{1A}$ receptors
• Partial agonism at 5HT$_{1A}$ receptors increases serotonergic neurotransmission and may hasten antidepressant effect

C. PLASMA CONCENTRATIONS AND TREATMENT RESPONSE [1, 3, 4]

Initial Target Range
- No established plasma therapeutic range

Range for Treatment Resistance
- No established plasma therapeutic range

Typical Time to Response
- May be sooner than other antidepressants, improvement in mood occurring at week two

Time-Course of Improvement
- If no response by six to eight weeks at maximum tolerated dose, switch to an alternate antidepressant or augment with a second medication, e.g. lithium, triiodothyronine, second-generation antipsychotic, etc.

D. TYPICAL TREATMENT RESPONSE [1, 5, 6]

Usual Target Symptoms
- Affective symptoms
- Anxiety
- Mood-related cognitive symptoms
- Suicidality and suicidal behavior

Common Short-Term Adverse Effects
- Diarrhea
- Nausea
- Vomiting
- Insomnia

Rare Adverse Effects
- Acute angle closure glaucoma
- Agitation
- Akathisia
- Hyponatremia (mostly in elderly patients and reversible with drug discontinuation)
- Treatment-emergent suicidal ideation and suicide in young patients

- Increased risk of upper gastrointestinal (GI) bleed
- May trigger switch to hypomania or mania in bipolar disorder
- Seizures
- Serotonin syndrome
- Type 1 hypersensitivity reactions (anaphylaxis, angioedema, hypotension, tachycardia, swollen tongue, difficulty breathing, wheezing, rash)
- Third trimester fetal exposure may result in lower birth weight and premature delivery
- Rare pulmonary hypertension or discontinuation syndrome in exposed neonates

Long-Term Effects
- Discontinuation syndrome
- Sexual dysfunction (<other SSRIs)

E. PRE-TREATMENT WORKUP AND INITIAL LABORATORY TESTING [7]

History
- General history
- Personal history of GI bleed

Physical
- Vital signs
- General physical examination

Blood Tests
- Basic metabolic panel
- Liver function panel

Pregnancy Test
- Pregnancy test (premenopausal females)
- Classified as risk not ruled out

F. MONITORING [7]

In healthy patients
- None

Initial Dosing
- Administer an initial dose of 10 mg daily with food

Titration
- After seven days, titrate to 20 mg once daily
- If tolerated and clinically indicated, increase to 40 mg once daily after seven days

Half-Life
- 25 hours

Bioavailability
- 96–99% protein-bound
- 72% bioavailable when administered with food
- In the fasted state, total drug exposure and maximal plasma concentration are decreased by at least 50%

Adjustment for Hepatic Dysfunction (by Child-Pugh Criteria)
- No dose adjustment is necessary

Adjustment for Renal Dysfunction
- No dose adjustment necessary

Contraindicated in patients treated with monoamine oxidase inhibitors (MAOIs) due to risk of serotonin syndrome (either with concomitant treatment or treatment within 14 days of stopping an MAOI)

Do not start an MAOI for at least 14 days after discontinuing vilazodone
- MAOIs, including linezolid and intravenous methylene blue

Possible increased risk of bleeding when combined with drugs that interfere with hemostasis
- Aspirin
- NSAIDs
- Warfarin

Precautions with other drugs that are highly protein-bound
- Vilazodone is highly bound to plasma proteins and may displace other drugs that are highly protein-bound, e.g. warfarin

Precautions with strong cyp 3A4 inducers. Consider increasing the dose of vilazodone when co-administered with strong cyp 3A4 inducers
- Carbamazepine
- Phenytoin
- Rifampin

Precautions with strong cyp 3A4 inhibitors. Limit the dose of vilazodone to 20 mg once daily in patients co-administered a cyp 3A4 inhibitor
- Itraconazone
- Clathromycin
- Voriconazole

Precautions with digoxin as vilazodone has increased digoxin plasma concentrations in some patients
- Obtain a baseline digoxin plasma concentration and monitor digoxin plasma concentrations periodically. Reduce digoxin dose as necessary

ART OF PSYCHOPHARMACOLOGY: TAKE-HOME PEARLS [4, 5, 6]

- The combination of 5HT reuptake inhibition and 5HT$_{1A}$ partial agonism may hasten the onset of therapeutic effect with studies demonstrating an improvement in mood at two weeks.

- The incidence of drug-induced sexual side effects appears to be lower with vilazodone compared to the SSRIs.
- Vilazodone is generally well tolerated, is safe in patients with renal and hepatic impairments, and has few drug-drug interactions.

References

1. Allergan USA Inc. (2020). *Vilazodone Package Insert*. Madison, New Jersey.
2. Schwartz, T. L., Siddiqui, U. A., Stahl, S. M. (2011). Vilazodone: a brief pharmacological and clinical review of the novel serotonin partial agonist and reuptake inhibitor. *Ther Adv Psychopharmacol*, 1, 81–87.
3. Gaynes, B. N., Rush, A. J., Trivedi, M. H., et al. (2008). The STAR*D study: treating depression in the real world. *Clevel Clin J Med*, 75, 57–66.
4. Croft, H. A., Pomara, N., Gommoll, C., et al. (2014). Efficacy and safety of vilazodone in major depressive disorder: a randomized, double-blind, placebo-controlled trial. *J Clin Psychiatry*, 75, e1291–e1298.
5. Citrome, L. (2012). Vilazodone for major depressive disorder: a systematic review of the efficacy and safety profile for this newly approved antidepressant – what is the number needed to treat, number needed to harm and likelihood to be helped or harmed? *Int J Clin Pract*, 66, 356–368.
6. Mathews, M., Gommoll, C., Chen, D., et al. (2015). Efficacy and safety of vilazodone 20 and 40 mg in major depressive disorder: a randomized, double-blind, placebo-controlled trial. *Int Clin Psychopharmacol*, 30, 67–74.
7. California Department of State Hospitals. (2019). *DSH Psychotropic Medication Policy: SSRI Protocol*. Sacramento, California.

2.36 Vortioxetine

A. BASIC INFORMATION [1]

Principle Trade Names
- Trintellix®

Legal Status
- Prescription only
- Not controlled

Classifications
- Multimodal serotonin agent
- Antidepressant

Generics Available
- No

Formulations
- Tablet: 5 mg; 10 mg; 15 mg; 20 mg

FDA Indications
- Major depressive disorder

Other Data-Supported Indications
- Generalized anxiety disorder
- Depression in elderly patients
- Cognitive dysfunction associated with major depressive disorder

B. MECHANISMS OF ACTION

Serotonin
- Binds directly to 5HT transporter, potently and selectively inhibits 5HT reuptake
- Direct modulation of multiple G-protein linked presynaptic and postsynaptic 5HT receptors enhances serotonergic activity
- Antagonism at $5HT_3$ receptors may, via enhancement of multiple other neurotransmitters, contribute to procognitive effects
- Agonism at $5HT_{1A}$ receptors may diminish SSRI-induced sexual dysfunction

Other
- May overcome mood-related changes in synaptic plasticity and neurogenesis by increasing brain derived neurotrophic factor (BDNF) and inducing signaling through certain BDNF receptors

C. PLASMA CONCENTRATIONS AND TREATMENT RESPONSE [4]

Initial Target Range
• No established plasma therapeutic range

Range for Treatment Resistance
• No established plasma therapeutic range

Typical Time to Response
• Due to its long half-life, vortioxetine reaches steady state in two weeks. At least four weeks to attain response with six weeks needed to attain remission. Remission can take up to 12 weeks

Time-Course of Improvement
• If no response by six to eight weeks at maximum tolerated dose, switch to an alternate antidepressant or augment with a second medication, e.g. lithium, triiodothyronine, second-generation antipsychotic, etc.

D. TYPICAL TREATMENT RESPONSE [1, 5]

Usual Target Symptoms
• Affective symptoms
• Anxiety
• Mood-related cognitive symptoms
• Suicidality and suicidal behavior

Common Short-Term Adverse Effects
• Nausea
• Constipation
• Vomiting

Rare Adverse Effects
• Acute angle closure glaucoma
• Agitation
• Akathisia
• Hyponatremia (mostly in elderly patients and reversible with drug discontinuation)
• Treatment-emergent suicidal ideation and suicide in young patients
• Increased risk of upper gastrointestinal (GI) bleed

• May trigger switch to hypomania or mania in bipolar disorder
• Seizures
• Serotonin syndrome
• Type 1 hypersensitivity reactions (anaphylaxis, angioedema, hypotension, tachycardia, swollen tongue, difficulty breathing, wheezing, rash)
• When taken during pregnancy, rare hypertension and eclampsia during the third trimester
• Third trimester fetal exposure may result in lower birth weight and premature delivery
• Rare pulmonary hypertension or discontinuation syndrome in exposed neonates

Long-Term Effects
• Discontinuation syndrome, although less common than with certain SSRIs
• Sexual dysfunction, although less commonly observed when compared to the SSRIs and SNRIs

E. PRE-TREATMENT WORKUP AND INITIAL LABORATORY TESTING [6]

History
• General history
• Personal history of GI bleed

Physical
• Vital signs
• General physical examination

Blood Tests
• Basic metabolic panel
• Liver function panel

Pregnancy Test
• Pregnancy test (premenopausal females)
• Classified as risk not ruled out

F. MONITORING [6]

In healthy patients
• None

G. DOSING AND KINETICS [1]

Initial Dosing
- Administer an initial dose of 10 mg daily

Titration
- Titrate to 20 mg daily based on tolerability and clinical effect

Half-Life
- 66 hours

Bioavailability
- 75%
- 98% protein-bound

Adjustment for Hepatic Dysfunction (by Child-Pugh Criteria)
- Child-Pugh category A-C (mild to severe hepatic impairment): no dose adjustment necessary

Adjustment for Renal Dysfunction
- No dose adjustment necessary

H. MEDICATIONS TO AVOID IN COMBINATION/WARNINGS [1]

 Contraindicated in patients treated with monoamine oxygenase inhibitors (MAOIs) due to risk of serotonin syndrome (either with concomitant treatment or treatment within 14 days of stopping an MAOI)

Do not start an MAOI for at least 21 days after discontinuing vortioxetine
- MAOIs, including linezolid and intravenous methylene blue

 Possible increased risk of bleeding when combined with drugs that interfere with hemostasis
- Aspirin
- NSAIDs
- Warfarin

Precautions in known cyp 2D6 poor metabolizers and patients co-prescribed a strong cyp 2D6 inhibitor, e.g. bupropion, fluoxetine, paroxetine, quinidine
- In cyp 2D6 poor metabolizers, the maximum recommended dose is 10 mg/day
- In patients co-prescribed a strong cyp 2D6 inhibitor, reduce the dose by one-half

 Precautions in patients co-prescribed cyp 3A4 inducers, e.g. rifampin, carbamazepine, phenytoin
- Consider increasing the dose of vortioxetine if the inducer is co-administered for >14 days. The maximum dose should not exceed three times the original dose

 Possible decreased efficacy of triptans
- Due to vortioxetine's $5HT_{1D}$ antagonism and $5HT_{1B}$ partial agonism, when it is maximally dosed, triptans may be less effective

 Precautions with other highly protein-bound drugs
- Vortioxetine is highly protein-bound and while it was not found to displace warfarin, theoretically, it could displace highly protein-bound drugs

2.36 Vortioxetine (Continued)

- Vortioxetine has a favorable side effect profile with few drug-drug interactions and a lower incidence of sexual side effects when compared to SSRIs and SNRIs.
- There is a dose-dependent effect on improving depressive symptoms with higher doses demonstrating better effects in US trials.

- Vortioxetine has a multi-domain effect on improving executive function, attention, processing speed and memory which appears to be independent of its effect on improving depressive symptoms.

 References

1. Takeda Pharmaceuticals America Inc. (2019). *Vorioxetine Package Insert*. Deerfield, Illinois.
2. Stahl, S. M. (2015). Modes and nodes explain the mechanism of action of vortioxetine, a multimodal agent (MMA): enhancing serotonin release by combining serotonin (5HT) transporter inhibition with actions at 5HT receptors (5HT$_{1A}$, 5HT$_{1B}$, 5HT$_{1D}$, 5HT$_7$ receptors). *CNS Spectr*, 20, 93–97.
3. Sagud, M., Nikolac Perkovic, M., Vuksan-Cusa, B., et al. (2016). A prospective, longitudinal study of platelet serotonin and plasma brain-derived neurotrophic factor concentrations in major depression: effects of vortioxetine treatment. *Psychopharmacology (Berl)*, 233, 3259–3267.
4. Gaynes, B. N., Rush, A. J., Trivedi, M. H., et al. (2008). The STAR*D study: treating depression in the real world. *Clevel Clin J Med*, 75, 57–66.
5. Thase, M. E., Danchenko, N., Brignone, M., et al. (2017). Comparative evaluation of vortioxetine as a switch therapy in patients with major depressive disorder. *Eur Neuropsychopharmacol*, 27, 773–781.
6. California Department of State Hospitals. (2019). *DSH Psychotropic Medication Policy: SSRI Protocol*. Sacramento, California.
7. Harrison, J. E., Lophaven, S., Olsen, C. K. (2016). Which cognitive domains are improved by treatment with vortioxetine? *Int J Neuropsychopharmacol*, 19, pyw054.

Serotonin/Norepinephrine Reuptake Inhibitor Antidepressants
2.37 Desvenlafaxine

A. BASIC INFORMATION [1]

Principle Trade Names
- Pristiq®
- Khedezla®

Legal Status
- Prescription only
- Not controlled

Classifications
- Selective serotonin-norepinephrine reuptake inhibitor
- Antidepressant

Generics Available
- Yes

Formulations
- Tablet (extended-release): 50 mg; 100 mg

FDA Indications
- Major depressive disorder

Other Data-Supported Indications
- Generalized anxiety disorder
- Social anxiety disorder
- Panic disorder
- Fibromyalgia
- Post-traumatic stress disorder
- Premenstrual dysphoric disorder
- Vasomotor symptoms

Serotonin
- Binds directly to 5HT transporter, potently and selectively inhibits 5HT reuptake
- Desvenlafaxine has a ten-fold higher affinity for the 5HT transporter than it does for the NE transporter

Norepinephrine
- Binds directly to the NE transporter, inhibiting reuptake

Dopamine
- Weakly inhibits dopamine reuptake at higher doses

C. PLASMA CONCENTRATIONS AND TREATMENT RESPONSE [3, 4]

Initial Target Range
• No established plasma therapeutic range

Range for Treatment Resistance
• No established plasma therapeutic range

Typical Time to Response
• Certain patients demonstrate a response at two weeks
• At least four weeks to attain response with six weeks needed to attain remission. Remission can take up to 12 weeks

Time-Course of Improvement
• If no response by six to eight weeks to maximum tolerated dose, augment with an antidepressant with a different mechanism, e.g. mirtazapine or a second medication, e.g. lithium, triiodothyronine, second-generation antipsychotic, etc.

D. TYPICAL TREATMENT RESPONSE [1]

Usual Target Symptoms
• Affective symptoms
• Anxiety
• Mood-related cognitive symptoms
• Suicidality and suicidal behavior

Common Short-Term Adverse Effects
• Nausea
• Dry mouth
• Hyperhydrosis
• Dizziness
• Constipation
• Somnolence
• Fatigue
• Insomnia

Rare Adverse Effects
• Acute angle closure glaucoma
• Elevated blood pressure
• Orthostatic hypotension in patients ≥65 years
• Agitation
• Akathisia
• Hyponatremia (mostly in elderly patients and reversible with drug discontinuation)

• Interstitial lung disease and eosinophilic pneumonia
• Treatment-emergent suicidal ideation and suicide in young patients
• Increased risk of upper gastrointestinal (GI) bleed
• Seizures
• May trigger switch to hypomania or mania in bipolar disorder
• Serotonin syndrome
• Type 1 hypersensitivity reactions, e.g. anaphylaxis, angioedema, hypotension, tachycardia, swollen tongue, difficulty breathing, wheezing, rash
• Third trimester fetal exposure may result in lower birth weight and premature delivery
• Rare pulmonary hypertension or discontinuation syndrome in exposed neonates

Long-Term Effects
• Discontinuation syndrome following abrupt discontinuation or dose reduction
• Sexual dysfunction

E. PRE-TREATMENT WORKUP AND INITIAL LABORATORY TESTING [1]

History
• General history
• Personal history of GI bleed

Physical
• General physical examination
• Vital signs, with baseline blood pressure
• Treat and control hypertension before starting desvenlafaxine

Blood Tests
• Basic metabolic panel
• Liver function panel

Pregnancy Test
• Test premenopausal females
• Classified as risk not ruled out

Regular monitoring
• Blood pressure

Initial Dosing
• Desvenlafaxine ER: administer an initial dose of 50 mg once daily at the same time each day, with or without food
• Tablets must be swallowed whole. If crushed, chewed or dissolved, the controlled-release properties will be lost

Titration
• The 50 mg dose is both a starting dose and a therapeutic dose. In studies, no additional benefit was observed with doses >50 mg/day

Half-Life
• 10 hours

Bioavailability
• Oral bioavailability is 100%

Adjustment for Hepatic Dysfunction (by Child-Pugh Criteria)
• Child-Pugh category A (mild hepatic impairment): no dose adjustment
• Child-Pugh category B–C (moderate-severe hepatic impairment): 50 mg/day is the recommended dose. Doses >100 mg/day are not recommended

Adjustment for Renal Dysfunction
• Moderate renal impairment: 50 mg/day is the maximum recommended dose
• Severe renal impairment or end-stage renal disease: 25 mg/day or 50 mg every other day is the maximum recommended dose. Doses should not be given after dialysis

  Contraindicated in patients treated with monoamine oxidase inhibitors (MAOIs) due to risk of serotonin syndrome (either concomitant treatment or treatment within 14 days of stopping an MAOI)

Do not start an MAOI for at least seven days after discontinuing desvenlafaxine
• MAOIs, including linezolid and intravenous methylene blue

 Possible increased risk of bleeding when combined with drugs that interfere with hemostasis
• Aspirin
• NSAIDs
• Warfarin

2.37 Desvenlafaxine (Continued)

- Desvenlafaxine is characterized by predominantly serotonergic effects; however, in contrast to venlafaxine, it has a slightly greater effect on the norepinephrine transporter.
- Unlike venlafaxine, desvenlafaxine metabolism is not dependent on cyp 2D6 and is not impacted by cyp 2D6 genetic polymorphisms or inhibitors/inducers of this enzyme. This may allow a more predictable clinical effect.

- The 25 mg dose is intended to be used when tapering in order to avoid or ameliorate discontinuation symptoms.

References

1. Alembic Pharmaceuticals Limited. (2019). *Desvenlafaxine Package Insert.* Vadodara (India).
2. Deecher, D. C., Beyer, C. E., Johnston, G., et al. (2006). Desvenlafaxine succinate: a new serotonin and norepinephrine reuptake inhibitor. *J Pharmacol Exp Ther*, 318, 657–665.
3. Gaynes, B. N., Rush, A. J., Trivedi, M. H., et al. (2008). The STAR*D study: treating depression in the real world. *Clevel Clin J Med*, 75, 57–66.
4. Soares, C. N., Endicott, J., Boucher, M., et al. (2014). Predictors of functional response and remission with desvenlafaxine 50 mg/d in patients with major depressive disorder. *CNS Spectr*, 19, 519–527.
5. Preskorn, S., Patroneva, A., Silman, H., et al. (2009). Comparison of the pharmacokinetics of venlafaxine extended release and desvenlafaxine in extensive and poor cytochrome P450 2D6 metabolizers. *J Clin Psychopharmacol*, 29, 39–43.

A. BASIC INFORMATION [1]

Principle Trade Names
- Cymbalta®
- Irenka®

Legal Status
- Prescription only
- Not controlled

Classifications
- Selective serotonin-norepinephrine reuptake inhibitor (SNRI)
- Antidepressant
- Analgesic

Generics Available
- Yes

Formulations
- Capsule (extended-release): 20 mg; 30 mg; 60 mg

FDA Indications
- Major depressive disorder
- Diabetic peripheral neuropathic pain
- Fibromyalgia
- Generalized anxiety disorder, acute and maintenance
- Chronic musculoskeletal pain

Other Data-Supported Indications
- Stress urinary incontinence
- Neuropathic pain and certain other chronic pain conditions, e.g. chronic low back pain
- Other anxiety disorders

Serotonin
- Binds directly to 5HT transporter, potently and selectively inhibits 5HT reuptake
- Duloxetine has a ten-fold higher affinity for the 5HT transporter than it does for the NE transporter

Norepinephrine
- Binds directly to the NE transporter, inhibiting reuptake

Dopamine
- Weakly inhibits dopamine reuptake at higher doses, unlikely to be clinically relevant

2.38 Duloxetine (Continued)

C. PLASMA CONCENTRATIONS AND TREATMENT RESPONSE [3]

Initial Target Range
- No established plasma therapeutic range

Range for Treatment Resistance
- No established plasma therapeutic range

Typical Time to Response
- Improvements in depressed mood and pain beginning after one week of treatment with duloxetine 60 mg/day

- Response was observed at two weeks with five weeks needed to attain remission. Remission can take up to 12 weeks

Time-Course of Improvement
- If no response by six to eight weeks at maximum tolerated dose, augment with an antidepressant with a different mechanism, e.g. mirtazapine or a second medication, e.g. lithium, triiodothyronine, second-generation antipsychotic, etc.

D. TYPICAL TREATMENT RESPONSE [1]

Usual Target Symptoms
- Affective symptoms
- Anxiety
- Mood-related cognitive symptoms
- Suicidality and suicidal behavior
- Pain

Common Short-Term Adverse Effects
- Nausea
- Dry mouth
- Somnolence
- Constipation
- Decreased appetite
- Hyperhydrosis

Rare Adverse Effects
- Hepatotoxicity
- Severe skin reactions, e.g. Stevens-Johnson Syndrome
- Urinary hesitation and retention
- Small increases in fasting blood glucose and hemoglobin A1c have been observed in patients with diabetes
- Acute angle closure glaucoma
- Orthostatic hypotension, falls, syncope, more common in first week of treatment

- Agitation
- Akathisia
- Hyponatremia (mostly in elderly patients and reversible with drug discontinuation)
- Treatment-emergent suicidal ideation and suicide in young patients
- Increased risk of upper gastrointestinal (GI) bleed
- Seizures
- May trigger switch to hypomania or mania in bipolar disorder
- Serotonin syndrome
- Type 1 hypersensitivity reactions, e.g. anaphylaxis, angioedema, hypotension, tachycardia, swollen tongue, difficulty breathing, wheezing, rash
- Third trimester fetal exposure may result in lower birth weight and premature delivery
- Rare pulmonary hypertension or discontinuation syndrome in exposed neonates

Long-Term Effects
- Discontinuation syndrome
- Sexual dysfunction

E. PRE-TREATMENT WORKUP AND INITIAL LABORATORY TESTING

History
- General history
- Personal history of GI bleed

Physical
- General physical examination
- Vital signs, with baseline blood pressure measurement

Blood Tests
- Basic metabolic panel
- Liver function panel

Pregnancy Test
- Test premenopausal females
- Classified as risk not ruled out

F. MONITORING

In all patients
• Blood pressure

Initial Dosing
• Depression or anxiety: administer 40–60 mg/day given either as a single dose or divided doses, with or without food
• Neuropathic pain, chronic pain or fibromyalgia: administer 30–60 mg once daily
• Stress urinary incontinence: 40 mg twice daily
• Tablets must be swallowed whole. If crushed, chewed or dissolved, the controlled-release properties will be lost

Titration
• Depression and anxiety: while studies do not support doses >60 mg/day, if clinically indicated, the dose can be increased in 30 mg/day increments to a maximum dose of 120 mg/day
• Neuropathic pain, chronic pain or fibromyalgia: data do not support the use of doses >60 mg/day

Half-Life
• 12 hours

Bioavailability
• Incompletely absorbed with wide variability in bioavailability
• Bioavailability reduced by one-third in smokers. Dose adjustment is not recommended
• >90% bound to plasma proteins

Adjustment for Elderly Patients
• Initiate duloxetine at 30 mg daily for two weeks.
• If clinically indicated, titrate to 60 mg/day. Further increases may proceed in 30 mg/day increments to a maximum dose of 120 mg/day

Adjustment for Hepatic Dysfunction (by Child-Pugh Criteria)
• Hepatic insufficiency results in substantial decrease in duloxetine metabolism
• Use of duloxetine in patients with clinically significant hepatic impairment is not recommended

Adjustment for Renal Dysfunction
• Mild-moderate renal impairment: no dose adjustment
• Severe renal impairment: duloxetine is not recommended

Contraindicated in patients treated with monoamine oxidase inhibitors (MAOIs) due to risk of serotonin syndrome (either concomitant treatment or treatment within 14 days of stopping an MAOI)

Do not start an MAOI for at least seven days after discontinuing duloxetine

- MAOIs, including linezolid and intravenous methylene blue

 Possible increased risk of bleeding when combined with drugs that interfere with hemostasis

- Aspirin
- NSAIDs
- Warfarin

 Avoid co-prescription with potent cyp 1A2 inhibitors

- Fluvoxamine
- Cimetidine
- Quinolone antimicrobials, e.g. ciprofloxacin, enoxacin

 Potent cyp 2D6 inhibitors increase duloxetine plasma concentrations

- Bupropion
- Fluoxetine
- Paroxetine
- Quinidine

 Duloxetine is a moderate inhibitor of cyp 2D6. Use with caution in patients co-prescribed drugs metabolized by cyp 2D6 with a narrow therapeutic index

- TCAs, e.g. nortriptyline, amitriptyline
- Type IC antiarrhythmics, e.g. flecainide

 Certain QT prolonging dopamine antagonists

- Pimozide
  - Pimozide can prolong the QT interval. Duloxetine's inhibition of cyp 2D6 can increase the level of pimozide resulting in increased risk of QT prolongation
- Thioridazine
  - Thioridazine can prolong the QT interval. Duloxetine's inhibition of cyp 2D6 can increase the level of thioridazine resulting in increased risk of QT prolongation
  - Co-prescription of duloxetine and thioridazine is contraindicated

 Alcohol and duloxetine may interact to cause liver injury

- Avoid prescribing duloxetine to patients with substantial alcohol use

 Precautions with other highly protein-bound drugs

- Duloxetine is highly protein-bound and while it was not found to displace warfarin, theoretically, it could displace highly protein-bound drugs

- Duloxetine is generally well tolerated and is considered a balanced SNRI given its high affinity for both serotonin and norepinephrine reuptake transporters.
- At a dose of 60 mg daily, duloxetine demonstrates an early appearing analgesic effect independent of its effect on treating depression.

- Although duloxetine does not provide a significant advantage over other antidepressants in treating major depression, it is advantageous in treating comorbid pain and depression.

References

1. Aurobindo Pharma Limited. (2019). *Duloxetine Package Insert.* East Windsor, New Jersey.
2. Stahl, S. M., Grady, M. M., Moret, C., et al. (2005). SNRIs: the pharmacology, clinical efficacy, and tolerability in comparison with other classes of antidepressants. *CNS Spectr*, 10, 732–747.
3. Hirschfeld, R. M., Mallinckrodt, C., Lee, T. C., et al. (2005). Time course of depression-symptom improvement during treatment with duloxetine. *Depress Anxiety*, 21, 170–177.
4. Brannan, S. K., Mallinckrodt, C. H., Brown, E. B., et al. (2005). Duloxetine 60 mg once-daily in the treatment of painful physical symptoms in patients with major depressive disorder. *J Psychiatr Res*, 39, 43–53.
5. Cipriani, A., Koesters, M., Furukawa, T. A., et al. (2012). Duloxetine versus other anti-depressive agents for depression. *Cochrane Database Syst Rev*, 10, CD006533.

2.39 Levomilnacipran

A. BASIC INFORMATION [1]

Principle Trade Names
• Fetzima®

Generics Available
• No

Legal Status
• Prescription only
• Not controlled

Formulations
• Capsule (extended-release): 20 mg; 40 mg; 80 mg; 120 mg

FDA Indications
• Major depressive disorder

Classifications
• Selective serotonin-norepinephrine reuptake inhibitor (SNRI)
• Antidepressant
• Analgesic

Other Data-Supported Indications
• Fibromyalgia
• Neuropathic and chronic pain

B. MECHANISMS OF ACTION [2]

Serotonin
• Binds directly to 5HT transporter, potently and selectively inhibits 5HT reuptake

Norepinephrine
• Binds directly to NE transporter, inhibiting reuptake
• Two-fold greater affinity for the NE transporter than for the 5HT transporter

C. PLASMA CONCENTRATIONS AND TREATMENT RESPONSE [3]

Initial Target Range
• No established plasma therapeutic range

Range for Treatment Resistance
• No established plasma therapeutic range

Typical Time to Response
• Onset of symptom improvement has been observed within the first two weeks. Remission can take up to 12 weeks

Time-Course of Improvement
• If no response by six to eight weeks at maximum tolerated dose, augment with an antidepressant with a different mechanism, e.g. mirtazapine or a second medication, e.g. lithium, triiodothyronine, second-generation antipsychotic, etc.

D. TYPICAL TREATMENT RESPONSE [1]

Usual Target Symptoms
- Affective symptoms
- Anxiety
- Mood-related cognitive symptoms
- Suicidality and suicidal behavior
- Pain

Common Short-Term Adverse Effects
- Nausea
- Constipation
- Hyperhydrosis
- Increased heart rate, tachycardia
- Erectile dysfunction
- Vomiting
- Palpitations

Rare Adverse Effects
- Urinary hesitation and retention
- Elevated blood pressure
- Elevated heart rate
- Acute angle closure glaucoma
- Orthostatic hypotension
- Agitation

- Akathisia
- Hyponatremia (mostly in elderly patients and reversible with drug discontinuation)
- Treatment-emergent suicidal ideation and suicide in young patients
- Increased risk of upper gastrointestinal (GI) bleed
- Seizures
- May trigger switch to hypomania or mania in bipolar disorder
- Serotonin syndrome
- Type 1 hypersensitivity reactions, e.g. anaphylaxis, angioedema, hypotension, tachycardia, swollen tongue, difficulty breathing, wheezing, rash
- Third trimester fetal exposure may result in lower birth weight and premature delivery
- Rare pulmonary hypertension or discontinuation syndrome in exposed neonates

Long-Term Effects
- Discontinuation syndrome
- Sexual dysfunction

E. PRE-TREATMENT WORKUP AND INITIAL LABORATORY TESTING

History
- General history
- Personal history of GI bleed

Physical
- General physical examination
- Vital signs, with baseline blood pressure and heart rate measurement

Blood Tests
- Basic metabolic panel
- Liver function panel

Pregnancy Test
- Test premenopausal females
- Classified as risk not ruled out

F. MONITORING [1]

In all patients
- Periodic heart rate and blood pressure measurements

Initial Dosing

- Administer 20 mg once daily, at the same time each day, with or without food
- Tablets must be swallowed whole. If crushed, chewed or dissolved, the controlled-release properties will be lost

Titration

- After two days, increase to 40 mg once daily
- Based on clinical presentation and tolerability, titrate in increments of 40 mg daily every two or more days. The maximum recommended dose is 120 mg/day

Half-Life

- 12 hours

Bioavailability

- 92%

Dose adjustment with potent cyp 3A4 inhibitors, e.g. ketoconazole

- The dose should not exceed 80 mg/day

Adjustment for Hepatic Dysfunction (by Child-Pugh Criteria)

- No dose adjustment recommended for Child-Pugh Class A, B or C

Adjustment for Renal Dysfunction

- Renal excretion plays a major role in elimination of levomilnacipran
- Mild renal impairment (creatinine clearance of 60–89 ml/min): no dose adjustment recommended
- Moderate renal impairment (creatinine clearance of 30–59 ml/min): maintenance dose should not exceed 80 mg/day
- Severe renal impairment (creatinine clearance of 15–29 ml/min): maintenance dose should not exceed 40 mg/day
- Levomilnacipran is not recommended for patients with end-stage renal disease

H. MEDICATIONS TO AVOID IN COMBINATION/WARNINGS [1]

 Contraindicated in patients treated with monoamine oxidase inhibitors (MAOIs) due to risk of serotonin syndrome (either concomitant treatment or treatment within 14 days of stopping an MAOI)

Do not start an MAOI for at least seven days after discontinuing levomilnacipran

- MAOIs, including linezolid and intravenous methylene blue

 Possible increased risk of bleeding when combined with drugs that interfere with hemostasis

- Aspirin
- NSAIDs
- Warfarin

ART OF PSYCHOPHARMACOLOGY: TAKE-HOME PEARLS [3, 4]

- Levomilnacipran is well tolerated, has few drug-drug interactions, and is safe in patients with mild-severe hepatic impairment.
- It is the more active enantiomer of milnacipran and compared to the other SNRIs, levomilnacipran is the only drug to preferentially inhibit the NE reuptake transporter which could contribute to effects in treating pain.

- Although milnacipran (levomilnacipran's enantiomer) and the SSRIs are comparable in overall efficacy in treating depression, fatigue and cognition-related symptoms are particularly responsive to levomilnacipran.

References

1. Amneal Pharmaceuticals LLC. (2019). *Levomilnacipran Package Insert*. Bridgewater, New Jersey.
2. Auclair, A., Martel, J., Assié, M., et al. (2013). Levomilnacipran (F2695), a norepinephrine-preferring SNRI: profile in vitro and in models of depression and anxiety. *Neuropharmacol*, 70, 338–347.
3. McIntyre, R. S., Gommoll, C., Chen, C., et al. (2016). The efficacy of levomilnacipran ER across symptoms of major depressive disorder: a post hoc analysis of 5 randomized, double-blind, placebo-controlled trials. *CNS Spectr*, 21, 385–392.
4. Papakostas, G. I., Fava, M. (2007). A meta-analysis of clinical trials comparing milnacipran, a serotonin–norepinephrine reuptake inhibitor, with a selective serotonin reuptake inhibitor for the treatment of major depressive disorder. *Eur Neuropsychopharmacol*, 17, 32–36.

2.40 Venlafaxine

A. BASIC INFORMATION [1, 2]

Principle Trade Names
- Effexor®
- Effexor XR®

Legal Status
- Prescription only
- Not controlled

Classifications
- Selective serotonin-norepinephrine reuptake inhibitor (SNRI)
- Antidepressant

Generics Available
- Yes

Formulations
- Venlafaxine tablet: 25 mg; 37.5 mg; 50 mg; 75 mg; 100 mg
- Venlafaxine XR (extended-release) tablet: 37.5 mg; 75 mg; 150 mg; 225 mg
- Venlafaxine XR (extended-release) capsule: 37.5 mg; 75 mg; 150 mg

FDA Indications
- Major depressive disorder
- Generalized anxiety disorder
- Social anxiety disorder
- Panic disorder

Other Data-Supported Indications
- Post-traumatic stress disorder
- Premenstrual dysphoric disorder
- Migraine prophylaxis
- Vasomotor symptoms

B. MECHANISMS OF ACTION [3]

Serotonin
- Binds directly to 5HT transporter, potently and selectively inhibits 5HT reuptake
- Venlafaxine has a 30-fold higher affinity for the 5HT transporter than it does for the NE transporter
- Reuptake inhibition is sequential with 5HT reuptake initially inhibited, followed by the inhibition of NE reuptake

Norepinephrine
- Binds directly to NE transporter, inhibiting reuptake
- Clinically meaningful NE reuptake occurs at venlafaxine doses greater than 150 mg/day

Dopamine
- Weakly inhibits dopamine reuptake at higher doses, e.g. >375 mg/day

Initial Target Range
• No established plasma therapeutic range

Range for Treatment Resistance
• No established plasma therapeutic range

Typical Time to Response
• Certain patients demonstrate a response at two weeks

• At least four weeks to attain response with six weeks needed to attain remission. Remission can take up to 12 weeks

Time-Course of Improvement
• If no response by six to eight weeks at maximum tolerated dose, augment with an antidepressant with a different mechanism, e.g. mirtazapine or a second medication, e.g. lithium, triiodothyronine, second-generation antipsychotic, etc.

Usual Target Symptoms
• Affective symptoms
• Anxiety
• Mood-related cognitive symptoms
• Suicidality and suicidal behavior

Common Short-Term Adverse Effects
• Dry mouth
• Diarrhea or constipation
• Headache
• Nausea
• Nervousness
• Somnolence or insomnia
• Tremor
• Anorexia, weight loss

Rare Adverse Effects
• Acute angle closure glaucoma
• Dose-dependent sustained hypertension defined as supine diastolic blood pressure ≥90 mm Hg and ≥10 mm Hg above baseline for three consecutive visits, with the greatest incidence (13%) appearing in patients treated with >300 mg/day
• Agitation
• Akathisia

• Hyponatremia (mostly in elderly patients and reversible with drug discontinuation)
• Interstitial lung disease and eosinophilic pneumonia
• Treatment-emergent suicidal ideation and suicide in young patients
• Increased risk of upper gastrointestinal (GI) bleed
• Seizures
• May trigger switch to hypomania or mania in bipolar disorder
• Serotonin syndrome
• Type 1 hypersensitivity reactions, e.g. anaphylaxis, angioedema, hypotension, tachycardia, swollen tongue, difficulty breathing, wheezing, rash
• Third trimester fetal exposure may result in lower birth weight and premature delivery
• Rare pulmonary hypertension or discontinuation syndrome in exposed neonates

Long-Term Effects
• Discontinuation syndrome following abrupt discontinuation or dose reduction is common
• Sexual dysfunction

History
• General history
• Personal history of GI bleed

Physical
• General physical examination
• Vital signs, with baseline blood pressure

Blood Tests
• Basic metabolic panel
• Liver function panel

Pregnancy Test
• Test premenopausal females
• Classified as risk not ruled out

All patients after dose increase to 225 mg/day
• Periodic blood pressure monitoring

Initial Dosing
• Venlafaxine: administer an initial dose of 25–37.5 mg, two to three times daily, with food
• Venlafaxine extended-release (ER): administer an initial dose of 37.5–75 mg once daily with food
• ER tablets must be swallowed whole. If crushed, chewed or dissolved, the controlled-release properties will be lost

Titration
• If clinically indicated and tolerated venlafaxine and venlafaxine ER can be titrated to a maximum dose of 225 mg daily, per the package insert
• In clinical practice, 375 mg once daily is considered the maximum dose

Half-Life
• Venlafaxine: 5 ± 2 hours
• Venlafaxine ER: 11 ± 2 hours

Bioavailability
• 98%
• Bioavailability is not affected by food
• 27% ± 2% protein-bound

Adjustment for Hepatic Dysfunction (by Child-Pugh Criteria)
• Child-Pugh category A or B (mild-moderate hepatic impairment): decrease the initial and maintenance doses by 50%
• Child-Pugh category C (severe hepatic impairment): decrease the initial and maintenance doses by at least 50%

Adjustment for Renal Dysfunction
• Mild-moderate renal impairment: decrease the initial and maintenance doses by 25–50%
• Severe renal impairment/hemodialysis: decrease initial and maintenance doses by 50% or more

 Contraindicated in patients treated with monoamine oxidase inhibitors (MAOIs) due to risk of serotonin syndrome (either concomitant treatment or treatment within 14 days of stopping an MAOI)

Do not start an MAOI for at least seven days after discontinuing venlafaxine
• MAOIs, including linezolid and intravenous methylene blue

 Possible increased risk of bleeding when combined with drugs that interfere with hemostasis
• Aspirin
• NSAIDs
• Warfarin

 Possible false-positive urine immunoassay drug screen
• False-positive tests for phencyclidine and amphetamine have been reported in patients taking venlafaxine. Confirm with gas chromatography/mass spectrometry

- Venlafaxine demonstrates a dose-response relationship in treating major depression.
- Venlafaxine is converted to its active metabolite, O-desmethylvenlafaxine (ODV), via cyp 2D6. Individuals who are cyp 2D6 poor metabolizers, i.e. have two inactive copies of the allele, will have high plasma concentrations of venlafaxine, low plasma concentrations of ODV, and are more likely to be nonresponders.
- While venlafaxine may be superior to fluoxetine, there is no evidence that it is superior to all members of the SSRI class.

- There is a modest benefit when switching a patient to venlafaxine from an SSRI.
- If slowing the taper doesn't reduce symptoms of venlafaxine discontinuation, consider switching the patient to an SSRI with a long half-life, e.g. fluoxetine.
- Venlafaxine (a.k.a. red dragon) is prone to diversion and abuse in forensic settings.

References

1. Aurobindo Pharma Limited. (2019). *Venlafaxine Package Insert. East Windsor*, New Jersey.
2. Aurobindo Pharma Limited. (2019). *Venlafaxine Extended Release Package Insert.* East Windsor, New Jersey.
3. Stahl, S. M., Grady, M. M., Moret, C., et al. (2005). SNRIs: the pharmacology, clinical efficacy, and tolerability in comparison with other classes of antidepressants. *CNS Spectr*, 10, 732–747.
4. Benkert, O., Gründer, G., Wetzel, H., et al. (1996). A randomized, double-blind comparison of a rapidly escalating dose of venlafaxine and imipramine in inpatients with major depression and melancholia. *J Psychiatr Res*, 30, 441–451.
5. Gaynes, B. N., Rush, A. J., Trivedi, M. H., et al. (2008). The STAR*D study: treating depression in the real world. *Clevel Clin J Med*, 75, 57–66.
6. Cipriani, A., Furukawa, T. A., Salanti, G., et al. (2009). Comparative efficacy and acceptability of 12 new-generation antidepressants: a multiple-treatments meta-analysis. *Lancet*, 373, 746–758.
7. Preskorn, S. H. (2010). Understanding outliers on the usual dose-response curve: venlafaxine as a way to phenotype patients in terms of their CYP 2D6 status and why it matters. *J Psychiatr Prac*, 16, 46–49.

Mixed Mechanism Antidepressants
2.41 Bupropion

A. BASIC INFORMATION [1–3]

Principle Trade Names
• Wellbutrin®
• Wellbutrin SR®
• Wellbutrin XL®
• Zyban®
• Aplenzin®
• Aplenzin ER®

Legal Status
• Prescription only
• Not controlled

Classifications
• Nonselective norepinephrine and dopamine reuptake inhibitor
• Antidepressant
• Smoking cessation pharmacotherapy

Generics Available
• Yes

Formulations
• Bupropion tablet: 75 mg; 100 mg
• Bupropion sustained-release (SR) tablet: 100 mg; 150 mg; 200 mg
• Bupropion XL extended-release (ER) tablet: 150 mg; 300 mg; 450 mg
• Bupropion hydrobromide ER tablet: 174 mg; 378 mg; 522 mg

FDA Indications
• Major depressive disorder (all formulations)
• Seasonal affective disorder (Bupropion XL)
• Tobacco use disorder (Bupropion SR)

Other Data-Supported Indications
• Attention deficit hyperactivity disorder
• Antidepressant-related sexual dysfunction

B. MECHANISMS OF ACTION [4]

Dopamine
• Binds directly to DA transporter, non-selectively inhibits DA reuptake and increases DA concentration in the synaptic cleft
• Increases intracellular vesicular DA reuptake resulting in an increased pool of presynaptic DA

Norepinephrine
• Binds directly to NE transporter, non-selectively inhibits reuptake

Acetylcholine
• Antagonist at nicotinic acetylcholine receptors

C. PLASMA CONCENTRATIONS AND TREATMENT RESPONSE [4, 5]

Initial Target Range
• No established plasma therapeutic range

Range for Treatment Resistance
• No established plasma therapeutic range

Typical Time to Response
• Certain patients demonstrate a response at two weeks

• At least four weeks to attain response with six weeks needed to attain remission. Remission can take up to 12 weeks

Time-Course of Improvement
• If no response by six to eight weeks at maximum tolerated dose, augment with an antidepressant with a different mechanism, e.g. mirtazapine or a second medication, e.g. lithium, triiodothyronine, second-generation antipsychotic, etc.

D. TYPICAL TREATMENT RESPONSE [1, 2]

Usual Target Symptoms
• Affective symptoms
• Mood-related cognitive symptoms
• Suicidality and suicidal behavior
• Reduction of nicotine withdrawal symptoms and cravings
• Medication-induced sexual dysfunction

Common Short-Term Adverse Effects
• Headache
• Dizziness
• Dry mouth
• Anorexia, weight loss
• Nausea
• Abdominal pain
• Constipation or diarrhea
• Sweating
• Tinnitus
• Anxiety, nervousness
• Tremor
• Insomnia

Rare Adverse Effects
• Acute angle closure glaucoma
• Psychosis and other neuropsychiatric reactions
• Hypertension
• Treatment-emergent suicidal ideation and suicide in young patients
• Seizures
• May trigger switch to hypomania or mania in bipolar disorder
• Type 1 hypersensitivity reactions, e.g. anaphylaxis, angioedema, hypotension, tachycardia, swollen tongue, difficulty breathing, wheezing, rash
• Third trimester fetal exposure may result in lower birth weight and premature delivery
• Rare pulmonary hypertension or discontinuation syndrome in exposed neonates (less common with bupropion compared to selective serotonin reuptake inhibitors (SSRIs))

Long-Term Effects
• Possible weight loss
• Drug interactions, e.g. bupropion is a potent inhibitor of cyp 2D6

E. PRE-TREATMENT WORK-UP AND INITIAL LABORATORY TESTING [1, 2]

History
• General history
• Personal history of seizure disorder; bulimia; anorexia nervosa; alcohol use disorder; sedative, hypnotic, or anxiolytic use disorder

Physical
• General physical examination
• Vital signs, with baseline blood pressure

Blood Tests
• Basic metabolic panel
• Liver function panel

Pregnancy Test
• Test premenopausal females
• Classified as risk not ruled out

In healthy patients
• Periodically monitor blood pressure

Initial Dosing
• Bupropion: 100 mg twice daily
• Bupropion SR (depression): 100 mg twice daily
• Bupropion SR (smoking cessation): initiate treatment one to two weeks prior to planned quit date starting with 150 mg daily
• Bupropion XL: 150 mg once daily
• In extended-release formulations, tablets must be swallowed whole. If crushed, chewed or dissolved, the controlled-release properties will be lost

Titration
• Bupropion: after at least three days, increase to 100 mg three times daily with at least six hours between doses. Maximum dose 450 mg/day given as 150 mg three times daily
• Bupropion SR (depression): after at least three days, increase dose to 150 mg twice daily. Maximum dose 400 mg/day
• Bupropion SR (smoking cessation): after at least three days, increase dose to 150 mg twice daily. Maximum dose 300 mg/day
• Bupropion XL: after at least four days, increase the dose to 300 mg once daily. Maximum dose 450 mg/day

Half-Life
• 21 ± 9 hours

Bioavailability
• 84%
• Bioavailability is not affected by food

Adjustment for Hepatic Dysfunction (by Child-Pugh Criteria)
• Child-Pugh category A (mild hepatic impairment): consider dose reduction or decrease dosing frequency
• Child-Pugh category B–C (moderate-severe hepatic impairment): decrease dose as follows: Bupropion 75 mg once daily; Bupropion SR 100 mg daily or 150 mg every other day; Bupropion XL 150 mg every other day. Maximum dose of the SR or XL formulations should not exceed 150 mg every other day

Adjustment for Renal Dysfunction
• Bupropion and metabolites are renally cleared
• Consider dose reduction or decrease dosing frequency in patients with renal impairment (eGFR <90 ml/min)

Contraindicated in patients treated with monoamine oxidase inhibitors (MAOIs) due to increased risk of hypertensive reactions. Risk is present either during concomitant treatment or within 14 days of stopping an MAOI

Do not start an MAOI for at least 14 days after discontinuing bupropion

- MAOIs, including linezolid and intravenous methylene blue

 Seizure

- Contraindicated in patients with seizure disorder
- Risk of seizure is dose-related
- Minimize risk by gradually increasing dose and titrating slowly
- Other factors may increase risk of seizure. These include: CNS pathology (brain injury, tumor, infection); concomitant medications that lower seizure threshold (antipsychotics, TCAs, theophylline, corticosteroids); metabolic disorders; electrolyte abnormalities and illicit drug use

 Bupropion inhibits cyp 2D6 and can increase the plasma concentration of certain cyp 2D6 substrates

- Antidepressants, e.g. venlafaxine, nortriptyline, paroxetine, fluoxetine, sertraline

- Antipsychotics, e.g. haloperidol, risperidone, thioridazine
- Beta blockers, e.g. metoprolol
- Type IC antiarrhythmics, e.g. flecainide, propafenone
- Codeine
- Atomoxetine
- Tamoxifen

 Bupropion is a substrate of cyp 2B6

Bupropion dose increase may be necessary if co-administered with a cyp 2B6 inducer

- Antiretroviral HIV medications, e.g. ritonavir, lopinavir, efavirenz
- Antiepileptics, e.g. carbamazepine, phenytoin, phenobarbital
- Estradiol
- Rifampin

 CNS toxicity can occur when bupropion is co-administered with other dopaminergic drugs

- Amantadine
- Levodopa

 Possible false-positive immunoassay urine drug screen

- False-positive tests for amphetamine have been reported in patients taking bupropion. Confirm with gas chromatography/mass spectrometry

- Bupropion's efficacy in treating depression and anxiety associated with depression is comparable to that of the SSRIs.
- Bupropion is associated with modest weight loss which is proportional to body mass index.
- In patients with antidepressant-induced sexual side effects, switching to bupropion OR augmenting with bupropion can reduce or resolve sexual dysfunction.

- Treating tobacco use disorder with bupropion in patients with treatment-resistant psychosis is effective and tends not to worsen psychotic symptoms in stable patients.
- Given structural and neurochemical similarities to amphetamines, bupropion (a.k.a. wellbies) is a substance of abuse in forensic populations. Some correctional systems have removed bupropion from the formulary. Forensic patients treated with bupropion should be monitored carefully.

2.41 Bupropion (Continued)

References

1. BluePoint Laboratories. (2020). *Bupropion Extended Release (XL) Package Insert*. Ridgewood, New Jersey.
2. Dr. Reddy's Laboratories Inc. (2020). *Bupropion Extended Release (SR) Package Insert*. Princeton, New Jersey.
3. Heritage Pharmaceuticals Inc. (2020). *Bupropion Package Insert*. East Brunswick, New Jersey.
4. Stahl, S. M., Pradko, J. F., Haight, B. R., et al. (2004). A review of the neuropharmacology of bupropion, a dual norepinephrine and dopamine reuptake inhibitor. *Prim Care Companion J Clin Psychiatry*, 6, 159.
5. Gaynes, B. N., Rush, A. J., Trivedi, M. H., et al. (2008). The STAR*D study: treating depression in the real world. *Clevel Clin J Med*, 75, 57–66.
6. Tsoi, D. T-Y., Porwal, M., Webster, A. C. (2010). Efficacy and safety of bupropion for smoking cessation and reduction in schizophrenia: systematic review and meta-analysis. *Br J Psychiatry*, 196, 346–353.
7. Hilliard, W. T., Barloon, L., Farley, P., et al. (2013). Bupropion diversion and misuse in the correctional facility. *J Correct Health Care*, 19, 211–217.

2.42 Mirtazapine

A. BASIC INFORMATION [1]

Principle Trade Names
• Remeron®

Legal Status
• Prescription only
• Not controlled

Classifications
• Noradrenergic and selective serotonin receptor antagonist antidepressant
• Alpha 2 antagonist
• Antidepressant

Generics Available
• Yes

Formulations
• Tablet: 7.5 mg; 15 mg; 30 mg; 45 mg
• Orally disintegrating tablet: 15 mg; 30 mg; 45 mg

FDA Indications
• Major depressive disorder

Other Data-Supported Indications
• Generalized anxiety disorder
• Panic disorder
• Post-traumatic stress disorder
• Insomnia
• Akathisia

B. MECHANISMS OF ACTION [2]

Serotonin
• Antagonist at $5HT_2$ and $5HT_3$ receptors results in an increase in $5HT_{1A}$ receptor-mediated neurotransmission

Norepinephrine
• Blocks presynaptic α_2-adrenergic receptors on both NE and 5HT neurons, increasing release of both 5HT and NE
• Moderate peripheral α_1-adrenergic antagonist resulting in orthostatic hypotension in certain patients

Acetylcholine
• Low affinity for muscarinic cholinergic receptors may rarely result in mild anticholinergic effects

Histamine
• Potent H_1 antagonist resulting in sedation, increased appetite and weight gain

2.42 Mirtazapine (Continued)

Initial Target Range
- No established plasma therapeutic range

Range for Treatment Resistance
- No established plasma therapeutic range

Typical Time to Response
- Onset in treating insomnia is immediate
- Certain patients demonstrate early improvement in depressive symptoms occurring by week two
- At least four weeks to attain response with six weeks needed to attain remission. Remission can take up to 12 weeks

Time-Course of Improvement
- If no response by six to eight weeks at maximum tolerated dose, augment with an antidepressant with a different mechanism, e.g. venlafaxine or a second medication, e.g. lithium, triiodothyronine, second-generation antipsychotic, etc.

Usual Target Symptoms
- Affective symptoms
- Anxiety
- Mood-related cognitive symptoms
- Suicidality and suicidal behavior
- Insomnia
- Akathisia symptoms

Common Short-Term Adverse Effects
- Dry mouth
- Constipation
- Somnolence
- Dizziness
- Increased appetite/weight gain

Rare Adverse Effects
- Acute angle closure glaucoma
- Agranulocytosis
- Hyponatremia (mostly in elderly patients and reversible with drug discontinuation)
- Treatment-emergent suicidal ideation and suicide in young patients

- Lipid abnormalities
- Transaminitis
- Seizure
- May trigger switch to hypomania or mania in bipolar disorder
- Serotonin syndrome
- Type 1 hypersensitivity reactions, e.g. anaphylaxis, angioedema, hypotension, tachycardia, swollen tongue, difficulty breathing, wheezing, rash
- Third trimester fetal exposure may result in lower birth weight and premature delivery
- Rare pulmonary hypertension or discontinuation syndrome in exposed neonates

Long-Term Effects
- Weight gain
- Discontinuation syndrome following abrupt discontinuation or dose reduction
- Sexual dysfunction, although less common than with the SSRIs

History
- General history
- Personal history of GI bleed
- Alcohol use

Physical
- General physical examination
- Vital signs, with baseline weight, BMI and waist circumference

Blood Tests
- Basic metabolic panel
- Liver function panel
- Complete blood count
- Fasting lipid panel

Pregnancy Test
- Test premenopausal females
- Classified as risk not ruled out

All patients
- Body weight, BMI and waist circumference
- Fasting lipid panel, complete blood count, liver function panel as clinically indicated

Initial Dosing
- Administer an initial dose of 15 mg in the evening at bedtime

Titration
- Effective dose range is 15–45 mg/day
- Due to half-life, wait one to two weeks before titrating in 15 mg increments
- Due to increasing adrenergic effects at higher doses, consider moving the dosing time to the morning

Half-Life
- 20–40 hours

Bioavailability
- 85%
- Bioavailability is minimally affected by food. No dose adjustment is required

Adjustment for Hepatic Dysfunction (by Child-Pugh Criteria)
- Child-Pugh category A–C: may require dose adjustment based on measurement of plasma concentration or clinical effects

Adjustment for Renal Dysfunction
- Mild renal impairment: no dose adjustment per the package insert
- Moderate-severe renal impairment reduces clearance by 30–50%. Decrease initial and maintenance doses

Elderly Populations
- Clearance is reduced in the elderly
- Consider dose reduction

 Contraindicated in patients treated with monoamine oxidase inhibitors (MAOIs) due to risk of serotonin syndrome (either concomitant treatment or treatment within 14 days of stopping an MAOI)

Do not start an MAOI for at least 14 days after discontinuing mirtazapine
- MAOIs, including linezolid and intravenous methylene blue

 Precautions with strong cyp 3A4 inducers

May require higher dose of mirtazapine
- Carbamazepine
- Phenytoin
- Rifampin

 Precautions with strong cyp 3A4 inhibitors. Mirtazapine plasma level may be increased. Monitor patients carefully
- Ketoconazole
- Ritonavir
- Itraconazole
- Clarithromycin
- Voriconazole

 Alcohol

- Mirtazapine's effect on motor skills and cognition is additive with alcohol's effect
- Advise patients to avoid drinking alcohol while taking mirtazapine

2.42 Mirtazapine (Continued)

- Mirtazapine is a dual action antidepressant that is well tolerated, as effective as the SSRIs, and has a lower incidence of sexual side effects.
- Mirtazapine's effect on appetite and body weight is considerable and due to this, some consider it a second-line medication.
- Mirtazapine has multiple effects on sleep including shortening of sleep-onset latency, increasing total sleep time, and improving sleep architecture. At low doses it can be helpful to augment SSRIs in the treatment of depression-related insomnia or as a solo agent in the treatment of insomnia. Note that due to increased NE activity, higher doses are less sedating.
- Low-dose mirtazapine (15 mg/day) is a first-line treatment for antipsychotic-induced akathisia.

References

1. RemedyRepack Inc. (2020). *Mirtazapine Package Insert*. Indiana, Pennsylvania.
2. Stimmel, G. L., Dopheide, J. A., Stahl, S. M. (1997). Mirtazapine: an antidepressant with noradrenergic and specific serotonergic effects. *Pharmacotherapy*, 17, 10–21.
3. Benkert, O., Muller, M., Szegedi, A. (2002). An overview of the clinical efficacy of mirtazapine. *Hum Psychopharm Clin*, 17, S23–S26.
4. Gaynes, B. N., Rush, A. J., Trivedi, M. H., et al. (2008). The STAR*D study: treating depression in the real world. *Clevel Clin J Med*, 75, 57–66.
5. Thase, M. E. (1999). Antidepressant treatment of the depressed patient with insomnia. *J Clin Psychiatry*, 60 Suppl. 17, 28–31.
6. Poyurovsky, M. (2010). Acute antipsychotic-induced akathisia revisited. *Br J Psychiatry*, 196, 89–91.

A. BASIC INFORMATION [1]

Principle Trade Names
• Desyrel®
• Oleptro®

Legal Status
• Prescription only
• Not controlled

Classifications
• Serotonin 2A receptor antagonist and serotonin reuptake inhibitor
• Antidepressant
• Hypnotic

Generics Available
• Yes

Formulations
• Tablet: 50 mg; 100 mg; 150 mg; 300 mg

FDA Indications
• Major depressive disorder

Other Data-Supported Indications
• Anxiety
• Insomnia

B. MECHANISMS OF ACTION [2]

Serotonin
• Potent antagonist at $5HT_{2A}$ receptors
• Binds directly to 5HT transporter, inhibiting 5HT reuptake
• Partial agonist at $5HT_{1A}$ receptors
• Trazodone's active metabolite is an agonist at multiple 5HT receptors

Norepinephrine
• Moderate peripheral α_1-adrenergic antagonist resulting in orthostatic hypotension in certain patients
• Weak antagonism of α_2-adrenergic receptors

Histamine
• Potent H_1 antagonist resulting in sedation, increased appetite and weight gain

C. PLASMA CONCENTRATIONS AND TREATMENT RESPONSE [1]

Initial Target Range
• No established plasma therapeutic range

Range for Treatment Resistance
• No established plasma therapeutic range

Typical Time to Response
• Onset in treating insomnia is immediate
• At least two to four weeks to attain response with six weeks needed to attain remission. Remission can take up to 12 weeks

Time-Course of Improvement
• If no response by six to eight weeks at maximum tolerated dose, augment with an antidepressant with a different mechanism, e.g. SSRI or a second medication, e.g. lithium, triiodothyronine, second-generation antipsychotic, etc.

D. TYPICAL TREATMENT RESPONSE [1]

Usual Target Symptoms
• Affective symptoms
• Anxiety
• Mood-related cognitive symptoms
• Suicidality and suicidal behavior
• Insomnia

Common Short-Term Adverse Effects
• Somnolence/sedation
• Dry mouth
• Dizziness

Rare Adverse Effects
• Acute angle closure glaucoma
• Cardiac arrhythmias
• Increased risk of bleeding
• Priapism (1/500 cases)
• Hyponatremia (mostly in elderly patients and reversible with drug discontinuation)
• Treatment-emergent suicidal ideation and suicide in young patients

• May trigger switch to hypomania or mania in bipolar disorder
• Serotonin syndrome
• Type 1 hypersensitivity reactions, e.g. anaphylaxis, angioedema, hypotension, tachycardia, swollen tongue, difficulty breathing, wheezing, rash
• Third trimester fetal exposure may result in lower birth weight and premature delivery
• Rare pulmonary hypertension or discontinuation syndrome in exposed neonates

Long-Term Effects
• Discontinuation syndrome following abrupt discontinuation or dose reduction

E. PRE-TREATMENT WORKUP AND INITIAL LABORATORY TESTING [1]

History
• General history
• Personal history of cardiovascular disease, GI bleed

Physical
• General physical examination
• ECG in patients with cardiovascular disease

Blood Tests
• Basic metabolic panel
• Liver function panel

Pregnancy Test
• Test premenopausal females
• Classified as risk not ruled out

Healthy patients
- None

Patients with cardiovascular disease
- Periodic ECG

Initial Dosing
- Depression: administer an initial dose of 150 mg in divided doses with the larger dose after an evening meal or with a bedtime snack
- Insomnia: administer an initial dose of 25–50 mg at bedtime

Titration
- Depression: increase by 50 mg/day every three to four days. Maximum dose is 400 mg/day (outpatients) or 600 mg/day (inpatients)
- Insomnia: effective hypnotic dose ranges from 25–100 mg

Half-Life
- 20–40 hours

Bioavailability
- 85%
- Bioavailability is minimally affected by food. No dose adjustment is required

Adjustment for Hepatic Dysfunction (by Child-Pugh Criteria)
- Child-Pugh category A–C: may require dose adjustment based on measurement of plasma concentration or clinical effects

Adjustment for Renal Dysfunction
- Mild renal impairment: no dose adjustment per the package insert
- Moderate-severe renal impairment reduces clearance by 30–50%. Decrease initial and maintenance doses

Elderly Populations
- Clearance is reduced in the elderly
- Consider dose reduction

Contraindicated in patients treated with monoamine oxidase inhibitors (MAOIs) due to risk of serotonin syndrome (either concomitant treatment or treatment within 14 days of stopping an MAOI)

Do not start an MAOI for at least 14 days after discontinuing trazodone

• MAOIs, including linezolid and intravenous methylene blue

 Trazodone may be arrhythmogenic and prolongs the QT interval. Avoid in certain cardiovascular diseases or when prescribing drugs that potently inhibit HERG potassium channels

• History of cardiac arrhythmia
• During initial recovery after myocardial infarction
• Chronic electrolyte abnormalities
• Symptomatic bradycardia
• Known QT prolongation
• In combination with other drugs known to prolong the QT interval, e.g. certain antipsychotics, class IA antiarrhythmics, class III antiarrhythmics and certain antibiotics
• In combination with drugs that are cyp 3A4 inhibitors, e.g. itraconazole, clarithromycin, voriconazole and others

 Precautions with strong cyp 3A4 inducers

May require higher dose of trazodone

• Carbamazepine
• Phenytoin
• Rifampin

 Precautions with strong cyp 3A4 inhibitors. Trazodone plasma level may be increased. Monitor patients carefully

• Itraconazole
• Clarithromycin
• Voriconazole
• Ketoconazole
• Ritonavir

 Precautions in patients taking antihypertensives

• Trazodone can cause orthostatic hypotension and syncope
• Concomitant prescription of antihypertensive may increase risk. Consider reducing dose of antihypertensive

 Possible increased risk of bleeding when combined with drugs that interfere with hemostasis

• Aspirin
• NSAIDs
• Warfarin

 Precautions in treating men with risk factors for priapism

• Sickle cell anemia
• Multiple myeloma
• Leukemia
• Anatomical deformation of the penis

 Precautions with narrow therapeutic index drugs. Trazodone can increase plasma concentrations

• Phenytoin
• Digoxin

- Trazodone's antidepressant activity is comparable to the SSRIs, SNRIs and TCAs. It is generally well tolerated, tends to be weight neutral, and tends not to cause sexual side effects.

- Low-dose trazodone primarily targets $5HT_{2A}$, H_1 and α_1-adrenergic receptors promoting sleep onset and sleep maintenance without causing dependence or physiological tolerance. Because of its long half-life, however, it may cause morning drowsiness.

References

1. Apotex Corp. (2019). *Trazodone: Package Insert and Label Information.* Weston, Florida
2. Stahl, S. M. (2009). Mechanism of action of trazodone: a multifunctional drug. *CNS Spectr*, 14, 536–546.

Tricyclic Antidepressants
2.44 Amitriptyline

A. BASIC INFORMATION [1–3]

Principle Trade Names
• Elavil®

Legal Status
• Prescription only
• Not controlled

Classifications
• Tricyclic antidepressant (TCA)

Generics Available
• Yes

Formulations
• Tablets: 10 mg; 25 mg; 50 mg; 75 mg; 100 mg; 150 mg
• A combination of low-dose amitriptyline and perphenazine is available but has no use in modern psychiatry
• A combination of low-dose amitriptyline and chlordiazepoxide is available but has no use in modern psychiatry

FDA Indications
• Depression

Other Data-Supported Indications
• Neuropathic pain
• Interstitial cystitis/painful bladder (second-line)
• Irritable bowel (third-line)

B. MECHANISMS OF ACTION [4, 5]

Norepinephrine
• Inhibition of norepinephrine reuptake

Serotonin
• Inhibition of serotonin reuptake

Alpha$_1$-adrenergic
• Moderate inhibitor (associated with dizziness/orthostasis)

Histamine
• High affinity for H$_1$ (associated with sedation)

Muscarinic cholinergic
• High affinity for M$_1$ (associated with anticholinergic adverse effects)

C. PLASMA CONCENTRATIONS AND TREATMENT RESPONSE [6]

Initial Target Range
- Optimal initial target range is 80–150 ng/ml for the combined total of amitriptyline + nortriptyline

Range for Treatment Resistance
- May consider levels (combined amitriptyline + nortriptyline) up to 250 ng/ml if tolerated

Typical Time to Response
- In responders to a given dose, some therapeutic improvement can be seen in two weeks

Time-Course of Improvement
- If no response after two weeks of a given dose, verify adherence and plasma level. Consider dose increase if no adverse effects and plasma level (combined amitriptyline + nortriptyline) is <80 ng/ml
- If no response after four weeks at maximum tolerated plasma concentration, withdraw treatment

D. TYPICAL TREATMENT RESPONSE [7]

Usual Target Symptoms
- Depression

Common Short-Term Adverse Effects
- Somnolence
- Dry mouth
- Constipation
- Gastroesophageal reflux, dyspepsia
- Blurred vision
- Urinary retention (males)
- Tachycardia
- Dizziness/orthostasis

Rare Adverse Effects
- Prolonged QTc interval

Long-Term Effects
- None

E. PRE-TREATMENT WORKUP AND INITIAL LABORATORY TESTING [7, 8, 9]

History
- Obtain personal and family histories of sudden death or cardiac arrhythmia
- Use with caution in patients with urinary retention, benign prostatic hypertrophy

Physical
- Vital signs

Blood Tests
- Consider cyp 2D6 genotyping. Consensus recommendation is 25% initial dose reduction for intermediate metabolizers, and a 50% initial dose reduction for poor metabolizers
- Consider cyp 2C19 genotyping. Consensus recommendation is a 50% initial dose reduction for poor metabolizers

Cardiac Tests
- Baseline ECG required

Urine Tests
- None required

Pregnancy Test
- Pregnancy test (premenopausal females)
- Classified as risk not ruled out

F. MONITORING [8]

Annually
- Plasma amitriptyline level
- ECG

Initial Dosing
• Initial oral dose for major depression 25 mg qhs

Titration
• Based on tolerance of anticholinergic effects and sedation, may proceed by 25 mg every four to seven days until 100 mg qhs reached, and a plasma level obtained one week later
• Expected range for response in major depression is 100–200 mg qhs, but higher doses may be needed based on plasma levels. Maximum recommended dose is 300 mg qhs

Half-Life
• Oral: 12.5–15.7 hours (the half-life for the active metabolite nortriptyline is 33–44 hours)

Bioavailability
• 33–62%

Adjustment for Hepatic Dysfunction (by Child-Pugh Criteria)
• Not studied. Use plasma levels to guide treatment, with extreme caution when treating Child-Pugh C patients.

Adjustment for Renal Dysfunction
• Limited effects, even with hemodialysis. Plasma levels should be obtained to document safety, and to examine any changes from baseline if renal function has declined significantly

⚠ H. MEDICATIONS TO AVOID IN COMBINATION/WARNINGS [15–18]

Precautions with metabolic inducers (may require higher doses)
• Limited data
• Plasma levels should be obtained if strong inducers (carbamazepine, phenobarbital, phenytoin) are used >14 days
• Plasma levels should be obtained seven days and 14 days after an inducer is stopped

Precautions with metabolic inhibitors (may require lower doses)
• Significant interactions with strong 2D6 inhibitors (bupropion, fluoxetine, paroxetine) and moderate 2D6 inhibitors (duloxetine). Concomitant use should be avoided
• Kinetic interactions are possible with strong cyp 2C19 inhibitors (omeprazole, esomeprazole, possibly fluvoxamine). Monitor plasma levels

Precautions with other protein-bound drugs
• None known

Precautions when transitioning to or from a monoamine oxidase inhibitor (MAOI)
• Allow a medication-free interval of at least 14 days after stopping the MAOI before starting amitriptyline
• Allow a medication-free interval of at least 14 days after stopping amitriptyline and before starting the MAOI

ART OF PSYCHOPHARMACOLOGY: TAKE-HOME PEARLS [19]

- Amitriptyline should not be used for major depression due to its adverse effect profile (especially anticholinergic effects) and lethality in overdose due to slowing of cardiac conduction, thereby producing widening of the QRS interval and prolongation of the QT interval.
- Previous evidence suggesting superior benefits of TCAs over SSRIs for acute major depression is probably an artifact of recent declines in placebo response. No difference is found in a large series of direct comparisons.

- Amitriptyline has compelling evidence for low dose use in pain syndromes, but is largely supplanted by its less sedating metabolite nortriptyline for these uses.

References

1. Trinkley, K. E., Nahata, M. C. (2014). Medication management of irritable bowel syndrome. *Digestion*, 89, 253–267.
2. Moore, R. A., Derry, S., Aldington, D., et al. (2015). Amitriptyline for neuropathic pain in adults. *Cochrane Database Syst Rev*, 2015, CD008242.
3. Scheiner, D. A., Perucchini, D., Fink, D., et al. (2015). Interstitial cystitis/bladder pain syndrome (IC/BPS). *Praxis (Bern 1994)*, 104, 909–918.
4. Gillman, P. K. (2007). Tricyclic antidepressant pharmacology and therapeutic drug interactions updated. *Br J Pharmacol*, 151, 737–748.
5. Rheker, J., Rief, W., Doering, B. K., et al. (2018). Assessment of adverse events in clinical drug trials: identifying amitriptyline's placebo- and baseline-controlled side effects. *Exp Clin Psychopharmacol*, 26, 320–326.
6. Perry, P. J., Zeilmann, C., Arndt, S. (1994). Tricyclic antidepressant concentrations in plasma: an estimate of their sensitivity and specificity as a predictor of response. *J Clin Psychopharmacol*, 14, 230–240.
7. Brueckle, M. S., Thomas, E. T., Seide, S. E., et al. (2020). Adverse drug reactions associated with amitriptyline – protocol for a systematic multiple-indication review and meta-analysis. *Syst Rev*, 9, 59.
8. Guy, S., Silke, B. (1990). The electrocardiogram as a tool for therapeutic monitoring: a critical analysis. *J Clin Psychiatry*, 51 Suppl. B, 37–39.
9. Hicks, J. K., Sangkuhl, K., Swen, J. J., et al. (2017). Clinical pharmacogenetics implementation consortium guideline (CPIC) for CYP2D6 and CYP2C19 genotypes and dosing of tricyclic antidepressants: 2016 update. *Clin Pharmacol Ther*, 102, 37–44.
10. Lieberman, J. A., Cooper, T. B., Suckow, R. F., et al. (1985). Tricyclic antidepressant and metabolite levels in chronic renal failure. *Clin Pharmacol Ther*, 37, 301–307.
11. Gupta, S. K., Shah, J. C., Hwang, S. S. (1999). Pharmacokinetic and pharmacodynamic characterization of OROS and immediate-release amitriptyline. *Br J Clin Pharmacol*, 48, 71–78.
12. Hayasaka, Y., Purgato, M., Magni, L. R., et al. (2015). Dose equivalents of antidepressants: evidence-based recommendations from randomized controlled trials. *J Affect Disord*, 180, 179–184.
13. Constantino, J. L., Fonseca, V. A. (2019). Pharmacokinetics of antidepressants in patients undergoing hemodialysis: a narrative literature review. *Braz J Psychiatry*, 41, 441–446.
14. Cheng, Q., Huang, J., Xu, L., et al. (2020). Analysis of time-course, dose-effect, and influencing factors of antidepressants in the treatment of acute adult patients with major depression. *Int J Neuropsychopharmacol*, 23, 76–87.
15. Olesen, O. V., Linnet, K. (1997). Metabolism of the tricyclic antidepressant amitriptyline by cDNA-expressed human cytochrome P450 enzymes. *Pharmacology*, 55, 235–243.
16. Rasmussen, B. B., Nielsen, T. L., Brøsen, K. (1998). Fluvoxamine inhibits the CYP2C19-catalysed metabolism of proguanil in vitro. *Eur J Clin Pharmacol*, 54, 735–740. doi: 710.1007/s002280050544
17. Venkatakrishnan, K., Greenblatt, D. J., von Moltke, L. L., et al. (1998). Five distinct human cytochromes mediate amitriptyline N-demethylation in vitro: dominance of CYP 2C19 and 3A4. *J Clin Pharmacol*, 38, 112–121.
18. Patroneva, A., Connolly, S. M., Fatato, P., et al. (2008). An assessment of drug-drug interactions: the effect of desvenlafaxine and duloxetine on the pharmacokinetics of the CYP2D6 probe desipramine in healthy subjects. *Drug Metab Dispos*, 36, 2484–2491.
19. Undurraga, J., Baldessarini, R. J. (2017). Direct comparison of tricyclic and serotonin-reuptake inhibitor antidepressants in randomized head-to-head trials in acute major depression: systematic review and meta-analysis. *J Psychopharmacol*, 31, 1184–1189.

2.45 Clomipramine

A. BASIC INFORMATION

Principle Trade Names
• Anafranil®

Generics Available
• Yes

Legal Status
• Prescription only
• Not controlled

Formulations
• Capsules: 25 mg; 50 mg; 75 mg

FDA Indications
• Obsessive-compulsive disorder (OCD)

Classifications
• Tricyclic antidepressant (TCA)

Other Data-Supported Indications
• Major depression

B. MECHANISMS OF ACTION [1]

Norepinephrine
• Inhibition of norepinephrine reuptake

Histamine
• High affinity for H₁ (associated with sedation)

Serotonin
• Inhibition of serotonin reuptake

Muscarinic cholinergic
• High affinity for M₁ (associated with anticholinergic adverse effects)

Alpha₁-adrenergic
• Moderate inhibitor (associated with dizziness/orthostasis)

C. PLASMA CONCENTRATIONS AND TREATMENT RESPONSE [2–4]

Initial Target Range
- Optimal initial target is 150 ng/ml for the combined total of clomipramine + desmethylclomipramine

Range for Treatment Resistance
- A threshold level of approximately 230 ng/ml for the combined total of clomipramine (55 ng/ml) + desmethylclomipramine (179 ng/ml) is the next target. This corresponds to a dose of approximately 100 mg/day, but there is marked interindividual variability
- Maximum clomipramine level is 150 ng/ml. The desmethylclomipramine level will be two- to four-fold higher (300–600 ng/ml)

Typical Time to Response
- In responders to a given dose, some therapeutic improvement can be seen in two weeks

Time-Course of Improvement
- If no response after two weeks of a given dose, verify adherence and plasma level. Consider dose increase if no adverse effects and plasma level (combined clomipramine + desmethylclomipramine) is <150 ng/ml
- If no response after four weeks at maximum tolerated plasma concentration, withdraw treatment

 D. TYPICAL TREATMENT RESPONSE

Usual Target Symptoms
- Obsessions/compulsions
- Depression

Common Short-Term Adverse Effects
- Somnolence
- Dry mouth
- Constipation
- Gastroesophageal reflux, dyspepsia
- Blurred vision
- Urinary retention (males)
- Tachycardia
- Dizziness/orthostasis

Rare Adverse Effects
- Seizures
- Prolonged QTc interval

Long-Term Effects
- None

 E. PRE-TREATMENT WORKUP AND INITIAL LABORATORY TESTING [5]

History
- Obtain personal and family histories of sudden death or cardiac arrhythmia
- Use with caution in patients with urinary retention, benign prostatic hypertrophy

Physical
- Vital signs

Blood Tests
- Consider cyp 2D6 genotyping. Consensus recommendation is 25% initial dose reduction for intermediate metabolizers, and a 50% initial dose reduction for poor metabolizers

- Consider cyp 2C19 genotyping. Consensus recommendation is a 50% initial dose reduction for poor metabolizers

Cardiac Tests
- Baseline ECG required

Urine Tests
- None required

Pregnancy Test
- Pregnancy test (premenopausal females)
- Classified as risk not ruled out

Annually
- Plasma clomipramine level
- ECG

Initial Dosing
- Initial oral dose for OCD or major depression 25 mg qhs

Titration
- Based on tolerance of anticholinergic effects and sedation, may proceed by 25 mg every four to seven days until 100 mg qhs reached by day 14 or slightly later. A plasma level should be obtained 14 days later when at steady state
- Expected range for response in OCD or major depression is 75–150 mg qhs. As the kinetics are nonlinear at doses ≥150 mg, higher doses should only be pursued based on steady state plasma levels and acceptable tolerability. Maximum recommended dose is 250 mg qhs

Half-Life
- Oral: 32 hours (range 19–37 hours). The half-life for the active metabolite desmethylclomipramine is 69 hours (range 54–77 hours)

Bioavailability
- 48%

Adjustment for Hepatic Dysfunction (by Child-Pugh Criteria)
- Not studied. Use plasma levels to guide treatment, with extreme caution when treating Child-Pugh C patients

Adjustment for Renal Dysfunction
- Not studied. Use plasma levels to guide treatment

Precautions with metabolic inducers (may require higher doses)
- Limited data
- Plasma levels should be obtained if strong inducers (carbamazepine, phenobarbital, phenytoin) are used > 14 days
- Plasma levels should be obtained seven days and 14 days after an inducer is stopped

Precautions with metabolic inhibitors (may require lower doses)
- Significant interactions with strong 2D6 inhibitors (bupropion, fluoxetine, paroxetine) and moderate 2D6 inhibitors (duloxetine)
- Kinetic interactions are possible with strong cyp 2C19 inhibitors (omeprazole, esomeprazole, possibly fluvoxamine). Concomitant use should be avoided

Precautions with other protein-bound drugs
- None known.

Precautions when transitioning to or from a monoamine oxidase inhibitor (MAOI)
- Allow a medication-free interval of at least 14 days after stopping the MAOI before starting clomipramine
- Allow a medication-free interval of at least 14 days after stopping clomipramine and before starting the MAOI

ART OF PSYCHOPHARMACOLOGY: TAKE-HOME PEARLS [10–12]

- Clomipramine should generally not be used for OCD treatment due to its adverse effect profile (especially anticholinergic effects), lethality in overdose due to slowing of cardiac conduction resulting in widening of the QRS interval and prolongation of the QT interval, and nonlinear kinetics at doses ≥150 mg. The non-tricyclic SSRI and SNRI agents approved since 1986 provide more potent serotonin reuptake inhibition and significant safety advantages.
- Clomipramine should not be used for major depression due to its adverse effect profile (especially anticholinergic effects), lethality in overdose due to slowing of cardiac conduction resulting in widening of the QRS interval and prolongation of the QT interval, and nonlinear kinetics at doses ≥150 mg.
- Previous evidence suggesting superior benefits of TCAs over SSRIs for acute major depression is probably an artifact of recent declines in placebo response. No difference is found in a large series of direct comparisons.

 References

1. Kelly, M. W., Myers, C. W. (1990). Clomipramine: a tricyclic antidepressant effective in obsessive compulsive disorder. *Ann Pharmacother*, 24, 739–744.
2. Gex-Fabry, M., Balant-Gorgia, A. E., Balant, L. P. (1999). Clomipramine concentration as a predictor of delayed response: a naturalistic study. *Eur J Clin Pharmacol*, 54, 895–902.
3. Charlier, C., Pinto, E., Ansseau, M., et al. (2000). Relationship between clinical effects, serum drug concentration, and concurrent drug interactions in depressed patients treated with citalopram, fluoxetine, clomipramine, paroxetine or venlafaxine. *Hum Psychopharmacol*, 15, 453–459.
4. Herrera, D., Mayet, L., Galindo, M. C., et al. (2000). Pharmacokinetics of a sustained-release dosage form of clomipramine. *J Clin Pharmacol*, 40, 1488–1493.
5. Hicks, J. K., Sangkuhl, K., Swen, J. J., et al. (2017). Clinical pharmacogenetics implementation consortium guideline (CPIC) for CYP2D6 and CYP2C19 genotypes and dosing of tricyclic antidepressants: 2016 update. *Clin Pharmacol Ther*, 102, 37–44.
6. Evans, L. E., Bett, J. H., Cox, J. R., et al. (1980). The bioavailability of oral and parenteral chlorimipramine (Anafranil). *Prog Neuropsychopharmacol*, 4, 293–302.
7. Balant-Gorgia, A. E., Gex-Fabry, M., Balant, L. P. (1991). Clinical pharmacokinetics of clomipramine. *Clin Pharmacokinet*, 20, 447–462.
8. Vandel, S., Bertschy, G., Baumann, P., et al. (1995). Fluvoxamine and fluoxetine: interaction studies with amitriptyline, clomipramine and neuroleptics in phenotyped patients. *Pharmacol Res*, 31, 347–353.
9. Rasmussen, B. B., Nielsen, T. L., Brøsen, K. (1998). Fluvoxamine inhibits the CYP2C19-catalysed metabolism of proguanil in vitro. *Eur J Clin Pharmacol*, 54, 735–740. doi: 710.1007/s002280050544
10. Pigott, T. A., Seay, S. M. (1999). A review of the efficacy of selective serotonin reuptake inhibitors in obsessive-compulsive disorder. *J Clin Psychiatry*, 60, 101–106. doi: 110.4088/jcp.v4060n0206
11. Albert, U., Aguglia, E., Maina, G., et al. (2002). Venlafaxine versus clomipramine in the treatment of obsessive-compulsive disorder: a preliminary single-blind, 12-week, controlled study. *J Clin Psychiatry*, 63, 1004–1009. doi: 1010.4088/jcp.v1063n1108
12. Undurraga, J., Baldessarini, R. J. (2017). Direct comparison of tricyclic and serotonin-reuptake inhibitor antidepressants in randomized head-to-head trials in acute major depression: systematic review and meta-analysis. *J Psychopharmacol*, 31, 1184–1189.

2.46 Desipramine

A. BASIC INFORMATION [1, 2]

Principle Trade Names
- Norpramin®
- Pertofrane®

Legal Status
- Prescription only
- Not controlled

Classifications
- Tricyclic antidepressant (TCA)

Generics Available
- Yes

Formulations
- Tablets: 10 mg; 25 mg; 50 mg; 75 mg; 100 mg; 150 mg

FDA Indications
- Depression

Other Data-Supported Indications
- Neuropathic pain (low-quality evidence)

B. MECHANISMS OF ACTION [3]

Norepinephrine
- Inhibition of norepinephrine reuptake (extremely high affinity)

Serotonin
- Inhibition of serotonin reuptake (low affinity)

Alpha$_1$-adrenergic
- Low affinity (lower risk of dizziness/orthostasis than other TCAs)

Histamine
- Low affinity for H$_1$ (lower risk of sedation than other TCAs)

Muscarinic cholinergic
- Low affinity for M$_1$ (lower risk of anticholinergic adverse effects than other TCAs)

C. PLASMA CONCENTRATIONS AND TREATMENT RESPONSE [1]

Initial Target Range
- Optimal initial target range is 116–150 ng/ml

Range for Treatment Resistance
- May consider levels up to 300 ng/ml if tolerated

Typical Time to Response
- In responders to a given dose, some therapeutic improvement can be seen in two weeks

Time-Course of Improvement
- If no response after two weeks of a given dose, verify adherence and plasma level. Consider dose increase if no adverse effects and plasma level is < 116 ng/ml
- If no response after four weeks at maximum tolerated plasma concentration, withdraw treatment

D. TYPICAL TREATMENT RESPONSE

Usual Target Symptoms
- Depression

Common Short-Term Adverse Effects
- Somnolence
- Dry mouth
- Constipation
- Gastroesophageal reflux, dyspepsia
- Blurred vision
- Urinary retention (males)
- Tachycardia
- Dizziness/orthostasis

Rare Adverse Effects
- Prolonged QTc interval

Long-Term Effects
- None

E. PRE-TREATMENT WORKUP AND INITIAL LABORATORY TESTING [4]

History
- Obtain personal and family histories of sudden death or cardiac arrhythmia
- Use with caution in patients with urinary retention, benign prostatic hypertrophy

Physical
- Vital signs

Blood Tests
- Consider cyp 2D6 genotyping. Consensus recommendation is 25% initial dose reduction for intermediate metabolizers, and a 50% initial dose reduction for poor metabolizers

Cardiac Tests
- Baseline ECG required

Urine Tests
- None required

Pregnancy Test
- Pregnancy test (premenopausal females)
- Classified as risk not ruled out

F. MONITORING

Annually
- Plasma desipramine level
- ECG

Initial Dosing
• Initial oral dose for major depression 25 mg qhs

Titration
• Based on tolerance of anticholinergic effects and sedation, may proceed by 25 mg every four to seven days until 100 mg qhs reached, and a plasma level obtained one week later
• Expected range for response in major depression is 100–200 mg qhs, but higher doses may be needed based on plasma levels. Maximum recommended dose is 300 mg qhs

Half-Life
• Oral: 22 hours

Bioavailability
• 40–60%

Adjustment for Hepatic Dysfunction (by Child-Pugh Criteria)
• Not studied. Use plasma levels to guide treatment with extreme caution when treating Child-Pugh C patients

Adjustment for Renal Dysfunction
• Limited effects, even with hemodialysis. Plasma levels should be obtained to document safety, and to examine any changes from baseline if renal function has declined significantly

---

H. MEDICATIONS TO AVOID IN COMBINATION/WARNINGS [8–10]

Precautions with metabolic inducers (may require higher doses)
• Plasma levels should be obtained if strong inducers (carbamazepine, phenobarbital, phenytoin) are used >14 days
• Plasma levels should be obtained seven days and 14 days after an inducer is stopped

Precautions with metabolic inhibitors (may require lower doses)
• Significant interactions with strong 2D6 inhibitors (bupropion, fluoxetine, paroxetine) and moderate 2D6 inhibitors (duloxetine). Concomitant use should be avoided

Precautions with other protein-bound drugs
• None known

Precautions when transitioning to or from a monoamine oxidase inhibitor (MAOI)
• Allow a medication-free interval of at least 14 days after stopping the MAOI before starting desipramine
• Allow a medication-free interval of at least 14 days after stopping desipramine and before starting the MAOI

Children
• Desipramine has been reported to cause sudden death in children, avoid use

ART OF PSYCHOPHARMACOLOGY: TAKE-HOME PEARLS [2, 11]

- Desipramine should not be used for major depression due to its adverse effect profile (especially anticholinergic effects) and lethality in overdose due to slowing of cardiac conduction resulting in widening of the QRS interval and QT prolongation.
- Previous evidence suggesting superior benefits of TCAs over SSRIs for acute major depression is probably an artifact of recent declines in placebo response. No difference is found in a large series of direct comparisons.

- Desipramine has limited evidence for low dose use in pain syndromes and is largely supplanted by newer medications with stronger evidence (e.g. milnacipran, levomilnacipran, gabapentin, duloxetine).

 References

1. Perry, P. J., Zeilmann, C., Arndt, S. (1994). Tricyclic antidepressant concentrations in plasma: an estimate of their sensitivity and specificity as a predictor of response. *J Clin Psychopharmacol*, 14, 230–240.
2. Hearn, L., Moore, R. A., Derry, S., et al. (2014). Desipramine for neuropathic pain in adults. *Cochrane Database Syst Rev*, 2014, CD011003.
3. Gillman, P. K. (2007). Tricyclic antidepressant pharmacology and therapeutic drug interactions updated. *Br J Pharmacol*, 151, 737–748.
4. Hicks, J. K., Sangkuhl, K., Swen, J. J., et al. (2017). Clinical pharmacogenetics implementation consortium guideline (CPIC) for CYP2D6 and CYP2C19 genotypes and dosing of tricyclic antidepressants: 2016 update. *Clin Pharmacol Ther*, 102, 37–44.
5. Nagy, A., Johansson, R. (1975). Plasma levels of imipramine and desipramine in man after different routes of administration. *Naunyn Schmiedebergs Arch Pharmacol*, 290, 145–160.
6. Lieberman, J. A., Cooper, T. B., Suckow, R. F., et al. (1985). Tricyclic antidepressant and metabolite levels in chronic renal failure. *Clin Pharmacol Ther*, 37, 301–307.
7. Sallee, F. R., Pollock, B. G. (1990). Clinical pharmacokinetics of imipramine and desipramine. *Clin Pharmacokinet*, 18, 346–364.
8. von Ammon Cavanaugh, S. (1990). Drug-drug interactions of fluoxetine with tricyclics. *Psychosomatics*, 31, 273–276.
9. Spina, E., Avenoso, A., Campo, G. M., et al. (1995). The effect of carbamazepine on the 2-hydroxylation of desipramine. *Psychopharmacology (Berl)*, 117, 413–416.
10. Spina, E., Avenoso, A., Campo, G. M., et al. (1996). Phenobarbital induces the 2-hydroxylation of desipramine. *Ther Drug Monit*, 18, 60–64.
11. Undurraga, J., Baldessarini, R. J. (2017). Direct comparison of tricyclic and serotonin-reuptake inhibitor antidepressants in randomized head-to-head trials in acute major depression: systematic review and meta-analysis. *J Psychopharmacol*, 31, 1184–1189.

2.47 Doxepin

A. BASIC INFORMATION

Principle Trade Names
- Tofranil®
- Sinequan®
- Silenor®
- Zonalon® (a topical 5% cream for pruritus)

Legal Status
- Prescription only
- Not controlled

 ### Classifications
- Tricyclic antidepressant (TCA)

Generics Available
- Yes

Formulations
- Tablets: 3 mg; 6 mg (for insomnia)
- Capsules: 10 mg; 25 mg; 50 mg; 75 mg; 100 mg; 150 mg
- Concentrate: 10 mg/ml
- Topical: 5% cream

FDA Indications
- Depression
- Insomnia

Other Data-Supported Indications
- Pruritus (topical)
- Irritable bowel syndrome (largely anecdotal data)

B. MECHANISMS OF ACTION (FIG. 2)

Norepinephrine
- Inhibition of norepinephrine reuptake

Serotonin
- Inhibition of serotonin reuptake

Alpha$_1$-adrenergic
- Moderate affinity (associated with dizziness/orthostasis)

Histamine
- Very high affinity for H$_1$ (higher risk of sedation than other TCAs)
- Antagonist at H$_2$ receptors (reports of use to treat irritable bowel syndrome)

Muscarinic cholinergic
- Moderate affinity for M$_1$ (associated with anticholinergic adverse effects)

C. PLASMA CONCENTRATIONS AND TREATMENT RESPONSE [1]

Initial Target Range
- Initial target for major depression is 50 ng/ml for the combined total of doxepin + desmethyldoxepin levels

Range for Treatment Resistance
- A combined total level of 150 ng/ml (doxepin + desmethyldoxepin) is the next target
- Maximum combined total level of 250 ng/ml (doxepin + desmethyldoxepin) can be pursued if tolerated

Typical Time to Response
- In responders to a given dose, some therapeutic improvement can be seen in two weeks

Time-Course of Improvement
- If no response after two weeks of a given dose, verify adherence and plasma level. Consider dose increase if no adverse effects and combined plasma level (doxepin + desmethyldoxepin) is <50 ng/ml
- If no response after four weeks at maximum tolerated plasma concentration, withdraw treatment

D. TYPICAL TREATMENT RESPONSE [3, 4]

Usual Target Symptoms
- Depression
- Insomnia
- Pruritis (topical)
- Irritable bowel symptoms

Common Short-Term Adverse Effects
- Somnolence
- Dry mouth
- Constipation

- Gastroesophageal reflux, dyspepsia
- Blurred vision
- Urinary retention (males)
- Tachycardia
- Dizziness/orthostasis

Rare Adverse Effects
- Prolonged QTc interval

Long-Term Effects
- None

E. PRE-TREATMENT WORKUP AND INITIAL LABORATORY TESTING [3, 5]

History
- Obtain personal and family histories of sudden death or cardiac arrhythmia
- Use with caution in patients with urinary retention, benign prostatic hypertrophy

Physical
- Vital signs

Blood Tests
- Consider cyp 2D6 genotyping. Consensus recommendation is 25% initial dose reduction for intermediate metabolizers, and a 50% initial dose reduction for poor metabolizers
- Consider cyp 2C19 genotyping. Consensus recommendation is a 50% initial dose reduction for poor metabolizers

Cardiac Tests
- Baseline ECG required

Urine Tests
- None required

Pregnancy Test
- Pregnancy test (premenopausal females)
- Classified as no risk in nonhuman studies

F. MONITORING

Annually
- Plasma doxepin level
- ECG

G. DOSING AND KINETICS [5, 9]

Initial Dosing
- Initial oral dose for major depression 25 mg qhs
- For insomnia 3 mg within 30 minutes of bedtime. For adults <65 years old, the maximum dose is 6 mg 30 minutes before bedtime

Titration
- Based on tolerance of anticholinergic effects and sedation, may proceed by 25 mg every four to seven days until 100 mg qhs reached, and a plasma level obtained one week later
- Expected range for response in major depression is 75–150 mg qhs, but higher doses may be needed based on plasma levels. Maximum recommended dose is 300 mg qhs

Half-Life
- Oral: 17 hours (range 8–24 hours). The half-life for the active metabolite desmethyldoxepin is 31 hours (range 33–80 hours)

Bioavailability
- 29%

Adjustment for Hepatic Dysfunction (by Child-Pugh Criteria)
- Not studied. Use plasma levels to guide treatment, with extreme caution when treating Child-Pugh C patients

Adjustment for Renal Dysfunction
- Limited effects, even with hemodialysis. Plasma levels should be obtained to document safety, and to examine any changes from baseline if renal function has declined significantly

H. MEDICATIONS TO AVOID IN COMBINATION/WARNINGS [5, 9]

 Precautions with metabolic inducers (may require higher doses)
- Plasma levels should be obtained if strong inducers (carbamazepine, phenobarbital, phenytoin) are used >14 days. Expected reduction in combined serum level (doxepin + desmethyldoxepin) is 45%
- Plasma levels should be obtained seven days and 14 days after an inducer is stopped

 Precautions with metabolic inhibitors (may require lower doses)
- Significant interactions with strong 2D6 inhibitors (bupropion, fluoxetine, paroxetine) and moderate 2D6 inhibitors (duloxetine). Concomitant use should be avoided

- Kinetic interactions are possible with strong cyp 2C19 inhibitors (omeprazole, esomeprazole, possibly fluvoxamine). Concomitant use should be avoided

 Precautions with other protein-bound drugs
- None known

 Precautions when transitioning to or from a monoamine oxidase inhibitor (MAOI)
- Allow a medication-free interval of at least 14 days after stopping the MAOI before starting doxepin
- Allow a medication-free interval of at least 14 days after stopping doxepin and before starting the MAOI

ART OF PSYCHOPHARMACOLOGY: TAKE-HOME PEARLS [10]

• Doxepin should not be used for major depression due to its adverse effect profile (especially anticholinergic effects) and lethality in overdose due to slowing of cardiac conduction resulting in widening of the QRS interval and QT prolongation.
• Previous evidence suggesting superior benefits of TCAs over SSRIs for acute major depression is probably an artifact of recent declines in placebo response. No difference is found in a large series of direct comparisons.

• Low-dose doxepin can be considered for insomnia using 3 mg or 6 mg tablets. Due to lethality in overdose, the quantity dispensed should be limited.

References

1. Leucht, S., Steimer, W., Kreuz, S., et al. (2001). Doxepin plasma concentrations: is there really a therapeutic range? *J Clin Psychopharmacol*, 21, 432–439.
2. Wang, W. A., Qian, J. M., Pan, G. Z. (2003). Treatment of refractory irritable bowel syndrome with subclinical dosage of antidepressants. *Zhongguo Yi Xue Ke Xue Yuan Xue Bao*, 25, 74–78.
3. Rodriguez de la Torre, B., Dreher, J., Malevany, I., et al. (2001). Serum levels and cardiovascular effects of tricyclic antidepressants and selective serotonin reuptake inhibitors in depressed patients. *Ther Drug Monit*, 23, 435–440.
4. Müller, M. J., Dragicevic, A., Fric, M., et al. (2003). Therapeutic drug monitoring of tricyclic antidepressants: how does it work under clinical conditions? *Pharmacopsychiatry*, 36, 98–104.
5. Hicks, J. K., Sangkuhl, K., Swen, J. J., et al. (2017). Clinical pharmacogenetics implementation consortium guideline (CPIC) for CYP2D6 and CYP2C19 genotypes and dosing of tricyclic antidepressants: 2016 update. *Clin Pharmacol Ther*, 102, 37–44.
6. Ziegler, V. E., Biggs, J. T., Wylie, L. T., et al. (1978). Doxepin kinetics. *Clin Pharmacol Ther*, 23, 573–579.
7. Faulkner, R. D., Senekjian, H. O., Lee, C. S. (1984). Hemodialysis of doxepin and desmethyldoxepin in uremic patients. *Artif Organs*, 8, 151–155.
8. Yan, J. H., Hubbard, J. W., McKay, G., et al. (2002). Absolute bioavailability and stereoselective pharmacokinetics of doxepin. *Xenobiotica*, 32, 615–623.
9. Leinonen, E., Lillsunde, P., Laukkanen, V., et al. (1991). Effects of carbamazepine on serum antidepressant concentrations in psychiatric patients. *J Clin Psychopharmacol*, 11, 313–318.
10. Undurraga, J., Baldessarini, R. J. (2017). Direct comparison of tricyclic and serotonin-reuptake inhibitor antidepressants in randomized head-to-head trials in acute major depression: systematic review and meta-analysis. *J Psychopharmacol*, 31, 1184–1189.

2.48 Imipramine

A. BASIC INFORMATION

Principle Trade Names
- Tofranil®
- Tofranil-PM®

Legal Status
- Prescription only
- Not controlled

Classifications
- Tricyclic antidepressant (TCA)

Generics Available
- Yes

Formulations
- Tablets: 10 mg; 25 mg; 50 mg

FDA Indications
- Major depression

Other Data-Supported Indications
- Panic disorder
- Childhood enuresis

B. MECHANISMS OF ACTION [1, 2]

Norepinephrine
- Inhibition of norepinephrine reuptake

Serotonin
- Inhibition of serotonin reuptake

Alpha$_1$-adrenergic
- Moderate inhibitor (associated with dizziness/orthostasis)

Histamine
- High affinity for H$_1$ (associated with sedation)

Muscarinic cholinergic
- High affinity for M$_1$ (associated with anticholinergic adverse effects)

C. PLASMA CONCENTRATIONS AND TREATMENT RESPONSE [3]

Initial Target Range
• Optimal initial target is 175 ng/ml for the combined total of imipramine + desipramine

Range for Treatment Resistance
• Maximum combined imipramine + desipramine level is 350 ng/ml

Typical Time to Response
• In responders to a given dose, some therapeutic improvement can be seen in two weeks

Time-Course of Improvement
• If no response after two weeks of a given dose, verify adherence and plasma level. Consider dose increase if no adverse effects and plasma level (combined imipramine + desipramine) is <175 ng/ml
• If no response after four weeks at maximum tolerated plasma concentration, withdraw treatment

D. TYPICAL TREATMENT RESPONSE [4]

Usual Target Symptoms
• Depression

Common Short-Term Adverse Effects
• Somnolence
• Dry mouth
• Constipation
• Gastroesophageal reflux, dyspepsia
• Blurred vision
• Urinary retention (males)
• Tachycardia
• Dizziness/orthostasis

Rare Adverse Effects
• Seizures
• Prolonged QTc interval

Long-Term Effects
• None

E. PRE-TREATMENT WORKUP AND INITIAL LABORATORY TESTING [5, 6]

History
• Obtain personal and family histories of sudden death or cardiac arrhythmia
• Use with caution in patients with urinary retention, benign prostatic hypertrophy

Physical
• Vital signs

Blood Tests
• Consider cyp 2D6 genotyping. Consensus recommendation is 25% initial dose reduction for intermediate metabolizers, and a 50% initial dose reduction for poor metabolizers
• Consider cyp 2C19 genotyping. Consensus recommendation is a 50% initial dose reduction for poor metabolizers

Cardiac Tests
• Baseline ECG required

Urine Tests
• None required

Pregnancy Test
• Pregnancy test (premenopausal females)
• Pregnancy risk not classified

F. MONITORING

Annually
- Plasma imipramine level
- ECG

Initial Dosing
- Initial oral dose for major depression or panic disorder 25 mg qhs

Titration
- Based on tolerance of anticholinergic effects and sedation, may proceed by 25 mg every four to seven days until 100 mg qhs reached by day 14 or slightly later. A plasma level should be obtained seven days later when at steady state
- Expected range for response in outpatients with major depression is 50–150 mg qhs. Maximum recommended dose is 300 mg qhs for inpatients, and 200 mg qhs for outpatients

Half-Life
- Oral: 20 ± 5.5 hours. The half-life for the active metabolite desipramine is 30 ± 8.6 hours

Bioavailability
- 38%

Adjustment for Hepatic Dysfunction (by Child-Pugh Criteria)
- Not studied. Use plasma levels to guide treatment, with extreme caution when treating Child-Pugh C patients

Adjustment for Renal Dysfunction
- Limited effects, even with hemodialysis. Plasma levels should be obtained to document safety, and to examine any changes from baseline if renal function has declined significantly

H. MEDICATIONS TO AVOID IN COMBINATION/WARNINGS [10]

Precautions with metabolic inducers (may require higher doses)
- Limited data
- Plasma levels should be obtained if strong inducers (carbamazepine, phenobarbital, phenytoin) are used >14 days
- Plasma levels should be obtained seven days and 14 days after an inducer is stopped

Precautions with metabolic inhibitors (may require lower doses)
- Significant interactions with strong 2D6 inhibitors (bupropion, fluoxetine, paroxetine) and moderate 2D6 inhibitors (duloxetine). Concomitant use should be avoided
- Kinetic interactions are possible with strong cyp 2C19 inhibitors (omeprazole, esomeprazole, possibly fluvoxamine). Concomitant use should be avoided

Precautions with other protein-bound drugs
- None known

Precautions when transitioning to or from a monoamine oxidase inhibitor (MAOI)
- Allow a medication-free interval of at least 14 days after stopping the MAOI before starting imipramine
- Allow a medication-free interval of at least 14 days after stopping imipramine and before starting the MAOI

ART OF PSYCHOPHARMACOLOGY: TAKE-HOME PEARLS [11, 12]

• Imipramine should not be used for major depression or panic disorder due to its adverse effect profile (especially anticholinergic effects) and lethality in overdose due to slowing of cardiac conduction resulting in widening of the QRS interval and QT prolongation. The non-tricyclic SSRI and SNRI agents approved since 1986 provide more potent serotonin reuptake inhibition and significant safety advantages.

• Previous evidence suggesting superior benefits of TCAs over SSRIs for acute major depression is probably an artifact of recent declines in placebo response. No difference is found in a large series of direct comparisons.

References

1. Deupree, J. D., Montgomery, M. D., Bylund, D. B. (2007). Pharmacological properties of the active metabolites of the antidepressants desipramine and citalopram. *Eur J Pharmacol*, 576, 55–60.
2. Lopez-Munoz, F., Alamo, C. (2009). Monoaminergic neurotransmission: the history of the discovery of antidepressants from 1950s until today. *Curr Pharm Des*, 15, 1563–1586.
3. Perry, P. J., Zeilmann, C., Arndt, S. (1994). Tricyclic antidepressant concentrations in plasma: an estimate of their sensitivity and specificity as a predictor of response. *J Clin Psychopharmacol*, 14, 230–240.
4. Rief, W., Nestoriuc, Y., von Lilienfeld-Toal, A., et al. (2009). Differences in adverse effect reporting in placebo groups in SSRI and tricyclic antidepressant trials: a systematic review and meta-analysis. *Drug Saf*, 32, 1041–1056.
5. Rodriguez de la Torre, B., Dreher, J., Malevany, I., et al. (2001). Serum levels and cardiovascular effects of tricyclic antidepressants and selective serotonin reuptake inhibitors in depressed patients. *Ther Drug Monit*, 23, 435–440.
6. Hicks, J. K., Sangkuhl, K., Swen, J. J., et al. (2017). Clinical pharmacogenetics implementation consortium guideline (CPIC) for CYP2D6 and CYP2C19 genotypes and dosing of tricyclic antidepressants: 2016 update. *Clin Pharmacol Ther*, 102, 37–44.
7. Nagy, A., Johansson, R. (1975). Plasma levels of imipramine and desipramine in man after different routes of administration. *Naunyn Schmiedebergs Arch Pharmacol*, 290, 145–160.
8. Lieberman, J. A., Cooper, T. B., Suckow, R. F., et al. (1985). Tricyclic antidepressant and metabolite levels in chronic renal failure. *Clin Pharmacol Ther*, 37, 301–307.
9. Sallee, F. R., Pollock, B. G. (1990). Clinical pharmacokinetics of imipramine and desipramine. *Clin Pharmacokinet*, 18, 346–364.
10. Rasmussen, B. B., Nielsen, T. L., Brøsen, K. (1998). Fluvoxamine inhibits the CYP2C19-catalysed metabolism of proguanil in vitro. *Eur J Clin Pharmacol*, 54, 735–740. doi: 710.1007/s002280050544
11. Undurraga, J., Baldessarini, R. J. (2017). Direct comparison of tricyclic and serotonin-reuptake inhibitor antidepressants in randomized head-to-head trials in acute major depression: systematic review and meta-analysis. *J Psychopharmacol*, 31, 1184–1189.
12. Bighelli, I., Castellazzi, M., Cipriani, A., et al. (2018). Antidepressants versus placebo for panic disorder in adults. *Cochrane Database Syst Rev*, 4, CD010676.

2.49 Nortriptyline

A. BASIC INFORMATION [1, 2]

Principle Trade Names
• Pamelor®

Legal Status
• Prescription only
• Not controlled

Classifications
• Tricyclic antidepressant (TCA)

Generics Available
• Yes

Formulations
• Capsules: 10 mg; 25 mg; 50 mg; 75 mg

FDA Indications
• Depression

Other Data-Supported Indications
• Neuropathic pain (low-quality evidence)

B. MECHANISMS OF ACTION [3]

Norepinephrine
• Inhibition of norepinephrine reuptake (high affinity)

Serotonin
• Inhibition of serotonin reuptake (moderate affinity)

Alpha$_1$-adrenergic
• Low affinity (lower risk of dizziness/ orthostasis than other TCAs)

Histamine
• Low affinity for H$_1$ (lower risk of sedation than other TCAs)

Muscarinic cholinergic
• Low affinity for M$_1$ (lower risk of anticholinergic adverse effects than other TCAs)

C. PLASMA CONCENTRATIONS AND TREATMENT RESPONSE [1, 4]

Initial Target Range
• Optimal initial target range is 50–150 ng/ml

Range for Treatment Resistance
• May consider levels up to 170 ng/ml if tolerated

Typical Time to Response
• In responders to a given dose, some therapeutic improvement can be seen in two weeks

Time-Course of Improvement
• If no response after two weeks of a given dose, verify adherence and plasma level. Consider dose increase if no adverse effects and plasma level is <50 ng/ml
• If no response after four weeks at maximum tolerated plasma concentration, withdraw treatment

D. TYPICAL TREATMENT RESPONSE [4]

Usual Target Symptoms
• Depression

Common Short-Term Adverse Effects
• Somnolence
• Dry mouth
• Constipation
• Gastroesophageal reflux, dyspepsia
• Blurred vision
• Urinary retention (males)
• Tachycardia
• Dizziness/orthostasis

Rare Adverse Effects
• Prolonged QTc interval

Long-Term Effects
• None

E. PRE-TREATMENT WORKUP AND INITIAL LABORATORY TESTING [5]

History
• Obtain personal and family histories of sudden death or cardiac arrhythmia
• Use with caution in patients with urinary retention, benign prostatic hypertrophy

Physical
• Vital signs

Blood Tests
• Consider cyp 2D6 genotyping. Consensus recommendation is 25% initial dose reduction for intermediate metabolizers, and a 50% initial dose reduction for poor metabolizers

Cardiac Tests
• Baseline ECG required

Urine Tests
• None required

Pregnancy Test
• Pregnancy test (premenopausal females)
• Classified as evidence of risk

F. MONITORING

Annually
• Plasma nortriptyline level
• ECG

G. DOSING AND KINETICS [6–10]

Initial Dosing

- Initial oral dose for major depression 25 mg qhs

Titration

- Based on tolerance of anticholinergic effects and sedation, may proceed by 25 mg every four to seven days until 50 mg qhs reached, and a plasma level obtained one week later
- Expected range for response in major depression is 50–100 mg qhs, but higher doses may be needed based on plasma levels. Maximum recommended dose is 150 mg qhs

Half-Life

- Oral: 27 hours (may be 52 hours or longer in cyp 2D6 poor metabolizers)

Bioavailability

- 49% (71% in cyp 2D6 poor metabolizers)

Adjustment for Hepatic Dysfunction (by Child-Pugh Criteria)

- Not studied. Use plasma levels to guide treatment, with extreme caution when treating Child-Pugh C patients

Adjustment for Renal Dysfunction

- Limited effects, even with hemodialysis. Plasma levels should be obtained to document safety, and to examine any changes from baseline if renal function has declined significantly

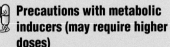

H. MEDICATIONS TO AVOID IN COMBINATION/WARNINGS [11]

Precautions with metabolic inducers (may require higher doses)

- Plasma levels should be obtained if strong inducers (carbamazepine, phenobarbital, phenytoin) are used >14 days
- Plasma levels should be obtained seven days and 14 days after an inducer is stopped

Precautions with metabolic inhibitors (may require lower doses)

- Significant interactions with strong 2D6 inhibitors (bupropion, fluoxetine, paroxetine) and moderate 2D6 inhibitors (duloxetine). Concomitant use should be avoided

Precautions with other protein-bound drugs

- None known

Precautions when transitioning to or from a monoamine oxidase inhibitor (MAOI)

- Allow a medication-free interval of at least 14 days after stopping the MAOI before starting nortriptyline
- Allow a medication-free interval of at least 14 days after stopping nortriptyline and before starting the MAOI

ART OF PSYCHOPHARMACOLOGY: TAKE-HOME PEARLS [2, 12]

- Nortriptyline should not be used for major depression due to its adverse effect profile (especially anticholinergic effects) and lethality in overdose due to slowing of cardiac conduction resulting in widening of the QRS interval and QT prolongation.
- Previous evidence suggesting superior benefits of TCAs over SSRIs for acute major depression is probably an artifact of recent declines in placebo response. No difference is found in a large series of direct comparisons.

- Nortriptyline has limited evidence for low dose use in pain syndromes, and is largely supplanted by newer medications with stronger evidence (e.g. duloxetine, gabapentin, milnacipran, levomilnacipran).

References

1. Perry, P. J., Zeilmann, C., Arndt, S. (1994). Tricyclic antidepressant concentrations in plasma: an estimate of their sensitivity and specificity as a predictor of response. *J Clin Psychopharmacol*, 14, 230–240.
2. Derry, S., Wiffen, P. J., Aldington, D., et al. (2015). Nortriptyline for neuropathic pain in adults. *Cochrane Database Syst Rev*, 1, CD011209.
3. Gillman, P. K. (2007). Tricyclic antidepressant pharmacology and therapeutic drug interactions updated. *Br J Pharmacol*, 151, 737–748.
4. Macaluso, M., Preskorn, S. H. (2011). CYP 2D6 PM status and antidepressant response to nortriptyline and venlafaxine: is it more than just drug metabolism? *J Clin Psychopharmacol*, 31, 143–145.
5. Hicks, J. K., Sangkuhl, K., Swen, J. J., et al. (2017). Clinical pharmacogenetics implementation consortium guideline (CPIC) for CYP2D6 and CYP2C19 genotypes and dosing of tricyclic antidepressants: 2016 update. *Clin Pharmacol Ther*, 102, 37–44.
6. Alexanderson, B. (1972). Pharmacokinetics of nortriptyline in man after single and multiple oral doses: the predictability of steady-state plasma concentrations from single-dose plasma-level data. *Eur J Clin Pharmacol*, 4, 82–91.
7. Dawling, S., Lynn, K., Rosser, R., et al. (1981). The pharmacokinetics of nortriptyline in patients with chronic renal failure. *Br J Clin Pharmacol*, 12, 39–45.
8. Tasset, J. J., Singh, S., Pesce, A. J. (1985). Evaluation of amitriptyline pharmacokinetics during peritoneal dialysis. *Ther Drug Monit*, 7, 255–257.
9. Yue, Q. Y., Zhong, Z. H., Tybring, G., et al. (1998). Pharmacokinetics of nortriptyline and its 10-hydroxy metabolite in Chinese subjects of different CYP2D6 genotypes. *Clin Pharmacol Ther*, 64, 384–390.
10. Kvist, E. E., Al-Shurbaji, A., Dahl, M. L., et al. (2001). Quantitative pharmacogenetics of nortriptyline: a novel approach. *Clin Pharmacokinet*, 40, 869–877.
11. von Ammon Cavanaugh, S. (1990). Drug-drug interactions of fluoxetine with tricyclics. *Psychosomatics*, 31, 273–276.
12. Undurraga, J., Baldessarini, R. J. (2017). Direct comparison of tricyclic and serotonin-reuptake inhibitor antidepressants in randomized head-to-head trials in acute major depression: systematic review and meta-analysis. *J Psychopharmacol*, 31, 1184–1189.

Monoamine Oxidase Inhibitor Antidepressants
2.50 Isocarboxazid

A. BASIC INFORMATION [1]

Principle Trade Names
- Marplan®

Legal Status
- Prescription only
- Not controlled

Classifications
- Monoamine oxidase inhibitor (MAOI), irreversible

Generics Available
- Yes

Formulations
- Tablets: 10 mg

FDA Indications
- Depression

Other Data-Supported Indications
- None

B. MECHANISMS OF ACTION [1, 2]

Norepinephrine
- Via inhibition of monoamine oxidase A

Serotonin
- Via inhibition of monoamine oxidase A

Alpha$_1$-adrenergic
- No affinity

Histamine
- No affinity

Muscarinic cholinergic
- No affinity

C. PLASMA CONCENTRATIONS AND TREATMENT RESPONSE

Initial Target Range
• Not used for MAOIs

Range for Treatment Resistance
• Not used for MAOIs

Typical Time to Response
• In responders to a given dose, some therapeutic improvement can be seen in two weeks

Time-Course of Improvement
• If no response after two weeks of a given dose, verify adherence. Consider dose increase if no adverse effects
• If no response after four weeks at maximum tolerated dose (30 mg BID), withdraw treatment

D. TYPICAL TREATMENT RESPONSE [3, 4]

Usual Target Symptoms
• Depression

Common Short-Term Adverse Effects
• Dizziness/orthostasis
• Headache
• Dry mouth
• Insomnia
• Agitation
• Sedation
• Constipation
• Peripheral edema
• Vitamin B6 deficiency

Rare Adverse Effects
• Serotonin syndrome
• Hypertensive crisis
• Hepatotoxicity

Long-Term Effects
• None

E. PRE-TREATMENT WORKUP AND INITIAL LABORATORY TESTING [3]

History
• None required

Physical
• Vital signs

Blood Tests
• Liver function tests
• Vitamin B6

Cardiac Tests
• None required

Urine Tests
• None required

Pregnancy Test
• Pregnancy test (premenopausal females)
• Classified as risk not ruled out

F. MONITORING [3]

Annually
• Liver function tests
• Vitamin B6

Initial Dosing
• Initial oral dose for major depression 10 mg BID

Titration
• Based on tolerance of orthostasis and other adverse effects, may increase by 5 mg BID after seven days to 15 mg BID. Most respond in the range of 30–50 mg/day. Maximum dose is 30 mg BID

Half-Life
• Oral: <4 hours

Bioavailability
• Not reported

Adjustment for Hepatic Dysfunction (by Child-Pugh Criteria)
• Contraindicated

Adjustment for Renal Dysfunction
• Contraindicated with severe renal impairment (creatinine clearance <30 ml/min)

Precautions with serotonin agonist medications
• See Appendix 3.10

Precautions with other protein-bound drugs
• None known

Dietary precautions
• See Appendix 3.09

Precautions when transitioning to or from isocarboxazid
• See Appendix 3.10

• Isocarboxazid should only be used for major depression in individuals capable of adhering to the dietary and medication precautions.

References

1. Shulman, K. I., Herrmann, N., Walker, S. E. (2013). Current place of monoamine oxidase inhibitors in the treatment of depression. *CNS Drugs*, 27, 789–797.
2. Kennedy, S. H. (1997). Continuation and maintenance treatments in major depression: the neglected role of monoamine oxidase inhibitors. *J Psychiatry Neurosci*, 22, 127–131.
3. Zisook, S. (1984). Side effects of isocarboxazid. *J Clin Psychiatry*, 45, 53–58.
4. Larsen, J. K., Bendsen, B. B., Bech, P. (2011). Vitamin B6 treatment of oedema induced by mirtazapine and isocarboxazid. *Acta Psychiatr Scand*, 124, 76–77; discussion 77.
5. Koechlin, B. A., Schwartz, M. A., Oberhaensli, W. E. (1962). Metabolism of C-14-iproniazid and C-14-isocarboxazid in man. *J Pharmacol Exp Ther*, 138, 11–20.
6. Davidson, J. R., Giller, E. L., Zisook, S., et al. (1988). An efficacy study of isocarboxazid and placebo in depression, and its relationship to depressive nosology. *Arch Gen Psychiatry*, 45, 120–127.
7. Thase, M. E., Trivedi, M. H., Rush, A. J. (1995). MAOIs in the contemporary treatment of depression. *Neuropsychopharmacology*, 12, 185–219.

A. BASIC INFORMATION [1]

Principle Trade Names
• Aurorix®
• Amira®
• Clobemix®
• Depnil®
• Manerix®

Legal Status
• Prescription only (not available in the US)
• Not controlled

Classifications
• Monoamine oxidase inhibitor (MAOI), reversible

Generics Available
• Yes

Formulations
• Tablets: 150 mg; 300 mg

FDA Indications
• Depression

Other Data-Supported Indications
• Panic disorder
• Social phobia (low-quality evidence)

B. MECHANISMS OF ACTION [2-4]

Norepinephrine
• Via inhibition of monoamine oxidase A

Serotonin
• Via inhibition of monoamine oxidase A

Alpha$_1$-adrenergic
• No affinity

Histamine
• No affinity

Muscarinic cholinergic
• No affinity

C. PLASMA CONCENTRATIONS AND TREATMENT RESPONSE

Initial Target Range
• Not used for MAOIs

Range for Treatment Resistance
• Not used for MAOIs

Typical Time to Response
• In responders to a given dose, some therapeutic improvement can be seen in two weeks

Time-Course of Improvement
• If no response after two weeks of a given dose, verify adherence. Consider dose increase if no adverse effects
• If no response after four weeks at maximum tolerated dose (300 mg BID), withdraw treatment

D. TYPICAL TREATMENT RESPONSE [4]

Usual Target Symptoms
• Depression

Common Short-Term Adverse Effects
• Dizziness/orthostasis
• Insomnia
• Tremor
• Nausea
• Peripheral edema

Rare Adverse Effects
• Serotonin syndrome

Long-Term Effects
• None

E. PRE-TREATMENT WORKUP AND INITIAL LABORATORY TESTING

History
• None required

Physical
• Vital signs

Blood Tests
• None required

Cardiac Tests
• None required

Urine Tests
• None required

Pregnancy Test
• Pregnancy test (premenopausal females)
• Classified as no risk in human studies

F. MONITORING

Annually
• None required

Initial Dosing
- Initial oral dose for major depression 150 mg BID

Titration
- Based on tolerance of orthostasis and other adverse effects, may increase to 450 mg/day after two weeks. Maximum dose is 300 mg BID

Half-Life
- Oral: 1.6 hours

Bioavailability
- 60% (range: 44% for 50 mg; 86% for 200 mg)

Adjustment for Hepatic Dysfunction (by Child-Pugh Criteria)
- Patients with cirrhosis have two to three times greater drug exposure. Dosages must be reduced by 50% or 67%

Adjustment for Renal Dysfunction
- No differences were found for patients with renal dysfunction, with the exception of the mean absorption time which was significantly prolonged

 Precautions with serotonin agonist medications
- See Appendix 3.10

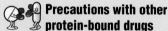 **Dietary precautions**
- None

Precautions with other protein-bound drugs
- None known

 Precautions when transitioning to or from moclobemide
- See Appendix 3.10

- Moclobemide should only be used for major depression in individuals capable of adhering to the medication precautions. It is not available in the US
- Moclobemide is a reversible MAOI, is well tolerated, and lacks the dietary restrictions mandated for the irreversible MAOIs. Efficacy appears at least comparable to dual mechanism antidepressants and may be superior to SSRI antidepressants.

- Moclobemide has moderate evidence for panic disorder, but limited evidence in social phobia. Newer agents with a stronger evidence base are used for these indications (e.g. SSRI or SNRI antidepressants).

2.51 Moclobemide (Continued)

 References

1. Bonnet, U. (2003). Moclobemide: therapeutic use and clinical studies. *CNS Drug Rev*, 9, 97–140.
2. Kennedy, S. H. (1997). Continuation and maintenance treatments in major depression: the neglected role of monoamine oxidase inhibitors. *J Psychiatry Neurosci*, 22, 127–131.
3. Shulman, K. I., Herrmann, N., Walker, S. E. (2013). Current place of monoamine oxidase inhibitors in the treatment of depression. *CNS Drugs*, 27, 789–797.
4. Macaluso, M., Preskorn, S. H. (2011). CYP 2D6 PM status and antidepressant response to nortriptyline and venlafaxine: is it more than just drug metabolism? *J Clin Psychopharmacol*, 31, 143–145.
5. Schoerlin, M. P., Horber, F. F., Frey, F. J., et al. (1990). Disposition kinetics of moclobemide, a new MAO-A inhibitor, in subjects with impaired renal function. *J Clin Pharmacol*, 30, 272–284.
6. Stoeckel, K., Pfefen, J. P., Mayersohn, M., et al. (1990). Absorption and disposition of moclobemide in patients with advanced age or reduced liver or kidney function. *Acta Psychiatr Scand Suppl*, 360, 94–97.
7. Mayersohn, M., Guentert, T. W. (1995). Clinical pharmacokinetics of the monoamine oxidase-A inhibitor moclobemide. *Clin Pharmacokinet*, 29, 292–332.
8. Amrein, R., Stabl, M., Henauer, S., et al. (1997). Efficacy and tolerability of moclobemide in comparison with placebo, tricyclic antidepressants, and selective serotonin reuptake inhibitors in elderly depressed patients: a clinical overview. *Can J Psychiatry*, 42, 1043–1050.
9. Papakostas, G. I., Thase, M. E., Fava, M., et al. (2007). Are antidepressant drugs that combine serotonergic and noradrenergic mechanisms of action more effective than the selective serotonin reuptake inhibitors in treating major depressive disorder? A meta-analysis of studies of newer agents. *Biol Psychiatry*, 62, 1217–1227.
10. Kriston, L., von Wolff, A., Westphal, A., et al. (2014). Efficacy and acceptability of acute treatments for persistent depressive disorder: a network meta-analysis. *Depress Anxiety*, 31, 621–630.
11. Bandelow, B., Reitt, M., Röver, C., et al. (2015). Efficacy of treatments for anxiety disorders: a meta-analysis. *Int Clin Psychopharmacol*, 30, 183–192.

2.52 Phenelzine

A. BASIC INFORMATION [1]

Principle Trade Names
• Nardil®

Legal Status
• Prescription only
• Not controlled

Classifications
• Monoamine oxidase inhibitor (MAOI), irreversible

Generics Available
• Yes

Formulations
• Tablets: 15 mg

FDA Indications
• Depression

Other Data-Supported Indications
• None

Norepinephrine
• Via inhibition of monoamine oxidase A

Serotonin
• Via inhibition of monoamine oxidase A

Alpha$_1$-adrenergic
• No affinity

Histamine
• No affinity

Muscarinic cholinergic
• No affinity

C. PLASMA CONCENTRATIONS AND TREATMENT RESPONSE [3]

Initial Target Range
• Not used for MAOIs

Range for Treatment Resistance
• Not used for MAOIs

Typical Time to Response
• In responders to a given dose, some therapeutic improvement can be seen in two weeks

Time-Course of Improvement
• If no response after two weeks of a given dose, verify adherence. Consider dose increase if no adverse effects
• If no response after four weeks at maximum tolerated dose (90 mg/day), withdraw treatment

D. TYPICAL TREATMENT RESPONSE [2, 4, 5]

Usual Target Symptoms
- Depression

Common Short-Term Adverse Effects
- Dizziness/orthostasis
- Headache
- Dry mouth
- Insomnia
- Sedation or fatigue
- Tremor
- Agitation
- Constipation
- Peripheral edema
- Sexual dysfunction
- Vitamin B6 deficiency

Rare Adverse Effects
- Serotonin syndrome
- Hypertensive crisis
- Hepatotoxicity

Long-Term Effects
- None

E. PRE-TREATMENT WORKUP AND INITIAL LABORATORY TESTING [4]

History
- None required

Physical
- Vital signs

Blood Tests
- Liver function tests
- Vitamin B6

Cardiac Tests
- None required

Urine Tests
- None required

Pregnancy Test
- Pregnancy test (premenopausal females)
- Classified as risk not ruled out

F. MONITORING [4]

Annually
- Liver function tests
- Vitamin B6

G. DOSING AND KINETICS [6, 7]

Initial Dosing
- Initial oral dose for major depression 15 mg qhs

Titration
- Based on tolerance of orthostasis and other adverse effects, may increase by 15 mg after seven days to 15 mg BID. Most respond in the range of 30–60 mg/day in divided doses. Maximum dose is 90 mg/day

Half-Life
- Oral: 1.5–4.0 hours

Bioavailability
- Not reported

Adjustment for Hepatic Dysfunction (by Child-Pugh Criteria)
- Contraindicated

Adjustment for Renal Dysfunction
- Contraindicated with severe renal impairment (creatinine clearance <30 ml/min)

H. MEDICATIONS TO AVOID IN COMBINATION/WARNINGS

 Precautions with serotonin agonist medications
• See Appendix 3.10

 Precautions with other protein-bound drugs
• None known

 Dietary precautions
• See Appendix 3.09

 Precautions when transitioning to or from phenelzine
• See Appendix 3.10

ART OF PSYCHOPHARMACOLOGY: TAKE-HOME PEARLS [8]

• Phenelzine should only be used for major depression in individuals capable of adhering to the dietary and medication precautions.

References

1. Shulman, K. I., Herrmann, N., Walker, S. E. (2013). Current place of monoamine oxidase inhibitors in the treatment of depression. *CNS Drugs*, 27, 789–797.
2. Kennedy, S. H. (1997). Continuation and maintenance treatments in major depression: the neglected role of monoamine oxidase inhibitors. *J Psychiatry Neurosci*, 22, 127–131.
3. Tyrer, P., Gardner, M., Lambourn, J., et al. (1980). Clinical and pharmacokinetic factors affecting response to phenelzine. *Br J Psychiatry*, 136, 359–365.
4. Malcolm, D. E., Yu, P. H., Bowen, R. C., et al. (1994). Phenelzine reduces plasma vitamin B6. *J Psychiatry Neurosci*, 19, 332–334.
5. Birkenhager, T. K., van den Broek, W. W., Mulder, P. G., et al. (2004). Efficacy and tolerability of tranylcypromine versus phenelzine: a double-blind study in antidepressant-refractory depressed inpatients. *J Clin Psychiatry*, 65, 1505–1510.
6. Robinson, D. S., Cooper, T. B., Jindal, S. P., et al. (1985). Metabolism and pharmacokinetics of phenelzine: lack of evidence for acetylation pathway in humans. *J Clin Psychopharmacol*, 5, 333–337.
7. Chiuccariello, L., Cooke, R. G., Miler, L., et al. (2015). Monoamine oxidase-A occupancy by moclobemide and phenelzine: implications for the development of monoamine oxidase inhibitors. *Int J Neuropsychopharmacol*, 19(1), pyv078.
8. Thase, M. E., Trivedi, M. H., Rush, A. J. (1995). MAOIs in the contemporary treatment of depression. *Neuropsychopharmacol*, 12, 185–219.

2.53 Transdermal Selegiline

A. BASIC INFORMATION [1]

Principle Trade Names
• Emsam®

Legal Status
• Prescription only
• Not controlled

Classifications
• Monoamine oxidase inhibitor (MAOI), irreversible

Generics Available
• Yes

Formulations
• Patches: 6 mg/24 hours; 9 mg/24 hours; 12 mg/24 hours

FDA Indications
• Depression
• Parkinson's disease (oral formulations more commonly used)

Other Data-Supported Indications
• None

B. MECHANISMS OF ACTION [1]

Norepinephrine
• Via inhibition of monoamine oxidase A

Serotonin
• Via inhibition of monoamine oxidase A

Dopamine
• Via inhibition of monoamine oxidase B
• Low-dose selegiline is relatively selective for monoamine oxidase B, but becomes non-selective at higher doses

Alpha₁-adrenergic
• No affinity

Histamine
• No affinity

Muscarinic cholinergic
• No affinity

Initial Target Range
• Not used for MAOIs

Range for Treatment Resistance
• Not used for MAOIs

Typical Time to Response
• In responders to a given dose, some therapeutic improvement can be seen in two weeks

Time-Course of Improvement
• If no response after two weeks of a given dose, verify adherence. Consider dose increase if no adverse effects
• If no response after four weeks at maximum tolerated dose (12 mg/24 hours), withdraw treatment

Usual Target Symptoms
• Depression

Common Short-Term Adverse Effects
• Application site reaction
• Headache
• Dry mouth
• Insomnia
• Diarrhea
• Dyspepsia
• Rash

Rare Adverse Effects
• Serotonin syndrome
• Hypertensive crisis

Long-Term Effects
• None

History
• None required

Physical
• Vital signs

Blood Tests
• None required

Cardiac Tests
• None required

Urine Tests
• None required

Pregnancy Test
• Pregnancy test (premenopausal females)
• Classified as risk not ruled out

Annually
• None required

Initial Dosing

- Initial dose for major depression 6 mg/24 hours (note: there are no dietary restrictions on this dose)

Titration

- Based on tolerance of orthostasis and other adverse effects, may increase by 3 mg after 14 days. Maximum dose is 12 mg/24 hours

Half-Life

- Transdermal: 18–25 hours (including metabolites)

Bioavailability

- Transdermal: 73% (protein binding: 94%)
- Oral formulations: 10%

Adjustment for Hepatic Dysfunction (by Child-Pugh Criteria)

- No dose adjustment for mild or moderate hepatic dysfunction (Child-Pugh A, B). Has not been studied in patients with severe liver impairment (Child-Pugh C)

Adjustment for Renal Dysfunction

- No dose adjustment is required for eGFR as low as 15 ml/min. It has not been studied in patients with eGFR <15 ml/min or in those requiring dialysis

 H. MEDICATIONS TO AVOID IN COMBINATION/WARNINGS [2, 5, 6]

 Precautions with serotonin agonist medications

- See Appendix 3.10

 Precaution against use with carbamazepine

- After carbamazepine 400 mg/day for 14 days there was a two-fold increase in systemic exposure to selegiline and its metabolites
- Carbamazepine is contraindicated as this kinetic interaction may increase the risk of a hypertensive crisis

 Dietary precautions

- Note: on the lowest dose (6 mg/24 hours) there are no dietary restrictions. Higher doses must follow the same considerations as for other MAOIs
- See Appendix 3.09

 Precautions with other protein-bound drugs

- None known

 Precautions when transitioning to or from transdermal selegiline

- See Appendix 3.10

 ART OF PSYCHOPHARMACOLOGY: TAKE-HOME PEARLS [2, 5, 6]

- Transdermal selegiline should only be used for major depression in individuals capable of adhering to the dietary and medication precautions.

- Transdermal selegiline has no dietary restrictions for the lowest dose (6 mg/24 hours) and may have tolerability advantages over other MAOIs.

References

1. Shulman, K. I., Herrmann, N., Walker, S. E. (2013). Current place of monoamine oxidase inhibitors in the treatment of depression. *CNS Drugs*, 27, 789–797.
2. Lee, K. C., Chen, J. J. (2007). Transdermal selegiline for the treatment of major depressive disorder. *Neuropsychiatr Dis Treat*, 3, 527–537.
3. Clarke, A., Brewer, F., Johnson, E. S., et al. (2003). A new formulation of selegiline: improved bioavailability and selectivity for MAO-B inhibition. *J Neural Transm (Vienna)*, 110, 1241–1255.
4. Goodnick, P. J. (2007). Seligiline transdermal system in depression. *Expert Opin Pharmacother*, 8, 59–64.
5. Patkar, A. A., Pae, C. U., Masand, P. S. (2006). Transdermal selegiline: the new generation of monoamine oxidase inhibitors. *CNS Spectr*, 11, 363–375.
6. Blob, L. F., Sharoky, M., Campbell, B. J., et al. (2007). Effects of a tyramine-enriched meal on blood pressure response in healthy male volunteers treated with selegiline transdermal system 6 mg/24 hour. *CNS Spectr*, 12, 25–34.

2.54 Tranylcypromine

A. BASIC INFORMATION [1]

Principle Trade Names
• Parnate®

Generics Available
• Yes

Legal Status
• Prescription only
• Not controlled

Formulations
• Tablets: 10 mg

FDA Indications
• Depression

Classifications
• Monoamine oxidase inhibitor (MAOI), irreversible

Other Data-Supported Indications
• None

B. MECHANISMS OF ACTION [1, 2]

Norepinephrine
• Via inhibition of monoamine oxidase A

Histamine
• No affinity

Serotonin
• Via inhibition of monoamine oxidase A

Muscarinic cholinergic
• No affinity

Alpha₁-adrenergic
• No affinity

C. PLASMA CONCENTRATIONS AND TREATMENT RESPONSE [3]

Initial Target Range
• Not used for MAOIs

Range for Treatment Resistance
• Not used for MAOIs

Typical Time to Response
• In responders to a given dose, some therapeutic improvement can be seen in two weeks

Time-Course of Improvement
• If no response after two weeks of a given dose, verify adherence. Consider dose increase if no adverse effects
• If no response after four weeks at maximum tolerated dose (30 mg BID), withdraw treatment

D. TYPICAL TREATMENT RESPONSE [4]

Usual Target Symptoms
• Depression

Common Short-Term Adverse Effects
• Dizziness/orthostasis
• Headache
• Dry mouth
• Insomnia
• Sedation or fatigue
• Tremor

• Agitation
• Constipation
• Peripheral edema

Rare Adverse Effects
• Serotonin syndrome
• Hypertensive crisis

Long-Term Effects
• None

E. PRE-TREATMENT WORKUP AND INITIAL LABORATORY TESTING

History
• None required

Physical
• Vital signs

Blood Tests
• None required

Cardiac Tests
• None required

Urine Tests
• None required

Pregnancy Test
• Pregnancy test (premenopausal females)
• Classified as risk not ruled out

F. MONITORING

Annually
• None required

G. DOSING AND KINETICS

Initial Dosing
• Initial oral dose for major depression 10 mg BID

Titration
• Based on tolerance of orthostasis and other adverse effects, may increase by 10 mg after seven days to 30 mg/day in divided doses. Most respond in the range of 30–45 mg/day in divided doses. Maximum dose is 30 mg BID

Half-Life
• Oral: 2.5 hours (range 1.54–3.15 hours)

Bioavailability
• 15% (estimated/not well established)

Adjustment for Hepatic Dysfunction (by Child-Pugh Criteria)
• Patients with cirrhosis have markedly increased adverse effects. Contraindicated

Adjustment for Renal Dysfunction
• No data. Consider other MAOIs

2.54 Tranylcypromine (Continued)

 Precautions with serotonin agonist medications

• See Appendix 3.10

 Dietary precautions

• See Appendix 3.09

 Precautions with other protein-bound drugs

• None known

 Precautions when transitioning to or from tranylcypromine

• See Appendix 3.10

ART OF PSYCHOPHARMACOLOGY: TAKE-HOME PEARLS [8]

• Tranylcypromine should only be used for major depression in individuals capable of adhering to the dietary and medication precautions.

 References

1. Shulman, K. I., Herrmann, N., Walker, S. E. (2013). Current place of monoamine oxidase inhibitors in the treatment of depression. *CNS Drugs*, 27, 789–797.
2. Kennedy, S. H. (1997). Continuation and maintenance treatments in major depression: the neglected role of monoamine oxidase inhibitors. *J Psychiatry Neurosci*, 22, 127–131.
3. Mallinger, A. G., Himmelhoch, J. M., Thase, M. E., et al. (1990). Plasma tranylcypromine: relationship to pharmacokinetic variables and clinical antidepressant actions. *J Clin Psychopharmacol*, 10, 176–183.
4. Ulrich, S., Ricken, R., Buspavanich, P., et al. (2020). Efficacy and adverse effects of tranylcypromine and tricyclic antidepressants in the treatment of depression: a systematic review and comprehensive meta-analysis. *J Clin Psychopharmacol*, 40, 63–74.
5. Morgan, M. H., Read, A. E. (1972). Antidepressants and liver disease. *Gut*, 13, 697–701.
6. Mallinger, A. G., Edwards, D. J., Himmelhoch, J. M., et al. (1986). Pharmacokinetics of tranylcypromine in patients who are depressed: relationship to cardiovascular effects. *Clin Pharmacol Ther*, 40, 444–450.
7. Ulrich, S., Ricken, R., Adli, M. (2017). Tranylcypromine in mind (part I): review of pharmacology. *Eur Neuropsychopharmacol*, 27, 697–713.
8. Thase, M. E., Trivedi, M. H., Rush, A. J. (1995). MAOIs in the contemporary treatment of depression. *Neuropsychopharmacol*, 12, 185–219.

A. BASIC INFORMATION [1–3]

Principle Trade Names
- Xanax®
- Xanax XR®

Legal Status
- Prescription only
- Controlled

Classifications
- Triazolobenzodiazepine
- Anxiolytic

Generics Available
- Yes

Formulations
- Immediate-release (IR) tablet: 0.25 mg scored; 0.4 mg (Japan); 0.5 mg scored; 0.8 mg (Japan); 1 mg scored; 2 mg multi-scored
- IR orally disintegrating tablet: 0.25 mg; 0.5 mg; 1 mg; 2 mg
- IR solution: 1 mg/ml
- XR (extended-release) tablet: 0.5 mg; 1 mg; 2 mg; 3 mg

FDA Indications
- Generalized anxiety disorder (IR)
- Panic disorder (IR and XR)

Other Data-Supported Indications
- Other anxiety disorders
- Anxiety associated with depression
- Premenstrual dysphoric disorder
- Irritable bowel syndrome and other somatic symptoms associated with anxiety disorders
- Chemotherapy-induced nausea
- Insomnia (rapid tolerance)
- Acute mania (adjunctive)
- Acute psychosis (adjunctive)
- Catatonia
- Akathisia
- Alcohol withdrawal
- Interruption of seizures
- Reserved as an adjunctive anticonvulsant for ongoing seizure disorder
- Note: benzodiazepines inhibit response prevention treatment in obsessive-compulsive disorder (OCD), increase the rate of conversion of acute stress disorder to post-traumatic stress disorder (PTSD), and have no overall beneficial effect in PTSD

Gamma-Aminobutyric Acid (GABA)

- Binds to benzodiazepine receptors at the GABA-A ligand-gated chloride channel complex
- Enhances the inhibitory effects of GABA
- Boosts chloride conductance through GABA-regulated channels
- Inhibits neuronal activity presumably in amygdala-centered fear circuits to provide therapeutic benefits in anxiety disorders
- Initially inhibits activity in the reticular activating system, producing sedation

Dopamine

- Associated with increased dopamine D_1 and D_2 receptor density in the striatum. This may be related to suppression of the hypothalamic-pituitary-adrenal axis and antidepressant effects

Initial Target Range

- No established plasma therapeutic range

Range for Treatment Resistance

- No established plasma therapeutic range

Typical Time to Response

- Some immediate relief with first dosing is common

Time-Course of Improvement

- Usually based on reducing psychotic symptoms. Chronic use not recommended
- For patients with schizophrenia, benzodiazepines only have scant supporting literature for use in akathisia and for very short-term use in acute agitation

- Tiihonen J, et al. found that in all combinations, current benzodiazepine use was associated with higher mortality compared to no benzodiazepine use. The study found that benzodiazepine use nearly doubled the mortality rate and increased suicide deaths by almost four-fold
- Dold M, et al. found no medium- to long-term benefits for adjunctive benzodiazepines in schizophrenia and only low-quality evidence to suggest that benzodiazepines are effective for very short-term sedation and could be considered for calming acutely agitated people with schizophrenia

Usual Target Symptoms

- Anxiety
- Psychomotor agitation

Common Short-Term Adverse Effects

- Sedation
- Fatigue
- Depression
- Dizziness
- Ataxia
- Slurred speech
- Weakness
- Amnesia
- Confusion
- Paradoxical anxiety
- Paradoxical agitation/disinhibition

Rare Adverse Effects

- Hallucinations
- Mania
- Hypotension
- Hypersalivation
- Dry mouth
- Hepatic dysfunction
- Renal dysfunction
- Blood dyscrasias

Long-Term Effects

- Dependence, tolerance and withdrawal
- Possible negative neurocognitive impact

History
• Substance abuse or dependence, neurodevelopmental disorder, angle closure glaucoma

Physical
• Pulmonary examination for chronic obstructive pulmonary disease (COPD)

Neurological
• Alertness, cognitive impairment

Blood Tests
• None

Cardiac Tests
• None

Urine Tests
• None

Pregnancy Test
• Pregnancy test (premenopausal females)
• May cause neonatal withdrawal in chronic users
• Other benzodiazepines have been associated with cleft palate (diazepam and related ketobenzodiazepines)

Other Tests (ECG, etc.)
• None

Monthly
• Assessment of alertness
• Assessment of immediate and recent recall
• Examination for ataxia
• Examination for lateral nystagmus

Initial Dosing
• For anxiety, alprazolam IR 0.75–1.5 mg/day divided into three doses
• Dose reduction in elderly

Titration
• Increase dose every three to four days until desired efficacy is reached; maximum dose generally 4 mg/day

Half-Life
• 12–15 hours

Bioavailability
• Metabolized by cyp 3A4 to inactive metabolites
• Food does not affect absorption

Adjustment for Hepatic Dysfunction (by Child-Pugh Criteria)
• Child-Pugh category A or B (mild-moderate hepatic impairment): no dosage adjustment necessary
• Child-Pugh category C (severe hepatic impairment): contraindicated

Adjustment for Renal Dysfunction
• No dosage adjustment necessary per the package insert
• However, dose reductions may be necessary in the presence of significant renal impairment

2.55 Alprazolam (Continued)

H. MEDICATIONS TO AVOID IN COMBINATION/WARNINGS [1, 3, 4]

 Central Nervous System (CNS) depressants

- Medications likely to worsen confusion, memory impairment or ataxia, e.g. carbamazepine, oxcarbazepine, valproic acid, divalproex, topiramate, phenobarbital, phenytoin, tiagabine, gabapentin, pregabalin, sedating antihistamines, sedating antidepressants, sedating antipsychotics and opioids

 cyp 3A4 inhibitors

- Inhibitors of cyp 3A, such as nefazodone, fluvoxamine, fluoxetine, azole antifungal agents, macrolide antibiotics, protease inhibitors and grapefruit juice may decrease clearance of alprazolam, raise alprazolam plasma levels and enhance sedative side effects; alprazolam dose may need to be lowered

 cyp 3A4 inducers

- Inducers of cyp 3A, such as carbamazepine, may increase clearance and lower alprazolam plasma levels
- Cigarette smoking can reduce plasma concentration

 Clozapine

- First week of clozapine treatment associated with rare severe orthostatic hypotension leading to respiratory arrest

 Warnings

- Prone to diversion and abuse, especially in forensic settings
- Contraindicated in currently impaired consciousness or coma
- Respiratory depression, especially combined with CNS depressants in overdose – administer flumazenil if severe or life-threatening
- Avoid in angle closure glaucoma
- Secreted in breast milk at concentrations sufficient to affect the infant
- Caution in COPD, especially if severe, and sleep apnea
- Caution in neurocognitive and amnestic disorders
- Caution with positive history of suicide attempts
- Caution in borderline personality disorder or impulse control disorders

 ### ART OF PSYCHOPHARMACOLOGY: TAKE-HOME PEARLS

- Treating psychosis is often the best treatment for anxiety.
- Increased agitation is a signal to reduce or eliminate, rather than increase dose in many cases as it often reflects decreased impulse control.
- Benzodiazepines may function well as acute "rescue" medications, but chronic use should be avoided whenever possible.

 ### References

1. Jonas, J. M., Cohon, M. S. (1993). A comparison of the safety and efficacy of alprazolam versus other agents in the treatment of anxiety, panic, and depression: a review of the literature. *J Clin Psychiatry*, 54 Suppl., 25–45; discussion 46–48.
2. Liver Toxicology. (2012). Benzodiazepines. In *LiverTox: Clinical and Research Information on Drug-Induced Liver Injury* (eds.). Bethesda, MD: National Institute of Diabetes and Digestive and Kidney Diseases.
3. Ait-Daoud, N., Hamby, A. S., Sharma, S., et al. (2018). A review of alprazolam use, misuse, and withdrawal. *J Addict Med*, 12, 4–10.
4. DeVane, C. L., Ware, M. R., Lydiard, R. B. (1991). Pharmacokinetics, pharmacodynamics, and treatment issues of benzodiazepines: alprazolam, adinazolam, and clonazepam. *Psychopharmacol Bull*, 27, 463–473.
5. Olivier, J. D. A., Olivier, B. (2020). Translational studies in the complex role of neurotransmitter systems in anxiety and anxiety disorders. *Adv Exp Med Biol*, 1191, 121–140.
6. Dold, M., Li, C., Tardy, M., et al. (2012). Benzodiazepines for schizophrenia. *Cochrane Database Syst Rev*, 11, CD006391.
7. Tiihonen, J., Suokas, J. T., Suvisaari, J. M., et al. (2012). Polypharmacy with antipsychotics, antidepressants, or benzodiazepines and mortality in schizophrenia. *Arch Gen Psychiatry*, 69, 476–483.

8. Dold, M., Li, C., Gillies, D., et al. (2013). Benzodiazepine augmentation of antipsychotic drugs in schizophrenia: a meta-analysis and Cochrane review of randomized controlled trials. *Eur Neuropsychopharmacol*, 23, 1023–1033.

9. Spiegel, D. A. (1998). Efficacy studies of alprazolam in panic disorder. *Psychopharmacol Bull*, 34, 191–195.

10. Klein, E. (2002). The role of extended-release benzodiazepines in the treatment of anxiety: a risk-benefit evaluation with a focus on extended-release alprazolam. *J Clin Psychiatry*, 63 Suppl. 14, 27–33.

11. No authors listed. (2019). Drugs for anxiety disorders. *Med Lett Drugs Ther*, 61, 121–126.

12. Greenblatt, D. J., Wright, C. E. (1993). Clinical pharmacokinetics of alprazolam. Therapeutic implications. *Clin Pharmacokinet*, 24, 453–471.

2.56 Buspirone

A. BASIC INFORMATION [1, 2]

Principle Trade Names
• BuSpar®

Legal Status
• Prescription only
• Not controlled

Classifications
• Anxiolytic
• Azapirone
• Serotonin 1A partial agonist
• Serotonin stabilizer

Generics Available
• Yes

Formulations
• Tablets: 5 mg scored; 10 mg scored; 15 mg multi-scored; 30 mg multi-scored

FDA Indications
• Management of anxiety disorders
• Short-term treatment of symptoms of anxiety

Other Data-Supported Indications
• Mixed anxiety and depression
• Treatment-resistant depression (adjunctive)

B. MECHANISMS OF ACTION [1]

Serotonin
• Binds to serotonin type 1A receptors
• Partial agonist actions postsynaptically may theoretically diminish serotonergic activity and contribute to anxiolytic actions
• Partial agonist actions at presynaptic somatodendritic serotonin autoreceptors may theoretically enhance serotonergic activity and contribute to antidepressant actions

Dopamine
• Moderate binding affinity with unknown impact

C. PLASMA CONCENTRATIONS AND TREATMENT RESPONSE [1]

Initial Target Range
• No established plasma therapeutic range

Range for Treatment Resistance
• No established plasma therapeutic range

Typical Time to Response
• Two to four weeks
• Primarily an augmenting agent

Time-Course of Improvement
• If not working within six to eight weeks at typical doses, it may require a dosage increase
• If no improvement after four weeks at maximum tolerated dose, then withdraw treatment

D. TYPICAL TREATMENT RESPONSE [1, 2, 3]

Usual Target Symptoms
• Anxiety

Common Short-Term Adverse Effects
• Dizziness
• Headache
• Nervousness
• Sedation
• Lightheadedness
• Excitement
• Nausea
• Fatigue
• Restlessness
• Disturbed dreams
• Nonspecific chest pain
• Tinnitus, sore throat, nasal congestion

Rare Adverse Effects
• Cardiac
• Weight gain
• Burning sensation of the tongue

• Galactorrhea
• Thyroid abnormality
• Inner ear abnormality
• Eye pain or pressure, photophobia
• Psychosis
• Feelings of claustrophobia
• Cold intolerance
• Stupor
• Slurred speech
• Involuntary movements, akathisia
• Amenorrhea, pelvic inflammatory disease, enuresis and nocturia
• Muscle pain, stiffness or weakness
• Acne, thinning of nails
• Nosebleed

Long-Term Effects
• None

E. PRE-TREATMENT WORKUP AND INITIAL LABORATORY TESTING [1, 2, 4]

History
• Substance abuse or dependence – especially in forensic settings

Physical
• None

Neurological
• Observe for involuntary movements or tremor

Blood Tests
• None

Cardiac Tests
• None

Urine Tests
• None

Pregnancy Test
• Pregnancy test (premenopausal females)
• Classified as no risk in nonhuman studies

Other Tests (ECG, etc.)
• None

F. MONITORING [1, 2]

Monthly
- Mental status exam and assessment of physical health for a brief period following initiation

Annually
- Assessment for involuntary movements

Other
- As clinically indicated

G. DOSING AND KINETICS [1, 2, 3]

Initial Dosing
- 15 mg twice a day
- Requires dosing two to three times a day for full effect

Titration
- Increase in 5 mg/day increments every two to three days until desired efficacy is reached; maximum dose generally 60 mg/day

Half-Life
- Two to three hours

Bioavailability
- 90%
- 86% protein-bound
- Increased by administration with food

Adjustment for Hepatic Dysfunction (by Child-Pugh Criteria)
- Child-Pugh category A or B (mild-moderate hepatic impairment): no dosage adjustment necessary
- Child-Pugh category C (severe hepatic impairment): contraindicated

Adjustment for Renal Dysfunction
- No dosage adjustment necessary per the package insert
- However, dose reductions may be necessary in the presence of significant renal impairment

H. MEDICATIONS TO AVOID IN COMBINATION/WARNINGS [1, 2, 3, 4]

 Monoamine oxidase inhibitors (MAOIs)
- Wait at least 14 days after stopping MAOIs to avoid possibility of hypertensive crisis or serotonin syndrome
- Avoid with linezolid or IV methylene blue

 cyp 3A4 inhibitors (may require lower doses)
- Fluoxetine
- Fluvoxamine
- Nefazodone
- Verapamil
- Diltiazem
- Erythromycin
- Grapefruit juice
- Azole antibiotics
- Ritonavir

 cyp 3A4 inducers (may require higher doses)
- Phenytoin
- Carbamazepine
- Phenobarbital
- Rifampin
- Dexamethasone

 Haloperidol
- Buspirone may increase levels of haloperidol

 Diazepam
- Buspirone may raise levels of nordiazepam, the active metabolite of diazepam, which may result in increased symptoms of dizziness, headache or nausea

 Warnings
- Abused and diverted – especially in forensic settings
- Could destabilize those with a bipolar diathesis
- Could exacerbate agitation or aggression
- Likely excreted in breast milk

ART OF PSYCHOPHARMACOLOGY: TAKE-HOME PEARLS

- Treating psychosis with adequate antipsychotic therapy is often the best treatment for anxiety in psychotic disorders.

- At best consider buspirone as an augmenting agent.
- Lacks withdrawal symptoms and does not cause sexual dysfunction.

References

1. Stahl, S. M. (2017). Buspirone. In *Stahl's Essential Psychopharmacology Prescriber's Guide* (eds.). Cambridge: Cambridge University Press, pp. 113–115.
2. Amneal Pharmaceuticals LLC. (2019). *Buspirone Package Insert*. Bridgewater, New Jersey.
3. Mahmood, I., Sahajwalla, C. (1999). Clinical pharmacokinetics and pharmacodynamics of buspirone, an anxiolytic drug. *Clin Pharmacokinet*, 36, 277–287.
4. Mezher, A. W., McKnight, C. A., Caplan, J. P. (2019). Buspirone abuse: no safe haven. *Psychosomatics*, 60, 534–535.

2.57 Clonazepam

A. BASIC INFORMATION [1–3]

Principle Trade Names
• Klonopin®

Legal Status
• Prescription only
• Controlled

Classifications
• Benzodiazepine
• Antiepileptic
• Anxiolytic

Generics Available
• Yes

Formulations
• Tablets: 0.5 mg scored; 1 mg; 2 mg
• Disintegrating (wafer): 0.125 mg; 0.25 mg; 0.5 mg; 1 mg; 2 mg

FDA Indications
• Panic disorder, with or without agoraphobia
• Lennox-Gastaut syndrome (petit mal variant)
• Akinetic seizure
• Myoclonic seizure
• Absence seizure (petit mal)

Other Data-Supported Indications
• Atonic seizures
• Other seizure disorders
• Other anxiety disorders
• Acute mania (adjunctive)
• Acute psychosis (adjunctive)
• Insomnia (slow onset, rapid tolerance)
• Catatonia
• Akathisia

B. MECHANISMS OF ACTION [2]

Gamma-Aminobutyric Acid (GABA)
• Binds to benzodiazepine receptors at the GABA-A ligand-gated chloride channel complex
• Enhances the inhibitory effects of GABA
• Boosts chloride conductance through GABA-regulated channels

• Inhibits neuronal activity presumably in amygdala-centered fear circuits to provide therapeutic benefits in anxiety disorders
• Inhibits activity in the reticular activating system, initially producing sedation

C. PLASMA CONCENTRATIONS AND TREATMENT RESPONSE [2, 4–10]

Initial Target Range
• No established plasma therapeutic range

Range for Treatment Resistance
• No established plasma therapeutic range

Typical Time to Response
• Some immediate relief with first dosing is common

Time-Course of Improvement
• Usually based on reducing affective response to psychotic symptoms
• For patients with schizophrenia, benzodiazepines only have scant supporting literature for use in akathisia and acute agitation. Chronic use is not recommended
• Benzodiazepine use is associated with higher mortality including increased suicide deaths

D. TYPICAL TREATMENT RESPONSE [2, 11]

Usual Target Symptoms
• Anxiety
• Psychomotor agitation
• Seizure activity

Common Short-Term Adverse Effects
• Sedation
• Fatigue
• Depression
• Dizziness
• Ataxia
• Slurred speech
• Weakness
• Amnesia
• Confusion
• Paradoxical anxiety
• Paradoxical agitation/disinhibition

Rare Adverse Effects
• Hallucinations
• Mania
• Hypotension
• Hypersalivation/impaired swallowing
• Dry mouth
• Hepatic dysfunction
• Renal dysfunction
• Blood dyscrasias

Long-Term Effects
• Dependence, tolerance and withdrawal
• Possible negative neurocognitive impact

E. PRE-TREATMENT WORKUP AND INITIAL LABORATORY TESTING [11, 12]

History
• Substance abuse or dependence, neurodevelopmental disorder, angle closure glaucoma

Physical
• Pulmonary examination for chronic obstructive pulmonary disease (COPD)

Neurological
• Alertness, cognitive impairment

Blood Tests
• None

Cardiac Tests
• None

Urine Tests
• None

Pregnancy Test
• Pregnancy test (premenopausal females)
• Classified as having evidence of risk
• May cause neonatal withdrawal in chronic users
• Other benzodiazepines have been associated with cleft palate (diazepam and related ketobenzodiazepines)

Other Tests (ECG, etc.)
• None

F. MONITORING [11]

Monthly
- Assessment of alertness
- Assessment of immediate and recent recall
- Examination for ataxia
- Examination for lateral nystagmus

G. DOSING AND KINETICS [2, 3, 10]

Initial Dosing
- Generally dosed half the dosage of alprazolam
- Panic: 1 mg/day; start at 0.25 mg divided into two doses, raise to 1 mg after three days; dose either twice daily or once at bedtime; maximum dose generally 4 mg/day
- Seizures: 1.5 mg divided into three doses, raise by 0.5 mg every three days until desired effect is reached; divide into three even doses or else give largest dose at bedtime; maximum dose generally 20 mg/day

Titration
- Start at lowest effective dose
- Due to tolerance upward titration likely needed once or twice in chronic use

Half-Life
- 30–40 hours

Bioavailability
- 90%
- 85% protein-bound
- Food does not affect absorption

Adjustment for Hepatic Dysfunction (by Child-Pugh Criteria)
- Child-Pugh category A or B (mild-moderate hepatic impairment): no dosage adjustment necessary
- Child-Pugh category C (severe hepatic impairment): 30–90% dose reduction or contraindicated

Adjustment for Renal Dysfunction
- No dosage adjustment necessary per the package insert
- However, dose reductions may be necessary in the presence of significant renal impairment

H. MEDICATIONS TO AVOID IN COMBINATION/WARNINGS [2, 3, 11]

 Central Nervous System (CNS) depressants
- Medications likely to worsen confusion, memory impairment or ataxia, e.g. carbamazepine, oxcarbazepine, valproic acid, divalproex, topiramate, phenobarbital, phenytoin, tiagabine, gabapentin, pregabalin, sedating antihistamines, sedating antidepressants, sedating antipsychotics and opioids

 cyp 3A4 inhibitors (may require lower doses)
- Oral azole antifungal agents

 cyp 3A4 inducers (may require higher doses)
- Phenytoin
- Carbamazepine
- Lamotrigine
- Phenobarbital

 Clozapine
- First week of clozapine treatment associated with rare severe orthostatic hypotension leading to respiratory arrest

 Warnings
- Prone to diversion and abuse, especially in forensic settings
- Contraindicated in currently impaired consciousness or coma
- Respiratory depression, especially combined with CNS depressants in overdose – administer flumazenil if severe or life-threatening
- Avoid in angle closure glaucoma
- Secreted in breast milk at concentrations sufficient to affect the infant
- Caution in COPD, especially if severe, and sleep apnea
- Caution in neurocognitive and amnestic disorders
- Caution with positive history of suicide attempts
- Caution in borderline personality disorder or impulse control disorders

ART OF PSYCHOPHARMACOLOGY: TAKE-HOME PEARLS

- Treating psychosis adequately with antipsychotics is often the best treatment for anxiety in psychotic disorders.
- Increased agitation is a signal to reduce or eliminate, rather than increase dose in many cases as it often reflects decreased impulse control.

- Benzodiazepines may function well as acute "rescue" medications, but chronic use should be avoided whenever possible.

References

1. Liver Toxicology. (2012). Benzodiazepines. In *LiverTox: Clinical and Research Information on Drug-Induced Liver Injury* (eds.). Bethesda, MD: National Institute of Diabetes and Digestive and Kidney Diseases.
2. Stahl, S. M. (2017). Clonazepam. In *Stahl's Essential Psychopharmacology Prescriber's Guide* (eds.). Cambridge: Cambridge University Press, pp. 159–163.
3. Sandoz Inc. (2019). *Clonazepam Package Insert*. Princeton, New Jersey.
4. Volz, A., Khorsand, V., Gillies, D., et al. (2007). Benzodiazepines for schizophrenia. *Cochrane Database Syst Rev*, 24(1), CD006391.
5. Dold, M., Li, C., Tardy, M., et al. (2012). Benzodiazepines for schizophrenia. *Cochrane Database Syst Rev*, 11, CD006391.
6. Tiihonen, J., Suokas, J. T., Suvisaari, J. M., et al. (2012). Polypharmacy with antipsychotics, antidepressants, or benzodiazepines and mortality in schizophrenia. *Arch Gen Psychiatry*, 69, 476–483.
7. Dold, M., Li, C., Gillies, D., et al. (2013). Benzodiazepine augmentation of antipsychotic drugs in schizophrenia: a meta-analysis and Cochrane review of randomized controlled trials. *Eur Neuropsychopharmacol*, 23, 1023–1033.
8. Gillies, D., Sampson, S., Beck, A., et al. (2013). Benzodiazepines for psychosis-induced aggression or agitation. *Cochrane Database Syst Rev*, 24(1), CD003079.
9. Dodds, T. J. (2017). Prescribed benzodiazepines and suicide risk: a review of the literature. *Prim Care Companion CNS Disord*, 19, doi 10.4088
10. Zaman, H., Sampson, S., Beck, A., et al. (2018). Benzodiazepines for psychosis-induced aggression or agitation. *Schizophr Bull*, 44, 966–969.
11. California Department of State Hospitals. (2019). *DSH Psychotropic Medication Policy: Benzodiazepine Protocol*. Sacramento, California.
12. DeVane, C. L., Ware, M. R., Lydiard, R. B. (1991). Pharmacokinetics, pharmacodynamics, and treatment issues of benzodiazepines: alprazolam, adinazolam, and clonazepam. *Psychopharmacol Bull*, 27, 463–473.
13. No authors listed. (2019). Drugs for anxiety disorders. *Med Lett Drugs Ther*, 61, 121–126.

2.58 Diazepam

A. BASIC INFORMATION [1–4]

Principle Trade Names
• Valium®
• Diastat®

Legal Status
• Prescription only
• Controlled

Classifications
• Ketobenzodiazepine
• Anxiolytic

Generics Available
• Yes

Formulations
• Tablets: 2 mg scored; 5 mg scored; 10 mg scored
• Liquid: 5 mg/5 ml; concentrate: 5 mg/ml
• Injection: 5 mg/ml; 10 ml, boxes of 1; 2 ml boxes of 10
• Rectal gel: 5 mg/ml: 2.5 mg, 5 mg; 10 mg; 15 mg; 20 mg

FDA Indications
• Anxiety disorder
• Symptoms of anxiety (short-term): acute agitation, tremor, impending or acute delirium tremens and hallucinosis in acute alcohol withdrawal
• Skeletal muscle spasm due to reflex spasm to local pathology
• Spasticity caused by upper motor neuron disorder
• Athetosis
• Stiffman syndrome
• Convulsive disorder (adjunctive)
• Anxiety during endoscopic procedures (adjunctive) (injection only)
• Preoperative anxiety (injection only)
• Anxiety relief prior to cardioversion (intravenous)
• Initial treatment of status epilepticus (injection only)

Other Data-Supported Indications
• Insomnia (rapid tolerance)
• Catatonia

B. MECHANISMS OF ACTION [2, 5]

Gamma-Aminobutyric Acid (GABA)
• Binds to benzodiazepine receptors at the GABA-A ligand-gated chloride channel complex
• Enhances the inhibitory effects of GABA
• Boosts chloride conductance through GABA-regulated channels

• Inhibits neuronal activity presumably in amygdala-centered fear circuits to provide therapeutic benefits in anxiety disorders
• Initially inhibits activity in the reticular activating system, producing sedation

C. PLASMA CONCENTRATIONS AND TREATMENT RESPONSE [2, 6–12]

Initial Target Range
• No established plasma therapeutic range

Range for Treatment Resistance
• No established plasma therapeutic range

Typical Time to Response
• Some immediate relief with first dosing is common

Time-Course of Improvement
• Usually based on reducing affective response to psychotic symptoms
• For patients with schizophrenia, benzodiazepines only have scant supporting literature for use in akathisia and acute agitation. Chronic use is not recommended
• Benzodiazepine use is associated with higher mortality including increased suicide deaths

D. TYPICAL TREATMENT RESPONSE [2, 13]

Usual Target Symptoms
• Anxiety
• Psychomotor agitation

Common Short-Term Adverse Effects
• Sedation
• Fatigue
• Depression
• Dizziness
• Ataxia
• Slurred speech
• Weakness
• Amnesia
• Confusion
• Anxiety
• Paradoxical agitation/disinhibition

Rare Adverse Effects
• Hallucinations
• Mania
• Hypotension
• Hypersalivation
• Dry mouth
• Hepatic dysfunction
• Renal dysfunction
• Blood dyscrasias

Long-Term Effects
• Dependence, tolerance and withdrawal
• Possible negative neurocognitive impact

E. PRE-TREATMENT WORKUP AND INITIAL LABORATORY TESTING [13, 14]

History
• Substance abuse or dependence, neurodevelopmental disorder, angle closure glaucoma

Physical
• Pulmonary examination for chronic obstructive pulmonary disease (COPD)

Neurological
• Alertness, cognitive impairment

Blood Tests
• None

Cardiac Tests
• None

Urine Tests
• None

Pregnancy Test
• Pregnancy test (premenopausal females)
• Classified as evidence of risk
• May cause neonatal withdrawal in chronic users
• Diazepam and related ketobenzodiazepines have been associated with cleft palate

Other Tests (ECG, etc.)
• None

F. MONITORING [13]

Monthly
• Assessment of alertness
• Assessment of immediate and recent recall
• Examination for ataxia
• Examination for lateral nystagmus

Initial Dosing

- Oral (anxiety, muscle spasm, seizure): 2–10 mg, two to four times/day
- Elderly: initial 2–2.5 mg, one to two times/day; increase gradually as needed
- Oral (alcohol withdrawal): initial 10 mg, three to four times/day for one day; reduce to 5 mg, three to four times/day; continue treatment as needed
- Intramuscular administration produces erratic absorption
- Intravenous (adults): 5 mg/min
- Liquid formulation should be mixed with water or fruit juice, applesauce or pudding
- Because of risk of respiratory depression, rectal diazepam treatment should not be given more than once in five days or more than twice during a treatment course, especially for alcohol withdrawal or status epilepticus

Titration

- Due to tolerance upward titration once or twice after initial dosing may be needed
- Titrate gradually in elderly patients

- Diazepam may accumulate in elderly patients or in patients with hepatic impairment

Half-Life

- 20–50 hours

Bioavailability

- 90%
- 97% protein-bound
- Food does not affect absorption

Adjustment for Hepatic Dysfunction (by Child-Pugh Criteria)

- Child-Pugh category A or B (mild-moderate hepatic impairment): no dosage adjustment necessary
- Child-Pugh category C (severe hepatic impairment): contraindicated

Adjustment for Renal Dysfunction

- No dosage adjustment necessary per the package insert
- However, dose reductions may be necessary in the presence of significant renal impairment

H. MEDICATIONS TO AVOID IN COMBINATION/WARNINGS [1–4, 13]

Central Nervous System (CNS) depressants

- Medications likely to worsen confusion, memory impairment or ataxia, e.g. carbamazepine, oxcarbazepine, valproic acid, divalproex, topiramate, phenobarbital, phenytoin, tiagabine, gabapentin, pregabalin, sedating antihistamines, sedating antidepressants, sedating antipsychotics and opioids

cyp 3A4 and cyp 2C19 inhibitors (may require lower doses)

- Cimetidine
- Ketoconazole
- Fluvoxamine
- Fluoxetine
- Omeprazole

Clozapine

- First week of clozapine treatment associated with rare severe orthostatic hypotension leading to respiratory arrest

Warnings

- Prone to diversion and abuse, especially in forensic settings
- Contraindicated in currently impaired consciousness or coma
- Respiratory depression, especially combined with CNS depressants in overdose – administer flumazenil if severe or life-threatening
- Avoid in angle closure glaucoma
- Secreted in breast milk at concentrations sufficient to affect the infant
- Caution in COPD, especially if severe, and sleep apnea
- Caution in neurocognitive and amnestic disorders
- Caution with positive history of suicide attempts
- Caution in borderline personality disorder or impulse control disorders

ART OF PSYCHOPHARMACOLOGY: TAKE-HOME PEARLS

- Treating psychosis with adequate antipsychotic therapy is often the best treatment for anxiety in psychotic disorders.
- Increased agitation is a signal to reduce or eliminate, rather than increase dose in many cases as it often reflects decreased impulse control.
- Benzodiazepines may function well as acute "rescue" medications, but chronic use should be avoided whenever possible.

References

1. Oceanside Pharmaceuticals Inc. (2017). *Diazepam Gel Package Insert.* Bridgewater, New Jersey.
2. Stahl, S. M. (2017). Diazepam. In *Stahl's Essential Psychopharmacology Prescriber's Guide* (eds.). Cambridge: Cambridge University Press, pp. 211–215.
3. Civica. (2019). *Diazepam Injection Package Insert.* London (UK).
4. Mayne Pharma. (2019). *Diazepam Tablets Package Insert.* London (UK).
5. Olivier, J. D. A., Olivier, B. (2020). Translational studies in the complex role of neurotransmitter systems in anxiety and anxiety disorders. *Adv Exp Med Biol*, 1191, 121–140.
6. Volz, A., Khorsand, V., Gillies, D., et al. (2007). Benzodiazepines for schizophrenia. *Cochrane Database Syst Rev*, 11 CD006391.
7. Dold, M., Li, C., Tardy, M., et al. (2012). Benzodiazepines for schizophrenia. *Cochrane Database Syst Rev*, 11, CD006391.
8. Tiihonen, J., Suokas, J. T., Suvisaari, J. M., et al. (2012). Polypharmacy with antipsychotics, antidepressants, or benzodiazepines and mortality in schizophrenia. *Arch Gen Psychiatry*, 69, 476–483.
9. Dold, M., Li, C., Gillies, D., et al. (2013). Benzodiazepine augmentation of antipsychotic drugs in schizophrenia: a meta-analysis and Cochrane review of randomized controlled trials. *Eur Neuropsychopharmacol*, 23, 1023–1033.
10. Gillies, D., Sampson, S., Beck, A., et al. (2013). Benzodiazepines for psychosis-induced aggression or agitation. *Cochrane Database Syst Rev*, 9, CD003079.
11. Dodds, T. J. (2017). Prescribed benzodiazepines and suicide risk: a review of the literature. *Prim Care Companion CNS Disord*, 19, doi 10.4088
12. Zaman, H., Sampson, S., Beck, A., et al. (2018). Benzodiazepines for psychosis-induced aggression or agitation. *Schizophr Bull*, 44, 966–969.
13. California Department of State Hospitals. (2019). *DSH Psychotropic Medication Policy: Benzodiazepine Protocol.* Sacramento, California
14. Liver Toxicology. (2012). Benzodiazepines. In *LiverTox: Clinical and Research Information on Drug-Induced Liver Injury* (eds.). Bethesda, MD: National Institute of Diabetes and Digestive and Kidney Diseases.

2.59 Hydroxyzine

A. BASIC INFORMATION [1, 2]

Principle Trade Names
• Vistaril®
• Atarax®
• Marax®

Legal Status
• Prescription only
• Not controlled

Classifications
• Histamine receptor antagonist
• Antihistamine
• Anxiolytic
• Hypnotic
• Antiemetic

Generics Available
• Yes

Formulations
• Tablets: 10 mg; 25 mg; 50 mg; 100 mg
• Capsules: 25 mg; 50 mg; 100 mg
• Oral liquid: 10 mg/5 ml; 25 mg/5 ml
• Intramuscular injection: 25 mg/ml; 50 mg/ml; 100 mg/2 ml

FDA Indications
• Anxiety and tension associated with psychoneurosis
• Adjunct in organic disease states in which anxiety is manifested
• Pruritus due to allergic conditions
• Histamine-mediated pruritus
• Premedication sedation
• Sedation following general anesthesia
• Acute disturbance/hysteria (injection)
• Anxiety withdrawal symptoms in alcoholics or patients with delirium tremens (injection)
• Adjunct in pre/postoperative and pre/postpartum patients to allay anxiety, control emesis and reduce narcotic dose (injection)
• Nausea and vomiting (injection)

Other Data-Supported Indications
• Insomnia

B. MECHANISMS OF ACTION [1, 2]

Histamine
• Blocks histamine$_1$ receptors

Acetylcholine
• Has no affinity for acetylcholine receptors and unlike diphenhydramine does not contribute to anticholinergic burden

C. PLASMA CONCENTRATIONS AND TREATMENT RESPONSE [1, 2]

Initial Target Range
• No established plasma therapeutic range

Range for Treatment Resistance
• No established plasma therapeutic range

Typical Time to Response
• 15–20 minutes (oral administration)

Time-Course of Improvement
• Some immediate relief with first dosing is common; can take several weeks with daily dosing for maximal therapeutic benefit in chronic conditions

D. TYPICAL TREATMENT RESPONSE [1, 2]

Usual Target Symptoms
• Anxiety
• Agitation
• Insomnia
• Skeletal muscle tension
• Itching
• Nausea, vomiting

Common Short-Term Adverse Effects
• Sedation
• Dry mouth
• Tremor

Rare Adverse Effects
• Acute generalized exanthematous pustulosis
• Convulsions (generally at high doses)
• Cardiac arrest, death (intramuscular formulation combined with central nervous system (CNS) depressants)
• Bronchodilation
• Respiratory depression
• Weight gain
• Hallucinations
• Headache

Long-Term Effects
• None

E. PRE-TREATMENT WORKUP AND INITIAL LABORATORY TESTING [1, 2]

History
• Risk factors for QT prolongation

Physical
• None

Neurological
• None

Blood Tests
• None for healthy individuals
• Hydroxyzine may cause falsely elevated urinary concentrations of 17-hydroxycorticosteroids in certain lab tests (e.g. Porter-Silber reaction, Glenn-Nelson method)

Cardiac Tests
• ECG if positive history of QT interval prolongation or if taking other medications that prolong the QT interval, as reflected by a warning in the package insert

Urine Tests
• None

Pregnancy Test
• Pregnancy test (premenopausal females)
• Classified as risk not ruled out

Other Tests (ECG, etc.)
• None

F. MONITORING [1, 2]

Monthly
• Mental status exam and assessment of physical health as clinically indicated

Annually
• Routine annual assessment including mental status examination and general health and possibly ECG

Initial Dosing
- Anxiety: 50–100 mg four times a day
- Sedative: 50–100 mg oral, 25–100 mg intramuscular injection
- Emergency intramuscular injection: initial 50–100 mg, repeat every four to six hours as needed
- Pruritus: 75 mg/day divided into three to four doses

Titration
- Oral dosing does not require titration
- May be administered intramuscularly initially, but should be changed to oral administration as soon as possible
- Tolerance usually develops to sedation, allowing higher dosing over time
- Intramuscular injection should not be given in the lower or mid-third of the arm and should only be given in the deltoid area if it is well developed
- In adults, intramuscular injections may be given in the upper outer quadrant of the buttock or in the midlateral thigh

Half-Life
- 20 hours

Bioavailability
- Rapidly absorbed from gastrointestinal (GI) tract

Adjustment for Hepatic Dysfunction (by Child-Pugh Criteria)
- Child-Pugh category A or B (mild-moderate hepatic impairment): no dosage adjustment necessary
- Child-Pugh category C (severe hepatic impairment): contraindicated

Adjustment for Renal Dysfunction
- No dosage adjustment necessary per the package insert
- However, dose reductions may be necessary in the presence of significant renal impairment

H. MEDICATIONS TO AVOID IN COMBINATION/WARNINGS [1, 2]

CNS depressants
- Caution when combining hydroxyzine with CNS depressants including alcohol, barbiturates and opiates

QT prolonging agents
- Caution with concomitant use of drugs known to prolong the QT interval

Warnings
- Contraindicated in patients with a prolonged QT interval
- Contraindicated in early pregnancy
- Can prolong QT at doses >200 mg/day
- Intramuscular hydroxyzine hydrochloride may result in severe injection site reactions

ART OF PSYCHOPHARMACOLOGY: TAKE-HOME PEARLS

- Treating psychosis with adequate antipsychotic therapy is often the best treatment for anxiety in psychotic disorders.
- Helpful for anxiety, agitation and sleep without anticholinergic impact or issues associated with benzodiazepines.
- Tablets, capsules, oral solution and injectable formulations provide flexibility.

References
1. Stahl, S. M. (2017). Hydroxyzine. In *Stahl's Essential Psychopharmacology Prescriber's Guide* (eds.). Cambridge: Cambridge University Press, pp. 331–334.
2. Avet Pharmaceuticals Inc. (2020). *Hydroxyzine Package Insert.* East Brunswick, New Jersey.
3. Paton, D. M., Webster, D. R. (1985). Clinical pharmacokinetics of H1-receptor antagonists (the antihistamines). *Clin Pharmacokinet*, 10, 477–497.

2.60 Lorazepam

A. BASIC INFORMATION [1–4]

Principle Trade Names
- Ativan®

Legal Status
- Prescription only
- Controlled

Classifications
- Hydroxybenzodiazepine
- Anxiolytic

Generics Available
- Yes

Formulations
- Tablets: 0.5 mg; 1 mg; 2 mg
- Liquid: 0.5 mg/5 ml; 2 mg/ml
- Injection: 1 mg/0.5 ml; 2 mg/ml; 4 mg/ml

FDA Indications
- Anxiety disorder (oral)
- Anxiety associated with depressive symptoms (oral)
- Initial treatment of status epilepticus (injection)
- Preanesthetic (injection)

Other Data-Supported Indications
- Insomnia (rapid tolerance)
- Muscle spasm
- Alcohol withdrawal psychosis
- Headache
- Panic disorder
- Acute mania (adjunctive)
- Acute psychosis (adjunctive)
- Delirium (with haloperidol)
- Catatonia

Gamma-Aminobutyric Acid (GABA)
- Binds to benzodiazepine receptors at the GABA-A ligand-gated chloride channel complex
- Enhances the inhibitory effects of GABA
- Boosts chloride conductance through GABA-regulated channels
- Inhibits neuronal activity presumably in amygdala-centered fear circuits to provide therapeutic benefits in anxiety disorders
- Initially inhibits activity in the reticular activating system, producing sedation

C. PLASMA CONCENTRATIONS AND TREATMENT RESPONSE [1, 5–11]

Initial Target Range
• No established plasma therapeutic range

Range for Treatment Resistance
• No established plasma therapeutic range

Typical Time to Response
• Some immediate relief with first dosing is common

Time-Course of Improvement
• Usually based on reducing psychotic symptoms
• For patients with schizophrenia, benzodiazepines only have scant supporting literature for use in akathisia and acute agitation. Chronic use not recommended
• Benzodiazepine use is associated with higher mortality including increased suicide deaths

D. TYPICAL TREATMENT RESPONSE [1, 12, 13]

Usual Target Symptoms
• Anxiety
• Psychomotor agitation

Common Short-Term Adverse Effects
• Sedation
• Fatigue
• Depression
• Dizziness
• Ataxia
• Slurred speech
• Weakness
• Amnesia
• Confusion
• Paradoxical anxiety
• Paradoxical agitation/disinhibition

Rare Adverse Effects
• Hallucinations
• Mania
• Hypotension
• Hypersalivation/impaired swallowing
• Dry mouth
• Hepatic dysfunction
• Renal dysfunction
• Blood dyscrasias

Long-Term Effects
• Dependence, tolerance and withdrawal
• Possible negative neurocognitive impact

E. PRE-TREATMENT WORKUP AND INITIAL LABORATORY TESTING [13]

History
• Substance abuse or dependence, neurodevelopmental disorder, angle closure glaucoma

Physical
• Pulmonary examination for chronic obstructive pulmonary disease (COPD)

Neurological
• Alertness, cognitive impairment

Blood Tests
• None

Cardiac Tests
• None

Urine Tests
• None

Pregnancy Test
• Pregnancy test (premenopausal females)
• May cause neonatal withdrawal in chronic users
• Other benzodiazepines have been associated with cleft palate (diazepam and related ketobenzodiazepines)

Other Tests (ECG, etc.)
• None

Monthly

- Assessment of alertness
- Assessment of immediate and recent recall
- Examination for ataxia
- Examination for lateral nystagmus

Initial Dosing ORAL

- Oral: initial 1–3 mg/day in two to three doses; increase as needed, starting with evening dose; maximum generally 10 mg/day
- For elderly or debilitated patients, an initial dosage of 1–2 mg/day in divided doses is recommended, to be adjusted as needed and tolerated
- Injection: initial 1–4 mg administered slowly; after 10–15 minutes may administer again
- Intramuscular administration is reliably absorbed
- Take liquid formulation with water, soda, applesauce or pudding
- Catatonia: initial 1–2 mg; can repeat in three hours and then again in another three hours if necessary

Titration

- Increase dose gradually to help avoid adverse effects
- The evening dose should be increased before the daytime doses
- Due to tolerance dosing may need to be increased once or twice after initial dosing

Half-Life

- 12 hours
- No active metabolites

Bioavailability

- 90%
- 85% protein-bound
- Food does not affect absorption

Adjustment for Hepatic Dysfunction (by Child-Pugh Criteria)

- Child-Pugh category A or B (mild-moderate hepatic impairment): no dosage adjustment necessary
- Child-Pugh category C (severe hepatic impairment): requires only conjugation, unlikely to accumulate

Adjustment for Renal Dysfunction

- No dosage adjustment necessary per the package insert
- However, dose reductions may be necessary in the presence of significant renal impairment

H. MEDICATIONS TO AVOID IN COMBINATION/WARNINGS [1–4, 13]

 Central Nervous System (CNS) depressants

- Increased CNS-depressant effects when administered with other CNS depressants such as alcohol, barbiturates, antipsychotics, sedative/hypnotics, anxiolytics, antidepressants, narcotic analgesics, sedative antihistamines, anticonvulsants and anesthetics

 Valproate or probenecid

- Valproate and probenecid may reduce clearance and raise plasma concentrations of lorazepam
- Lorazepam dosage should be reduced by approximately 50% when co-administered with either valproate or probenecid

 Oral contraceptives

- Oral contraceptives may increase clearance and lower plasma concentrations of lorazepam

 Clozapine

- First week of clozapine treatment associated with rare severe orthostatic hypotension leading to respiratory arrest

Warnings

- Black box: concomitant use of benzodiazepines and opioids may result in profound sedation, respiratory depression, coma and death
- Prone to diversion and abuse, especially in forensic settings
- Contraindicated in currently impaired consciousness or coma
- Respiratory depression, especially combined with CNS depressants in overdose – administer flumazenil if severe or life-threatening
- Avoid in angle closure glaucoma
- Secreted in breast milk at concentrations sufficient to affect the infant
- Caution in COPD, especially if severe, and sleep apnea
- Caution in neurocognitive and amnestic disorders
- Caution with positive history of suicide attempts
- Caution in borderline personality disorder or impulse control disorders

 ### ART OF PSYCHOPHARMACOLOGY: TAKE-HOME PEARLS

- Treating psychosis with adequate antipsychotic therapy is often the best treatment for anxiety in psychotic disorders.
- Increased agitation is a signal to reduce or eliminate, rather than increase dose in many cases as it often reflects decreased impulse control.
- Benzodiazepines may function well as acute "rescue" medications, but chronic use should be avoided whenever possible.

References

1. Stahl, S. M. (2017). Lorazepam. In *Stahl's Essential Psychopharmacology Prescriber's Edition* (eds.). Cambridge: Cambridge University Press, pp. 403–407.
2. Qualitest Pharmaceuticals Inc. (2018). *Lorazepam Tablets Package Insert*. Huntsville, Alabama.
3. Amneal Pharmaceuticals LLC. (2019). *Lorazepam Concentrate Package Insert*. Bridgewater, New Jersey.
4. International Medication Systems. (2019). *Lorazepam Injection Package Insert*. South El Monte, California.
5. Volz, A., Khorsand, V., Gillies, D., et al. (2007). Benzodiazepines for schizophrenia. *Cochrane Database Syst Rev*, 11, CD006391.
6. Dold, M., Li, C., Tardy, M., et al. (2012). Benzodiazepines for schizophrenia. *Cochrane Database Syst Rev*, 11, CD006391.
7. Tiihonen, J., Suokas, J. T., Suvisaari, J. M., et al. (2012). Polypharmacy with antipsychotics, antidepressants, or benzodiazepines and mortality in schizophrenia. *Arch Gen Psychiatry*, 69, 476–483.
8. Dold, M., Li, C., Gillies, D., et al. (2013). Benzodiazepine augmentation of antipsychotic drugs in schizophrenia: a meta-analysis and Cochrane review of randomized controlled trials. *Eur Neuropsychopharmacol*, 23, 1023–1033.
9. Gillies, D., Sampson, S., Beck, A., et al. (2013). Benzodiazepines for psychosis-induced aggression or agitation. *Cochrane Database Syst Rev*, 9, CD003079.
10. Dodds, T. J. (2017). Prescribed benzodiazepines and suicide risk: a review of the literature. *Prim Care Companion CNS Disord*, 19, doi: 10.4088
11. Zaman, H., Sampson, S., Beck, A., et al. (2018). Benzodiazepines for psychosis-induced aggression or agitation. *Schizophr Bull*, 44, 966–969.
12. Liver Toxicology. (2012). Benzodiazepines. In *LiverTox: Clinical and Research Information on Drug-Induced Liver Injury* (eds.). Bethesda, MD: National Institute of Diabetes and Digestive and Kidney Diseases.
13. California Department of State Hospitals. (2019). *DSH Psychotropic Medication Policy: Benzodiazepine Protocol*. Sacramento, California.

Sedatives
2.61 Diphenhydramine

*Please see Chapter 2.23 "Diphenhydramine".

A. BASIC INFORMATION [1, 2]

Principle Trade Names
• Lunesta®
• Eszop®

Legal Status
• Prescription only
• Controlled

Classifications
• Gamma-aminobutyric acid positive allosteric modulator (GABA-PAM)
• Non-benzodiazepine hypnotic
• Alpha₁ isoform selective agonist of GABA-A/ benzodiazepine receptors

Generics Available
• Yes

Formulations
• Tablets: 1 mg; 2 mg; 3 mg

FDA Indications
• Insomnia

Other Data-Supported Indications
• Primary insomnia
• Chronic insomnia
• Transient insomnia
• Insomnia secondary to psychiatric or medical conditions
• Residual insomnia following treatment with antidepressants

Gamma-Aminobutyric Acid (GABA)
• May bind selectively to a subtype of the benzodiazepine receptor, the alpha 1 isoform
• May enhance GABA inhibitory actions that provide sedative hypnotic effects more selectively than other actions of GABA
• Boosts chloride conductance through GABA-regulated channels
• Inhibitory actions in sleep centers may provide sedative hypnotic effects

C. PLASMA CONCENTRATIONS AND TREATMENT RESPONSE [1]

Initial Target Range
• No established plasma therapeutic range

Range for Treatment Resistance
• No established plasma therapeutic range

Typical Time to Response
• Less than one hour

Time-Course of Improvement
• Seven to ten days

D. TYPICAL TREATMENT RESPONSE [1]

Usual Target Symptoms
• Time to sleep onset
• Nighttime awakenings
• Total sleep time

Common Short-Term Adverse Effects
• Unpleasant taste
• Sedation
• Dizziness
• Dose-dependent amnesia
• Nervousness
• Dry mouth
• Headache

Rare Adverse Effects
• Respiratory depression, especially when taken with other central nervous system (CNS) depressants in overdose
• Angioedema

Long-Term Effects
• Some patients could develop dependence and/or tolerance with drugs of this class; risk may be theoretically greater with higher doses
• History of drug addiction may theoretically increase risk of dependence

E. PRE-TREATMENT WORKUP AND INITIAL LABORATORY TESTING [1]

History
• Depression, suicidal ideation
• Sleep apnea
• Restless leg syndrome
• Breastfeeding

Physical
• Pulmonary examination for chronic obstructive pulmonary disease (COPD)

Neurological
• Alertness, cognitive impairment

Blood Tests
• None in healthy individuals

Cardiac Tests
• None

Urine Tests
• None

Pregnancy Test
• Pregnancy test (premenopausal females)
• Classified as risk not ruled out

Other Tests (ECG, etc.)
• None

F. MONITORING

Monthly
• Assessment of alertness
• Assessment of immediate and recent recall
• Examination for ataxia

Initial Dosing

- 1–3 mg at bedtime (start at 1 mg in elderly patients)

Titration

- Adjust dose based on clinical response, take dose at bedtime
- Usual maximum dose is 3 mg q bedtime
- In treatment-resistant cases may be titrated to 8 mg q bedtime (monitor carefully for common adverse effects at higher doses)
- If taken for more than a few weeks, taper to reduce chances of withdrawal effects if discontinued

Half-Life

- Six hours

Bioavailability

- Metabolized by cyp 3A4 and 2E1

- Bioavailability: circa 80% (52–59% protein-bound)
- Heavy high-fat meal slows absorption, which could reduce effect on sleep latency

Adjustment for Hepatic Dysfunction (by Child-Pugh Criteria)

- Child-Pugh category A or B (mild-moderate hepatic impairment): no dosage adjustment necessary
- Child-Pugh category C (severe hepatic impairment): contraindicated

Adjustment for Renal Dysfunction

- No dosage adjustment necessary per the package insert
- However, dose reductions may be necessary in the presence of significant renal impairment

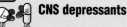
H. MEDICATIONS TO AVOID IN COMBINATION/WARNINGS [1, 2]

CNS depressants

- Increased depressive effects when taken with other CNS depressants

cyp 3A4 inhibitors (may require lower doses)

- Nefazodone
- Fluvoxamine
- Fluoxetine
- Azole antifungal agents
- Macrolide antibiotics
- Protease inhibitors
- Grapefruit juice

cyp 3A4 inducers (may require higher doses)

- Rifampicin
- Phenytoin
- Carbamazepine
- Phenobarbital

Warnings

- Insomnia may be a symptom of a primary disorder, rather than a primary disorder itself
- Eszopiclone actions at benzodiazepine receptors that carry over to the next day can cause daytime sedation, amnesia and ataxia
- Doses higher than 3 mg may be associated with carryover effects, hallucinations or other CNS adverse effects

- Some patients may exhibit abnormal thinking or behavioral changes similar to those caused by other CNS depressants (i.e. either depressant actions or disinhibiting actions)
- Some depressed patients may experience a worsening of suicidal ideation
- Use only with caution in patients with impaired respiratory function or obstructive sleep apnea
- Unknown if eszopiclone is secreted in human breast milk, but all psychotropics assumed to be secreted in breast milk; recommended either to discontinue drug or bottle feed
- Eszopiclone should only be administered at bedtime
- Rare angioedema has occurred with sedative hypnotic use and could potentially cause fatal airway obstruction if it involves the throat, glottis or larynx; thus, if angioedema occurs treatment should be discontinued
- Sleep driving and other complex behaviors, such as eating and preparing food and making phone calls, have been reported in patients taking sedative hypnotics
- Infants whose mothers took sedative hypnotics during pregnancy may experience some withdrawal symptoms
- Neonatal flaccidity has been reported in infants whose mothers took sedative hypnotics during pregnancy

2.62 Eszopiclone (Continued)

- Safe for long-term use and may be preferred over benzodiazepines because of its rapid onset of action, short duration of effect, and safety profile without notable tolerance or dependence developing over time.

- To avoid problems with memory, take eszopiclone only if planning to have a full night's sleep.
- Rebound insomnia does not appear to be common.

 References

1. Stahl, S. M. (2017). Eszopiclone. In *Stahl's Essential Psychopharmacology Prescriber's Guide* (eds.). Cambridge: Cambridge University Press, pp. 261–264.
2. West-Ward Pharmaceuticals Corp. (2020). *Eszopiclone Package Insert*. West Eatontown, New Jersey.

2.63 Hydroxyzine

*Please see Chapter 2.59 "Hydroxyzine".

2.64 Lorazepam

*Please see Chapter 2.60 "Lorazepam".

2.65 Oxazepam

A. BASIC INFORMATION [1–3]

Principle Trade Names
• Serax®

Legal Status
• Prescription only
• Controlled

Classifications
• Benzodiazepine
• Hydroxybenzodiazepine
• Sedative
• Anxiolytic

Generics Available
• Yes

Formulations
• Capsules: 10 mg; 15 mg; 30 mg
• Tablets: 15 mg
• Note: tablets contain tartrazine, which may cause allergic reactions in certain patients, particularly those who are sensitive to aspirin

FDA Indications
• Anxiety
• Anxiety associated with depression
• Alcohol withdrawal

Other Data-Supported Indications
• Catatonia
• Insomnia (rapid tolerance)

Gamma-Aminobutyric Acid (GABA)
• Binds to benzodiazepine receptors at the GABA-A ligand-gated chloride channel complex
• Enhances the inhibitory effects of GABA
• Boosts chloride conductance through GABA-regulated channels
• Inhibits neuronal activity presumably in amygdala-centered fear circuits to provide therapeutic benefits in anxiety disorders
• Increased GABA activity in the reticular activating system produces sedation; however, rapid tolerance develops

C. PLASMA CONCENTRATIONS AND TREATMENT RESPONSE [1, 4–10]

Initial Target Range
- No established plasma therapeutic range

Range for Treatment Resistance
- No established plasma therapeutic range

Typical Time to Response
- Some immediate relief with first dosing is common

- Usually based on reducing fear response to psychotic symptoms
- For patients with schizophrenia, benzodiazepines only have scant supporting literature for use in akathisia and acute agitation. Chronic use is not recommended
- Benzodiazepine use is associated with higher mortality including increased suicide deaths

D. TYPICAL TREATMENT RESPONSE [1, 2, 11]

Usual Target Symptoms
- Anxiety
- Insomnia
- Psychomotor agitation

Common Short-Term Adverse Effects
- Sedation
- Fatigue
- Depression
- Dizziness
- Ataxia
- Slurred speech
- Weakness
- Amnesia
- Confusion
- Anxiety
- Paradoxical agitation/disinhibition

Rare Adverse Effects
- Hallucinations
- Mania
- Hypotension
- Hypersalivation
- Dry mouth
- Hepatic dysfunction
- Renal dysfunction
- Blood dyscrasias

Long-Term Effects
- Dependence, tolerance and withdrawal
- Possible negative neurocognitive impact

E. PRE-TREATMENT WORKUP AND INITIAL LABORATORY TESTING [11]

History
- Substance abuse or dependence, neurodevelopmental disorder, angle closure glaucoma

Physical
- Pulmonary examination for chronic obstructive pulmonary disease (COPD)

Neurological
- Alertness, cognitive impairment

Blood Tests
- None

Cardiac Tests
- None

Urine Tests
- None

Pregnancy Test
- Pregnancy test (premenopausal females)
- Classified as risk not ruled out
- May cause neonatal withdrawal, seizures in chronic users
- Other benzodiazepines have been associated with cleft palate (diazepam and related ketobenzodiazepines)

Other Tests (ECG, etc.)
- None

F. MONITORING [11]

Monthly
- Assessment of alertness
- Assessment of immediate and recent recall
- Examination for ataxia
- Examination for lateral nystagmus

Initial Dosing
- Mild-moderate anxiety: 30–60 mg/day in three to four divided doses
- Severe anxiety, anxiety associated with alcohol withdrawal: 45–120 mg/day in three to four divided doses
- Insomnia: 15–30 mg at bedtime (brief use only)

Titration
- Titration generally not necessary

Half-Life
- 5–11 hours
- No active metabolites

Bioavailability
- 93%
- 96% protein-bound
- Food does not affect absorption

Adjustment for Hepatic Dysfunction (by Child-Pugh Criteria)
- Child-Pugh category A or B (mild-moderate hepatic impairment): no dosage adjustment necessary
- Child-Pugh category C (severe hepatic impairment): contraindicated

Adjustment for Renal Dysfunction
- No dosage adjustment necessary per the package insert
- However, dose reductions may be necessary in the presence of significant renal impairment

H. MEDICATIONS TO AVOID IN COMBINATION/WARNINGS [1, 3, 11]

Central Nervous System (CNS) depressants
- Increased CNS-depressant effects when administered with other CNS depressants such as alcohol, barbiturates, antipsychotics, sedative/hypnotics, anxiolytics, antidepressants, narcotic analgesics, sedative antihistamines, anticonvulsants and anesthetics

Clozapine
- First week of clozapine treatment associated with rare severe orthostatic hypotension leading to respiratory arrest

Warnings
- Black box: concomitant use of benzodiazepines and opioids may result in profound sedation, respiratory depression, coma and death
- Prone to diversion and abuse, especially in forensic settings
- Contraindicated in currently impaired consciousness or coma
- Respiratory depression, especially combined with CNS depressants in overdose – administer flumazenil if severe or life-threatening
- Avoid in angle closure glaucoma
- Secreted in breast milk at concentrations sufficient to affect the infant
- Caution in COPD, especially if severe, and sleep apnea
- Caution in neurocognitive and amnestic disorders
- Caution with positive history of suicide attempts
- Caution in borderline personality disorder or impulse control disorders

2.65 Oxazepam (Continued)

References

1. Stahl, S. M. (2017). Oxazepam. In *Stahl's Essential Psychopharmacology Prescriber's Guide* (eds.). Cambridge: Cambridge University Press, pp. 537–541.
2. Frase, L., Nissen, C., Riemann, D., et al. (2018). Making sleep easier: pharmacological interventions for insomnia. *Expert Opin Pharmacother*, 19, 1465–1473.
3. Aphena Pharma Solutions LLC. (2019). *Oxazepam Package Insert*. Cookville, Tennesee.
4. Volz, A., Khorsand, V., Gillies, D., et al. (2007). Benzodiazepines for schizophrenia. *Cochrane Database Syst Rev*, 11, CD006391.
5. Dold, M., Li, C., Tardy, M., et al. (2012). Benzodiazepines for schizophrenia. *Cochrane Database Syst Rev*, 11, CD006391.
6. Tiihonen, J., Suokas, J. T., Suvisaari, J. M., et al. (2012). Polypharmacy with antipsychotics, antidepressants, or benzodiazepines and mortality in schizophrenia. *Arch Gen Psychiatry*, 69, 476–483.
7. Dold, M., Li, C., Gillies, D., et al. (2013). Benzodiazepine augmentation of antipsychotic drugs in schizophrenia: a meta-analysis and Cochrane review of randomized controlled trials. *Eur Neuropsychopharmacol*, 23, 1023–1033.
8. Gillies, D., Sampson, S., Beck, A., et al. (2013). Benzodiazepines for psychosis-induced aggression or agitation. *Cochrane Database Syst Rev*, 9, CD003079.
9. Dodds, T. J. (2017). Prescribed benzodiazepines and suicide risk: a review of the literature. *Prim Care Companion CNS Disord*, 19, doi: 10.4088
10. Zaman, H., Sampson, S., Beck, A., et al. (2018). Benzodiazepines for psychosis-induced aggression or agitation. *Schizophr Bull*, 44, 966–969.
11. California Department of State Hospitals. (2019). *DSH Psychotropic Medication Policy: Benzodiazepine Protocol*. Sacramento, California.
12. Greenblatt, D. J. (1981). Clinical pharmacokinetics of oxazepam and lorazepam. *Clin Pharmacokinet*, 6, 89–105.
13. Sonne, J., Loft, S., Døssing, M., et al. (1988). Bioavailability and pharmacokinetics of oxazepam. *Eur J Clin Pharmacol*, 35, 385–389.
14. Ayd, F. J., Jr. (1990). Oxazepam: update 1989. *Int Clin Psychopharmacol*, 5, 1–15.
15. Sonne, J., Boesgaard, S., Poulsen, H. E., et al. (1990). Pharmacokinetics and pharmacodynamics of oxazepam and metabolism of paracetamol in severe hypothyroidism. *Br J Clin Pharmacol*, 30, 737–742.

2.66 Temazepam

A. BASIC INFORMATION [1, 2]

Principle Trade Names
• Restoril®

Legal Status
• Prescription only
• Controlled

Classifications
• Hydroxybenzodiazepine
• Anxiolytic
• Sedative

Generics Available
• Yes

Formulations
• Capsules: 7.5 mg; 15 mg; 22.5 mg; 30 mg

FDA Indications
• Short-term treatment of insomnia (rapid tolerance)

Other Data-Supported Indications
• Anxiety
• Catatonia

B. MECHANISMS OF ACTION

Gamma-Aminobutyric Acid (GABA)
• Binds to benzodiazepine receptors at the GABA-A ligand-gated chloride channel complex
• Enhances the inhibitory effects of GABA
• Boosts chloride conductance through GABA-regulated channels
• Inhibits neuronal activity presumably in amygdala-centered fear circuits to provide therapeutic benefits in anxiety disorders
• Inhibits activity in the reticular activating system, providing sedation

C. PLASMA CONCENTRATIONS AND TREATMENT RESPONSE [1, 3–9]

Initial Target Range
- No established plasma therapeutic range

Range for Treatment Resistance
- No established plasma therapeutic range

Typical Time to Response
- Some immediate relief with first dosing is common

- Usually based on reducing affective response to psychotic symptoms
- For patients with schizophrenia, benzodiazepines only have scant supporting literature for use in akathisia and acute agitation. Chronic use is not recommended
- Benzodiazepine use is associated with higher mortality including increased suicide deaths

D. TYPICAL TREATMENT RESPONSE [1, 10]

Usual Target Symptoms
- Insomnia
- Anxiety
- Psychomotor agitation

Common Short-Term Adverse Effects
- Sedation
- Fatigue
- Depression
- Dizziness
- Ataxia
- Slurred speech
- Weakness
- Amnesia
- Confusion
- Paradoxical anxiety
- Paradoxical agitation/disinhibition

Rare Adverse Effects
- Hallucinations
- Mania
- Hypotension
- Hypersalivation
- Dry mouth
- Hepatic dysfunction
- Renal dysfunction
- Blood dyscrasias

Long-Term Effects
- Dependence, tolerance and withdrawal
- Possible negative neurocognitive impact

E. PRE-TREATMENT WORKUP AND INITIAL LABORATORY TESTING [10]

History
- Substance abuse or dependence, neurodevelopmental disorder, angle closure glaucoma

Physical
- Pulmonary examination for chronic obstructive pulmonary disease (COPD)

Neurological
- Alertness, cognitive impairment

Blood Tests
- None

Cardiac Tests
- None

Urine Tests
- None

Pregnancy Test
- Pregnancy test (premenopausal females)
- Classified as evidence of risk
- May cause neonatal withdrawal in chronic users
- Other benzodiazepines have been associated with cleft palate (diazepam and related ketobenzodiazepines)

Other Tests (ECG, etc.)
- None

F. MONITORING [10]

Monthly
- Assessment of alertness
- Assessment of immediate and recent recall
- Examination for ataxia
- Examination for lateral nystagmus

Initial Dosing
- 15 mg/day at bedtime; may increase to 30 mg/day at bedtime if ineffective

Titration
- Titration generally not necessary but may become ineffective for chronic insomnia

Half-Life
- 4–18 hours
- No active metabolites

Bioavailability
- 92%
- 96% protein-bound
- Food does not affect absorption

Adjustment for Hepatic Dysfunction (by Child-Pugh Criteria)
- Child-Pugh category A or B (mild-moderate hepatic impairment): no dosage adjustment necessary
- Child-Pugh category C (severe hepatic impairment): requires conjugation only, unlikely to accumulate

Adjustment for Renal Dysfunction
- No dosage adjustment necessary per the package insert
- However, dose reductions may be necessary in the presence of significant renal impairment

H. MEDICATIONS TO AVOID IN COMBINATION/WARNINGS [1, 2, 12]

 Central Nervous System (CNS) depressants
- Increased CNS-depressant effects when administered with other CNS depressants such as alcohol, barbiturates, antipsychotics, sedative/hypnotics, anxiolytics, antidepressants, narcotic analgesics, sedative antihistamines, anticonvulsants and anesthetics

 Oral contraceptives
- Can lower temazepam plasma levels

 Clozapine
- First week of clozapine treatment associated with rare severe orthostatic hypotension leading to respiratory arrest

 Warnings
- Black box: concomitant use of benzodiazepines and opioids may result in profound sedation, respiratory depression, coma and death

- Prone to diversion and abuse, especially in forensic settings
- Contraindicated in currently impaired consciousness or coma
- Respiratory depression, especially combined with CNS depressants in overdose – administer flumazenil if severe or life-threatening
- Avoid in angle closure glaucoma
- Secreted in breast milk at concentrations sufficient to affect the infant
- Caution in COPD, especially if severe, and sleep apnea
- Caution in neurocognitive and amnestic disorders
- Caution with positive history of suicide attempts
- Caution in borderline personality disorder or impulse control disorders

2.66 Temazepam (Continued)

ART OF PSYCHOPHARMACOLOGY: TAKE-HOME PEARLS

- Treating psychosis with adequate antipsychotic therapy is often the best treatment for anxiety in psychotic disorders.
- Increased agitation is a signal to reduce or eliminate, rather than increase dose in many cases as it often reflects decreased impulse control.

- Benzodiazepines may function well as acute "rescue" medications, but chronic use should be avoided whenever possible.

References

1. Stahl, S. M. (2017). Temazepam. In *Stahl's Essential Psychopharmacology Prescriber's Guide* (eds.). Cambridge: Cambridge University Press, pp. 703–706.
2. SpecGx LLC. (2020). *Restoril Package Insert*. Webster Groves, Montana.
3. Volz, A., Khorsand, V., Gillies, D., et al. (2007). Benzodiazepines for schizophrenia. *Cochrane Database Syst Rev*, 11, CD006391.
4. Dold, M., Li, C., Tardy, M., et al. (2012). Benzodiazepines for schizophrenia. *Cochrane Database Syst Rev*, 11, CD006391.
5. Tiihonen, J., Suokas, J. T., Suvisaari, J. M., et al. (2012). Polypharmacy with antipsychotics, antidepressants, or benzodiazepines and mortality in schizophrenia. *Arch Gen Psychiatry*, 69, 476–483.
6. Dold, M., Li, C., Gillies, D., et al. (2013). Benzodiazepine augmentation of antipsychotic drugs in schizophrenia: a meta-analysis and Cochrane review of randomized controlled trials. *Eur Neuropsychopharmacol*, 23, 1023–1033.
7. Gillies, D., Sampson, S., Beck, A., et al. (2013). Benzodiazepines for psychosis-induced aggression or agitation. *Cochrane Database Syst Rev*, 9, CD003079.
8. Dodds, T. J. (2017). Prescribed benzodiazepines and suicide risk: a review of the literature. *Prim Care Companion CNS Disord*, 19, doi: 10.4088
9. Zaman, H., Sampson, S., Bec, A., et al. (2018). Benzodiazepines for psychosis-induced aggression or agitation. *Schizophr Bull*, 44, 966–969.
10. California Department of State Hospitals. (2019). *DSH Psychotropic Medication Policy: Benzodiazepine Protocol*. Sacramento, California.
11. Liver Toxicology. (2012). Benzodiazepines. In *LiverTox: Clinical and Research Information on Drug-Induced Liver Injury* (eds.). Bethesda, MD: National Institute of Diabetes and Digestive and Kidney Diseases.
12. Stoehr, G. P., Kroboth, P. D., Juhl, R. P., et al. (1984). Effect of oral contraceptives on triazolam, temazepam, alprazolam, and lorazepam kinetics. *Clin Pharmacol Ther*, 36, 683–690.

A. BASIC INFORMATION [1, 2]

Principle Trade Names
• Sonata®

Legal Status
• Prescription only
• Controlled

Classifications
• GABA positive allosteric modulator (GABA-PAM)
• Non-benzodiazepine hypnotic
• Alpha 1 isoform selective agonist of GABA-A/benzodiazepine receptors

Generics Available
• Yes

Formulations
• Capsules: 5 mg; 10 mg

FDA Indications
• Short-term treatment of insomnia

Other Data-Supported Indications
• Middle of the night awakenings
• Short-term sedation, e.g. during travel

Gamma-Aminobutyric Acid (GABA)
• Binds selectively to a subtype of the benzodiazepine receptor, the alpha 1 isoform
• May enhance GABA inhibitory actions that provide sedative hypnotic effects more selectively than other actions of GABA
• Boosts chloride conductance through GABA-regulated channels
• Inhibitory actions in sleep centers may provide sedative hypnotic effects

2.67 Zaleplon (Continued)

C. PLASMA CONCENTRATIONS AND TREATMENT RESPONSE [1]

Initial Target Range
• No established plasma therapeutic range

Range for Treatment Resistance
• No established plasma therapeutic range

Typical Time to Response
• Less than one hour

Time-Course of Improvement
• Seven to ten days

D. TYPICAL TREATMENT RESPONSE [1, 2]

Usual Target Symptoms
• Time to sleep onset
• Total sleep time
• Nighttime awakenings

Common Short-Term Adverse Effects
• Sedation
• Dizziness
• Ataxia
• Dose-dependent amnesia
• Hyperexcitability, nervousness
• Decreased appetite
• Headache

Rare Adverse Effects
• Hallucinations
• Respiratory depression, especially when taken with other CNS depressants in overdose
• Angioedema

Long-Term Effects
• Not generally intended for long-term use
• Increased wakefulness during the latter part of the night (wearing off) or an increase in daytime anxiety (rebound) may occur because of short half-life
• Some patients could develop dependence and/or tolerance with drugs of this class; risk may be theoretically greater with higher doses
• History of drug addiction may theoretically increase risk of dependence

E. PRE-TREATMENT WORKUP AND INITIAL LABORATORY TESTING [1]

History
• Sleep hygiene
• Depression, suicidal ideation
• Sleep apnea
• Restless leg syndrome
• Breastfeeding

Physical
• Pulmonary examination for chronic obstructive pulmonary disease (COPD)

Neurological
• Alertness, cognitive impairment

Blood Tests
• None in healthy individuals

Cardiac Tests
• None

Urine Tests
• None

Pregnancy Test
• Pregnancy test (premenopausal females)
• Classified as risk not ruled out

Other Tests (ECG, etc.)
• None

386

Monthly

- Assessment of alertness
- Assessment of immediate and recent recall
- Examination for ataxia

Initial Dosing

- 10 mg/day at bedtime

Titration

- May increase to 20 mg/day at bedtime if 10 mg/day ineffective
- Maximum dose generally 20 mg/day
- Patients with lower body weights may require only a 5 mg dose
- Elderly recommended initial dose: 5 mg
- Rebound insomnia may occur the first night after stopping
- If taken for more than a few weeks, taper to reduce chances of withdrawal effects
- Zaleplon should not generally be prescribed in quantities greater than a one-month supply

Half-Life

- One hour – ultra-short

Bioavailability

- 30%
- 60% protein-bound
- Zaleplon is not absorbed as quickly if taken with high-fat foods, which may reduce onset of action

Adjustment for Hepatic Dysfunction (by Child-Pugh Criteria)

- Child-Pugh category A or B (mild-moderate hepatic impairment): recommended dose 5 mg
- Child-Pugh category C (severe hepatic impairment): contraindicated

Adjustment for Renal Dysfunction

- No dosage adjustment necessary per the package insert
- However, dose reductions may be necessary in the presence of significant renal impairment

H. MEDICATIONS TO AVOID IN COMBINATION/WARNINGS [1, 2]

Central Nervous System (CNS) depressants

- Increased depressive effects when taken with other CNS depressants

cyp 3A4 inhibitors (may require lower doses)

- Cimetidine: lower initial dose of zaleplon (5 mg/day)
- Nefazodone
- Fluvoxamine
- Azole antifungal agents
- Macrolide antibiotics
- Protease inhibitors

cyp 3A4 inducers (may require higher doses)

- Rifampicin
- Phenytoin
- Carbamazepine
- Phenobarbital
- St. John's Wort

Warnings

- Insomnia may be a symptom of a primary disorder, rather than a primary disorder itself
- Zaleplon should only be administered at bedtime
- Actions at benzodiazepine receptors that carry over to the next day can cause daytime sedation, amnesia and ataxia
- Elderly may have increased risk for falls, confusion
- History of drug addiction may increase risk of dependence
- Risk of dependence may increase with dose and duration of treatment. However, treatment with alpha 1 selective non-benzodiazepine hypnotics may cause less tolerance or dependence than benzodiazepine hypnotics
- Some patients may exhibit abnormal thinking or behavioral changes similar to those caused by other CNS depressants (i.e. either depressant actions or disinhibiting actions)
- Some depressed patients may experience a worsening of suicidal ideation
- Use only with extreme caution in patients with impaired respiratory function or obstructive sleep apnea
- Some drug is found in mother's breast milk; recommended either to discontinue drug or bottle feed
- Rare angioedema has occurred with sedative hypnotic use and could potentially cause fatal airway obstruction if it involves the throat, glottis or larynx; thus if angioedema occurs treatment should be discontinued
- Sleep driving and other complex behaviors, such as eating and preparing food and making phone calls have been reported in patients taking sedative hypnotics
- Infants whose mothers took sedative hypnotics during pregnancy may experience some withdrawal symptoms
- Neonatal flaccidity has been reported in infants whose mothers took sedative hypnotics during pregnancy

ART OF PSYCHOPHARMACOLOGY: TAKE-HOME PEARLS

- Consider for uses requiring short half-life (e.g. dosing in the middle of the night, sleeping on airplanes, jet lag).
- Safe for long-term use and may be preferred over benzodiazepines because of its rapid onset of action, short duration of effect, and safety profile without notable tolerance or dependence developing over time.
- To avoid problems with memory, do not take zaleplon if planning to sleep for less than four hours.

References

1. Stahl, S. M. (2017). Zaleplon. In *Stahl's Essential Psychopharmacology Prescriber's Guide* (eds.). Cambridge: Cambridge University Press, pp. 803–806.
2. OrchidPharma Ltd. (2019). *Zaleplon Package Insert*. Chennai (India).

2.68 Zolpidem

 A. BASIC INFORMATION [1, 2]

Principle Trade Names
• Ambien®
• Ambien CR®
• Intermezzo®

Legal Status
• Prescription only
• Controlled

 Classifications
• GABA positive allosteric modulator (GABA-PAM)
• Non-benzodiazepine hypnotic
• Alpha 1 isoform selective agonist of GABA-A/benzodiazepine receptors

Generics Available
• Yes

Formulations
• Immediate-release (IR) tablet: 5 mg
• Controlled-release (CR) tablets: 6.25 mg; 12.5 mg
• Sublingual tablet (Intermezzo®): 1.75 mg; 3.5 mg; 5 mg; 10 mg
• Oral spray: 5 mg

FDA Indications
• Short-term treatment of insomnia (CR indication is not restricted to short-term)
• Intermezzo as needed for the treatment of insomnia when a middle-of-the-night awakening is followed by difficulty returning to sleep and there are at least four hours of bedtime remaining before the planned time of awakening

Other Data-Supported Indications
• None

 B. MECHANISMS OF ACTION

Gamma-Aminobutyric Acid (GABA)
• Binds selectively to a subtype of the benzodiazepine receptor, the alpha 1 isoform
• May enhance GABA inhibitory actions that provide sedative hypnotic effects more selectively than other actions of GABA
• Boosts chloride conductance through GABA-regulated channels

• Inhibitory actions in sleep centers may provide sedative hypnotic effects
• CR formulation may allow sufficient drug to persist at receptors to improve total sleep time and to prevent early morning awakenings that can be associated with the immediate-release formulation

Initial Target Range
- No established plasma therapeutic range

Typical Time to Response
- Less than one hour

Range for Treatment Resistance
- No established plasma therapeutic range

Time-Course of Improvement
- Seven to ten days

Usual Target Symptoms
- Time to sleep onset
- Total sleep time
- Nighttime awakenings

Common Short-Term Adverse Effects
- Sedation
- Dizziness
- Ataxia
- Dose-dependent amnesia
- Hyperexcitability, nervousness
- Diarrhea, nausea
- Headache

Rare Adverse Effects
- Hallucinations
- Dissociation (more likely if wakefulness maintained after dosing)

- Respiratory depression, especially when taken with other CNS depressants in overdose
- Angioedema

Long-Term Effects
- Some patients could develop dependence and/or tolerance with drugs of this class; risk may be theoretically greater with higher doses
- History of drug addiction may theoretically increase risk of dependence

History
- Depression, suicidal ideation
- Sleep apnea
- Restless leg syndrome
- Breastfeeding

Physical
- Pulmonary examination for chronic obstructive pulmonary disease (COPD)

Neurological
- Alertness, cognitive impairment

Blood Tests
- None in healthy individuals

Cardiac Tests
- None

Urine Tests
- None

Pregnancy Test
- Pregnancy test (premenopausal females)
- Classified as risk not ruled out

Other Tests (ECG, etc.)
- None

Monthly
- Assessment of alertness
- Assessment of immediate and recent recall
- Examination for ataxia

Initial Dosing
- 10 mg/day at bedtime for seven to ten days (IR)
- 12.5 mg/day at bedtime (CR)

Titration
- Men: 10 mg at bedtime for seven to ten days (IR); 12.5 mg at bedtime for seven to ten days (CR); 3.5 mg sublingually in the middle of the night if more than four hours of bedtime remain (Intermezzo)
- Women: 5 mg at bedtime for seven to ten days (IR); 6.25 mg at bedtime for seven to ten days (CR); 1.75 mg sublingually in the middle of the night if more than four hours of bedtime remain (Intermezzo)
- Patients with lower body weights may require only a 5 mg dose (IR) or 6.25 mg (CR)
- Elderly recommended initial dose: 5 mg (IR); 6.25 mg (CR); 1.75 mg (Intermezzo)
- Intermezzo formulation is administered sublingually in the middle of the night; it should be placed under the tongue and allowed to dissolve completely before swallowing
- Intermezzo formulation should not be taken more than once per night and only if the patient has greater than four hours of bedtime remaining before the planned time of waking
- Increased wakefulness during the latter part of the night (wearing off) or an increase in daytime anxiety (rebound) may occur with IR and be less common with CR

- CR tablets should be swallowed whole and should not be divided, crushed or chewed
- Zolpidem should generally not be prescribed in quantities greater than a one-month supply; however, zolpidem CR is not restricted to short-term use
- If taken for more than a few weeks, taper to reduce chances of withdrawal effects if discontinued

Half-Life
- 2.5 hours

Bioavailability
- 93% protein-bound
- Zolpidem is not absorbed as quickly if taken with food, which could delay onset of action

Adjustment for Hepatic Dysfunction (by Child-Pugh Criteria)
- Child-Pugh category A or B (mild-moderate hepatic impairment): no dosage adjustment necessary
- Child-Pugh category C (severe hepatic impairment): contraindicated

Adjustment for Renal Dysfunction
- No dosage adjustment necessary per the package insert
- However, dose reductions may be necessary in the presence of significant renal impairment

Central Nervous System (CNS) depressants

- Increased depressive effects when taken with other CNS depressants

cyp 3A4 inhibitors (may require lower doses)

- Nefazodone
- Fluvoxamine
- Azole antifungal agents
- Macrolide antibiotics
- Protease inhibitors

cyp 3A4 inducers (may require higher doses)

- Rifampicin
- Phenytoin
- Carbamazepine
- Phenobarbital
- St. John's Wort

Warnings

- Insomnia may be a symptom of a primary disorder, rather than a primary disorder itself
- Zolpidem and zolpidem CR should only be administered at bedtime
- Actions at benzodiazepine receptors that carry over to the next day can cause daytime sedation, amnesia and ataxia
- Temporary memory loss may occur at doses above 10 mg/night
- Elderly may have increased risk for falls, confusion

- History of drug addiction may increase risk of dependence
- Risk of dependence may increase with dose and duration of treatment. However, treatment with alpha 1 selective non-benzodiazepine hypnotics may cause less tolerance or dependence than benzodiazepine hypnotics
- Some patients may exhibit abnormal thinking or behavioral changes similar to those caused by other CNS depressants (i.e. either depressant actions or disinhibiting actions)
- Some depressed patients may experience a worsening of suicidal ideation
- Use only with caution in patients with impaired respiratory function or obstructive sleep apnea
- Some drug is found in mother's breast milk; recommended either to discontinue drug or bottle feed
- Rare angioedema has occurred with sedative hypnotic use and could potentially cause fatal airway obstruction if it involves the throat, glottis or larynx; thus if angioedema occurs treatment should be discontinued
- Sleep driving and other complex behaviors, such as eating and preparing food and making phone calls, (dissociated mental state) have been reported in patients taking sedative hypnotics
- Infants whose mothers took sedative hypnotics during pregnancy may experience some withdrawal symptoms
- Neonatal flaccidity has been reported in infants whose mothers took sedative hypnotics during pregnancy

- Zolpidem has been shown to increase the total time asleep and to reduce the amount of nighttime awakenings.
- Safe for long-term use and may be preferred over benzodiazepines because of its rapid onset of action, short duration of effect, and safety profile without notable tolerance or dependence developing over time.

- To avoid problems with memory, take zolpidem only if planning to have a full night's sleep.

References

1. Stahl, S. M. (2017). Zolpidem. In *Stahl's Essential Psychopharmacology Prescriber's Guide* (eds.). Cambridge: Cambridge University Press, pp. 815–818.
2. ACI Healthcare USA. (2020). *Zolpidem Package Insert*. Colorado Springs, Florida

A. BASIC INFORMATION [1–6]

Principle Trade Names
• N/A

Legal Status
• Prescription only in some countries and non-prescription nutraceutical and dietary supplement in the US and other countries
• Not controlled

Classifications
• Melatonin receptor agonist

Generics Available
• Yes

Formulations
• Immediate-release (IR) and various extended-release (ER) formulations
• Solid tablets, rapid dissolving tablets and strips, capsules, flavored liquids, liquid gel, and transdermal patches among others

• Wide range of doses
• The US Food and Drug Administration (FDA) does not regulate melatonin manufacturing and good manufacturing practices are not monitored by regulatory authorities in many countries resulting in a variation in melatonin dose, formulation and purity

FDA Indications
• None

Other Data-Supported Indications
• Reducing sleep latency in primary insomnia
• Chronic insomnia
• Transient insomnia
• Insomnia associated with shift work, jet lag or circadian rhythm disturbances
• REM-behavior disorder
• Perioperative anxiety

Melatonin
• Full agonist
• Theoretically, stimulation of melatonin 1 receptors mediates the suppressive effects of melatonin on the suprachiasmatic nucleus

• Theoretically, stimulation of melatonin 2 receptors mediates the phase shifting effect of melatonin

C. PLASMA CONCENTRATIONS AND TREATMENT RESPONSE

Initial Target Range
• No established plasma therapeutic range

Range for Treatment Resistance
• No established plasma therapeutic range

Typical Time to Response
• Less than one hour

Time-Course of Improvement
• Varies

D. TYPICAL TREATMENT RESPONSE [3, 6, 8]

Usual Target Symptoms
• Time to sleep onset
• Total sleep time

Common Short-Term Adverse Effects
• Headache
• Dizziness
• Nausea, vomiting
• Diarrhea
• Somnolence

Rare Adverse Effects
• Possible glucose intolerance at doses >5 mg/day
• No reports of dependence, tolerance or abuse liability
• No hangover effect and no adverse impact on alertness or mood the following day

Long-Term Effects
• Inadequate number of quality long-term studies

E. PRE-TREATMENT WORKUP AND INITIAL LABORATORY TESTING

History
• Sleep hygiene
• Depression, suicidal ideation
• Sleep apnea
• Pregnancy
• Breastfeeding

Physical
• None

Neurological
• None

Blood Tests
• None in healthy individuals

Cardiac Tests
• None

Urine Tests
• None

Pregnancy Test
• Pregnancy test (premenopausal females)
• Risk undefined

Other Tests (ECG, etc.)
• None

F. MONITORING [3]

Quarterly
• For patients presenting with unexplained amenorrhea, galactorrhea, decreased libido, or problems with fertility, could consider measuring prolactin and testosterone levels

G. DOSING AND KINETICS [1, 8, 9, 11]

Initial Dosing
- Optimal dosing varies as melatonin physiology varies between individuals
- Elderly: doses between 1–6 mg/day may be most effective
- For most patients dosing at bedtime is optimal
- Evening administration of melatonin 0.3–5 mg between 19:00–20:00 shifts circadian rhythms to earlier time

Titration
- No strong correlation between dose and maximum improvements in sleep
- IR melatonin formulations may be superior to slow-release (SR) formulations for improving sleep latency
- SR melatonin formulations may be superior to IR formulations for improving total sleep time and overall sleep efficiency
- Does not appear to suppress or delay onset of REM sleep

- No evidence of rebound insomnia the first night after stopping
- No need to taper dose

Half-Life
- 30–60 minutes

Bioavailability
- 3%

Adjustment for Hepatic Dysfunction (by Child-Pugh Criteria)
- Child-Pugh category A or B (mild-moderate hepatic impairment): no dosing adjustment necessary
- Child-Pugh category C (severe hepatic impairment): dose reduction may be necessary

Adjustment for Renal Dysfunction
- Dosing adjustment generally not necessary
- However, dose reductions may be necessary in the presence of significant renal impairment

H. MEDICATIONS TO AVOID IN COMBINATION/WARNINGS [1, 8, 10, 11]

Central Nervous System (CNS) depressants
- Caution when combined with alcohol and other CNS depressants

cyp 1A2 inhibitors (may require lower doses)
- Fluvoxamine
- Oral contraceptives
- Caffeine

cyp 3A4 inhibitors (may require lower doses)
- Cimetidine
- Donepezil
- Azole antifungal agents
- Macrolide antibiotics
- Protease inhibitors

cyp 3A4 inducers (may require higher doses)
- Rifampicin
- Phenytoin
- Carbamazepine
- Phenobarbital
- St. John's Wort

cyp 2C9 inhibitors (may require lower doses)
- Fluconazole

Warnings

- Insomnia may be a symptom of a primary disorder, rather than a primary disorder itself
- Daytime melatonin administration can cause significant drowsiness, fatigue and performance decrements
- Avoid melatonin during pregnancy
- Avoid melatonin during breastfeeding
- People with epilepsy or those taking warfarin (or another oral anticoagulant) should only use melatonin under medical supervision

2.69 Melatonin (Continued)

- Rebound insomnia does not appear to be common and may have fewer carryover side effects than some other sedative hypnotics.
- Lack of actions on GABA systems may be related to lack of apparent abuse liability and melatonin may be preferred over

benzodiazepines because of its rapid onset of action, short duration of effect and safety profile.
- High-quality product sourcing necessary in countries without regulation over good manufacturing processes.

References

1. Herxheimer, A. (2014). Jet lag. *BMJ Clin Evid*, 2014, 2303.
2. Hansen, M. V., Halladin, N. L., Rosenberg, J., et al. (2015). Melatonin for pre- and postoperative anxiety in adults. *Cochrane Database Syst Rev*, 2015(4), CD009861.
3. Auld, F., Maschauer, E. L., Morrison, I., et al. (2017). Evidence for the efficacy of melatonin in the treatment of primary adult sleep disorders. *Sleep Med Rev*, 34, 10–22.
4. Erland, L. A., Saxena, P. K. (2017). Melatonin natural health products and supplements: presence of serotonin and significant variability of melatonin content. *J Clin Sleep Med*, 13, 275–281.
5. Posadzki, P. P., Bajpai, R., Kyaw, B. M., et al. (2018). Melatonin and health: an umbrella review of health outcomes and biological mechanisms of action. *BMC Med*, 16, 18.
6. Pierce, M., Linnebur, S. A., Pearson, S. M., et al. (2019). Optimal melatonin dose in older adults: a clinical review of the literature. *Sr Care Pharm*, 34, 419–431.
7. Tordjman, S., Chokron, S., Delorme, R., et al. (2017). Melatonin: pharmacology, functions and therapeutic benefits. *Curr Neuropharmacol*, 15, 434–443.
8. Riha, R. L. (2018). The use and misuse of exogenous melatonin in the treatment of sleep disorders. *Curr Opin Pulm Med*, 24, 543–548.
9. Andersen, L. P., Werner, M. U., Rosenkilde, M. M., et al. (2016). Pharmacokinetics of oral and intravenous melatonin in healthy volunteers. *BMC Pharmacol Toxicol*, 17, 8.
10. Costello, R. B., Lentino, C. V., Boyd, C. C., et al. (2014). The effectiveness of melatonin for promoting healthy sleep: a rapid evidence assessment of the literature. *Nutr J*, 13, 106.
11. Andersen, L. P., Gogenur, I., Rosenberg, J., et al. (2016). The safety of melatonin in humans. *Clin Drug Investig*, 36, 169–175.

QUICK CHECK

A. BASIC INFORMATION [1, 2]

Principle Trade Names
• Rozerem®

Legal Status
• Prescription only
• Not controlled

Classifications
• Melatonin 1 and 2 receptor agonist
• Circadian modulator

Generics Available
• No

Formulations
• Tablet: 8 mg

FDA Indications
• Insomnia (difficulty with sleep onset)

Other Data-Supported Indications
• Primary insomnia
• Chronic insomnia
• Transient insomnia
• Insomnia associated with shift work, jet lag or circadian rhythm disturbances

Melatonin
• Binds selectively to melatonin 1 and melatonin 2 receptors as a full agonist

• Theoretically, stimulation of melatonin 1 receptors mediates the suppressive effects of melatonin on the suprachiasmatic nucleus
• Theoretically, stimulation of melatonin 2 receptors mediates the phase shifting effect of melatonin

C. PLASMA CONCENTRATIONS AND TREATMENT RESPONSE [1]

Initial Target Range
• No established plasma therapeutic range

Range for Treatment Resistance
• No established plasma therapeutic range

Typical Time to Response
• Less than one hour

Time-Course of Improvement
• Seven to ten days

D. TYPICAL TREATMENT RESPONSE [1–3]

Usual Target Symptoms
• Time to sleep onset
• Phase shifted sleep-wake cycle

Common Short-Term Adverse Effects
• Sedation
• Dizziness
• Fatigue
• Headache

Rare Adverse Effects
• Respiratory depression, especially when taken with other CNS depressants in overdose
• Angioedema

Long-Term Effects
• Not restricted to short-term use but few long-term studies
• No reports of dependence, tolerance or abuse liability
• May decrease testosterone levels or increase prolactin levels, but the clinical significance of this is unknown

E. PRE-TREATMENT WORKUP AND INITIAL LABORATORY TESTING [3]

History
• Sleep hygiene
• Depression, suicidal ideation
• Sleep apnea
• Restless leg syndrome
• Breastfeeding

Physical
• None

Neurological
• None

Blood Tests
• None in healthy individuals

Cardiac Tests
• None

Urine Tests
• None

Pregnancy Test
• Pregnancy test (premenopausal females)
• Classified as risk not ruled out
• Classified as risk not ruled out

Other Tests (ECG, etc.)
• None

F. MONITORING [3]

Quarterly
• For patients presenting with unexplained amenorrhea, galactorrhea, decreased libido, or problems with fertility, could consider measuring prolactin and testosterone levels

Initial Dosing
• 8 mg at bedtime

Titration
• Unusual lack of apparent dose response curve
• Doses between 4 mg and 64 mg may have similar effects on sleep and similar side effects
• Doses up to 160 mg were studied without apparent abuse liability
• Suggests therapeutic effects may be mediated by an "on-off" type of therapeutic effect on a sleep switch that works at any dose over a certain threshold
• Since ramelteon has very low oral bioavailability and thus highly variable absorption, a substantial dose range may be required to generate sufficient absorption in various patients
• Suggest increasing dose before concluding lack of efficacy
• No evidence of rebound insomnia the first night after stopping
• No need to taper dose

Half-Life
• Parent drug mean is 1–2.6 hours
• Active metabolite (M-II) mean is 2–5 hours

Bioavailability
• 2%
• 82% protein-bound
• Do not administer with or immediately after a high-fat meal as this may delay its onset of action or diminish its efficacy

Adjustment for Hepatic Dysfunction (by Child-Pugh Criteria)
• Child-Pugh category A or B (mild-moderate hepatic impairment): use with caution in patients with moderate hepatic impairment
• Child-Pugh category C (severe hepatic impairment): contraindicated

Adjustment for Renal Dysfunction
• Dosing adjustment generally not necessary
• However, dose reductions may be necessary in the presence of significant renal impairment

---

H. MEDICATIONS TO AVOID IN COMBINATION/WARNINGS [1, 2]

 Central Nervous System (CNS) depressants
• Caution when combined with alcohol and other CNS depressants

 cyp 1A2 inhibitors (may require lower doses)
• Fluvoxamine – contraindicated

 cyp 3A4 inhibitors (may require lower doses)
• Cimetidine
• Donepezil
• Azole antifungal agents
• Macrolide antibiotics
• Protease inhibitors

 cyp 3A4 inducers (may require higher doses)
• Rifampicin
• Phenytoin
• Carbamazepine
• Phenobarbital
• St. John's Wort

 cyp 2C9 inhibitors (may require lower doses)
• Fluconazole

 Warnings

• Insomnia may be a symptom of a primary disorder, rather than a primary disorder itself
• Ramelteon should only be administered at bedtime
• Alcohol and ramelteon may have additive effects when used in conjunction
• No evidence that ramelteon worsens apnea/hypopnea index in chronic obstructive pulmonary disease (COPD) or in obstructive sleep apnea, but not recommended in severe cases
• Patients who develop angioedema after treatment with ramelteon should not be rechallenged
• Unknown if ramelteon is secreted in human breast milk, but all psychotropics assumed to be secreted in breast milk. Recommended either to discontinue drug or bottle feed

ART OF PSYCHOPHARMACOLOGY: TAKE-HOME PEARLS

- Rebound insomnia does not appear to be common and may have fewer carryover side effects than some other sedative hypnotics.
- Lack of actions on GABA systems may be related to lack of apparent abuse liability and ramelteon may be preferred over

benzodiazepines because of its rapid onset of action, short duration of effect and safety profile.
- To avoid problems with memory, only take ramelteon if planning to have a full night's sleep.

References

1. Borja, N. L., Daniel, K. L. (2006). Ramelteon for the treatment of insomnia. *Clin Ther*, 28, 1540–1555.
2. Low, T. L., Choo, F. N., Tan, S. M. (2020). The efficacy of melatonin and melatonin agonists in insomnia – an umbrella review. *J Psychiatr Res*, 121, 10–23.
3. Erman, M., Seiden, D., Zammit, G., et al. (2006). An efficacy, safety, and dose-response study of Ramelteon in patients with chronic primary insomnia. *Sleep Med*, 7, 17–24.

2.71 Tasimelteon

A. BASIC INFORMATION [1, 2]

Principle Trade Names
• Hetlioz®

Legal Status
• Prescription only
• Not controlled

Classifications
• Melatonin 1 and 2 receptor agonist
• Circadian modulator

Generics Available
• No

Formulations
• Capsule: 20 mg

FDA Indications
• Non-24-hour Sleep-Wake Disorder

Other Data-Supported Indications
• Insomnia associated with shift work, jet lag or circadian rhythm disturbances

B. MECHANISMS OF ACTION

Melatonin
• Binds selectively to melatonin 1 and melatonin 2 receptors as a full agonist
• Greater affinity for melatonin 2 receptors

• Theoretically, stimulation of melatonin 1 receptors mediates the suppressive effects of melatonin on the suprachiasmatic nucleus
• Theoretically, stimulation of melatonin 2 receptors mediates the phase shifting effect of melatonin

C. PLASMA CONCENTRATIONS AND TREATMENT RESPONSE [1, 2]

Initial Target Range
• No established plasma therapeutic range

Range for Treatment Resistance
• No established plasma therapeutic range

Typical Time to Response
• Because of individual differences in circadian rhythms, daily use for several weeks or months may be necessary before efficacy is observed

D. TYPICAL TREATMENT RESPONSE [1–3]

Usual Target Symptoms
• Total nighttime sleep time

Common Short-Term Adverse Effects
• Headache
• Nightmares or unusual dreams
• Increased alanine aminotransferase
• Upper respiratory infection
• Urinary infection

Rare Adverse Effects
• None reported

Long-Term Effects
• Not restricted to short-term use but few long-term studies
• No reports of dependence, tolerance or abuse liability

E. PRE-TREATMENT WORKUP AND INITIAL LABORATORY TESTING [1, 2]

History
• Sleep hygiene
• Breastfeeding

Physical
• None

Neurological
• None

Blood Tests
• None in healthy individuals

Cardiac Tests
• None

Urine Tests
• None

Pregnancy Test
• Pregnancy test (premenopausal females)
• Classified as risk not ruled out

Other Tests (ECG, etc.)
• None

F. MONITORING [1, 2]

• None specific

G. DOSING AND KINETICS [1, 2]

Initial Dosing
• 20 mg at bedtime

Titration
• No data to support higher doses
• Take at the same time nightly without food
• If tasimelteon cannot be taken at its usual time on a given night, the dose for that night should be skipped
• Swallow capsule whole
• No need to taper dose

Half-Life
• Parent drug mean is 1–2.6 hours
• Active metabolite (M-II) mean is 2–5 hours

Bioavailability
• 38%
• 90% protein-bound
• Should be taken without food

Adjustment for Hepatic Dysfunction (by Child-Pugh Criteria)
• Child-Pugh category A or B (mild-moderate hepatic impairment): dose adjustment not necessary
• Child-Pugh category C (severe hepatic impairment): contraindicated

Adjustment for Renal Dysfunction
• Dosing adjustment generally not necessary
• However, dose reductions may be necessary in the presence of significant renal impairment

H. MEDICATIONS TO AVOID IN COMBINATION/WARNINGS [1, 2]

Central Nervous System (CNS) depressants

• Caution when combined with alcohol and other CNS depressants

cyp 1A2 inhibitors

• Fluvoxamine – contraindicated
• Others may require lower doses

cyp 1A2 inducers (may require higher doses)

• Smoking tobacco

cyp 3A4 inhibitors (may require lower doses)

• Azole antifungal agents
• Macrolide antibiotics
• Protease inhibitors

cyp 3A4 inducers (contraindicated)

• Rifampicin
• Phenytoin
• Carbamazepine
• Phenobarbital
• St. John's Wort

Warnings

• Insomnia may be a symptom of a primary disorder, rather than a primary disorder itself
• Should only be administered at bedtime
• Elderly – exposure to tasimelteon is increased by approximately two-fold
• Alcohol and tasimelteon may have additive effects when used in conjunction
• Unknown if tasimelteon is secreted in human breast milk, but all psychotropics assumed to be secreted in breast milk. Use caution if patient is breastfeeding
• Controlled studies have not been conducted in pregnant women
• In animal studies, administration during pregnancy resulted in developmental toxicity (embryofetal mortality, neurobehavioral impairment, decreased growth and development in offspring)

ART OF PSYCHOPHARMACOLOGY: TAKE-HOME PEARLS

• Tasimelteon may be beneficial for patients suffering from insomnia associated with shift work, jet lag or circadian rhythm disturbances.
• Tasimelteon can be used long-term and its lack of actions on GABA systems may be related to lack of apparent abuse liability.
• To avoid problems with memory, only take tasimelteon if planning to have a full night's sleep.

References

1. Stahl, S. M. (2017). Tasimelteon. In *Stahl's Essential Psychopharmacology Prescriber's Guide* (eds.). Cambridge: Cambridge University Press, pp. 699–701.
2. Vanda Pharmaceuticals Inc. (2019). *Tasimelteon Package Insert*. Washington, D.C.
3. Low, T. L., Choo, F. N., Tan, S. M. (2020). The efficacy of melatonin and melatonin agonists in insomnia – an umbrella review. *J Psychiatr Res*, 121, 10–23.

Stimulants
2.72 Atomoxetine

A. BASIC INFORMATION [1, 2]

Principle Trade Names
• Strattera®

Legal Status
• Prescription only
• Not controlled

Classifications
• Norepinephrine reuptake inhibitor
• Stimulant

Generics Available
• Yes

Formulations
• Capsules: 10 mg; 18 mg; 25 mg; 40 mg; 60 mg; 80 mg; 100 mg

FDA Indications
• Attention deficit hyperactivity disorder (ADHD) in adults and children over six

Other Data-Supported Indications
• Treatment-resistant depression

B. MECHANISMS OF ACTION [1, 2]

Norepinephrine
• Increases norepinephrine in prefrontal cortex
• Blocks norepinephrine reuptake transporters
• Presumed increased noradrenergic transmission

Dopamine
• May also increase dopamine in prefrontal cortex
• Decreases dopamine inactivation in prefrontal cortex

Initial Target Range
- 0.5–1.2 mg/kg/day in children up to 70 kg; 40–100 mg/day in adults
- No established plasma concentration range

Range for Treatment Resistance
- Maximum dose 1.4 mg/kg per day or 100 mg/day in children and adults
- No established plasma concentration range

Typical Time to Response
- The onset of action in ADHD can be the first day of dosing
- Therapeutic improvement can be seen for eight to twelve weeks

Time-Course of Improvement
- If no response by six to eight weeks at maximum tolerated dose, it may not be effective and therapy should be withdrawn

Usual Target Symptoms
- Reduction of symptoms of inattentiveness, motor hyperactivity and/or impulsiveness
- Improvement of depressive symptoms

Common Short-Term Adverse Effects
- Sedation, fatigue, decreased appetite, rare priapism, increased heart rate (6–9 bpm), increased blood pressure (2–4 mm Hg), insomnia, dizziness, anxiety, agitation, aggression, irritability, dry mouth, constipation, nausea, vomiting, abdominal pain, dyspepsia, urinary hesitancy, urinary retention (older men), dysmenorrhea, sweating, sexual dysfunction, orthostatic hypotension

Rare Adverse Effects
- Severe liver damage, hypomania, induction of mania, activation of suicidal ideation and behavior

Long-Term Effects
- Safe, not habit forming

History
- Use with caution in patients with hypertension, tachycardia, cardiovascular disease or cerebrovascular disease
- Use with caution in patients with bipolar disorder
- Use with caution in patients with urinary retention, benign prostatic hypertrophy
- Do not use in patients with pheochromocytoma or history of pheochromocytoma
- Do not use in severe cardiovascular disorders that may deteriorate with increases in heart rate and blood pressure
- Do not use in closed angle glaucoma
- Do not use if there is a proven allergy to atomoxetine

Physical
- Monitor height and weight. For patients who are not growing or gaining weight normally, cessation of drug should be considered
- Rare association with hepatotoxicity though no causation established
- Stop medication in patients with jaundice or other severe liver dysfunction symptoms

Neurological
- Avoid use if poorly controlled seizure disorder is present

Blood Tests
- Baseline liver function tests recommended if indicated by history or examination

Cardiac Tests
- Pulse, blood pressure and ECG (if indicated by history)

Urine Tests
- Residual urine volume if history of benign prostatic hypertrophy (BPH) present

Pregnancy Test
- Pregnancy test (premenopausal females)
- Classified as risk not ruled out
- Atomoxetine should generally be stopped before anticipated pregnancies
- Probably secreted in breast milk

Other Tests (ECG, etc.)
- Monitor heart rate and blood pressure periodically

F. MONITORING [2, 3]

During Titration or After Dose Adjustment

- Once daily dosing may increase gastrointestinal (GI) side effects
- Lower starting doses in patients sensitive to side effects such as tachycardia and increased blood pressure

Maintenance

- Height, weight, heart rate and blood pressure
- Hypomania/mania, suicidality, aggression

G. DOSING AND KINETICS [3]

Initial Dosing

- For children 70 kg or less: initial dose 0.5 mg/kg/day
- For adults and children over 70 kg: initial dose 40 mg/day

Titration

- For children 70 kg or less: after seven days can increase to 1.2 mg/kg/day either once in the morning or divided
- Maximum dose is 1.4 mg/kg/day or 100 mg/day, whichever is less
- For adults and children over 70 kg: after seven days can increase to 80 mg/day once in the morning or divided; after two to four weeks can increase to 100 mg/day if needed
- Maximum dose 100 mg/day

Half-Life

- ~5 hours

Bioavailability

- 63–94%
- Food does not affect absorption

Adjustment for Hepatic Dysfunction (by Child-Pugh Criteria)

- In those with moderate liver impairment (category B), reduce to 50% of the normal dose
- In those with severe liver impairment (category C), reduce to 25% of the normal dose

Adjustment for Renal Dysfunction

- Dose adjustment not generally necessary

H. MEDICATIONS TO AVOID IN COMBINATION/WARNINGS [2, 3]

Tramadol

- Tramadol increases risk of seizures in patients taking antidepressants

Albuterol

- Albuterol co-administration may lead to increased heart rate and blood pressure

Monoamine oxidase inhibitors (MAOIs)

- Avoid or co-administer with extreme caution. Do not use within 14 days after MAOIs are stopped

Antihypertensives or Pressor Agents

- Because of possible effects on blood pressure, atomoxetine capsules should be used cautiously with antihypertensive drugs and pressor agents (e.g. dopamine, dobutamine) or other drugs that increase blood pressure

P450 2D6 Inhibitors

- Atomoxetine plasma concentrations can be increased when combined with drugs that inhibit cyp 2D6 such as bupropion, paroxetine and fluoxetine. In conjunction with these agents, may need to decrease atomoxetine dose

P450 2D6 Poor Metabolizers (PM)

- Atomoxetine plasma concentrations can be increased when taken by those who metabolize P450 2D6 substrates poorly

Warnings

- Use with caution in patients with hypertension, tachycardia, cardiovascular disease or cerebrovascular disease
- Use with caution in patients with bipolar disorder
- Use with caution in patients with urinary retention, benign prostatic hypertrophy
- Use with caution with antihypertensive drugs
- Increased risk of sudden death in children with structural cardiac abnormalities or other serious heart conditions
- Monitor for activation of suicidal ideation
- Do not use in patients with pheochromocytoma or history of pheochromocytoma
- Do not use in severe cardiovascular disorders that may deteriorate with increases in heart rate and blood pressure
- Do not use in closed angle glaucoma
- Do not use if there is a proven allergy to atomoxetine

ART OF PSYCHOPHARMACOLOGY: TAKE-HOME PEARLS

- No known abuse potential and is not a controlled substance.
- Atomoxetine enhances both norepinephrine and dopamine in the frontal cortex leading to therapeutic effects for attention deficit hyperactivity disorder (ADHD).
- Pro-noradrenergic actions suggest efficacy as an antidepressant and may be useful in chronic pain.

References

1. Garnock-Jones, K. P., Keating, G. M. (2009). Atomoxetine: a review of its use in attention-deficit hyperactivity disorder in children and adolescents. *Paediatr Drugs*, 11, 203–226.
2. Stahl, S. M., Grady, M. M., Munter, N. (2017). *Prescriber's Guide: Stahl's Essential Psychopharmacology*. Cambridge: Cambridge University Press.
3. Prasco Laboratories. (2020). *Atomoxetine Package Insert*. Mason, Ohio.
4. Michelson, D., Adler, L., Spencer, T., et al. (2003). Atomoxetine in adults with ADHD: two randomized, placebo-controlled studies. *Biol Psychiatry*, 53, 112–120.
5. Kelsey, D. K., Sumner, C. R., Casat, C. D., et al. (2004). Once-daily atomoxetine treatment for children with attention-deficit/hyperactivity disorder, including an assessment of evening and morning behavior: a double-blind, placebo-controlled trial. *Pediatrics*, 114, e1–e8.
6. Stiefel, G., Besag, F. M. (2010). Cardiovascular effects of methylphenidate, amphetamines and atomoxetine in the treatment of attention-deficit hyperactivity disorder. *Drug Saf*, 33, 821–842.

2.73 Dextroamphetamine

A. BASIC INFORMATION [1–3]

Principle Trade Names
- Dexedrine®
- Dexedrine Spansules®
- Zenzedi®
- ProCentra®

Legal Status
- Prescription only
- Controlled, Schedule II

⬤ Classifications
- Dopamine and norepinephrine reuptake inhibitor and releaser (DN-RIRe)
- Stimulant

Generics Available
- Yes

Formulations
- Immediate-release (IR) tablet: 2.5 mg; 5 mg; 7.5 mg; 10 mg; 15 mg; 20 mg; 30 mg
- Extended-release (ER) capsule: 5 mg; 10 mg; 15 mg
- Oral solution: 5 mg/5 ml

FDA Indications
- Attention deficit hyperactivity disorder (ADHD) in adults and children over three and over six depending on formulation
- Narcolepsy

Other Data-Supported Indications
- Treatment-resistant anergic depression

B. MECHANISMS OF ACTION [2, 3]

Dopamine
- Potently increases dopamine actions by blocking its reuptake and facilitating its release (displacement from axon terminal vesicles)

Norepinephrine
- Increases norepinephrine in certain brain regions (e.g. dorsolateral prefrontal cortex), may improve attention, concentration, executive dysfunction and wakefulness in addition to effects of increased dopamine

Dopamine (collateral effects)
- Increased dopamine in other brain areas (e.g. basal ganglia) may improve hyperactivity

Combined Effects
- Increased dopamine and norepinephrine in other brain areas (e.g. medial prefrontal cortex, hypothalamus) may improve depression, fatigue and sleepiness

Initial Target Range
- ADHD: 5–40 mg/day divided doses for tablet, once daily morning dose for Spansule capsule
- Narcolepsy: 5–60 mg/day divided doses for tablet, once daily morning dose for Spansule capsule
- No established plasma concentration range

Range for Treatment Resistance
- ADHD maximum dose 40 mg/day
- Narcolepsy maximum dose 60 mg/day
- No established plasma concentration range

Typical Time to Response
- The onset of clinical effects is often the first day of dosing
- Can take several weeks for maximal therapeutic benefits

Time-Course of Improvement
- If no response in a few weeks at maximum tolerated dose, it may not be effective and should be withdrawn

Usual Target Symptoms
- Concentration, attention span
- Motor hyperactivity
- Impulsivity
- Physical and mental fatigue
- Daytime sleepiness
- Depression (anergia/apathy)

Common Short-Term Adverse Effects
- Tremor, tachycardia, hypertension, cardiac arrhythmias, insomnia, agitation, psychosis, substance abuse, headache, exacerbation of tics, nervousness, irritability, overstimulation, dizziness, anorexia, nausea, dry mouth, constipation, diarrhea, weight loss, can temporarily slow growth in children (controversial), can improve sexual function short-term

Rare Adverse Effects
- Psychotic episodes, seizures, palpitations, tachycardia, hypertension, activation of hypomania, mania, or suicidal ideation (controversial), sudden death in patients with pre-existing cardiac structural abnormalities
- Overdose: rarely fatal; panic, hyperreflexia, rhabdomyolysis, rapid respiration, confusion, coma, hallucinations, convulsions, arrhythmia, change in blood pressure, circulatory collapse

Long-Term Effects
- Growth suppression in children (controversial)
- Impotence, libido changes
- Prolonged use should be avoided or done with close monitoring due to marked tolerance and drug dependence, including psychological dependence with variable degrees of abnormal behavior

History
- Assess for history of cardiac disease including family history of sudden death or ventricular arrhythmia
- Use with caution in patients with recent myocardial infarction or other conditions that could be negatively affected by increased blood pressure
- Use with caution in hypertension, hyperthyroidism
- Use with caution in patients with history of substance abuse, alcoholism or in emotionally unstable patients
- Pay attention to the possibility of patients obtaining stimulants for nontherapeutic use or distribution to others. Drugs should be prescribed sparingly
- May lower seizure threshold
- Use with caution in patients with bipolar disorder. Emergence or worsening agitation or activation may represent induction of a bipolar disorder
- Monitor for activation of suicidal ideation
- Do not use in patients with arteriosclerosis, cardiovascular disease or severe hypertension
- Do not use in patients with glaucoma
- Do not use in patients with structural cardiac abnormalities
- Tablets contain tartrazine which may cause allergic reactions, especially in patients allergic to aspirin
- Do not use in patients with proven allergy to sympathomimetic agents

Physical
- Monitor height and weight. For patients who are not growing or gaining weight normally, cessation of drug should be considered
- Monitor blood pressure regularly
- Assess for presence of cardiac disease
- Physical exam to assess for the presence of cardiac disease and should receive further cardiac evaluation if findings suggest such disease (e.g. electrocardiogram and echocardiogram)

Neurological
- May worsen motor and phonic tics
- May worsen symptoms of thought disorder and behavior disturbance in psychotic patients

Blood Tests
- In long-term use consider periodic monitoring of CBC, platelet counts and liver function

Cardiac Tests
- American Heart Association recommends ECG prior to starting stimulants in children though all experts do not agree

Urine Tests
Pregnancy Test
- Pregnancy test (premenopausal females)
- Classified as risk not ruled out
- In mothers taking d-amphetamine there is greater risk of premature birth and low birth weight
- In infants of mothers taking d-amphetamine, may have withdrawal symptoms as demonstrated by dysphoria, including agitation, and significant lassitude
- In animal studies, d-amphetamine caused delayed skeletal ossification and decreased post-weaning weight gain in rats. In rat and rabbit studies there were no major malformations seen
- Dextroamphetamine should generally be stopped before anticipated pregnancies
- Some drug is found in breast milk
- Thus, It Is recommended to stop the drug or bottle feed
- If infant is irritable, drug should be stopped

Other Tests (ECG, etc.)
- Before treatment assess for cardiac disease or family history of cardiac disease
- In long-term use consider periodic monitoring of weight, blood pressure, CBC, platelet counts and liver function

During Titration or After Dose Adjustment

- Monitor heart rate and blood pressure
- Patients who develop symptoms such as exertional chest pain, unexplained syncope, or other symptoms suggestive of cardiac disease during stimulant treatment should undergo prompt cardiac evaluation

Maintenance

- In pediatrics, monitor height and weight
- In adults, monitor for weight loss to BMI <20
- Monitor heart rate and blood pressure periodically as well as for hypomania/ mania, aggression, suicidality, abuse and dependence regularly
- Stop treatment, at least temporarily in children not growing or gaining weight

Initial Dosing/Titration

- ADHD, ages 6+ (Spansule capsule or tablet): initial 5 mg/day when waking; can increase by 5 mg/week
- ADHD, ages 3–5 (tablet IR): initial 2.5 mg/ day; can increase by 2.5 mg/week. Administer in divided doses
- Narcolepsy, ages 12+ (Spansule capsule or tablet): initial 10 mg/day; can increase by 10 mg/week; give first dose on waking; tablet administered in divided dose
- Narcolepsy, ages 6–12 (tablet IR): initial 5 mg/day; can increase by 5 mg each week; administered in divided doses
- May be able to dose only during school week for some ADHD patients
- May give drug holidays for ADHD patients over the summer to reassess therapeutic utility and side effects such as growth suppression to help decide whether to continue

Half-Life

- 9–12 hours

Bioavailability

- 75–100%
- 15–40% protein-bound
- Can be taken with or without food
- Taking with food may delay peak action two to three hours

Adjustment for Hepatic Dysfunction (by Child-Pugh Criteria)

- Use with caution for categories B or C (moderate-severe impairment)

Adjustment for Renal Dysfunction

- No dose adjustment necessary

H. MEDICATIONS TO AVOID IN COMBINATION/WARNINGS [2, 3]

 Gastrointestinal (GI) and urinary acidifying agents

- GI acidifying agents (e.g. ascorbic acid, fruit juice, glutamic acid, guanethidine, reserpine, etc.) and urinary acidifying agents (e.g. ammonium chloride, sodium phosphate, etc.) can lower amphetamine plasma levels. May be useful to administer in overdose

 GI and urinary alkalinizing agents

- GI alkalinizing agents (e.g. sodium bicarbonate) and urinary alkalinizing agents (e.g. acetazolamide, some thiazides) can increase amphetamine plasma levels and potentiate the action of amphetamine. Co-administration of dextroamphetamine and alkalinizing agents should be avoided

 Norepinephrine reuptake blockers (e.g. venlafaxine, duloxetine, atomoxetine, milnacipran, reboxetine)

- Norepinephrine reuptake blockers (e.g. venlafaxine, duloxetine, atomoxetine, milnacipran, reboxetine) could add to amphetamine's central nervous system (CNS) and cardiovascular effects

 cyp 2D6 Inhibitors (e.g. paroxetine, fluoxetine)

- Concomitant use of dextroamphetamine and cyp 2D6 inhibitors may increase the exposure of dextroamphetamine compared to use of the drug alone and increases the risk of serotonin syndrome. Initiate with lower doses and monitor patients for signs and symptoms of serotonin syndrome particularly during initiation and after a dosage increase. If serotonin syndrome occurs, discontinue dextroamphetamine and the cyp 2D6 inhibitor

 Serotonergic drugs (e.g. selective serotonin reuptake inhibitors (SSRIs), serotonin norepinephrine reuptake inhibitors (SNRIs), triptans, tricyclic antidepressants, fentanyl, lithium, tramadol, tryptophan, buspirone, St. John's Wort)

- The concomitant use of dextroamphetamine and serotonergic drugs increases the risk of serotonin syndrome. Initiate with lower doses and monitor patients for signs and symptoms of serotonin syndrome, particularly during dextroamphetamine initiation or dosage increase. If serotonin syndrome occurs, discontinue dextroamphetamine and the concomitant serotonergic drug(s)

 Desipramine and protryptiline

- Can cause substantial and sustained increases in d-amphetamine brain concentrations and may add to the cardiovascular effects of d-amphetamine

 Monoamine oxidase inhibitors (MAOIs)

- MAOIs slow absorption of amphetamines, thus potentiating their actions. This can cause headache, hypertension and rarely hypertensive crisis and malignant hyperthermia and sometimes death
- Use with MAOIs and within 14 days of MAOIs is not advised

 Adrenergic blockers

- Amphetamines inhibit adrenergic blockers and enhance adrenergic effects of norepinephrine

 Corticosteroids

- Amphetamines can raise corticosteroid levels. This increase is greatest in the evening
- Amphetamines may interfere with urinary steroid determinations

 Propoxyphene

- Amphetamines contribute to excessive CNS stimulation when used with large doses of propoxyphene

 Meperidine

- Amphetamines increase the analgesic effects of meperidine

 Veratrum alkaloids, other antihypertensives

- Amphetamines may antagonize hypotensive effects of antihypertensives

Phenobarbital, phenytoin, ethosuximide

• Amphetamines delay absorption of phenobarbital, phenytoin and ethosuximide

Proton Pump Inhibitors

• Time to maximum concentration (T) of amphetamine is decreased compared to when administered alone. Monitor patients for changes in clinical effect and adjust therapy based on clinical response

Chlorpromazine

• Chlorpromazine blocks dopamine and norepinephrine reuptake, thus inhibiting the central stimulant effects of amphetamines, and can be used to treat amphetamine poisoning

Warnings

• Serious cardiovascular events can occur with amphetamine use
• Sudden death in patients with pre-existing structural cardiac abnormalities or other serious heart problems can occur in those taking amphetamines

• Amphetamines can be associated with peripheral vasculopathy, including Raynaud's phenomenon
• Stop treatment, at least temporarily in children not growing or gaining weight
• Do not use in patients with motor tics, Tourette's or a family history of Tourette's
• Should not be administered with an MAOI or within 14 days of MAOI use
• Do not use in patients with glaucoma
• Do not use in patients with proven allergy to sympathomimetic agents
• Do not use in patients with severe anxiety or agitation
• May lower seizure threshold
• Difficulties with accommodation and blurring of vision have been reported with stimulant treatment
• Amphetamines may counteract sedating effects of antihistamines
• Amphetamines' stimulatory effect may be inhibited by antipsychotics and mood stabilizers
• Amphetamines could inhibit the antipsychotic effects of antipsychotics
• Amphetamines could inhibit mood stabilizing properties of mood stabilizers

• Dexedrine Spansules are controlled-release and should not be chewed, only swallowed whole.
• Controlled-release delivery of dextroamphetamine may be long enough in duration to eliminate the need for lunch-time dosing.
• May be more effective or tolerable in patients unresponsive to other stimulants.
• Immediate-release and Spansule formulations have established long-term efficacy.
• May be useful in depressive symptoms in medically ill elderly patients and in post-stroke patients.
• May be useful for residual major depressive disorder symptoms including cognitive dysfunction and fatigue/apathy/anergia that did not respond to prior treatments.

• Classical augmentation strategy for major depressive disorder.
• Can help treat cognitive impairment, depressive symptoms and severe fatigue in HIV and cancer patients.
• Can potentiate opioid analgesia and decrease sedation in end-of-life management.
• Can reverse sexual dysfunction (decreased libido, erectile dysfunction, delayed ejaculation and anorgasmia) due to psychiatric illness and some drugs including SSRIs.
• Atypical antipsychotics can treat stimulant overdose or psychosis due to stimulant use/abuse.
• Half-life and duration of clinical action tend to be shorter in younger children.
• Drug abuse may be lower in ADHD adolescents treated with stimulants compared to those not treated.

2.73 Dextroamphetamine (Continued)

 References

1. Fry, J. M. (1998). Treatment modalities for narcolepsy. *Neurology*, 50, S43–48.
2. Stahl, S. M., Grady, M. M., Munter, N. (2017). *Prescriber's Guide: Stahl's Essential Psychopharmacology*. Cambridge: Cambridge University Press.
3. SpecGx LLC. (2020). *Dextroamphetamine Package Insert*. Webster Groves, Missouri.
4. Vinson, D. C. (1994). Therapy for attention-deficit hyperactivity disorder. *Arch Fam Med*, 3, 445–451.
5. Jadad, A. R., Boyle, M., Cunningham, C., et al. (1999). Treatment of attention-deficit/hyperactivity disorder. *Evid Rep Technol Assess (Summ)*, i–viii, 1–341.
6. Wender, P. H., Wolf, L. E., Wasserstein, J. (2001). Adults with ADHD. An overview. *Ann N Y Acad Sci*, 931, 1–16.
7. Greenhill, L. L., Pliszka, S., Dulcan, M. K., et al. (2002). Practice parameter for the use of stimulant medications in the treatment of children, adolescents, and adults. *J Am Acad Child Adolesc Psychiatry*, 41, 26S–49S.
8. Stiefel, G., Besag, F. M. (2010). Cardiovascular effects of methylphenidate, amphetamines and atomoxetine in the treatment of attention-deficit hyperactivity disorder. *Drug Saf*, 33, 821–842.

2.74 Lisdexamfetamine

A. BASIC INFORMATION [1]

Principle Trade Names
- Vyvanse®
- Tyvense®
- Elvanse®

Legal Status
- Prescription only
- Controlled, Schedule II

Classifications
- Dopamine and norepinephrine reuptake inhibitor and releaser (DN-RIRe)
- Stimulant

Generics Available
- No

Formulations
- Capsules: 10 mg; 20 mg; 30 mg; 40 mg; 50 mg; 60 mg; 70 mg
- Chewable tablets: 10 mg; 20 mg; 30 mg; 40 mg; 50 mg; 60 mg

FDA Indications
- Attention deficit hyperactivity disorder (ADHD) in adults and children over six
- Binge eating disorder

Other Data-Supported Indications
- Treatment-resistant anergic depression
- Narcolepsy

Prodrug
- Lisdexamfetamine is a prodrug of dextroamphetamine, thus it is not active until absorbed by the intestine and converted to dextroamphetamine (active component) and l-lysine

Dopamine
- Once converted to dextroamphetamine, it potently increases dopamine actions by blocking its reuptake and facilitating its release

Dopamine/Norepinephrine
- Increased dopamine and norepinephrine in certain brain regions (e.g. dorsolateral prefrontal cortex), may improve attention, concentration, executive dysfunction and wakefulness

Dopamine (collateral)
- Increased dopamine in other brain areas (e.g. basal ganglia) may improve hyperactivity

Dopamine/Norepinephrine (collateral)
- Increased dopamine and norepinephrine in other brain areas (e.g. medial prefrontal cortex, hypothalamus) may improve depression, fatigue and sleepiness

C. PLASMA CONCENTRATIONS AND TREATMENT RESPONSE [1]

Initial Target Range
- 30–70 mg/day
- Binge eating disorder: 50–70 mg/day
- No established plasma concentration range

Range for Treatment Resistance
- Maximum dose 70 mg/day
- No established plasma concentration range

Typical Time to Response
- The onset of action often is the first day of dosing
- Can take several weeks for maximal therapeutic benefits

Time-Course of Improvement
- If no response in a few weeks at maximum tolerated dose, it may not be effective

D. TYPICAL TREATMENT RESPONSE [1, 2]

Usual Target Symptoms
- Concentration, attention span
- Motor hyperactivity
- Impulsivity
- Binge eating
- Physical and mental fatigue/anergia
- Daytime sleepiness
- Depression

Common Short-Term Adverse Effects
- Tremor, tachycardia, hypertension, cardiac arrhythmias, insomnia, agitation, psychosis, substance abuse, headache, exacerbation of tics, nervousness, irritability, anxiety, feeling jittery, overstimulation, dizziness, anorexia, nausea, vomiting, dry mouth, abdominal pain, constipation, diarrhea, weight loss, can temporarily slow growth in children

Rare Adverse Effects
- Psychotic episodes, seizures, palpitations, activation of hypomania, mania, or suicidal ideation, sudden death in patients with pre-existing cardiac structural abnormalities

Long-Term Effects
- Impotence, libido changes
- Prolonged use should be avoided or done with close monitoring due to marked tolerance and drug dependence, including psychological dependence with variable degrees of abnormal behavior

History

- Use with caution in patients with hypertension, hyperthyroidism
- Use with caution in patients with history of substance abuse, alcoholism or in emotionally unstable patients
- Pay attention to the possibility of patients obtaining stimulants for nontherapeutic use or distribution to others
- May lower seizure threshold
- Use with caution in patients with bipolar disorder. Emergence or worsening agitation or activation may represent induction of a bipolar disorder
- Monitor for activation of suicidal ideation
- Do not use in patients with motor tics, Tourette's or a family history of Tourette's
- Should not be administered with monoamine oxidase inhibitors (MAOIs) or within 14 days of MAOI use
- Do not use in patients with arteriosclerosis, cardiovascular disease or severe hypertension
- Do not use in patients with glaucoma
- Do not use in patients with structural cardiac abnormalities
- Do not use in those with known hypersensitivity or proven allergy to amphetamine products or other ingredients in lisdexamfetamine

Physical

- Monitor height and weight. For patients who are not growing or gaining weight normally, cessation of drug should be considered
- Monitor blood pressure regularly
- Assess for presence of cardiac disease

Neurological

- May worsen motor and phonic tics
- May worsen symptoms of thought disorder and behavior disturbance in psychotic patients

Blood Tests

- In long-term use consider periodic monitoring of CBC, platelet counts and liver function

Cardiac Tests

- American Heart Association recommends ECG prior to starting stimulants in children though all experts do not agree

Urine Tests

- No specific test

Pregnancy Test

- Pregnancy test (premenopausal females)
- Classified as risk not ruled out
- In mothers taking d-amphetamine there is greater risk of premature birth and low birth weight
- In infants of mothers taking d-amphetamine, may have withdrawal symptoms
- In animal studies, d-amphetamine caused delayed skeletal ossification and decreased post-weaning weight gain in rats. In rat and rabbit studies there were no major malformations seen
- Lisdexamfetamine should generally be stopped before anticipated pregnancies
- Some drug is found in breast milk
- Thus, it is recommended to stop the drug or bottle feed
- If infant is irritable, drug should be stopped

Other Tests (ECG, etc.)

- Before treatment assess for cardiac disease or family history of cardiac disease
- In long-term use consider periodic monitoring of weight, blood pressure, CBC, platelet counts and liver function

During Titration or After Dose Adjustment

- Monitor heart rate and blood pressure

Maintenance

- In pediatrics, monitor height and weight
- In adults, monitor for weight loss (BMI <20)

- In adults, monitor heart rate and blood pressure periodically as well as for hypomania/mania, suicidality, aggression, abuse and dependence regularly

Initial Dosing
- Initial 30 mg/day in the morning; can increase by 10–20 mg/week
- Binge eating disorder: initial 30 mg/day; can increase by 20 mg/week

Titration
- Can increase by 20 mg each week to a maximum dose of 70 mg/day
- May be able to dose only during school week for some ADHD patients
- May give drug holidays for ADHD patients over the summer to reassess therapeutic utility and side effects such as growth suppression to help decide whether to continue

Half-Life
- One hour for lisdexamfetamine
- 9–12 hours for dextroamphetamine

Bioavailability
- 96.4%
- Can be taken with or without food
- 3.5 hours until maximum concentration of dextroamphetamine

Adjustment for Hepatic Dysfunction (by Child-Pugh Criteria)
- Use with caution in categories B or C (moderate-severe impairment)

Adjustment for Renal Dysfunction
- Severe impairment: maximum dose 50 mg/day
- End-stage renal disease: maximum dose 30 mg/day

H. MEDICATIONS TO AVOID IN COMBINATION/WARNINGS [1]

Gastrointestinal (GI) and urinary acidifying agents
- GI acidifying agents (e.g. ascorbic acid, fruit juice, glutamic acid, guanethidine, reserpine, etc.) and urinary acidifying agents (e.g. ammonium chloride, sodium phosphate, etc.) can lower amphetamine plasma levels. May be useful to administer in overdose

GI and urinary alkalinizing agents
- GI alkalinizing agents (e.g. sodium bicarbonate) and urinary alkalinizing agents (e.g. acetazolamide, some thiazides) can increase amphetamine plasma levels and potentiate the action of amphetamine. Co-administration of lisdexamfetamine and alkalinizing agents should be avoided

Desipramine and protryptiline
- Can cause substantial and sustained increases in d-amphetamine brain concentrations and may add to the cardiovascular effects of d-amphetamine

MAOIs
- MAOIs slow absorption of amphetamines, thus potentiating their actions. This can cause headache, hypertension and rarely hypertensive crisis and malignant hyperthermia and sometimes death
- Use with MAOIs and within 14 days of MAOIs is not advised

Norepinephrine reuptake blockers (e.g. venlafaxine, duloxetine, atomoxetine, milnacipran, reboxetine)
- Norepinephrine reuptake blockers (e.g. venlafaxine, duloxetine, atomoxetine, milnacipran, reboxetine) could add to amphetamine's central nervous system (CNS) and cardiovascular effects

Corticosteroids
- Amphetamines can raise corticosteroid levels

Propoxyphene
- Amphetamines contribute to excessive CNS stimulation when used with large doses of propoxyphene

Meperidine
- Amphetamines increase the analgesic effects of meperidine

Phenobarbital, phenytoin, ethosuximide

- Amphetamines delay absorption of phenobarbital, phenytoin and ethosuximide

Warnings

- Sudden death has been reported in association with CNS stimulant treatment at recommended doses in pediatric patients with structural cardiac abnormalities or other serious heart problems. In adults, sudden death, stroke and myocardial infarction have been reported. Avoid use in patients with known structural cardiac abnormalities, cardiomyopathy, serious heart arrhythmia or coronary artery disease
- Lisdexamfetamine may increase blood pressure and heart rate. Monitor blood pressure and pulse
- May cause psychotic or manic symptoms in patients with no prior history, or exacerbation of symptoms in patients with pre-existing psychosis. Evaluate for bipolar disorder prior to stimulant use
- Stimulants are associated with peripheral vasculopathy, including Raynaud's phenomenon. Careful observation for digital changes is necessary during treatment with stimulants
- Increased risk of serotonin syndrome when co-administered with serotonergic agents (e.g. SSRIs, SNRIs, triptans), but also during overdosage situations. If it occurs, discontinue lisdexamfetamine and other serotonergic agents and initiate supportive treatment
- Cases of painful and prolonged penile erections, and priapism have been reported with amphetamines. Seek immediate medical attention if signs or symptoms of prolonged penile erections or priapism are observed
- Amphetamines may counteract sedating effects of antihistamines
- Amphetamine stimulatory effects may be inhibited by antipsychotics and mood stabilizers
- Amphetamines could inhibit the antipsychotic effects of antipsychotics
- Amphetamines could inhibit mood stabilizing properties of mood stabilizers
- Amphetamines inhibit adrenergic blockers and enhance adrenergic effects of norepinephrine

ART OF PSYCHOPHARMACOLOGY: TAKE-HOME PEARLS

- Lisdexamfetamine is a prodrug and thus may have fewer propensities for intoxication, abuse or dependence compared to other stimulants.
- Only approved treatment for binge eating disorder.
- Efficacy in binge eating disorder theoretically due to controlled release of stimulant enhancing tonic over phasic dopamine neuronal firing.
- Theoretically binge eating in binge eating disorder could be due to a shift from reward-related eating to habit and from impulsivity to compulsivity from a shift in control of dopamine from dorsal to ventral striatum which lisdexamfetamine can reverse.
- May be useful in depressive symptoms in medically ill elderly patients and in post-stroke patients.
- May be useful for residual major depressive disorder symptoms including cognitive dysfunction and fatigue/anergia that did not respond to prior treatments.
- Classical augmentation strategy for major depressive disorder.
- Can help treat cognitive impairment, depressive symptoms, and severe fatigue in HIV and cancer patients.
- Can potentiate opioid analgesia and decrease sedation in end-of-life management.
- Atypical antipsychotics can treat stimulant overdose or psychosis due to stimulant use/abuse.
- Half-life and duration of clinical action tend to be shorter in younger children.
- Drug abuse may be lower in ADHD adolescents treated with stimulants compared to those not treated.

References

1. Shire US Inc. (2019). *Lisdexamfetamine Package Insert.* Lexington, Massachusetts.
2. Biederman, J., Krishnan, S., Zhang, Y., et al. (2007). Efficacy and tolerability of lisdexamfetamine dimesylate (NRP-104) in children with attention-deficit/hyperactivity disorder: a phase III, multicenter, randomized, double-blind, forced-dose, parallel-group study. *Clin Ther,* 29, 450–463.
3. Stahl, S. M. (2020). *Stahl's Essential Psychopharmacology Prescriber's Guide.* 7th ed. New York: Cambridge University Press.

2.75 Methylphenidate

A. BASIC INFORMATION [1, 2]

Principle Trade Names
- Focalin®
- Focalin XR®
- Ritalin®
- Concerta®
- Daytrana®

Legal Status
- Prescription only
- Controlled, Schedule II

Classifications
- Dopamine, norepinephrine reuptake inhibitor and releaser (DN-RIRe)
- Stimulant

Generics Available
- Yes

Formulations
- Immediate-release tablet (Focalin®): 2.5 mg; 5 mg; 10 mg
- Extended-release capsule (Focalin XR): 5 mg; 10 mg; 15 mg; 20 mg; 25 mg; 30 mg; 35 mg; 40 mg
- Tablet, immediate-release (Ritalin): 5 mg; 10 mg; 20 mg
- Tablet, controlled-release (Concerta®): 18 mg; 27 mg; 36 mg; 54 mg
- Transdermal: 27.5 mg; 41.3 mg; 55 mg; 82.5 mg

FDA Indications
- Attention deficit hyperactivity disorder (ADHD) in children ages 6–17 (immediate-release, extended-release) and in adults (extended-release)

Other Data-Supported Indications
- Treatment-resistant depression
- Narcolepsy

Norepinephrine

- Increases norepinephrine by blocking reuptake
- Enhances norepinephrine in the dorsolateral prefrontal cortex, may improve attention, concentration, executive function and wakefulness
- Enhances norepinephrine in the medial prefrontal cortex and hypothalamus which may improve depression, fatigue and sleepiness

Dopamine

- Increases dopamine actions by blocking reuptake
- Enhances dopamine in the dorsolateral prefrontal cortex, may improve attention, concentration, executive function and wakefulness
- Enhances dopamine in the basal ganglia which may improve hyperactivity
- Enhances dopamine in the medial prefrontal cortex and hypothalamus which may improve depression, fatigue and sleepiness

Initial Target Range (For specific brands please see package insert)

- Immediate-release tablet: 2.5 mg twice per day in children ages four to five
- Immediate-release tablet: 2.5–5 mg twice per day in children six years and older
- Immediate-release tablet: 5–15 mg twice or three times per day in adults
- Extended-release capsule: 20–60 mg PO QAM in children ages six and older and adults
- Extended-release tablet: 18–54 mg PO QAM in children ages six to twelve
- Extended-release tablet: 18–72 mg PO QAM in children ages 13 and older and adults
- Plasma concentration range not established

Range for Treatment Resistance

- Immediate-release maximum dose is 30 mg/day for children ages four to five and 60 mg/day for children six years and older and adults

- Extended-release maximum dose is 30 mg for children and 60 mg for adults
- Extended-release tab maximum dose is 54 mg/day in children ages six to twelve
- Extended-release tab maximum dose is 72 mg/day in children ages 13 years and older
- Plasma concentration range not established

Typical Time to Response

- The onset of action is often the first day of dosing
- Can take several weeks for maximal therapeutic benefits

Time-Course of Improvement

- If no response in a few weeks at maximum tolerated dose, it may not be effective and should be withdrawn

Usual Target Symptoms

- Concentration, attention span
- Motor hyperactivity
- Impulsivity
- Binge eating
- Physical and mental fatigue/anergia
- Daytime sleepiness
- Depression

Common Short-Term Adverse Effects

- Insomnia, headache, exacerbation of tics, nervousness, irritability, overstimulation, tremor, dizziness, anorexia, nausea, abdominal pain, weight loss, blurred vision, can temporarily slow normal growth in children (controversial), palpitations, tachycardia, hypertension
- Side effects are generally dose related

Rare Adverse Effects

- Psychotic episodes, priapism, seizures, neuroleptic malignant syndrome, activation of hypomania, mania, or suicidal ideation (controversial), sudden cardiac death in patients with pre-existing cardiac structural abnormalities

Long-Term Effects

- Dependence and/or abuse, tolerance to therapeutic effects, growth suppression in children (controversial)

History

- Use with caution in patients with hypertension, hyperthyroidism
- Use with caution in patients with history of substance abuse, alcoholism or in emotionally unstable patients
- Pay attention to the possibility of patients obtaining stimulants for nontherapeutic use or distribution to others
- May lower seizure threshold
- Use with caution in patients with bipolar disorder. Emergence or worsening agitation or activation may represent induction of a bipolar disorder
- Monitor for activation of suicidal ideation
- Do not use in patients with Tourette's or a family history of Tourette's
- May worsen motor or phonic tics
- Should not be administered with a monoamine oxidase inhibitor (MAOI) or within 14 days of MAOI use
- Do not use in patients with extreme anxiety or agitation
- Do not use in patients with angioedema or anaphylaxis
- Do not use in patients with glaucoma
- Do not use in patients with structural cardiac abnormalities. Usual doses have been associated with death in children with cardiac structural abnormalities
- Not an appropriate first-line treatment for depression or fatigue
- Do not use in patients with proven allergy or hypersensitivity to methylphenidate or product components

Physical

- Monitor height and weight. For patients who are not growing or gaining weight normally, cessation of drug should be considered at least temporarily
- Monitor pulse and blood pressure regularly
- Assess for presence of cardiac disease

Neurological

- May worsen motor and phonic tics
- May worsen symptoms of thought disorder and behavior disturbance in psychotic patients

Blood Tests

- In long-term use consider periodic monitoring of CBC, platelet counts and liver function

Cardiac Tests

- American Heart Association recommends ECG prior to starting stimulants in children though all experts do not agree
- Use with caution in patients with recent myocardial infarction or other conditions that could be negatively affected by increased blood pressure
- Do not use in patients with structural cardiac abnormalities

Urine Tests

- No specific test

Pregnancy Test

- Pregnancy test (premenopausal females)
- Classified as risk not ruled out
- Infants of mothers taking methylphenidate may have withdrawal symptoms
- Racemic methylphenidate has been shown to have teratogenic effects in rabbits when given in very high doses of 200 mg/kg/day throughout organogenesis
- For ADHD patients, methylphenidate should generally be stopped before anticipated pregnancies
- Use in women of childbearing potential requires weighing potential benefits for the mother against potential risks to the fetus
- Unknown if methylphenidate is secreted in human breast milk, but all psychotropics are assumed to be secreted in breast milk
- Thus, it is recommended to stop the drug or bottle feed
- If infant is irritable, drug should be stopped

Other Tests (ECG, etc.)

- Before treatment assess for cardiac disease or family history of cardiac disease
- In long-term use consider periodic monitoring of weight

F. MONITORING [2]

During Titration or After Dose Adjustment
- Monitor heart rate and blood pressure

Maintenance
- In children, monitor height and weight

- In adults, monitor for weight loss (BMI <20)
- In adults, monitor heart rate and blood pressure periodically as well as for hypomania/mania, suicidality, aggression, abuse and dependence regularly

G. DOSING AND KINETICS [1, 9]

Initial Dosing/ Titration
- Immediate-release: for patients not taking racemic d,l-methylphenidate, initial 2.5 mg twice a day in four-hour intervals; may adjust by 2.5–5 mg/day per week; maximum dose generally 10 mg twice a day
- Immediate-release: for patients currently taking racemic d,l-methylphenidate, initial dose should be half the current dose of racemic d,l-methylphenidate; maximum dose generally 60 mg/day
- Extended-release: for children, same titration schedule as immediate-release but dosed once in the morning; maximum dose 30 mg/ day, swallow capsules whole or open and sprinkle on applesauce. Should not be crushed, chewed or divided
- Extended-release: for adults not taking racemic d,l-methylphenidate, initial 10 mg/ day in the morning; may adjust by 10 mg/ day per week; maximum dose generally 60 mg/day, swallow capsules whole or open and sprinkle on applesauce. Should not be crushed, chewed or divided

Dosing Tips
- Immediate-release d-methylphenidate has the same onset of action and duration of action as immediate-release racemic d,l-methylphenidate (i.e. two to four hours) but at half the dose
- Extended-release d-methylphenidate contains half the dose as immediate-release beads and half as delayed-release beads so the dose is released in two pulses
- D-methylphenidate is generally considered twice as potent as racemic d,l-methylphenidate though some studies suggest that the d-isomer is more than twice as effective as racemic d,l-methylphenidate
- Off-label uses are dosed the same as for ADHD

- May dose only during the school week in some ADHD patients
- May give drug holidays over the summer to reassess therapeutic use and effect on growth and to allow for catch-up of any growth suppression
- Avoid dosing late in the day due to risk of insomnia

Half-Life
- 2.2 hours

Bioavailability
- 11–52%
- Food may delay peak actions for two to three hours

Adjustment for Hepatic Dysfunction (by Child-Pugh Criteria)
- No dose adjustment necessary

Adjustment for Renal Dysfunction
- No dose adjustment necessary

Elderly
- Some may tolerate lower doses better

H. MEDICATIONS TO AVOID IN COMBINATION/WARNINGS [1, 2]

 Selective serotonin reuptake inhibitors (SSRIs), anticonvulsants (phenobarbital, phenytoin, primidone), tricyclic antidepressants (TCAs), coumarin anticoagulants

- Methylphenidate may inhibit metabolism, thus requiring a downward dose adjustment of these drugs

 Albuterol

- Oral or IV albuterol co-administration may lead to increased heart rate and blood pressure

 Norepinephrine reuptake blockers (TCAs, desipramine, protriptyline, venlafaxine, duloxetine, atomoxetine, milnacipran, reboxetine)

- Methylphenidate in combination with these can enhance central nervous system (CNS) and cardiovascular actions

 Clonidine

- Serious adverse effects may occur in combination (controversial)

 MAOIs

- Use with MAOIs, including 14 days after MAOIs are stopped is not advised (for the expert)

 Antacids or acid suppressants

- Could alter release of extended-release formulation

 Halogenated anesthetics (e.g. halothane, isoflurane, enflurane, desflurane, sevoflurane)

- Avoid use of methylphenidate on the day of surgery if halogenated anesthetics are used as when combined they may increase the risk of sudden blood pressure and heart rate increase during surgery

 cyp enzymes

- Does not inhibit

 Warnings

- Sudden death has been reported in association with CNS stimulant treatment at recommended doses in pediatric patients with structural cardiac abnormalities or other serious heart problems. In adults, sudden death, stroke and myocardial infarction have been reported. Avoid use in patients with known structural cardiac abnormalities, cardiomyopathy, serious heart arrhythmia or coronary artery disease
- Cases of painful and prolonged penile erections, and priapism have been reported with methylphenidate products. Seek immediate medical attention if signs or symptoms of prolonged penile erections or priapism are observed
- Methylphenidate may increase blood pressure and heart rate. Monitor blood pressure and pulse
- May cause psychotic or manic symptoms in patients with no prior history, or exacerbation of symptoms in patients with pre-existing psychosis. Evaluate for bipolar disorder prior to stimulant use
- Stimulants are associated with peripheral vasculopathy, including Raynaud's phenomenon. Careful observation for digital changes is necessary during treatment with stimulants
- Increased risk of serotonin syndrome when co-administered with serotonergic agents (e.g. SSRIs, SNRIs, triptans), but also during overdosage situations. If it occurs, discontinue methylphenidate and other serotonergic agents and initiate supportive treatment

- The active d-enantiomer of methylphenidate may be slightly more than twice as efficacious as racemic d,l-methylphenidate.
- May be useful in depressive symptoms in medically ill elderly patients and in post-stroke patients.
- May be useful for residual major depressive disorder symptoms including cognitive dysfunction and fatigue/anergia that did not respond to prior treatments.
- Classical augmentation strategy for major depressive disorder.
- Can help treat cognitive impairment, depressive symptoms, and severe fatigue in HIV and cancer patients.
- Can potentiate opioid analgesia and decrease sedation in end-of-life management.
- Atypical antipsychotics can treat stimulant overdose or psychosis due to stimulant use/abuse.

- Some patients respond to or tolerate methylphenidate better than amphetamine and vice versa.
- Half-life and duration of clinical action tend to be shorter in younger children.
- Drug abuse may be lower in ADHD adolescents treated with stimulants compared to those not treated.
- Extended-release formulation requires only once a day dosing.
- Extended-release capsule can be sprinkled over applesauce for those unable to swallow a capsule.
- Some may benefit from an occasional addition of an immediate-release dose of d-methylphenidate to the daily base dose of extended-release d-methylphenidate.

References

1. Stahl, S. M., Grady, M. M., Munter, N. (2017). *Prescriber's Guide: Stahl's Essential Psychopharmacology*. Cambridge: Cambridge University Press.
2. Sandoz Inc. (2019). *Methylphenidate Package Insert*. Princeton, New Jersey.
3. Keating, G. M., Figgitt, D. P. (2002). Dexmethylphenidate. *Drugs*, 62, 1899–1904; discussion 1905–1908.

2.76 Mixed Amphetamine Salts

A. BASIC INFORMATION [1–3]

Principle Trade Names
- Adderall®
- Adderall XR®
- Evekeo®
- Adzenys-XR-ODT®
- Dyanavel
- Mydayis®

Legal Status
- Prescription only
- Controlled, Schedule II

Classifications
- Dopamine and norepinephrine reuptake inhibitor and releaser (DN-RIRe)
- Stimulant

Generics Available
- Yes

Formulations
- Immediate-release tablets (Adderall®): 5 mg; 7.5 mg; 10 mg; 12.5 mg; 15 mg; 20 mg; 30 mg double-scored
- Immediate-release tablet (Evekeo®): 5 mg; 10 mg double-scored
- Extended-release orally disintegrating tablet (Adzenys XR-ODT®): 3.1 mg; 6.3 mg; 9.4 mg; 12.5 mg; 15.7 mg; 18.8 mg
- Extended-release tablet (Adderall XR®): 5 mg; 10 mg; 15 mg; 20 mg; 25 mg; 30 mg
- Extended-release capsules (Mydayis®): 12.5 mg; 25 mg; 37.5 mg; 50 mg

FDA Indications
- Attention deficit hyperactivity disorder (ADHD) in adults (Adderall XR®, Evekeo®, Adzenys XR-ODT®, Mydayis® (13 years and older))
- ADHD in children over six (Adderall XR®, Eveko®, Dyanavel XR®, Adzenys XR-ODT®)
- ADHD in children over three (Adderall®, Evekeo®)
- Narcolepsy (Adderall®, Evekeo®)
- Exogenous obesity (Evekeo®)

Other Data-Supported Indications
- Treatment-resistant depression, especially with anergia/fatigue

B. MECHANISMS OF ACTION [2]

Dopamine
- Potently increases dopamine actions by blocking its reuptake and facilitating its release

Dopamine (collateral)
- Increased dopamine in other brain areas (e.g. basal ganglia) may improve hyperactivity

Dopamine/Norepinephrine
- Increased dopamine and norepinephrine in certain brain regions (e.g. dorsolateral prefrontal cortex) may improve attention, concentration, executive dysfunction and wakefulness

Dopamine/Norepinephrine (collateral)
- Increased dopamine and norepinephrine in other brain areas (e.g. medial prefrontal cortex, hypothalamus) may improve depression, fatigue and sleepiness

C. PLASMA CONCENTRATIONS AND TREATMENT RESPONSE [1–3]

Initial Target Range
- ADHD: 5–40 mg/day divided doses for immediate-release tablet, once daily morning dose for extended-release formulations
- Narcolepsy: 5–60 mg/day in divided doses
- Exogenous obesity: 30 mg/day in divided doses
- No established plasma concentration range

Range for Treatment Resistance
- ADHD maximum dose 40 mg/day
- Narcolepsy maximum dose 60 mg/day
- Exogenous obesity maximum dose 30 mg/day

- No established plasma concentration range

Typical Time to Response
- The onset of action often is the first day of dosing
- Can take several weeks for maximal therapeutic benefits

Time-Course of Improvement
- If no response in a few weeks at maximum tolerated dose, it may not be effective and should be withdrawn

D. TYPICAL TREATMENT RESPONSE [2, 3]

Usual Target Symptoms
- Concentration, attention span
- Motor hyperactivity
- Impulsivity
- Physical and mental fatigue/anergia
- Daytime sleepiness
- Depression

Common Short-Term Adverse Effects
- Insomnia, anorexia, weight loss, irritability, nausea, dry mouth, nervousness, headache, tremor, exacerbation of tics, overstimulation, tachycardia, hypertension, cardiac arrhythmias, agitation, psychosis, substance abuse, dizziness, constipation, diarrhea, can temporarily slow growth in children (controversial), can improve sexual function short-term

Rare Adverse Effects
- Psychotic episodes, seizures, palpitations, hypertension, activation of hypomania, mania, or suicidal ideation (controversial), sudden death in patients with pre-existing cardiac structural abnormalities
- Overdose: rarely fatal; panic, hyperreflexia, rhabdomyolysis, rapid respiration, confusion, coma, hallucinations, convulsions, arrhythmia, change in blood pressure, circulatory collapse

Long-Term Effects
- Growth suppression in children (controversial)
- Impotence, libido changes
- Prolonged use should be avoided or done with close monitoring due to marked tolerance and drug dependence, including psychological dependence with variable degrees of abnormal behavior

History
- Use with caution in patients with recent myocardial infarction or other conditions that could be negatively affected by increased blood pressure
- Use with caution in hypertension, hyperthyroidism
- Use with caution in patients with history of substance abuse, alcoholism or in emotionally unstable patients
- Pay attention to the possibility of patients obtaining stimulants for nontherapeutic use or distribution to others. Drugs should be prescribed or dispensed sparingly
- May lower seizure threshold
- Use with caution in patients with bipolar disorder. Emergence or worsening agitation or activation may represent induction of a bipolar disorder
- Monitor for activation of suicidal ideation
- Stop treatment, at least temporarily in children not growing or gaining weight
- Do not use in patients with motor tics, Tourette's or a family history of Tourette's
- Should not be administered with a monoamine oxidase inhibitor (MAOI) or within 14 days of MAOI use
- Do not use in patients with arteriosclerosis, coronary artery disease, cardiomyopathy, serious arrhythmia or severe hypertension
- Do not use in patients with glaucoma
- Do not use in patients with structural cardiac abnormalities
- Do not use in patients with proven allergy to sympathomimetic agents
- Do not use in patients with severe anxiety or agitation

Physical
- Monitor height and weight. For patients who are not growing or gaining weight normally, cessation of drug should be considered
- Monitor blood pressure regularly
- Assess for presence of cardiac disease
- Observe carefully for digital changes. Stimulants used to treat ADHD are associated with peripheral vasculopathy including Raynaud's phenomenon

Neurological
- May worsen motor and phonic tics
- May worsen symptoms of thought disorder and behavior disturbance in psychotic patients

Blood Tests
- In long-term use consider periodic monitoring of CBC, platelet counts, and liver function

Cardiac Tests
- American Heart Association recommends ECG prior to starting stimulants in children though all experts do not agree

Urine Tests
- No specific tests

Pregnancy Test
- Pregnancy test (premenopausal females)
- Classified as risk not ruled out
- In mothers taking d-amphetamine there is greater risk of premature birth and low birth weight
- In infants of mothers taking d-amphetamine, may have withdrawal symptoms
- In animal studies, d-amphetamine caused delayed skeletal ossification and decreased post-weaning weight gain in rats. In rat and rabbit studies there were no major malformations seen
- In rat and rabbit studies, d,l-amphetamine did not affect embryofetal development or survival throughout organogenesis at doses of approximately one-and-a-half and eight times the maximum recommended human dose of 30 mg/day (child)
- D,l-amphetamine should generally be stopped before anticipated pregnancies
- Some drug is found in breast milk
- Thus, it is recommended to stop the drug or bottle feed
- If infant is irritable, drug should be stopped

Other Tests (ECG, etc.)
- Before treatment assess for cardiac disease or family history of cardiac disease
- In long-term use consider periodic monitoring of weight, blood pressure, CBC, platelet counts and liver function

2.76 Mixed Amphetamine Salts (Continued)

During Titration or After Dose Adjustment
• Monitor heart rate and blood pressure

Maintenance
• In pediatrics, monitor height and weight
• In adults monitor for weight loss (BMI <20)
• In adults, monitor heart rate and blood pressure periodically as well as for hypomania/mania, suicidality, abuse and dependence regularly

Initial Dosing/Titration
• ADHD, ages 6+ (immediate-release Adderall® or Evekeo®): initial 5 mg once or twice a day on waking and every four to six hours thereafter; can increase by 5 mg/week
• ADHD, ages 3–5 (immediate-release Evekeo®): initial 2.5 mg/day; can increase by 2.5 mg/week. Administer in divided doses
• ADHD, ages 6–17 (extended-release tablet Adderall XR®): initial 10 mg/day upon waking; can increase by 5–10 mg/week. Maximum dose 30 mg/day
• ADHD, ages 18+ (extended-release tablet Adderall XR®): initial 20 mg/day upon waking. Maximum dose 30 mg/day
• ADHD, ages 18+ (extended-release orally disintegrating tablet Adzenys XR-ODT®): 12.5 mg/day upon waking
• ADHD, ages 6–17 (extended-release orally disintegrating tablet Adzenys XR-ODT®): 6.3 mg/day upon waking. Maximum dose for 6–12 years old 18.8 mg/day. Maximum dose for 13–17 years old 12.5 mg/day
• ADHD, ages 13–17 (extended-release capsule Mydayis®): 12.5 mg/day upon waking; can increase by 12.5 mg/week up to a maximum dose of 25 mg/day
• ADHD, ages 18+ (extended-release capsule Mydayis®): 12.5 mg/day upon waking; can increase by 12.5 mg/week up to a maximum dose of 50 mg/day
• ADHD, ages 6+ (extended-release oral suspension Dyanavel XR®): 2.5–5 mg/day upon waking; can increase by 2.5–10 mg/week up to a maximum dose of 20 mg/day
• Narcolepsy, ages 6–12 (immediate-release Evekeo®): initial 5 mg/day in divided dose; can increase by 5 mg/week
• Narcolepsy, ages 12+ (immediate-release Evekeo®): initial 10 mg/day in divided doses; can increase by 10 mg/week

• Exogenous obesity, ages 12+ (immediate-release Evekeo®): usual daily dose 30 mg taken in divided doses of 5–10 mg, 30–60 minutes before meals
• May be able to dose only during school week for some ADHD patients
• May give drug holidays for ADHD patients over the summer to reassess therapeutic utility and side effects such as growth suppression to help decide whether to continue
• Extended-release tablets should not be chewed, rather they should be swallowed whole

Half-Life
• Adults: 9–12 hours for d-amphetamine
• Children (6–12): 9 hours for d-amphetamine and 11 hours for l-amphetamine

Bioavailability
• Can be taken with or without food
• Taking with food may delay peak action two to three hours

Adjustment for Hepatic Dysfunction (by Child-Pugh Criteria)
• Use with caution in categories B or C (moderate-severe impairment)

Adjustment for Renal Dysfunction
• (Mydayis®) Adults with severe renal impairment (GFR 15 to 30 ml/min/1.73 m²) start at 12.5 mg/day with maximum dose of 25 mg/day
• (Mydayis®) Children (13–17) with severe renal impairment, the maximum dose is 12.5 mg if tolerated
• (Mydayis®) Not recommended for use in patients with end-stage renal disease (ESRD <15 ml/min/1.73 m²)

H. MEDICATIONS TO AVOID IN COMBINATION/WARNINGS [2, 3]

 Gastrointestinal (GI) and urinary acidifying agents

- GI acidifying agents (e.g. ascorbic acid, fruit juice, glutamic acid, guanethidine, reserpine, etc.) and urinary acidifying agents (e.g. ammonium chloride, sodium phosphate, etc.) can lower amphetamine plasma levels. May be useful to administer in overdose

 GI and urinary alkalinizing agents

- GI alkalinizing agents (e.g. sodium bicarbonate) and urinary alkalinizing agents (e.g. acetazolamide, some thiazides) can increase amphetamine plasma levels and potentiate the action of amphetamine. Co-administration of amphetamines and alkalinizing agents should be avoided

 Norepinephrine reuptake blockers (e.g. venlafaxine, duloxetine, atomoxetine, milnacipran, reboxetine)

- Norepinephrine reuptake blockers (e.g. venlafaxine, duloxetine, atomoxetine, milnacipran, reboxetine) could add to amphetamine's central nervous system (CNS) and cardiovascular effects

 Desipramine and Protryptiline

- Can cause substantial and sustained increases in d-amphetamine brain concentrations and may add to the cardiovascular effects of d-amphetamine

 MAOIs

- MAOIs slow absorption of amphetamines, thus potentiating their actions. This can cause headache, hypertension and rarely hypertensive crisis and malignant hyperthermia and sometimes death
- Use with MAOIs and within 14 days of MAOIs is not advised

 Adrenergic blockers

- Amphetamines inhibit adrenergic blockers and enhance adrenergic effects of norepinephrine

 cyp 2D6 Inhibitors (e.g. paroxetine and fluoxetine (also serotonergic drugs), quinidine, ritonavir)

- The concomitant use of mixed amphetamine salts and cyp 2D6 inhibitors may increase the exposure of mixed amphetamine salts compared to the use of the drug alone and increase the risk of serotonin syndrome. Initiate with lower doses and monitor patients for signs and symptoms of serotonin syndrome particularly during mixed amphetamine salts initiation and after a dosage increase. If serotonin syndrome occurs, discontinue mixed amphetamine salts and the cyp 2D6 inhibitor

 Serotonergic drugs (e.g. selective serotonin reuptake inhibitors (SSRI), serotonin norepinephrine reuptake inhibitors (SNRI), triptans, tricyclic antidepressants (TCAs), fentanyl, lithium, tramadol, tryptophan, buspirone, St. John's Wort)

- The concomitant use of mixed amphetamine salts and serotonergic drugs increases the risk of serotonin syndrome. Initiate with lower doses and monitor patients for signs and symptoms of serotonin syndrome, particularly during mixed amphetamine salt initiation or dosage increase. If serotonin syndrome occurs, discontinue mixed amphetamine salts and the concomitant serotonergic drug(s)

 Corticosteroids

- Amphetamines can raise corticosteroid levels. This increase is greatest in the evening
- Amphetamines may interfere with urinary steroid determinations

 Propoxyphene

- Amphetamines contribute to excessive CNS stimulation when used with large doses of propoxyphene and fatal convulsions can occur

Meperidine

• Amphetamines increase the analgesic effects of meperidine

 Veratrum alkaloids, other antihypertensives

• Amphetamines may antagonize hypotensive effects of antihypertensives

 Phenobarbital, phenytoin, ethosuximide

• Amphetamines delay absorption of phenobarbital, phenytoin and ethosuximide

 Proton Pump Inhibitors

• Time to maximum concentration (T) of amphetamine is decreased compared to when administered alone. Monitor patients for changes in clinical effect and adjust therapy based on clinical response

 Chlorpromazine

• Chlorpromazine blocks dopamine and norepinephrine reuptake, thus inhibiting the central stimulant effects of amphetamines, and can be used to treat amphetamine poisoning

 Warnings

• Do not use in advanced arteriosclerosis, symptomatic cardiovascular disease, moderate to severe hypertension, hyperthyroidism, known hypersensitivity or idiosyncrasy to the sympathomimetic amines, glaucoma
• Do not use in agitated states
• Do not use in patients with a history of drug abuse
• Do not use during or within 14 days following the administration of MAOIs (hypertensive crisis may result)
• Serious cardiovascular events can occur with amphetamine use
• Sudden death in patients with pre-existing structural cardiac abnormalities or other serious heart problems can occur in those taking amphetamines
• Amphetamines can be associated with peripheral vasculopathy, including Raynaud's phenomenon.
• Difficulties with accommodation and blurring of vision have been reported with stimulant treatment
• Amphetamines may counteract sedating effects of antihistamines
• Amphetamine stimulatory effects may be inhibited by antipsychotics and mood stabilizers
• Amphetamines could inhibit the antipsychotic effects of antipsychotics
• Amphetamines could inhibit mood stabilizing properties of mood stabilizers

- Controlled-release delivery of some d,l-amphetamine formulations may be long enough in duration to eliminate the need for lunch-time dosing.
- D,l-amphetamine may be more effective or tolerable in patients unresponsive to other stimulants, including methylphenidate and vice versa.
- Adderall® and Adderall XR® have a mix of d- and l-amphetamine salts in a 3:1 ratio.
- Adderall® and Adderall XR® combine dextroamphetamine saccharate, dextroamphetamine sulfate, d,l-amphetamine aspartate and d,l-amphetamine sulfate. This mixture may have a different pharmacological profile including mechanism of action and duration of action, compared to pure dextroamphetamine which is a given as a sulfate salt.
- D-amphetamine may more profoundly work on dopamine than norepinephrine while l-amphetamine may have a more balanced action on dopamine and norepinephrine.
- Thus in theory, the Adderall® and Adderall XR® mixture of amphetamine salts may have more noradrenergic action as compared to pure dextroamphetamine sulfate, though this has not been proven and may not have clinical significance. However, some patients respond to or tolerate Adderall®/Adderall XR® differently than they do pure dextroamphetamine sulfate.
- Adderall XR® capsules contain two types of drug-containing beads which provide a double-pulsed amphetamine delivery to prolong their release.
- May be useful in depressive symptoms in medically ill elderly patients and in post-stroke patients.
- May be useful for residual major depressive disorder symptoms including cognitive dysfunction and fatigue/anergia that did not respond to prior treatments.
- Classical augmentation strategy for major depressive disorder.
- Can help treat cognitive impairment, depressive symptoms, and severe fatigue in HIV and cancer patients.
- Can potentiate opioid analgesia and decrease sedation in end-of-life management.
- Can reverse sexual dysfunction (decreased libido, erectile dysfunction, delayed ejaculation and anorgasmia) due to psychiatric illness and some drugs including SSRIs.
- Atypical antipsychotics can treat stimulant overdose or psychosis due to stimulant use/abuse.
- Half-life and duration of clinical action tend to be shorter in younger children.
- Drug abuse may be lower in ADHD adolescents treated with stimulants compared to those not treated.

References

1. Fry, J. M. (1998). Treatment modalities for narcolepsy. *Neurology*, 50, S43–48.
2. Stahl, S. M., Grady, M. M., Munter, N. (2017). *Prescriber's Guide: Stahl's Essential Psychopharmacology*. Cambridge: Cambridge University Press.
3. Teva Pharmaceuticals USA Inc. (2020). *Dextroamphetamine saccharate, amphetamine as partate, dextroamphetamine sulfate and amphetamine sulfate tablets (mixed salts of a single entity amphetamine product) Package Insert*. Parsippany, New Jersey.
4. Greenhill, L. L., Pliszka, S., Dulcan, M. K., et al. (2002). Practice parameter for the use of stimulant medications in the treatment of children, adolescents, and adults. *J Am Acad Child Adolesc Psychiatry*, 41, 26S–49S.
5. Stiefel, G., Besag, F. M. (2010). Cardiovascular effects of methylphenidate, amphetamines and atomoxetine in the treatment of attention-deficit hyperactivity disorder. *Drug Saf*, 33, 821–842.

Histaminic Stimulants
2.77 Armodafinil

A. BASIC INFORMATION [1]

Principle Trade Names
• Nuvigil

Legal Status
• Prescription only
• Controlled, Schedule IV

Classifications
• Histaminic stimulant
• Dopamine reuptake inhibitor (D-RI)
• Wake-promoting agent

Generics Available
• Yes

Formulations
• Tablets: 50 mg; 150 mg; 250 mg

FDA Indications
• Reducing excessive sleepiness in patients with narcolepsy and shift work sleep disorder
• Reducing excessive sleepiness in patients with obstructive sleep apnea/hypopnea syndrome (OSAHS) (adjunct to standard treatment for underlying airway obstruction)

Other Data-Supported Indications
• Attention deficit hyperactivity disorder (ADHD)
• Fatigue and sleepiness in depression
• Fatigue in multiple sclerosis
• Bipolar depression

B. MECHANISMS OF ACTION [1, 2]

Dopamine
• Binds to and requires presence of dopamine transporter. Also requires presence of α-adrenergic receptors
• Thought to act as an inhibitor of the dopamine transporter
• Selectively increases neuronal activity in the hypothalamus

Tuberomammillary Nucleus (TMN) Activity
• It is thought to enhance activity in the hypothalamic wakefulness center (TMN)

within the hypothalamic sleep-wake switch by an unknown mechanism

Histamine
• Activates TMN neurons that release histamine

Orexin/Hypocretin
• Activates other hypothalamic neurons that release orexin/hypocretin, increasing reticular activating network activity in the brainstem

C. PLASMA CONCENTRATIONS AND TREATMENT RESPONSE [1]

Initial Target Range
• 150–250 mg/day
• No established plasma concentration range

Range for Treatment Resistance
• Maximum dose 250 mg/day
• No established plasma concentration range

Typical Time to Response
• Can immediately decrease daytime sleepiness and improve cognitive task performance within two hours of first dose

Time-Course of Improvement
• Can take several days to optimize dosing and clinical improvement

 D. TYPICAL TREATMENT RESPONSE [1, 2]

Usual Target Symptoms
• Sleepiness
• Concentration
• Physical and mental fatigue

Common Short-Term Adverse Effects
• Headache, anxiety, dizziness, insomnia, dry mouth, diarrhea, nausea

Rare Adverse Effects
• Dyspepsia, fatigue, palpitations, rash, upper abdominal pain, agitation, anorexia, constipation, disturbance in attention, dyspnea, hyperhidrosis, increased gamma-glutamyltransferase, tachycardia, influenza-like illness, paresthesias, polyuria, pyrexia, seasonal allergy, thirst, tremor, vomiting
• Transient ECG ischemic changes in patients with mitral valve prolapse or left ventricular hypertrophy have been reported.
• Severe dermatologic reactions (Stevens-Johnson Syndrome and others)
• Angioedema, anaphylactoid reactions, drug reaction with eosinophilia and systemic symptoms (DRESS)/multi-organ hypersensitivity reactions have been reported

• Psychiatric symptoms: psychosis, mania, depression
• Post-marketing experience includes central nervous system (CNS) symptoms including restlessness, disorientation, confusion, excitation and hallucinations; digestive changes such as nausea and diarrhea; and cardiovascular changes such as tachycardia, bradycardia, hypertension and chest pain
• Overdose: agitation, insomnia, increase in hemodynamic parameters

Long-Term Effects
• The need for continued treatment should be re-evaluated periodically

History
- Monitor closely in patients with history of drug abuse
- Monitor for changes in mood, psychosis, mania or suicidal ideation especially in patients with underlying psychiatric illness
- Patients with abnormal levels of sleepiness should be advised that their level of wakefulness may not return to normal with use of armodafinil. Patients with excessive sleepiness should be frequently reassessed for their degree of sleepiness and, if appropriate, advised to avoid driving or any other potentially dangerous activity
- Use with caution in patients with cardiac impairment
- Do not use in patients with left ventricular hypertrophy, ischemic ECG changes, chest pain, arrhythmias or recent myocardial infarction
- Do not use if there is a proven allergy to armodafinil or modafinil
- Limited experience in patients over 65
- Armodafinil clearance may be reduced in elderly patients

Physical
- No specific examination

Neurological
- Assessment of drowsiness/fatigue

Blood Tests
- None for healthy individuals

Cardiac Tests
- Transient ECG ischemic changes have been reported in patients with mitral valve prolapse or left ventricular hypertrophy (rare)

Urine Tests
- No specific tests

Pregnancy Test
- Pregnancy test (premenopausal females)
- Classified as risk not ruled out
- Intrauterine growth restriction and spontaneous abortion have been reported with armodafinil and modafinil
- In animal studies, developmental toxicity was observed at clinically relevant plasma exposure of armodafinil and modafinil
- Armodafinil should generally be stopped before anticipated pregnancies
- It is not known if armodafinil is secreted in human breast milk. However, it is assumed that all psychotropics are secreted in breast milk
- Thus, it is recommended to stop the drug or bottle feed

Other Tests (ECG, etc.)
- None

During Titration or After Dose Adjustment

- May not completely normalize wakefulness
- If it does not work, change the dose. Some may do better with an increased dose, but others may do better with a decreased dose
- Higher doses may be better than lower doses for daytime sleepiness in sleep disorders
- Lower doses may be paradoxically better than higher doses in some patients with problems concentrating and fatigue

Maintenance

- Treat until improvement stabilizes then continue indefinitely as long as improvement persists (studies support at least 12 weeks of treatment)
- Dose may creep up in some patients with long-term treatment due to autoinduction. A drug holiday may restore efficacy at the original dose

Initial Dosing

- OSA and narcolepsy, start at 150 mg/day as a single dose in the morning
- Shift work sleep disorder, give 150 mg/day as a single dose one hour prior to the start of the work shift

Titration

- Titrate up or down only as necessary if not optimally efficacious at the standard starting dose of 150 mg/day

Half-Life

- 12–15 hours

Bioavailability

- Undetermined
- Can be taken with or without food
- Taking with food may delay peak action two to four hours

Adjustment for Hepatic Dysfunction (by Child-Pugh Criteria)

- Reduce dose in severely impaired patients

Adjustment for Renal Dysfunction

- Use with caution

H. MEDICATIONS TO AVOID IN COMBINATION/WARNINGS [1, 4]

 ### cyp 2C19 Substrates (e.g. diazepam, phenytoin, propranolol, omeprazole, clomipramine)

- Armodafinil may increase plasma levels of drugs metabolized by cyp 2C19

 ### cyp 3A4 Substrates (e.g. ethinyl estradiol, triazolam, midazolam, cyclosporine)

- Armodafinil may decrease plasma levels of cyp 3A4 substrates
- Due to induction of cyp 3A4 effectiveness of steroidal contraceptives may be reduced, including up to one month after discontinuation. It is advised to use alternative contraception while taking armodafinil and up to one month after its discontinuation

 ### cyp 3A4 Inducers (e.g. carbamazepine) and Inhibitors (e.g. fluvoxamine and fluoxetine)

- cyp 3A4 inducers may lower armodafinil plasma levels
- cyp 3A4 inhibitors may increase armodafinil plasma levels

 ### cyp 3A4 Autoinduction

- Armodafinil may slightly decrease its own plasma levels by autoinduction of cyp 3A4

 ### Warfarin

- Prothrombin times should be monitored in patients taking both warfarin and armodafinil

 ### Methylphenidate and Dextroamphetamine

- Armodafinil's absorption may be delayed by an hour if given in conjunction with methylphenidate and or dextroamphetamine
- However, co-administration of these agents does not significantly change the pharmacokinetics of armodafinil or either stimulant

 ### α1 Antagonists (e.g. prazosin)

- α1 antagonists may block the therapeutic actions of armodafinil

 ### Monoamine oxidase inhibitors (MAOIs)

- Interaction studies with MAOIs have not been done. MAOIs should only be given with armodafinil by experts with careful monitoring

 ### Warnings

- Serious rash, including Stevens-Johnson Syndrome: discontinue armodafinil at the first sign of rash, unless the rash is clearly not drug-related
- DRESS/multi-organ hypersensitivity reactions: if suspected, discontinue armodafinil
- Angioedema and anaphylaxis reactions: if suspected, discontinue armodafinil
- Persistent sleepiness: assess patients frequently for degree of sleepiness and, if appropriate, advise patients to avoid driving or engaging in any other potentially dangerous activity
- Psychiatric symptoms: use particular caution in treating patients with a history of psychosis, depression or mania. Consider discontinuing armodafinil if psychiatric symptoms develop
- Known cardiovascular disease: consider increased monitoring
- In OSAHS patients for whom continuous positive airway pressure (CPAP) is the treatment of choice, maximal effort should be made to treat with CPAP prior to starting armodafinil. CPAP should be continued after starting armodafinil
- Armodafinil is not a replacement for sleep

- Armodafinil is the longer lasting R-enantiomer of racemic modafinil.
- Armodafinil maintains high plasma concentrations later in the day than modafinil on a mg-to-mg basis. This could theoretically improve wakefulness throughout the day with armodafinil compared to modafinil.
- Armodafinil is selective for areas of the brain that promote sleep and wakefulness.
- Armodafinil has less activation and less potential for abuse than stimulants though may not work as well as stimulants in some patients.
- Armodafinil has a novel michanism of action and novel therapeutic uses compared to stimulants.
- Controlled studies suggest armodafinil improves attention in OSAHS and shift work sleep disorder, but controlled studies of attention have not been performed in ADHD or major depressive disorder.
- Controlled studies of racemic modafinil in ADHD suggest improvement in attention.
- May be useful to treat fatigue in patients with depression and other disorders such as multiple sclerosis, myotonic dystrophy and HIV/AIDS.
- May be useful in treating sleepiness associated with opioid analgesia especially in end-of-life management.
- Some controlled trials suggest efficacy in bipolar depression as an adjunct to atypical antipsychotics.
- The subjective sensation associated with armodafinil is usually normal wakefulness rather than stimulation. Though rarely jitteriness can occur.

References

1. Actavis Pharma Inc. (2019). *Armodafinil Package Insert.* Parsippany, New Jersey.
2. Murillo-Rodríguez, E., Barciela Veras, A., Barbosa Rocha, N., et al. (2018). An overview of the clinical uses, pharmacology, and safety of modafinil. *ACS Chem Neurosci,* 9, 151–158.
3. Darwish, M., Kirby, M., Hellriegel, E. T., et al. (2009). Armodafinil and modafinil have substantially different pharmacokinetic profiles despite having the same terminal half-lives: analysis of data from three randomized, single-dose, pharmacokinetic studies. *Clin Drug Investig,* 29, 613–623.
4. Darwish, M., Kirby, M., Robertson, P., Jr., et al. (2008). Interaction profile of armodafinil with medications metabolized by cytochrome P450 enzymes 1A2, 3A4 and 2C19 in healthy subjects. *Clin Pharmacokinet,* 47, 61–74.
5. Stahl, S. M., Grady, M. M., Munter, N. (2017). *Prescriber's Guide: Stahl's Essential Psychopharmacology.* Cambridge: Cambridge University Press.

2.78 Modafinil

A. BASIC INFORMATION [1–3]

Principle Trade Names
- Provigil®
- Alertec®

Legal Status
- Prescription only
- Controlled, Schedule IV

Classifications
- Dopamine reuptake inhibitor (D-RI)
- Histaminic stimulant
- Wake-promoting agent

Generics Available
- Yes

Formulations
- Tablets: 100 mg; 200 mg (scored)

FDA Indications
- Reducing excessive sleepiness in patients with narcolepsy and shift work sleep disorder
- Reducing excessive sleepiness in patients with obstructive sleep apnea/hypopnea syndrome (OSAHS) (adjunct to standard treatment for underlying airway obstruction)

Other Data-Supported Indications
- Attention deficit hyperactivity disorder (ADHD)
- Fatigue and sleepiness in depression
- Fatigue in multiple sclerosis
- Bipolar depression

B. MECHANISMS OF ACTION [3, 4]

Dopamine
- Binds to and requires presence of dopamine transporter. Also requires presence of α-adrenergic receptors
- Thought to act as an inhibitor of the dopamine transporter
- Selectively increases neuronal activity in the hypothalamus

Tuberomammillary Nucleus (TMN) Activity
- It is thought to enhance activity in the hypothalamic wakefulness center (TMN)

within the hypothalamic sleep-wake switch by an unknown mechanism

Histamine
- Activates TMN neurons that release histamine

Orexin/Hypocretin
- Activates other hypothalamic neurons that release orexin/hypocretin, increasing the activity level of the reticular activating system in the brainstem

C. PLASMA CONCENTRATIONS AND TREATMENT RESPONSE [3, 4, 5]

Initial Target Range
- 200 mg/day in the morning
- No established plasma concentration range

Range for Treatment Resistance
- Maximum dose usually 400 mg/day
- No established plasma concentration range

Typical Time to Response
- Can immediately decrease daytime sleepiness and improve cognitive task performance within two hours of first dose

Time-Course of Improvement
- Can take several days to optimize dosing and clinical improvement

D. TYPICAL TREATMENT RESPONSE [3, 4, 6]

Usual Target Symptoms
- Sleepiness
- Concentration
- Physical and mental fatigue

Common Short-Term Adverse Effects
- Headache (dose-dependent), nausea, nervousness, rhinitis, diarrhea, back pain, anxiety (dose-dependent), insomnia, dizziness, dyspepsia, dry mouth, anorexia, pharyngitis, infection, hypertension, palpitations

Rare Adverse Effects
- Chest pain, abnormal liver functions, constipation, depression, paresthesia, somnolence, tachycardia, vasodilation, abnormal vision, agitation, asthma, chills, confusion, dyskinesia, edema, emotional lability, eosinophilia, epistaxis, flatulence, hyperkinesia, hypertonia, mouth ulceration, sweating, taste perversion, thirst, tremor, urine abnormalities, vertigo
- Transient ECG ischemic changes in patients with mitral valve prolapse or left ventricular hypertrophy have been reported

- Severe dermatologic reactions (Stevens-Johnson Syndrome and others)
- Angioedema, anyphylactoid reactions, drug reaction with eosinophilia and systemic symptoms (DRESS)/multi-organ hypersensitivity reactions have been reported
- Psychiatric symptoms: psychosis, mania, depression
- Post-marketing experience includes central nervous system (CNS) symptoms including restlessness, disorientation, confusion, excitation and hallucinations; digestive changes such as nausea and diarrhea; and cardiovascular changes such as tachycardia, bradycardia, hypertension and chest pain
- Overdose: no fatalities; agitation, insomnia, increase in hemodynamic parameters

Long-Term Effects
- Unpublished data show safety for up to 136 weeks
- The need for continued treatment should be re-evaluated periodically

History

- Monitor closely in patients with history of drug abuse
- Monitor for changes in mood, psychosis, mania or suicidal ideation especially in patients with underlying psychiatric illness
- Patients with abnormal levels of sleepiness should be advised that their level of wakefulness may not return to normal with use of modafinil. Patients with excessive sleepiness should be frequently reassessed for their degree of sleepiness and, if appropriate, advised to avoid driving or any other potentially dangerous activity
- Use with caution in patients with cardiac impairment
- Do not use in patients with severe hypertension, left ventricular hypertrophy, ischemic ECG changes, chest pain, arrhythmias or recent myocardial infarction
- Do not use if there is a proven allergy to armodafinil or modafinil
- Limited experience in patients over 65
- Modafinil clearance may be reduced in elderly patients

Physical

- No specific examination

Neurological

- Assessment of drowsiness/fatigue

Blood Tests

- None for healthy individuals

Cardiac Tests

- Transient ECG ischemic changes have been reported in patients with mitral valve prolapse or left ventricular hypertrophy (rare)

Urine Tests

- No specific tests

Pregnancy Test

- Pregnancy test (premenopausal females)
- Classified as risk not ruled out
- Intrauterine growth restriction and spontaneous abortion have been reported with armodafinil and modafinil
- In animal studies, developmental toxicity was observed at clinically relevant plasma exposure of armodafinil and modafinil
- Modafinil should generally be stopped before anticipated pregnancies
- It is not known if modafinil is secreted in human breast milk. However, it is assumed that all psychotropics are secreted in breast milk
- Thus, it is recommended to stop the drug or bottle feed

Other Tests (ECG, etc.)

- None

During Titration or After Dose Adjustment
- May not completely normalize wakefulness
- If it does not work, change the dose. Some may do better with an increased dose but others may do better with a decreased dose
- Higher doses (200–800 mg/day) may be better than lower doses (50–200 mg/day) for daytime sleepiness in sleep disorders
- Lower doses (50–200 mg/day) may be paradoxically better than higher doses (200–800 mg/day) in some patients with problems concentrating and fatigue
- Dose may creep up in some patients with long-term treatment due to autoinduction. A drug holiday may restore efficacy at the original dose

Maintenance
- Treat until improvement stabilizes then continue indefinitely as long as improvement persists
- Efficacy in decreasing excessive sleepiness in sleep disorders has been demonstrated in nine- to twelve-week trials

Initial Dosing
- OSA and narcolepsy, start at 200 mg/day as a single dose in the morning
- Shift work sleep disorder, give 200 mg/day as a single dose one hour prior to the start of the work shift

Titration
- Titrate up or down only as necessary if not optimally efficacious at the standard starting dose of 200 mg/day

Half-Life
- 10–12 hours

Bioavailability
- Undetermined
- Can be taken with or without food
- Taking with food may delay peak action by one hour

Adjustment for Hepatic Dysfunction (by Child-Pugh Criteria)
- Reduce dose by half in severely impaired patients

Adjustment for Renal Dysfunction
- Use with caution, dose reduction is recommended

H. MEDICATIONS TO AVOID IN COMBINATION/WARNINGS [2, 3, 9]

 cyp 2C19 Substrates (e.g. diazepam, phenytoin, propranolol, omeprazole, clomipramine)

- Modafinil may increase plasma levels of drugs metabolized by cyp 2C19

 cyp 2D6 Substrates (e.g. tricyclic antidepressants (TCAs) and selective serotonin reuptake inhibitors (SSRIs))

- Modafinil may increase plasma levels of cyp 2D6 substrates, which may require a downward dose adjustment of these agents

 cyp 3A4 Substrates (e.g. ethinyl estradiol, triazolam, midazolam, cyclosporine)

- Modafinil may decrease plasma levels of cyp 3A4 substrates
- Due to induction of cyp 3A4, effectiveness of steroidal contraceptives may be reduced, including up to one month after discontinuation. It is advised to use alternative contraception while taking modafinil and up to one month after its discontinuation

 cyp 3A4 Inducers (e.g. carbamazepine) and Inhibitors (e.g. fluvoxamine and fluoxetine)

- cyp 3A4 inducers may lower modafinil plasma levels
- cyp 3A4 inhibitors may increase modafinil plasma levels

 cyp 3A4 Autoinduction

- Modafinil may slightly decrease its own plasma levels by autoinduction of cyp 3A4

 cyp 1A2 Substrates

- Modafinil may increase clearance of cyp 1A2 substrates which would reduce their plasma levels

 Warfarin

- Prothrombin times should be monitored in patients taking both warfarin and modafinil

 Methylphenidate

- Modafinil's absorption may be delayed by an hour if given in conjunction with methylphenidate and or dextroamphetamine
- Co-administration of methylphenidate and or dextroamphetamine does not significantly change the pharmacokinetics of modafinil or either stimulant

 α_1 **Antagonists (e.g. prazosin)**

- α_1 antagonists may block the therapeutic actions of modafinil

 Monoamine oxidase inhibitors (MAOIs)

- Interaction studies with MAOIs have not been done. MAOIs should only be given with modafinil by experts with careful monitoring

 Warnings

- Serious rash, including Stevens-Johnson Syndrome: discontinue modafinil at the first sign of rash, unless the rash is clearly not drug-related
- Angioedema and anaphylaxis reactions: if suspected, discontinue modafinil
- Multi-organ hypersensitivity reactions: if suspected, discontinue modafinil
- Persistent sleepiness: assess patients frequently for degree of sleepiness and, if appropriate, advise patients to avoid driving or engaging in any other potentially dangerous activity
- Psychiatric symptoms: use caution in patients with a history of psychosis, depression or mania. Consider discontinuing modafinil if psychiatric symptoms develop
- Known cardiovascular disease: consider increased monitoring
- In OSAHS patients for whom continuous positive airway pressure (CPAP) is the treatment of choice, maximal effort should be made to treat with CPAP prior to starting modafinil. CPAP should be continued after starting modafinil
- Modafinil is not a replacement for sleep

ART OF PSYCHOPHARMACOLOGY: TAKE-HOME PEARLS

- Can be used off label for jet lag, short-term.
- Modafinil is selective for areas of the brain involved in sleep and wakefulness.
- Modafinil has less activation and less potential for abuse than stimulants though may not work as well as stimulants in some patients.
- Modafinil has a novel mechanism of action and novel therapeutic uses compared to stimulants.
- Controlled studies suggest modafinil improves attention in OSAHS, shift work sleep disorder, and ADHD (both children and adults), but controlled studies of attention have not been performed in major depressive disorder.
- May be useful to treat fatigue in patients with depression and other disorders such as multiple sclerosis, myotonic dystrophy and HIV/AIDS.

- In depression, modafinil's actions on fatigue appear independent of actions on mood.
- In depression, modafinil's actions on sleepiness appear independent of actions on mood but may be linked to actions on fatigue or on global functioning.
- Several control studies in depression show improvement in sleepiness or global functioning, especially for depressed patients with sleepiness and fatigue.
- May be a useful adjunct to mood stabilizers for bipolar depression.
- May be useful in treating sleepiness associated with opioid analgesia especially in end-of-life management.
- The subjective sensation associated with modafinil is usually normal wakefulness rather than stimulation. Though rarely jitteriness can occur.

 References

1. Kumar, R. (2008). Approved and investigational uses of modafinil: an evidence-based review. *Drugs*, 68, 1803–1839.
2. Murillo-Rodríguez, E., Barciela Veras, A., Barbosa Rocha, N., et al. (2018). An overview of the clinical uses, pharmacology, and safety of modafinil. *ACS Chem Neurosci*, 9, 151–158.
3. Heritage Pharmaceuticals Inc. (2020). *Modafinil Package Insert*. East Brunswick, New Jersey.
4. Wesensten, N. J., Belenky, G., Kautz, M. A., et al. (2002). Maintaining alertness and performance during sleep deprivation: modafinil versus caffeine. *Psychopharmacology (Berl)*, 159, 238–247.
5. Cox, J. M., Pappagallo, M. (2001). Modafinil: a gift to portmanteau. *Am J Hosp Palliat Care*, 18, 408–410.
6. Batéjat, D. M., Lagarde, D. P. (1999). Naps and modafinil as countermeasures for the effects of sleep deprivation on cognitive performance. *Aviat Space Environ Med*, 70, 493–498.
7. Jasinski, D. R., Koyacevic-Ristanovic, R. (2000). Evaluation of the abuse liability of modafinil and other drugs for excessive daytime sleepiness associated with narcolepsy. *Clin Neuropharmacol*, 23, 149–156.
8. Darwish, M., Kirby, M., Hellriegel, E. T., et al. (2009). Armodafinil and modafinil have substantially different pharmacokinetic profiles despite having the same terminal half-lives: analysis of data from three randomized, single-dose, pharmacokinetic studies. *Clin Drug Investig*, 29, 613–623.
9. Bourdon, L., Jacobs, I., Bateman, W. A., et al. (1994). Effect of modafinil on heat production and regulation of body temperatures in cold-exposed humans. *Aviat Space Environ Med*, 65, 999–1004.
10. Stahl, S. M., Grady, M. M., Munter, N. (2017). *Prescriber's Guide: Stahl's Essential Psychopharmacology*. Cambridge: Cambridge University Press.

Cognitive Agents
2.79 Dextromethorphan/Quinidine

A. BASIC INFORMATION [1–3]

Principle Trade Names
• Nudexta®

Legal Status
• Prescription only
• Not controlled

Classifications
• Noncompetitive N-methyl-D-Aspartate (NMDA) receptor antagonist and σ_1 agonist

Generics Available
• No

Formulations
• Capsule: 20 mg/10 mg (dextromethorphan/quinidine)

FDA Indications
• Pseudobulbar affect

Other Data-Supported Indications
• Diabetic peripheral neuropathic pain
• Unstable mood and affect in post-traumatic stress disorder (PTSD) and mild traumatic brain injury (TBI)
• Third-line for treatment-resistant depression

B. MECHANISMS OF ACTION [2–4]

Glutamate
• By blocking NMDA receptors and acting as σ_1 receptor agonist dextromethorphan reduces glutamate neurotransmission

Serotonin
• May modulate serotonin levels as dextromethorphan has affinity for serotonin transporters

Quinidine
• Quinidine increases the availability of dextromethorphan by inhibiting its metabolism via cyp 2D6

Initial Target Range
• 20 mg/10 mg twice per day
• No established plasma concentration range

Range for Treatment Resistance
• Some patients may tolerate to and respond to higher than approved doses but there are few controlled studies of high doses
• No established plasma concentration range

Typical Time to Response
• In clinical trials the rate of pseudobulbar affect episodes was significantly decreased by day 15

Time-Course of Improvement
• If no response by six to eight weeks at maximum tolerated dose, it may not be effective and therapy should be withdrawn

Usual Target Symptoms
• Uncontrollable crying
• Uncontrollable laughter

Common Short-Term Adverse Effects
• Dizziness, asthenia, diarrhea, vomiting, cough, peripheral edema, urinary tract infection, euphoria, influenza, increased gamma-glutamyltransferase and flatulence

Rare Adverse Effects
• Immune-mediated thrombocytopenia, hepatotoxicity, dose-dependent QT prolongation, dissociative symptoms, sedation
• Cinchonism due to chronic quinidine toxicity is characterized by nausea, vomiting, diarrhea, headache tinnitus, hearing loss, vertigo, blurred vision, diplopia, photophobia, confusion and delirium

• Acute psychotic reactions have been reported after the first dose of quinidine, but this is extremely rare
• Other adverse reactions occasionally reported with quinidine include depression, mydriasis, disturbed color perception, night blindness, scotomata, optic neuritis and visual field loss photosensitivity, keratopathy, and abnormalities of skin pigmentation
• Overdose: nausea, dizziness, headache, ventricular arrhythmias, hypotension, coma, respiratory depression, seizures, tachycardia, hyperexcitability, toxic psychosis

Long-Term Effects
• The experience in open-label clinical trials is consistent with the safety profile observed in the placebo-controlled clinical trials

History

- Do not use in patients taking a monoamine oxidase inhibitor (MAOI)
- Do not use in patients taking another medication containing quinidine, quinine or mefloquine
- Do not use in patients with history of quinidine, quinine or mefloquine-induced thrombocytopenia, hepatitis, or other hypersensitivity reaction
- Do not use in patients with prolonged QT interval, congenital long QT syndrome, history suggestive of Torsades de Pointes or heart failure
- Do not use in patients with complete atrioventricular block (AV) without implanted pacemaker, or patients at high risk of complete AV block
- Do not use in patients taking a drug that prolongs QT interval and is metabolized by cyp 2D6 (e.g. thioridazine, pimozide)
- Do not use if there is a proven allergy or hypersensitivity to dextromethorphan or quinidine
- Cases of dextromethorphan abuse have been reported, predominantly in adolescents
- Patients with a history of drug abuse should be observed closely for signs of dextromethorphan/quinidine misuse or abuse (e.g. development of tolerance, increases in dose, drug-seeking behavior)

Physical

- If patients taking dextromethorphan/quinidine experience symptoms that could indicate the occurrence of cardiac arrhythmias, e.g. syncope or palpitations, dextromethorphan/quinidine should be discontinued and the patient further evaluated

Neurological

- No specific examination

Blood Tests

- None for healthy individuals

Cardiac Tests

- ECG should be monitored in patients who must take a QT interval prolonging agent or one that inhibits cyp 3A4
- Monitor ECG in patients with left ventricular hypertrophy or left ventricular dysfunction

Urine Tests

- No specific tests

Pregnancy Test

- Pregnancy test (premenopausal females)
- Controlled studies have not been conducted in pregnant women
- Some animal studies have shown adverse effects
- Dextromethorphan should generally be stopped before anticipated pregnancies
- Quinidine is excreted in human milk. Dextromethorphan is probably secreted in breast milk
- If child becomes irritable or sedated, breastfeeding or drug may need to be stopped
- Must weigh benefits of breastfeeding with risks and benefits of treatment versus nontreatment to both the infant and the mother

Other Tests (ECG, etc.)

- ECG should be monitored in patients who must take a QT interval prolonging agent or one that inhibits cyp 3A4
- Monitor ECG in patients with left ventricular hypertrophy or left ventricular dysfunction

During Titration or After Dose Adjustment

- When initiating dextromethorphan/quinidine in patients at risk of QT prolongation and Torsades de Pointes, ECG evaluation of QT interval should be conducted at baseline and three to four hours after the first dose. This includes patients concomitantly taking/initiating drugs that prolong the QT interval or that are strong or moderate cyp 3A4 inhibitors, and patients with left ventricular hypertrophy (LVH) or left ventricular dysfunction (LVD)
- Elderly patients may tolerate lower doses better

Maintenance

- ECG should be monitored in patients who must take a QT interval prolonging agent or one that inhibits cyp 3A4
- Re-evaluate ECG if risk factors for arrhythmia change during the course of treatment with dextromethorphan/quinidine (e.g. electrolyte abnormality (hypokalemia, hypomagnesemia), bradycardia, and family history of QT abnormality
- Hypokalemia and hypomagnesemia should be corrected prior to initiation of therapy with dextromethorphan/quinidine, and should be monitored during treatment

Initial Dosing

- 20 mg/10 mg once per day

Titration

- Increase to 20 mg/10 mg twice per day after seven days

Half-Life

- 13 hours for dextromethorphan
- Seven hours for quinidine

Bioavailability

- 11% for dextromethorphan
- Food does not affect absorption

Adjustment for Hepatic Dysfunction (by Child-Pugh Criteria)

- Dose adjustment not necessary in patients with mild to moderate impairment

Adjustment for Renal Dysfunction

- Dose adjustment not necessary in patients with mild to moderate impairment

cyp 2D6 Substrates (e.g. desipramine, tricyclic antidepressants (TCAs), paroxetine and fluoxetine)

- Quinidine may increase plasma levels of cyp 2D6 substrates, which may require a downward dose adjustment of these agents
- Desipramine plasma levels increased eight-fold in conjunction with dextromethorphan/quinidine. Reduce desipramine dose and adjust based on clinical response
- Paroxetine plasma levels increased two-fold in conjunction with dextromethorphan/quinidine. Reduce paroxetine dose and adjust based on clinical response

 Strong and moderate cyp 3A inhibitors (e.g. atazanavir, clarithromycin, indinavir, itraconazole, ketoconazole, nefazodone, nelfinavir, ritonavir, saquinavir, telithromycin, amprenavir, aprepitant, diltiazem, erythromycin, fluconazole, fosamprenavir, grapefruit juice and verapamil)

- cyp 3A4 inhibitors may increase plasma levels of quinidine, which may require a downward dose adjustment of dextromethorphan/quinidine

 Monoamine oxidase inhibitors (MAOIs)

- Can cause fatal serotonin syndrome. Do not use dextromethorphan/quinidine with MAOIs or for at least 14 days after MAOIs have been stopped
- Do not start a MAOI for at least five half-lives (five to seven days for most drugs) after stopping dextromethorphan/quinidine

 P-glycoprotein substrates (e.g. digoxin)

- Quinidine is a P-glycoprotein inhibitor, thus may increase plasma levels of P-glycoprotein substrates, which may require a downward dose adjustment of these agents

 Selective serotonin reuptake inhibitors (SSRIs)/TCAs

- Dextromethorphan/quinidine combined with SSRIs or TCAs can theoretically cause serotonin syndrome, but this is not well studied

 QT prolonging agents

- Dextromethorphan/quinidine can cause a dose-dependent and additive increase in QT intervals, especially when these agents are cyp 2D6 substrates (e.g. thioridazine, pimozide)

 Warnings

- Quinidine can cause immune-mediated thrombocytopenia that can be severe or fatal; dextromethorphan/quinidine should be stopped immediately if thrombocytopenia occurs unless it is clearly not drug-related, and should not be restarted in sensitized patients
- Quinidine has been associated with a lupus-like syndrome involving polyarthritis
- Hepatitis has been seen in patients taking quinidine. Stop quinidine if this occurs
- ECG should be monitored if patient must take an agent that prolongs QT interval or that inhibits cyp 3A4
- Monitor ECG in patients with LVH or LVD
- Do not use in patients taking another medication containing quinidine, quinine or mefloquine
- Do not use in patients with history of quinidine, quinine or mefloquine-induced thrombocytopenia, hepatitis, or other hypersensitivity reaction
- Do not use in patients with prolonged QT interval, congenital long QT syndrome, history suggestive of Torsades de Pointes or heart failure
- Do not use in patients with complete AV block without implanted pacemaker, or patients at high risk of complete AV block
- Anticholinergic effects of quinidine may lead to worsening in myasthenia gravis and other sensitive conditions
- Take precautions to reduce falls as dextromethorphan/quinidine may cause dizziness

ART OF PSYCHOPHARMACOLOGY: TAKE-HOME PEARLS

- Quinidine is intended to increase the actions of dextromethorphan by inhibiting its metabolism by cyp 2D6; thus, poor metabolizers of cyp 2D6 may not benefit as much from this treatment and may experience adverse effects associated with quinidine.
- Affective instability and agitation in Alzheimer's disease may be treatable with this agent, allowing antipsychotics to be avoided in this population.

- Some men express emotional lability as laughter and anger rather than laughter and crying.
- Affective instability in PTSD and in mild TBI may be improved by dextromethorphan/quinidine.
- Dextromethorphan/quinidine has similar binding properties to ketamine which suggests possible efficacy in treatment-resistant depression and chronic pain.

References

1. Garnock-Jones, K. P. (2011). Dextromethorphan/quinidine: in pseudobulbar affect. *CNS Drugs*, 25, 435–445.
2. Stahl, S. M., Grady, M. M., Munter, N. (2017). *Prescribers Guide: Stahl's Essential Psychopharmacology*. Cambridge: Cambridge University Press.
3. Avanir Pharmaceuticals Inc. (2019). *Nudexta Package Insert*. Aliso Viejo, California.
4. Pioro, E. P., Brooks, B. R., Cummings, J., et al. (2010). Dextromethorphan plus ultra low-dose quinidine reduces pseudobulbar affect. *Ann Neurol*, 68, 693–702.

2.80 Donepezil

A. BASIC INFORMATION [1–3]

Principle Trade Names
- Aricept®
- Memac®

Legal Status
- Prescription only
- Not controlled

Classifications
- Acetylcholine enzyme inhibitor (Ach-EI)
- Acetylcholinesterase inhibitor (selective)

Generics Available
- Yes

Formulations
- Tablets: 5 mg; 10 mg; 23 mg
- Orally disintegrating tablets: 5 mg; 10 mg

FDA Indications
- Alzheimer's disease (mild, moderate and severe)

Other Data-Supported Indications
- Memory disorders in other conditions
- Mild cognitive impairment

B. MECHANISM OF ACTION [1–3]

Acetylcholine
- Noncompetitively and reversibly inhibits central acting acetylcholinesterase increasing availability of acetylcholine
- Having more acetylcholine available compensates in part for degenerating cholinergic neurons in the nucleus basalis that regulate memory

Other
- Does not inhibit butylcholinesterase
- May release growth factors or interfere with amyloid deposition
- There is no evidence that donepezil alters the course of the underlying dementing process

C. PLASMA CONCENTRATIONS AND TREATMENT RESPONSE [2, 3]

Initial Target Range
- Mild to moderate Alzheimer's disease: 5 mg or 10 mg once daily at night
- Severe Alzheimer's disease: 10 mg once daily at night
- No established plasma concentration range

Range for Treatment Resistance
- Maximum dose: tablet 10 mg/day or 23 mg/day
- Probably best to utilize highest tolerated dose within the usual dosage range
- Cognitive improvement may be linked to substantial (>65%) inhibition of acetyl-cholinesterase
- No established plasma concentration range

Typical Time to Response
- May take up to six weeks before any evidence of improvement in baseline memory or behavior

Time-Course of Improvement
- May take months before any stabilization in degenerative course is evident
- What you see may depend upon how early you treat
- If discontinued, taper to avoid withdrawal effects
- Discontinuation may lead to notable deterioration in memory and behavior, which may not be restored when drug is restarted or another cholinesterase inhibitor is initiated

 D. TYPICAL TREATMENT RESPONSE [2, 3]

Usual Target Symptoms
- Memory loss in Alzheimer's disease
- Behavioral symptoms in Alzheimer's disease
- Memory loss in other neurocognitive disorders

Common Short-Term Adverse Effects
- Nausea, diarrhea, vomiting, appetite loss, increased gastric acid secretion, weight loss, insomnia, dizziness, muscle cramps, fatigue, depression, abnormal dreams
- The most prominent side effects of donepezil are gastrointestinal (GI) effects, which are usually mild and transient

Rare Adverse Effects
- Seizures, syncope

- Overdose: can be lethal; nausea, vomiting, excess salivation, sweating, hypotension, bradycardia, collapse, convulsions, muscle weakness (weakness of respiratory muscles can lead to death)

Long-Term Effects
- Must evaluate lack of efficacy and loss of efficacy over months, not weeks
- Drug may lose effectiveness in slowing degenerative course of Alzheimer's disease after six months
- Treat the patient but ask the caregiver about efficacy
- Can be effective in some patients for several years

History

- Should be used with caution in patients with cardiac impairment
- Syncopal episodes have been reported with the use of donepezil
- Do not use if there is a proven allergy or hypersensitivity to donepezil or to piperidine derivatives

Physical
Neurological

- No specific examination

Blood Tests

- None for healthy individuals

Cardiac Tests

- ECG if history of cardiac disease

Urine Tests

- No specific tests

Pregnancy Test

- Pregnancy test (premenopausal females)
- Classified as risk not ruled out
- Controlled studies have not been conducted in pregnant women
- Donepezil is not recommended for use in pregnant women or women of childbearing potential
- Probably secreted in breast milk
- Donepezil is not recommended for use in nursing women

Other Tests (ECG, etc.)

- None

During Titration or After Dose Adjustment

- Donepezil can cause vomiting so patients should be observed closely at initiation of treatment and after dose increases
- Some elderly patients may tolerate lower doses better
- Women over 85, particularly with low body weights, may experience more adverse effects
- Side effects occur more frequently at higher doses than at lower doses

- Slower titration (e.g. six weeks to 10 mg/day) may reduce the risk of side effects
- For patients with intolerable side effects, generally allow a washout period with resolution of side effects prior to switching to another cholinesterase inhibitor

Maintenance

- Must evaluate lack of efficacy and loss of efficacy over months, not weeks
- Treat the patient but ask the caregiver about efficacy

Initial Dosing

- 5 mg/day

Titration

- May increase to 10 mg/day after four to six weeks

Half-Life

- 70 hours

Bioavailability

- ~100%
- Food does not affect absorption

Adjustment for Hepatic Dysfunction (by Child-Pugh Criteria)

- Few data available; may need to lower dose

Adjustment for Renal Dysfunction

- Dose adjustment is most likely unnecessary

H. MEDICATIONS TO AVOID IN COMBINATION/WARNINGS [2, 3, 5]

Anesthetics

• Donepezil is likely to exaggerate succinylcholine-type muscle relaxation during anesthesia and should be discontinued prior to surgery

cyp 2D6 and cyp 3A4 Inhibitors

• cyp 2D6 and cyp 3A4 inhibitors may inhibit the metabolism of donepezil and increase its plasma levels

cyp 2D6 and cyp 3A4 Inducers

• cyp 2D6 and cyp 3A4 inducers may increase clearance of donepezil and decrease its plasma levels

Anticholinergic Agents

• Donepezil in combination with anticholinergic agents may decrease efficacy of both

Cholinergic Agents (e.g. bethanechol)

• Donepezil in combination with cholinergic agents may have a synergistic effect

Neuromuscular Blocking Agents (e.g. succinylcholine)

• Donepezil in combination with succinylcholine or similar neuromuscular blocking agents may have a synergistic effect

Beta-Blockers

• Donepezil in combination with beta-blockers may cause bradycardia

Levodopa

• Donepezil could theoretically reduce the efficacy of levodopa in Parkinson's disease

Cholinesterase Inhibitors

• It is not rational to combine donepezil with other cholinesterase inhibitors

Warnings

• Donepezil may exacerbate asthma or other pulmonary disease, prescribe with care in this population
• Donepezil may increase gastric acid secretion which may increase the risk of ulcers so monitor closely for symptoms of active or occult GI bleeding, especially those at increased risk for developing ulcers (e.g. those with a history of ulcer disease or those receiving concurrent nonsteroidal anti-inflammatory drugs (NSAIDs))
• Donepezil may have vagotonic effects on the sinoatrial and atrioventricular nodes manifesting as bradycardia or heart block in patients with or without cardiac impairment
• Cholinomimetics may cause bladder outflow obstructions
• Cholinomimetics are believed to have some potential to cause generalized convulsions
• Women over 85, particularly with low body weights, may experience more adverse effects
• Use with caution in underweight or frail patients
• Safety and efficacy have not been established in children or adolescents

2.80 Donepezil (Continued)

- Potential advantages of donepezil; once a day dosing, may be used in vascular dementia, may work in some patients who do not respond to other cholinesterase inhibitors, may work in some patients who do not tolerate other cholinesterase inhibitors.
- Fixed-dose combination of extended-release memantine and donepezil is approved for the treatment of moderate to severe Alzheimer's dementia in patients stabilized on memantine and donepezil.
- Dramatic reversal of symptoms of Alzheimer's disease is not generally seen with cholinesterase inhibitors which can lead to skepticism among prescribers and lack of an appropriate trial of a cholinesterase inhibitor.
- Treats behavioral and psychological symptoms of Alzheimer's dementia as well as cognitive symptoms (i.e. especially apathy, disinhibition, delusions, anxiety, cooperation, pacing).
- Patients who complain themselves of memory problems may have depression, whereas patients whose spouses or children complain of the patient's memory problems may have Alzheimer's disease.
- The first symptoms of Alzheimer's disease are generally mood changes; thus, Alzheimer's disease may initially be diagnosed as depression.
- What you see may depend upon how early you treat.
- Women may experience cognitive symptoms in perimenopause due to hormonal changes that are not a sign of dementia or Alzheimer's disease.
- Aggressively treat concomitant symptoms with augmentation (e.g. atypical antipsychotics for agitation, antidepressants for depression).
- If treatment with antidepressants fails to improve apathy and depressed mood in the elderly, it is possible that this may be early Alzheimer's disease and a cholinesterase inhibitor may be helpful.
- What to expect from a cholinesterase inhibitor; patients do not generally improve dramatically although this can be observed in a significant minority of patients, onset of behavioral problems and nursing home placement can be delayed, functional outcomes, including activities of daily living, can be preserved, caregiver burden and stress can be reduced.
- Delay in progression in Alzheimer's disease is not evidence of disease-modifying actions of cholinesterase inhibition.
- Cholinesterase inhibitors depend upon the presence of intact targets for acetylcholine for maximum effectiveness and therefore may be most effective in the early stages of Alzheimer's disease.
- Donepezil may cause more sleep disturbances than other cholinesterase inhibitors.
- Weight loss can be a problem in Alzheimer's patients with debilitation and muscle wasting.
- Women over 85, particularly with low body weights, may experience more adverse effects.
- Use with caution in underweight or frail patients.
- Cognitive improvement may be linked to substantial (>65%) inhibition of acetylcholinesterase.
- Donepezil has greater action on acetylcholinesterase in the CNS versus the periphery.
- Some Alzheimer's patients who fail to respond to donepezil may respond to another cholinesterase inhibitor and vice versa.
- To prevent potential clinical deterioration, switch from long-term treatment with one cholinesterase inhibitor to another without a washout period.
- Donepezil may slow the progression of mild cognitive impairment to Alzheimer's disease.
- Donepezil may be useful for dementia with Lewy bodies (DLB, constituted by early loss of attentiveness and visual perception with possible hallucinations, Parkinson-like movement problems, fluctuating cognition such as daytime drowsiness and lethargy, staring into space for long periods, episodes of disorganized speech).
- Donepezil may decrease delusions, apathy, agitation and hallucinations in dementia with Lewy bodies.
- Donepezil may be useful for vascular dementia (e.g. acute onset with slow stepwise progression that has plateaus,

often with gait abnormalities, focal signs, imbalance and urinary incontinence).
- Donepezil may be helpful for dementia in Down's syndrome.
- Donepezil may be useful in some cases of treatment-resistant bipolar disorder.
- Donepezil may theoretically be useful for ADHD, but not yet proven.
- Donepezil may theoretically be useful in any memory condition characterized by cholinergic deficiency (e.g. some cases of brain injury, cancer chemotherapy-induced cognitive changes, etc.).

References

1. Birks, J. S., Harvey, R. (2003). Donepezil for dementia due to Alzheimer's disease. *Cochrane Database Syst Rev*, CD001190, doi: 10.1002/14651858
2. Stahl, S. M., Grady, M. M., Munter, N. (2017). *Prescribers Guide: Stahl's Essential Psychopharmacology*. Cambridge: Cambridge University Press.
3. Camber Pharmaceuticals Inc. (2020). *Donepezil Package Insert*. Piscataway, New Jersey.
4. Jones, R. W. (2003). Have cholinergic therapies reached their clinical boundary in Alzheimer's disease? *Int J Geriatr Psychiatry*, 18, S7–S13.
5. Bentue-Ferrer, D., Tribut, O., Polard, E., et al. (2003). Clinically significant drug interactions with cholinesterase inhibitors: a guide for neurologists. *CNS Drugs*, 17, 947–963.

2.81 Galantamine

A. BASIC INFORMATION [1, 2]

Principle Trade Names
- Razadyne®
- Razadyne ER®

Legal Status
- Prescription only
- Not controlled

Classifications
- Acetylcholine multimodal; enzyme inhibitor; receptor PAM (Ach-MM)
- Cholinesterase inhibitor (acetyl-cholinesterase inhibitor); allosteric nicotinic cholinergic modulator

Generics Available
- Yes

Formulations
- Tablets: 4 mg; 8 mg; 12 mg
- Extended-release capsules: 8 mg; 16 mg; 24 mg
- Liquid: 4 mg/ml – 100 ml bottle

FDA Indications
- Alzheimer's disease (mild to moderate)

Other Data-Supported Indications
- Memory disturbances in other neurocognitive disorders
- Memory disturbances in other conditions
- Mild cognitive impairment

B. MECHANISMS OF ACTION [3-7]

Acetylcholine
- Reversibly and competitively inhibits central acting acetylcholinesterase (AChE), increasing availability of acetylcholine
- Having more acetylcholine available compensates in part for degenerating cholinergic neurons in the nucleus basalis that regulate memory
- Modulates nicotinic receptors which enhances actions of acetylcholine

Other
- Nicotinic modulation may also enhance actions of other neurotransmitters by increasing the release of dopamine, norepinephrine, serotonin, gamma-aminobutyric acid (GABA) and glutamate
- Does not inhibit butylcholinesterase
- May release growth factors or interfere with amyloid deposition
- There is no evidence that galantamine alters the course of the underlying dementing process

C. PLASMA CONCENTRATIONS AND TREATMENT RESPONSE [2, 8]

Initial Target Range
• 16–24 mg/day

Range for Treatment Resistance
• Maximum dose: 24 mg/day
• Probably best to utilize highest tolerated dose within the usual dosage range
• Cognitive improvement may be linked to substantial (>65%) inhibition of acetylcholinesterase
• No established plasma concentration range

Typical Time to Response
• May take up to six weeks before any evidence of improvement in baseline memory or behavior

Time-Course of Improvement
• May take months before any stabilization in degenerative course is evident
• What you see may depend upon how early you treat
• Discontinuation may lead to notable deterioration in memory and behavior, which may not be restored when drug is restarted, or another cholinesterase inhibitor is initiated

D. TYPICAL TREATMENT RESPONSE [2, 8]

Usual Target Symptoms
• Memory loss in Alzheimer's disease
• Behavioral symptoms in Alzheimer's disease
• Memory loss in other dementias

Common Short-Term Adverse Effects
• Nausea, diarrhea, vomiting, appetite loss, increased gastric acid secretion, weight loss, headache, dizziness, fatigue and depression
• The most prominent side effects of galantamine are gastrointestinal (GI) effects, which are usually mild and transient
• GI effects may be reduced if galantamine is titrated slowly and given with food

Rare Adverse Effects
• Seizures and syncope
• Overdose: can be lethal; nausea, vomiting, excess salivation, sweating, hypotension, bradycardia, collapse, convulsions, muscle weakness (weakness of respiratory muscles can lead to death)

Long-Term Effects
• Must evaluate lack of efficacy and loss of efficacy over months, not weeks
• Drug may lose effectiveness in slowing degenerative course of Alzheimer's disease after six months
• Treat the patient but ask the caregiver about efficacy
• Can be effective in some patients for several years

E. PRE-TREATMENT WORKUP AND INITIAL LABORATORY TESTING (6)

History
- Should be used with caution in patients with cardiac impairment
- Syncopal episodes have been reported with the use of galantamine
- Do not use if there is a proven allergy or hypersensitivity to galantamine

Physical
- During therapy, the patient's weight should be monitored

Neurological
- No specific examination

Blood Tests
- None for healthy individuals

Cardiac Tests
- ECG if history of cardiac disease

Urine Tests
- No specific tests

Pregnancy Test
- Pregnancy test (premenopausal females)
- Classified as risk not ruled out
- Controlled studies have not been conducted in pregnant women
- Animal studies have shown adverse effects
- Galantamine is not recommended for use in pregnant women or women of childbearing potential
- Probably secreted in breast milk
- Galantamine is not recommended for use in nursing women

Other Tests (ECG, etc.)
- None

 F. MONITORING (2)

During Titration or After Dose Adjustment
- GI effects may be reduced if galantamine is titrated slowly and given with food
- If therapy has been interrupted for more than three days, the patient should be restarted at the lowest dosage and retitrated to the current dose
- Galantamine can cause vomiting so patients should be observed closely at initiation of treatment and after dose increases
- Some elderly patients may tolerate lower doses better
- Women over 85, particularly with low body weights, may experience more adverse effects

- Side effects occur more frequently at higher doses than at lower doses
- Slower titration (e.g. six weeks to 16 mg BID) may reduce the risk of side effects
- For patients with intolerable side effects, generally allow a washout period with resolution of side effects prior to switching to another cholinesterase inhibitor

Maintenance
- During therapy, the patient's weight should be monitored
- Must evaluate lack of efficacy and loss of efficacy over months, not weeks
- Treat the patient but ask the caregiver about efficacy

Initial Dosing
- Immediate-release: 4 mg twice daily, take with meals; ensure adequate fluid intake during treatment
- Extended-release: 8 mg once a day in the morning, preferably with food

Titration
- Immediate-release: increase to 8 mg twice daily after four weeks; after four more weeks may increase to 12 mg twice daily
- Extended-release: increase to 16 mg once a day in the morning after four weeks; after four more weeks may increase to 24 mg once in the morning

Half-Life
- Seven hours

Bioavailability
- 90%

Adjustment for Hepatic Dysfunction (by Child-Pugh Criteria)
- Should not exceed 16 mg/day for moderate hepatic impairment
- Do not use in patients with severe hepatic impairment

Adjustment for Renal Dysfunction
- Should not exceed 16 mg/day for creatinine clearance 9–59 ml/min
- Do not use in patients with creatinine clearance less than 9 ml/min

2.81 Galantamine (Continued)

2.81 Galantamine (Continued)

H. MEDICATIONS TO AVOID IN COMBINATION/WARNINGS [2, 8, 9]

Anesthetics

- Galantamine is likely to exaggerate succinylcholine-type muscle relaxation during anesthesia and should be discontinued prior to surgery

cyp 2D6 and cyp 3A4 Inhibitors

- cyp 2D6 and cyp 3A4 inhibitors may inhibit the metabolism of galantamine and increase its plasma levels

cyp 2D6 and cyp 3A4 Inducers

- cyp 2D6 and cyp 3A4 inducers may increase clearance of galantamine and decrease its plasma levels

Anticholinergic Agents

- Galantamine in combination with anticholinergic agents may decrease efficacy of both

Cholinergic Agents (e.g. bethanechol)

- Galantamine in combination with cholinergic agents may have a synergistic effect

Neuromuscular Blocking Agents (e.g. succinylcholine)

- Galantamine in combination with succinylcholine or similar neuromuscular blocking agents may have a synergistic effect

Beta-Blockers

- Galantamine in combination with beta-blockers may cause bradycardia

Levodopa

- Galantamine could theoretically reduce the efficacy of levodopa in Parkinson's disease

Cholinesterase Inhibitors

- It is not rational to combine galantamine with other cholinesterase inhibitors

Cimetidine

- Cimetidine may increase the oral bioavailability of galantamine

Warnings

- Galantamine can cause serious skin reactions (Stevens-Johnson Syndrome and acute generalized exanthematous pustulosis), discontinue at first appearance of skin rash unless the rash is clearly not drug-related; if signs or symptoms suggest a serious skin reaction, do not resume galantamine, alternative therapy should be considered
- Galantamine may exacerbate asthma or other pulmonary disease, prescribe with care in this population
- Galantamine may increase gastric acid secretion which may increase the risk of ulcers so monitor closely for symptoms of active or occult GI bleeding, especially those at increased risk for developing ulcers (e.g. those with a history of ulcer disease or those receiving concurrent nonsteroidal anti-inflammatory drugs (NSAIDs))
- Galantamine may have vagotonic effects on the sinoatrial and atrioventricular nodes manifesting as bradycardia or heart block in patients with or without cardiac impairment
- Cholinomimetics may cause bladder outflow obstructions
- Cholinomimetics are believed to have some potential to cause generalized convulsions
- Women over 85, particularly with low body weights, may experience more adverse effects
- Use with caution in underweight or frail patients
- Use of cholinesterase inhibitors may be associated with increased rates of syncope, bradycardia, pacemaker insertion and hip fracture in older adults with dementia
- Safety and efficacy have not been established in children or adolescents

- Galantamine is a natural product present in daffodils and snowdrops.
- New extended-release formulation allows for once daily dosing.
- Novel dual action uniquely combines acetylcholinesterase inhibition with allosteric nicotine modulation.
- Novel dual action should theoretically enhance cholinergic actions but incremental clinical benefits have been difficult to demonstrate.
- Actions at nicotinic receptors enhance not only the release of acetylcholine but also other neurotransmitters, which may boost attention and improve behaviors caused by deficiencies in those neurotransmitters in Alzheimer's disease.
- Dramatic reversal of symptoms of Alzheimer's disease is not generally seen with cholinesterase inhibitors.
- Can lead to skepticism among prescribers and lack of an appropriate trial of a cholinesterase inhibitor.
- What you see may depend upon how early you treat.
- Women may experience cognitive symptoms in perimenopause due to hormonal changes that are not a sign of dementia or Alzheimer's disease.
- Aggressively treat concomitant symptoms with augmentation (e.g. atypical antipsychotics for agitation, antidepressants for depression).
- If treatment with antidepressants fails to improve apathy and depressed mood in the elderly, it is possible that this may be early Alzheimer's disease and a cholinesterase inhibitor may be helpful.
- What to expect from a cholinesterase inhibitor; patients do not generally improve dramatically although this can be observed in a significant minority of patients, onset of behavioral problems and nursing home placement can be delayed, functional outcomes, including activities of daily living, can be preserved, caregiver burden and stress can be reduced.
- Delay in progression in Alzheimer's disease is not evidence of disease-modifying actions of cholinesterase inhibition.
- Cholinesterase inhibitors depend upon the presence of intact targets for acetylcholine for maximum effectiveness and therefore

may be most effective in the early stages of Alzheimer's disease.
- Weight loss can be a problem in Alzheimer's patients with debilitation and muscle wasting.
- Women over 85, particularly with low body weights, may experience more adverse effects.
- Use with caution in underweight or frail patients.
- Cognitive improvement may be linked to substantial (>65%) inhibition of acetylcholinesterase.
- Some Alzheimer's patients who fail to respond to galantamine may respond to another cholinesterase inhibitor and vice versa.
- To prevent potential clinical deterioration, switch from long-term treatment with one cholinesterase inhibitor to another without a washout period.
- Galantamine may slow the progression of mild cognitive impairment to Alzheimer's disease.
- Galantamine may be useful for dementia with Lewy bodies (DLB, constituted by early loss of attentiveness and visual perception with possible hallucinations, Parkinson-like movement problems, fluctuating cognition such as daytime drowsiness and lethargy, staring into space for long periods, episodes of disorganized speech).
- Galantamine may decrease delusions, apathy, agitation and hallucinations in DLB.
- Galantamine may be useful for vascular dementia (e.g. acute onset with slow stepwise progression that has plateaus, often with gait abnormalities, focal signs, imbalance and urinary incontinence).
- Galantamine may be helpful for dementia in Down's syndrome.
- Galantamine may be useful in some cases of treatment-resistant bipolar disorder.
- Galantamine may theoretically be useful for ADHD, but not yet proven.
- Galantamine may theoretically be useful in any memory condition characterized by cholinergic deficiency (e.g. some cases of brain injury, cancer chemotherapy-induced cognitive changes, etc.).

2.81 Galantamine (Continued)

 References

1. Olin, J., Schneider, L. (2002). Galantamine for Alzheimer's disease. *Cochrane Database Syst Rev*, CD001747, doi: 10.1002/14651858
2. Stahl, S. M., Grady, M. M., Munter, N. (2017). *Prescribers Guide: Stahl's Essential Psychopharmacology*. Cambridge: Cambridge University Press.
3. Stahl, S. M. (2000). The new cholinesterase inhibitors for Alzheimer's disease, part 2: illustrating their mechanisms of action. *J Clin Psychiatry*, 61, 813–814.
4. Stahl, S. M. (2000). The new cholinesterase inhibitors for Alzheimer's disease, part 1: their similarities are different. *J Clin Psychiatry*, 61, 710–711.
5. Coyle, J., Kershaw, P. (2001). Galantamine, a cholinesterase inhibitor that allosterically modulates nicotinic receptors: effects on the course of Alzheimer's disease. *Biol Psychiatry*, 49, 289–299.
6. Bonner, L. T., Peskind, E. R. (2002). Pharmacologic treatments of dementia. *Med Clin North Am*, 86, 657–674.
7. Jones, R. W. (2003). Have cholinergic therapies reached their clinical boundary in Alzheimer's disease? *Int J Geriatr Psychiatry*, 18, S7–S13.
8. Zydus Pharmaceuticals USA Inc. (2020). *Galantamine Package Insert*. Pennington, New Jersey.
9. Bentue-Ferrer, D., Tribut, O., Polard, E., et al. (2003). Clinically significant drug interactions with cholinesterase inhibitors: a guide for neurologists. *CNS Drugs*, 17, 947–963.

2.82 Memantine

A. BASIC INFORMATION [1–3]

Principle Trade Names
- Namenda®
- Namenda XR®

Legal Status
- Prescription only
- Not controlled

Classifications
- Glutamate receptor antagonist
- N-methyl-D-aspartate (NMDA) receptor antagonist

Generics Available
- Yes

Formulations
- Tablets: 5 mg; 10 mg
- Oral solution: 2 mg/ml
- Extended-release capsules: 7 mg; 14 mg; 21 mg; 28 mg

FDA Indications
- Alzheimer's disease (moderate to severe)

Other Data-Supported Indications
- Alzheimer's disease (mild to moderate)
- Memory disorders in other conditions
- Mild cognitive impairment
- Chronic pain

B. MECHANISMS OF ACTION [1–4]

Glutamate
- Memantine is a noncompetitive antagonist with low to moderate affinity for the NMDA receptor
- Memantine binds preferentially to the NMDA receptor operated cation (calcium) channels

- Memantine is presumed to interfere with the postulated persistent activation of NMDA receptors by excessive glutamate release in Alzheimer's disease
- It is also thought to block calcium-influx-induced excitotoxicity

C. PLASMA CONCENTRATIONS AND TREATMENT RESPONSE [3, 5]

Initial Target Range
- 10 mg twice a day
- 28 mg once daily (extended-release)
- No established plasma concentration range

Range for Treatment Resistance
- Immediate-release maximum dose: 10 mg twice a day
- Extended-release maximum dose: 28 mg once a day
- No established plasma concentration range

Typical Time to Response
- Improvements in memory are not expected and it may take months before any stabilization in degenerative course is evident

Time-Course of Improvement
- Changes, e.g. behavioral improvement or slowing of cognitive decline, may occur over weeks to months

D. TYPICAL TREATMENT RESPONSE [3, 5]

Usual Target Symptoms
- Memory loss in Alzheimer's disease
- Behavioral symptoms in Alzheimer's disease
- Memory loss in other dementias

Common Short-Term Adverse Effects
- Dizziness, headache, confusion and constipation

Rare Adverse Effects
- Seizures

- Overdose: agitation, asthenia, bradycardia, confusion, coma, dizziness, ECG changes, increased blood pressure, lethargy, loss of consciousness, psychosis, restlessness, slowed movement, somnolence, stupor, unsteady gait, visual hallucinations, vertigo, vomiting and weakness

Long-Term Effects
- Drug may lose effectiveness in slowing degenerative course of Alzheimer's disease after six months

E. PRE-TREATMENT WORKUP AND INITIAL LABORATORY TESTING [5]

History
- Do not use if there is a proven allergy or hypersensitivity to memantine

Physical
- No specific examination

Neurological
- No specific examination

Blood Tests
- None for healthy individuals

Cardiac Tests
- None

Urine Tests
- No specific tests

Pregnancy Test
- Pregnancy test (premenopausal females)
- Classified as risk not ruled out
- Controlled studies have not been conducted in pregnant women
- Animal studies have shown adverse effects
- Memantine is not recommended for use in pregnant women or women of childbearing potential
- Probably secreted in breast milk
- Memantine is not recommended for use in nursing women

Other Tests (ECG, etc.)
- None

F. MONITORING [5]

During Titration or After Dose Adjustment
- Periodically re-evaluate mental status and cognitive performance

Maintenance
- If a patient fails to take memantine for several days, dosing may need to be resumed at lower doses and retitrated as described above

G. DOSING INFORMATION [5]

Initial Dosing
- Immediate-release: 5 mg/day
- Extended-release: 7 mg once daily

Titration
- Immediate-release: can increase by 5 mg each week; doses over 5 mg should be divided; maximum dose 10 mg twice daily
- Extended-release: can increase by 7 mg each week; maximum dose 28 mg once daily

Half-Life
- 60–80 hours

Bioavailability
- ~100%

- Food does not affect absorption

Adjustment for Hepatic Dysfunction (by Child-Pugh Criteria)
- Memantine should be administered with caution to patients with severe hepatic impairment

Adjustment for Renal Dysfunction
- Dose adjustment not necessary in patients with mild to moderate impairment
- Recommended dose is 5 mg twice a day in patients with severe impairment

H. MEDICATIONS TO AVOID IN COMBINATION/WARNINGS [3, 5]

 Drugs (e.g. carbonic anhydrase inhibitors, sodium bicarbonate) and clinical state of the patient (e.g. renal tubular acidosis or severe infections of the urinary tract) that raise urine pH)
- May reduce elimination of memantine and increase plasma levels of memantine
- Memantine should be used with caution under these conditions

 NMDA antagonists (amantadine, ketamine and dextromethorphan)
- Use memantine cautiously with other NMDA antagonists as their combined use has not been systematically evaluated

- Memantine is well tolerated with a low incidence of adverse effects.
- No interactions with drugs metabolized by cyp enzymes as mostly excreted unchanged in the urine.
- No interactions with cholinesterase inhibitors.
- Memantine has not been studied in children or adolescents.
- There is no evidence that memantine prevents or slows neurodegeneration in patients with Alzheimer's disease.
- Memantine's actions are somewhat like the natural inhibition of NMDA receptors by magnesium, and thus memantine is a sort of "artificial magnesium".
- Theoretically, NMDA antagonism of memantine is strong enough to block chronic low level overexcitation of glutamate receptors associated with Alzheimer's disease, but not strong enough to interfere with periodic high level utilization of glutamate for plasticity, learning and memory.
- Structurally related to the antiparkinsonian and anti-influenza agent amantadine, which is also a weak NMDA antagonist.

- Antagonist actions at $5HT_3$ receptors have unknown clinical consequences but may contribute to low incidence of GI side effects.
- A fixed-dose combination of memantine extended-release and donepezil has been approved for the treatment of moderate to severe Alzheimer's dementia in patients stabilized on memantine and donepezil.
- Delay in progression of Alzheimer's disease is not evidence of disease-modifying actions of NMDA antagonism.
- May or may not be effective in vascular dementia.
- Under investigation for dementia associated with HIV/AIDS.
- May or may not be effective in chronic neuropathic pain.
- Theoretically, could be useful in any condition characterized by moderate overactivation of NMDA glutamate receptors (possibly neurodegenerative conditions or even bipolar disorder, anxiety disorders or chronic neuropathic pain), but this is not proven.

References

1. Areosa, S. A., Sherriff, F. (2003). Memantine for dementia. *Cochrane Database Syst Rev*, CD003154, doi: 10.1002/14651858
2. Sani, G., Serra, G., Kotzalidis, G. D., et al. (2012). The role of memantine in the treatment of psychiatric disorders other than the dementias: a review of current preclinical and clinical evidence. *CNS Drugs*, 26, 663–690.
3. Stahl, S. M., Grady, M. M., Munter, N. (2017). *Prescribers Guide: Stahl's Essential Psychopharmacology*. Cambridge: Cambridge University Press.
4. Tariot, P. N., Federoff, H. J. (2003). Current treatment for Alzheimer disease and future prospects. *Alzheimer Dis Assoc Disord*, 17 Suppl. 4, S105–113.
5. Strides Pharma Inc. (2020). *Memantine Package Insert*. East Brunswick, New Jersey.

2.83 Rivastigmine

A. BASIC INFORMATION [1–4]

Principle Trade Names
• Exelon®

Legal Status
• Prescription only
• Not controlled

Classifications
• Acetylcholine enzyme inhibitor (Ach-EI)
• Cholinesterase inhibitor (acetylcholinesterase inhibitor and butylcholinesterase inhibitor)

Generics Available
• Yes

Formulations
• Capsules: 1.5 mg; 3 mg; 4.5 mg; 6 mg
• Liquid: 2 mg/ml – 120 ml bottle
• Transdermal: 9 mg/5 cm² (4.6 mg/24 hours); 18 mg/10 cm² (9.5 mg/24 hours); 27 mg/15 cm² (13.3 mg/24 hours)

FDA Indications
• Alzheimer's disease (mild to moderate)
• Parkinson's disease dementia (mild to moderate)

Other Data-Supported Indications
• Memory disturbances in other conditions
• Mild cognitive impairment

B. MECHANISMS OF ACTION [1–4]

Acetylcholine
• Pseudo-irreversibly inhibits central acting acetylcholinesterase (AChE), increasing availability of acetylcholine
• Having more acetylcholine available compensates in part for degenerating cholinergic neurons in the nucleus basalis that regulate memory

Other
• Inhibits butylcholinesterase (BuChE)
• May release growth factors or interfere with amyloid deposition
• There is no evidence that rivastigmine alters the course of the underlying dementing process

2.83 Rivastigmine (Continued)

C. PLASMA CONCENTRATIONS AND TREATMENT RESPONSE [3, 4]

Initial Target Range
- Oral: 6–12 mg/day in two doses, with meals
- Oral doses between 6–12 mg/day have been shown to be more effective than doses between 1–4 mg/day
- Transdermal: 4.6 mg/24 hours once daily
- No established plasma concentration range

Range for Treatment Resistance
- Oral: maximum dose generally 6 mg twice daily
- Transdermal: maximum recommended dose 13.3 mg/24 hours
- Probably best to utilize highest tolerated dose within the usual dosage range
- Cognitive improvement may be linked to substantial (>65%) inhibition of acetylcholinesterase
- No established plasma concentration range

Typical Time to Response
- May take up to six weeks before any evidence of improvement in baseline memory or behavior

Time-Course of Improvement
- May take months before any stabilization in degenerative course is evident
- What you see may depend upon how early you treat
- Discontinuation may lead to notable deterioration in memory and behavior, which may not be restored when drug is restarted, or another cholinesterase inhibitor is initiated

D. TYPICAL TREATMENT RESPONSE [3, 4]

Usual Target Symptoms
- Memory loss in Alzheimer's disease
- Behavioral symptoms in Alzheimer's disease
- Memory loss in other dementias

Common Short-Term Adverse Effects
- Nausea, diarrhea, vomiting, appetite loss, increased gastric acid secretion, dyspepsia, weight loss, headache, dizziness, fatigue, asthenia and sweating
- Incidence of nausea is generally higher during the titration phase than during maintenance treatment
- Theoretically, butyrylcholinesterase inhibition peripherally could enhance side effects
- The most prominent side effects of rivastigmine are gastrointestinal (GI) effects, which are usually mild and transient
- GI effects may be reduced if rivastigmine is titrated slowly and given with food
- May cause more GI side effects than some other cholinesterase inhibitors, especially if not slowly titrated
- At recommended doses, transdermal formulation may have lower incidence of GI side effects than oral formulation

Rare Adverse Effects
- Seizures and syncope
- Overdose: can be lethal; nausea, vomiting, excess salivation, sweating, hypotension, bradycardia, collapse, convulsions, muscle weakness (weakness of respiratory muscles can lead to death)

Long-Term Effects
- Must evaluate lack of efficacy and loss of efficacy over months, not weeks
- Drug may lose effectiveness in slowing degenerative course of Alzheimer's disease after six months
- Treat the patient but ask the caregiver about efficacy
- Can be effective in some patients for several years

History

- Should be used with caution in patients with cardiac impairment
- Syncopal episodes have been reported with the use of rivastigmine
- Do not use if there is a proven allergy or hypersensitivity to rivastigmine or other carbamates
- Do not use if history of application site reaction with rivastigmine transdermal patch suggestive of allergic contact dermatitis, in the absence of negative allergy testing

Physical

- No specific examination

Neurological

- No specific examination

Blood Tests

- None for healthy individuals

Cardiac Tests

- ECG if history of cardiac disease

Urine Tests

- No specific tests

Pregnancy Test

- Pregnancy test (premenopausal females)
- Classified as risk not ruled out
- Controlled studies have not been conducted in pregnant women
- Animal studies have not shown adverse effects
- Rivastigmine is not recommended for use in pregnant women or women of childbearing potential
- Probably secreted in breast milk
- Rivastigmine is not recommended for use in nursing women

Other Tests (ECG, etc.)

- No specific tests

During Titration or After Dose Adjustment

- Incidence of nausea is generally higher during the titration phase than during maintenance treatment
- Individuals with low body weight may be at greater risk for adverse effects
- GI effects may be reduced if rivastigmine is titrated slowly and given with food
- If therapy has been interrupted for more than three days, the patient should be restarted at the lowest dosage and retitrated to the current dose or there is risk of severe vomiting with possible esophageal rupture
- Some elderly patients may tolerate lower doses better
- Women over 85, particularly with low body weights, may experience more adverse effects
- Side effects occur more frequently at higher doses than at lower doses
- Slower titration may reduce the risk of side effects
- For patients with intolerable side effects, generally allow a washout period with resolution of side effects prior to switching to another cholinesterase inhibitor

Maintenance

- Dementia may cause gradual impairment of driving performance or compromise the ability to use machinery; rivastigmine may also result in adverse reactions that are detrimental to these functions, so routinely evaluate the patient's ability to continue driving or operating machinery
- Must evaluate lack of efficacy and loss of efficacy over months, not weeks
- Treat the patient but ask the caregiver about efficacy

Initial Dosing
- Oral: initial 1.5 mg twice daily
- Transdermal: initial 4.6 mg/24 hours

Titration
- Oral (Alzheimer's disease): increase by 3 mg every two weeks; give twice a day; titrate to tolerability; maximum dose generally 6 mg twice daily
- Oral (Parkinson's disease dementia): increase by 3 mg every four weeks; give twice a day; titrate to tolerability; maximum dose generally 6 mg twice daily
- Transdermal: initial 4.6 mg/24 hours; after four weeks increase to 9.5 mg/24 hours; maximum recommended dose 13.3 mg/24 hours
- For transdermal formulation, dose increases should occur after a minimum of four weeks at the previous dose and only if the previous dose was well tolerated

Half-Life
- 1.5 hours

Bioavailability
- 40%

Adjustment for Hepatic Dysfunction (by Child-Pugh Criteria)
- Patients with mild and moderate hepatic impairment may only be able to tolerate lower doses
- No data are available on the use of rivastigmine in patients with severe hepatic impairment

Adjustment for Renal Dysfunction
- Patients with moderate and severe renal impairment may only be able to tolerate lower doses

Neuromuscular Blocking Agents (e.g. succinylcholine)

- Rivastigmine in combination with succinylcholine or similar neuromuscular blocking agents may have a synergistic effect and should be discontinued prior to surgery

Anticholinergic Agents

- Rivastigmine in combination with anticholinergic agents may decrease efficacy of both

Cholinergic Agents (e.g. bethanechol)

- Rivastigmine in combination with cholinergic agents may have a synergistic effect

Beta-Blockers

- Rivastigmine in combination with beta-blockers may cause bradycardia

Levodopa

- Rivastigmine could theoretically reduce the efficacy of levodopa in Parkinson's disease

Cholinesterase Inhibitors

- It is not rational to combine rivastigmine with other cholinesterase inhibitors

Nicotine

- Nicotine may increase the clearance of rivastigmine

Metoclopramide

- Not recommended to combine rivastigmine with metoclopramide due to risk of additive extrapyramidal effects

Warnings

- Severe vomiting with esophageal rupture may occur if rivastigmine therapy is resumed without retitrating the drug to full dosing after interruption of more than three days
- Individuals with low body weight may be at greater risk for adverse effects
- GI adverse reactions may include significant nausea, vomiting, diarrhea, anorexia/ decreased appetite and weight loss, and may necessitate treatment interruption. Dehydration may result from prolonged vomiting or diarrhea and can be associated with serious outcomes
- Certain transdermal patches containing even small traces of aluminum or other metals in the adhesive backing can cause skin burns if worn during MRI, so warn patients taking the transdermal formulation about this possibility and advise them to disclose this information if they need an MRI
- Discontinue rivastigmine in case of disseminated allergic dermatitis, which may occur after oral or transdermal administration. In patients with suspected allergic contact dermatitis after transdermal rivastigmine use, switch to oral rivastigmine only after negative allergy testing
- It is possible that some patients sensitized to rivastigmine by exposure to rivastigmine patch may not be able to take rivastigmine in any form
- Rivastigmine may exacerbate asthma or other pulmonary disease, prescribe with care in this population
- Rivastigmine may increase gastric acid secretion which may increase the risk of ulcers so monitor closely for symptoms of active or occult GI bleeding, especially those at increased risk for developing ulcers (e.g. those with a history of ulcer disease or those receiving concurrent nonsteroidal anti-inflammatory drugs (NSAIDs))
- Rivastigmine may have vagotonic effects on the sinoatrial and atrioventricular nodes manifesting as bradycardia or heart block in patients with or without cardiac impairment
- Cholinomimetics may cause bladder outflow obstructions
- Cholinomimetics are believed to have some potential to cause generalized convulsions
- Cholinomimetics may exacerbate or induce extrapyramidal symptoms including worsening of Parkinsonian symptoms, particularly tremor
- Women over 85, particularly with low body weight, may experience more adverse effects
- Use with caution in underweight or frail patients
- Use of cholinesterase inhibitors may be associated with increased rates of syncope, bradycardia, pacemaker insertion and hip fracture in older adults with dementia
- Safety and efficacy have not been established in children or adolescents

- Potential advantages: butylcholinesterase's central inhibition could theoretically enhance therapeutic efficacy and may be useful in later stages or rapidly progressive Alzheimer's disease.
- Rivastigmine is not hepatically metabolized; no cyp-mediated pharmacokinetic drug interactions.
- Transdermal patch should only be applied to dry, intact skin on the upper torso or another area unlikely to rub against tight clothing.
- Plasma exposure with transdermal rivastigmine is 20–30% lower when applied to the abdomen or thigh as compared to the upper back, chest or upper arm.
- New application site should be selected for each day; patch should be applied at approximately the same time every day; only one patch should be applied at a time; patches should not be cut; new patch should not be applied to the same spot for at least 14 days.
- Avoid touching the exposed (sticky) side of the patch, and after application, wash hands with soap and water; do not touch eyes until after hands have been washed.
- At recommended doses, transdermal formulation may have lower incidence of GI side effects than oral formulation.
- Dramatic reversal of symptoms of Alzheimer's disease is not generally seen with cholinesterase inhibitors.
- This can lead to skepticism among prescribers and lack of an appropriate trial of a cholinesterase inhibitor.
- What you see may depend upon how early you treat.
- Women may experience cognitive symptoms in perimenopause due to hormonal changes that are not a sign of dementia or Alzheimer's disease.
- Aggressively treat concomitant symptoms with augmentation (e.g. atypical antipsychotics for agitation, antidepressants for depression).
- If treatment with antidepressants fails to improve apathy and depressed mood in the elderly, it is possible that this may be early Alzheimer's disease and a cholinesterase inhibitor may be helpful.
- What to expect from a cholinesterase inhibitor; patients do not generally improve dramatically although this can be observed in a significant minority of patients, onset

- of behavioral problems and nursing home placement can be delayed, functional outcomes, including activities of daily living, can be preserved, caregiver burden and stress can be reduced.
- Delay in progression in Alzheimer's disease is not evidence of disease-modifying actions of cholinesterase inhibition.
- Cholinesterase inhibitors depend upon the presence of intact targets for acetylcholine for maximum effectiveness and therefore may be most effective in the early stages of Alzheimer's disease.
- Weight loss can be a problem in Alzheimer's patients with debilitation and muscle wasting.
- Women over 85, particularly with low body weight, may experience more adverse effects.
- Use with caution in underweight or frail patients.
- Cognitive improvement may be linked to substantial (>65%) inhibition of acetylcholinesterase.
- Some Alzheimer's patients who fail to respond to rivastigmine may respond to another cholinesterase inhibitor and vice versa.
- To prevent potential clinical deterioration, switch from long-term treatment with one cholinesterase inhibitor to another without a washout period.
- Rivastigmine may be more selective for the form of acetylcholinesterase in the hippocampus (G1).
- More potent inhibitor of the G1 form of acetylcholinesterase enzyme, found in high concentrations in Alzheimer's patient brains, than the G4 form of the enzyme.
- Butylcholinesterase action in the brain may not be relevant in individuals without Alzheimer's disease or in early Alzheimer's disease; in the later stages of the disease, the enzyme actively increases as gliosis occurs.
- Rivastigmine's effects on butylcholinesterase may be more relevant in later stages of Alzheimer's disease or for more rapidly progressive forms of Alzheimer's disease, when gliosis is occurring and increasing butylcholinesterase.
- Butylcholinesterase actively could interfere with amyloid plaque formation, which contains this enzyme.

- Rivastigmine may slow the progression of mild cognitive impairment to Alzheimer's disease.
- Rivastigmine may be useful for dementia with Lewy bodies (DLB, constituted by early loss of attentiveness and visual perception with possible hallucinations, Parkinson-like movement problems, fluctuating cognition such as daytime drowsiness and lethargy, staring into space for long periods, episodes of disorganized speech).
- Rivastigmine may decrease delusions, apathy, agitation and hallucinations in DLB.
- Rivastigmine may be useful for vascular dementia (e.g. acute onset with slow stepwise progression that has plateaus, often with gait abnormalities, focal signs, imbalance and urinary incontinence).
- Rivastigmine may be helpful for dementia in Down's syndrome.
- Rivastigmine may be useful in some cases of treatment-resistant bipolar disorder.
- Rivastigmine may theoretically be useful for ADHD, but not yet proven.
- Rivastigmine may theoretically be useful in any memory condition characterized by cholinergic deficiency (e.g. some cases of brain injury, cancer chemotherapy-induced cognitive changes, etc.).

References

1. Birks, J., Grimley Evans, J., Iakovidou, V., et al. (2009). Rivastigmine for Alzheimer's disease. *Cochrane Database Syst Rev*, CD001191, doi: 10.100214651858
2. Dhillon, S. (2011). Rivastigmine transdermal patch: a review of its use in the management of dementia of the Alzheimer's type. *Drugs*, 71, 1209–1231.
3. Stahl, S. M., Grady, M. M., Munter, N. (2017). *Prescribers Guide: Stahl's Essential Psychopharmacology*. Cambridge: Cambridge University Press.
4. Nivagen Pharmaceuticals Inc. (2020). *Rivastigmine Package Insert*. Sacramento, California.
5. Jones, R. W. (2003). Have cholinergic therapies reached their clinical boundary in Alzheimer's disease? *Int J Geriatr Psychiatry*, 18, S7–S13.
6. Bentue-Ferrer, D., Tribut, O., Polard, E., et al. (2003). Clinically significant drug interactions with cholinesterase inhibitors: a guide for neurologists. *CNS Drugs*, 17, 947–963.

α₂-Adrenergic Agonists
2.84 Clonidine

A. BASIC INFORMATION [1–3]

Principle Trade Names
- Duraclon® (injection)
- Catapres®
- Kapvay® (extended-release)

Legal Status
- Prescription only
- Not controlled

Classifications
- Norepinephrine receptor agonist (N-RA)
- Central α_{2a} agonist
- Antihypertensive
- Non-stimulant for ADHD

Generics Available
- Yes (but not for transdermal)

Formulations
- Extended-release tablets: 0.1 mg; 0.2 mg
- Immediate-release tablets: 0.1 mg scored; 0.2 mg scored; 0.3 mg scored
- Transdermal (seven-day administration): 0.1 mg/24 hours; 0.2 mg/24 hours; 0.3 mg/24 hours
- Injection: 0.1 mg/ml; 0.5 mg/ml

FDA Indications
- Hypertension, alone or concomitantly with other antihypertensive agents
- Attention deficit hyperactivity disorder (ADHD) (Kapvay®)

Other Data-Supported Indications
- Oppositional defiant disorder
- Conduct disorder
- Pervasive developmental disorders
- Motor tics
- Tourette's syndrome
- Opioid and alcohol withdrawal
- Anxiety disorders, including post-traumatic stress disorder (PTSD) and social anxiety disorder
- Clozapine-induced hypersalivation
- Menopausal flushing
- Severe pain in cancer patients not adequately relieved by opioid analgesics alone (combination with opiates)

B. MECHANISM OF ACTION [1–5]

Norepinephrine
- Stimulates central α_2-adrenergic receptors
- In hypertension, by stimulating these receptors, clonidine reduces sympathetic nerve impulses from the vasomotor center to the heart and blood vessels. This results in a decrease in peripheral vascular resistance and a reduction in heart rate and blood pressure

Renin
- Studies in patients have provided evidence of a reduction in plasma renin activity and in the excretion of aldosterone and catecholamines. The exact relationship of these pharmacologic actions to the antihypertensive effect of clonidine has not been fully elucidated

Postsynaptic Adrenergic Effects
- Exact mechanism of action in ADHD is unknown
- For ADHD, clonidine theoretically has central actions on postsynaptic α_{2a} receptors in the prefrontal cortex which is thought to be responsible for modulating working memory, attention, impulse control and planning

Imidazoline
- Interacts at imidazoline receptors

C. PLASMA CONCENTRATIONS AND TREATMENT RESPONSE [4, 5]

Initial Target Range
- Extended-release for ADHD: 0.1–0.4 mg/day in divided doses
- Immediate-release for hypertension: 0.05–0.2 mg/day in divided doses
- Opioid withdrawal: 0.1 mg three times daily (can be higher in inpatient setting)
- No established plasma concentration range

Range for Treatment Resistance
- Oral (for ADHD): maximum dose generally 0.4 mg/day in divided doses
- For opioid withdrawal: 0.1 mg three times daily
- Oral (for hypertension): maximum dose generally 2.4 mg/day
- Transdermal (for hypertension): apply once every seven days in hairless area
- Injection (for hypertension): maximum 40 mcg/hour
- No established plasma concentration range

Typical Time to Response
- In ADHD, it can take a few weeks to see maximal therapeutic benefits
- Blood pressure can be lowered 30–60 minutes after the first dose with the greatest reduction seen in two to four hours
- May take several weeks to control blood pressure
- If ineffective, taper dose of no more than 0.1 mg every three to seven days to discontinue

Time-Course of Improvement
- Continue treatment until all symptoms are controlled or there is stable improvement and continue treatment indefinitely as long as there is persistent improvement
- Periodically re-evaluate the need for treatment
- Childhood ADHD treatment may need to be continued into adolescence and adulthood if there is documented continued benefit

2.84 Clonidine (Continued)

D. TYPICAL TREATMENT RESPONSE [1, 2, 3, 6, 7]

Usual Target Symptoms
- Concentration
- Motor hyperactivity
- Oppositional and impulsive behavior
- Elevated blood pressure

Common Short-Term Adverse Effects
- Adverse effects are dose-dependent and usually transient: dry mouth, dizziness, constipation, sedation, weakness, fatigue, impotence, loss of libido, insomnia, headache, major depression, dermatologic reactions (especially with transdermal clonidine), hypotension, occasional syncope, tachycardia, nervousness, agitation, nausea, vomiting
- Clonidine can slow the pulse rate but it does not alter the normal hemodynamic response to exercise

Rare Adverse Effects
- Sinus bradycardia, atrioventricular block during withdrawal; hypertensive encephalopathy, cerebrovascular accidents, and death (rare)
- Overdose: hypotension, hypertension, miosis, respiratory depression, seizures, bradycardia, hypothermia, coma, sedation, decreased reflexes, weakness, irritability, dysrhythmia
- Children may be more likely to experience central nervous system (CNS) depression with overdose and may exhibit signs of toxicity with 0.1 mg of clonidine

Long-Term Effects
- During long-term therapy, cardiac output tends to return to control values, while peripheral resistance remains decreased
- May develop tolerance to the antihypertensive effects
- There are no studies establishing clonidine's use for long-term CNS uses

E. PRE-TREATMENT WORKUP AND INITIAL LABORATORY TESTING [1–3, 8]

History
- Do not use in patients with known allergy to clonidine
- Use with caution in patients with severe coronary insufficiency, recent myocardial infarction, cerebrovascular disease
- Use with caution in patients at risk for hypotension, bradycardia, heart block or syncope
- Use with caution in patients with and without a history of addiction. Reports of some abuse by opiate addicts and by nonopioid-dependent patients
- Elderly patients may tolerate lower initial doses better
- Elderly patients may be more sensitive to sedative effects
- Children may be more sensitive to the hypertensive effects of withdrawing treatment
- Children may be more likely to experience CNS depression with overdose and may exhibit signs of toxicity with 0.1 mg of clonidine

Physical
- Heart rate, blood pressure

Neurological
- Assessment for CNS depression

Blood Tests
- None for healthy individuals

Cardiac Tests
- ECG if known coronary heart disease

Urine Tests
- No specific tests

Pregnancy Test
- Pregnancy test (premenopausal females)
- Classified as risk not ruled out
- Clonidine crosses the placental barrier
- Some animal studies have shown adverse effects
- For ADHD, clonidine should generally be stopped before anticipated pregnancies
- Some drug is found in human breast milk
- No adverse effects have been reported in nursing infants
- If irritability or sedation develop in a nursing infant, may need to discontinue the drug or bottle feed

Other Tests (ECG, etc.)
- None

During Titration or After Dose Adjustment
• Blood pressure and heart rate at baseline, after dose changes, then regularly during treatment
• Vital signs frequently if cardiac conduction disturbance

Maintenance
• Treat until improvement stabilizes, then continue indefinitely as long as improvement persists

Initial Dosing/Titration
• Oral (for ADHD): initial 0.05 mg at bedtime; can increase by 0.05 mg/day each week with dosing divided and larger dose at bedtime; maximum dose generally 0.4 mg/day in divided doses
• For opioid withdrawal: 0.1 mg three times daily; next dose should be withheld if blood pressure falls below 90/60 mm Hg; outpatients should not be given more than a three-day supply, detoxification can usually be achieved in four to six days for short-acting opioids
• Oral (for hypertension): initial 0.1 mg in two divided doses, morning and night; can increase by 0.1 mg/day each week; maximum dose generally 2.4 mg/day
• Topical (for hypertension): apply once every seven days in hairless area; change location with each application
• Injection (for hypertension): initial 30 mcg/hour; maximum 40 mcg/hour; 500 mg/ml must be diluted

Half-Life
• 12–16 hours

Bioavailability
• 70–80%
• Food does not influence the pharmacokinetics of clonidine

Adjustment for Hepatic Dysfunction (by Child-Pugh Criteria)
• Use with caution

Adjustment for Renal Dysfunction
• Use with caution and possibly reduce the dose
• A minimal amount of clonidine is removed during routine hemodialysis, thus there is no need to give supplemental clonidine following dialysis

2.84 Clonidine (Continued)

H. MEDICATIONS TO AVOID IN COMBINATION/WARNINGS [1–3]

Central Nervous System (CNS) Depressants (e.g. phenothiazines, barbiturates, benzodiazepines)

- Increased depressive and sedative effects may occur when clonidine is taken with other CNS-depressant drugs

Beta-Blockers

- There is increased likelihood of severe discontinuation reactions with CNS and cardiovascular symptoms when clonidine is given with a beta-blocker

Tricyclic Antidepressants (TCAs)

- TCAs may decrease hypotensive effects of clonidine

Neuroleptics

- Clonidine given with neuroleptics can cause or exacerbate orthostatic regulation disturbances (e.g. orthostatic hypotension, dizziness, fatigue)

Amitriptyline

- An increase in corneal lesions were found in rats when taking clonidine with amitriptyline

Agents that affect sinus node or atrioventricular (AV) node function (e.g. digitalis, calcium channel blockers, beta-blockers)

- Use of clonidine in conjunction with agents that affect sinus node or AV node function may result in severe bradycardia or AV block

Warnings

- Sudden discontinuation reactions are common and sometimes severe. This can result in nervousness, agitation, headaches, and tremor with rapid rise in blood pressure
- Because children commonly have gastrointestinal (GI) illnesses that lead to vomiting, they may be particularly susceptible to hypertensive episodes resulting from abrupt inability to take medication
- There have been cases of hypertensive encephalopathy, cerebrovascular accidents, and death after abrupt discontinuation
- Taper over two to four days or longer to avoid rebound effects (nervousness, increased blood pressure)
- If used with a beta-blocker, stop the beta-blocker several days before tapering clonidine
- Excessive rises in blood pressure after discontinuation of clonidine can be reversed by oral clonidine or intravenous phentolamine
- In hypertension caused by pheochromocytoma, no therapeutic effect of clonidine can be expected
- Exercise caution when operating dangerous machinery or driving motor vehicles until it is determined that there is no drowsiness or dizziness from the medication
- Sedative effects of clonidine may be increased by concomitant use of alcohol, barbiturates or other sedating drugs
- Do not substitute different clonidine products on a mg-per-mg basis as they have different pharmacokinetic properties
- Extended-release tablets should not be crushed, chewed or broken as this could alter the controlled-release properties
- In patients who develop localized contact sensitization to transdermal clonidine, continuing transdermal dosing on other skin areas or substituting with oral clonidine may be associated with the development of a generalized skin rash, urticaria or angioedema
- Injection is not recommended for use in managing obstetrical, postpartum or perioperative pain
- Some transdermal patches contain small traces of aluminum or other metals in the adhesive backing and can cause skin burns if worn during MRI. Warn patients using the transdermal formulation about this possibility and advise them to disclose this information if they need an MRI

- Clonidine extended-release is approved for ADHD in children ages 6–17.
- Clonidine as monotherapy or in combination with methylphenidate for ADHD with conduct disorder or oppositional defiant disorder may improve aggression, oppositional and conduct disorder symptoms.
- Clonidine is sometimes used in combination with stimulants to reduce side effects and enhance therapeutic effects on motor hyperactivity.
- Doses of 0.1 mg in three divided doses have been reported to reduce stimulant-induced insomnia as well as impulsivity.
- No known abuse potential. Not a controlled substance.
- Non-stimulant option to treat ADHD, though not well studied in adults.
- Sedation is often intolerable in various patients despite improvement in CNS symptoms and leads to discontinuation of treatment, especially for ADHD and Tourette's syndrome.
- Clonidine may be effective for treatment of tic disorders, including Tourette's syndrome.
- May suppress tics especially in severe Tourette's syndrome, and may be even better at reducing explosive violent behaviors in Tourette's syndrome.
- Considered an investigational treatment for most other CNS applications.
- May block autonomic symptoms in anxiety and panic disorders (e.g. palpitations, sweating) and improve subjective anxiety.
- May be useful in decreasing autonomic arousal of PTSD.
- May be useful as an as-needed medication for stage fright or other predictable socially phobic situations.
- May be useful when added to selective serotonin reuptake inhibitors (SSRIs) for reducing arousal and dissociative symptoms in PTSD.
- May block autonomic symptoms of opioid withdrawal (e.g. palpitations, sweating) but muscle aches, irritability and insomnia may not be well suppressed by clonidine.
- Can be prescribed with naltrexone to suppress opioid withdrawal symptoms; this requires monitoring of the patient for eight hours the first day due to the potential severity of naltrexone-induced withdrawal and the potential blood pressure effects of clonidine.
- May be useful in decreasing hypertension, tachycardia, and tremulousness associated with alcohol withdrawal, but not seizures or delirium tremens in complicated alcohol withdrawal.
- Clonidine may improve social relationships, affectual responses, and sensory responses in autistic disorder.
- Clonidine may reduce the incidence of menopausal flushing.
- Clonidine stimulates growth hormone secretion in adults and children (no chronic effects have been observed with long-term use).
- Growth hormone response to clonidine may be reduced during menses.
- Alcohol may reduce the effects of clonidine on growth hormone.
- Guanfacine is a related centrally acting alpha 2 agonist hypotensive agent that has been used for similar CNS applications but has not been as widely investigated or used as clonidine.
- Guanfacine may be tolerated better than clonidine (e.g. sedation) or it may work better in some patients for CNS applications than clonidine, but no head-to-head trials.

References

1. Stat RX USA LLC. (2010). *Clonidine Package Insert*. Gainsville, Georgia.
2. Actavis Pharma Inc. (2015). *Clonidine Transdermal System Package Insert*. Parsippany, New Jersey.
3. Amneal Pharmaceuticals LLC. (2020). *Clonidine Extended Release Package Insert*. Bridgewater, New Jersey.
4. Gavras, I., Manolis, A. J., Gavras, H. (2001). The alpha2-adrenergic receptors in hypertension and heart failure: experimental and clinical studies. *J Hypertens*, 19, 2115–2124.
5. Croxtall, J. D. (2011). Clonidine extended-release: in attention-deficit hyperactivity disorder. *Paediatr Drugs*, 13, 329–336.
6. Burris, J. F. (1993). The USA experience with the clonidine transdermal therapeutic system. *Clin Auton Res*, 3, 391–396.
7. Neil, M. J. (2011). Clonidine: clinical pharmacology and therapeutic use in pain management. *Curr Clin Pharmacol*, 6, 280–287.
8. American Psychiatric Association. (1995). Practice guideline for the treatment of patients with substance use disorders: alcohol, cocaine, opioids. *Am J Psychiatry*, 152, 1–59.

2.85 Guanfacine

A. BASIC INFORMATION [1–3]

Principle Trade Names
• Tenex®
• Intuniv ER®

Legal Status
• Prescription only
• Not controlled

Classifications
• Norepinephrine receptor agonist (N-RA)
• Central alpha$_{2a}$ agonist
• Antihypertensive
• Non-stimulant for ADHD

Generics Available
• Yes

Formulations
• Immediate-release (IR) tablets: 1 mg; 2 mg; 3 mg
• Extended-release (ER) tablets: 1 mg; 2 mg; 3 mg; 4 mg

FDA Indications
• Hypertension
• Attention deficit hyperactivity disorder (ADHD) in children ages 6–17 (Intuniv®, adjunct and monotherapy)

Other Data-Supported Indications
• Oppositional defiant disorder
• Conduct disorder
• Pervasive developmental disorders
• Motor tics
• Tourette's syndrome
• Opioid withdrawal
• Migraine headache prophylaxis

B. MECHANISMS OF ACTION [3]

Norepinephrine
• Stimulates central α_2-adrenergic receptors
• In hypertension, by stimulating these receptors, guanfacine reduces sympathetic nerve impulses from the vasomotor center to the heart and blood vessels. This results in a decrease in peripheral vascular resistance and a reduction in heart rate and blood pressure

Postsynaptic Adrenergic Effects
• Exact mechanism of action in ADHD is unknown

• For ADHD, guanfacine theoretically has central actions on postsynaptic α_{2a} receptors in the prefrontal cortex which is thought to be responsible for modulating working memory, attention, impulse control, and planning
• Guanfacine is 15–20 times more selective for α_{2A} versus α_{2B} or α_{2C} receptors

C. PLASMA CONCENTRATIONS AND TREATMENT RESPONSE [3, 4, 5]

Initial Target Range
- Hypertension: 0.5–2 mg PO qhs
- ADHD (Intuniv) (6–17 year olds): 0.05–0.12 mg/kg PO QD
- ADHD (Tenex) (6–17 year olds): 27–45 kg, 0.5 mg PO BID-QID
- ADHD (Tenex) (6–17 year olds): >45 kg, 1 mg PO BID-QID
- Opioid withdrawal: 3–4 mg PO divided TID
- Migraine headache prophylaxis: 1 mg PO QD
- Tourette syndrome (guanfacine): 0.5–2 mg PO BID
- Tourette syndrome (Tenex®) (6+ year olds): 1–4 mg/day PO divided BID-TID
- No established plasma concentration range

Range for Treatment Resistance
- Hypertension: maximum dose 3 mg/day
- ADHD (Tenex) (6–17 year olds): 27–40.5 kg maximum dose 2 mg/day
- ADHD (Tenex) (6–17 year olds): 40.5–45 kg maximum dose 3 mg/day
- ADHD (Tenex®) (6–17 year olds): >45 kg maximum dose 4 mg/day

- Tourette syndrome: maximum dose 4 mg/day
- No established plasma concentration range

Typical Time to Response
- In ADHD, it can take a few weeks to see maximal therapeutic benefits
- Blood pressure can be lowered 30–60 minutes after the first dose with the greatest reduction seen in two to four hours
- May take several weeks to control blood pressure
- If ineffective at maximum tolerated dose, taper dose over four to seven days to discontinue

Time-Course of Improvement
- Continue treatment until all symptoms are controlled or there is stable improvement and continue treatment indefinitely as long as there is persistent improvement
- Periodically re-evaluate the need for treatment
- Childhood ADHD treatment may need to be continued into adolescence and adulthood if there is documented continued benefit

D. TYPICAL TREATMENT RESPONSE [1, 3, 4]

Usual Target Symptoms
- Concentration
- Motor hyperactivity
- Oppositional and impulsive behavior
- Elevated blood pressure

Common Short-Term Adverse Effects
- Dose-dependent: sedation (somnolence), dizziness, fatigue, weakness (asthenia), dry mouth, constipation, hypotension, headache and impotence

Rare Adverse Effects
- Skin rash with exfoliation, syncope, bradycardia, palpitations, substernal pain, abdominal pain, diarrhea, dyspepsia, dysphagia, nausea, amnesia, confusion, depression, insomnia, libido decrease, rhinitis, taste perversion, tinnitus, conjunctivitis, iritis, vision disturbance, leg cramps, hypokinesia, dyspnea, dermatitis, pruritus, purpura, sweating, testicular disorder, urinary incontinence, malaise, paresthesia, paresis
- Post-marketing experience includes spontaneous reports of mania and aggressive behavioral changes in pediatric patients with ADHD receiving guanfacine. The reported cases were from a single center. All patients had medical or family risk factors for bipolar disorder. All patients recovered upon discontinuation of guanfacine HCl. Hallucinations have been reported in pediatric patients receiving guanfacine for treatment of ADHD
- Rare, serious disorders with no definitive cause and effect relationship to guanfacine have been reported spontaneously in post-marketing studies which include acute renal failure, cardiac fibrillation, cerebrovascular accident, congestive heart failure, heart block and myocardial infarction
- Overdose: drowsiness, lethargy, bradycardia and hypotension

Long-Term Effects
- Shown to be safe and effective to treat hypertension
- There are studies of use for up to two years in ADHD
- The need for continued treatment should be re-evaluated periodically

2.85 Guanfacine (Continued)

History
- Do not use in patients with known hypersensitivity/allergy to guanfacine
- Use with caution in patients with severe coronary insufficiency, recent myocardial infarction, cerebrovascular disease, or chronic renal or hepatic failure
- Use with caution in patients at risk for hypotension, bradycardia, heart block or syncope

Physical
- Heart rate, blood pressure

Neurological
- Assessment for central nervous system (CNS) depression

Blood Tests
- None for healthy individuals

Cardiac Tests
- ECG if known coronary artery disease

Urine Tests
- No specific test

Pregnancy Test
- Pregnancy test (premenopausal females)
- Classified as no evidence of risk in animal studies
- Administration of guanfacine to rats at 70 times the maximum recommended human dose and to rabbits at 20 times the maximum recommended human dose resulted in no evidence of harm to the fetus
- Higher doses (100 and 200 times the maximum recommended human dose in rabbits and rats respectively) were associated with reduced fetal survival and maternal toxicity. Rat experiments have shown that guanfacine crosses the placenta
- Guanfacine discontinuation should be considered before anticipated pregnancies
- Experiments with rats have shown that guanfacine is excreted in breast milk
- It is not known if guanfacine is secreted in human breast milk. However, it is assumed that all psychotropics are secreted in breast milk
- Thus, it is recommended to stop the drug or bottle feed

Other Tests (ECG, etc.)
- None

During Titration or After Dose Adjustment
- Blood pressure and heart rate at baseline, after dose changes, then regularly during treatment
- Vital signs frequently if cardiac conduction disturbance

Maintenance
- Treat until improvement stabilizes, then continue indefinitely as long as improvement persists
- Shown to be safe and effective to treat hypertension
- There are studies of use for up to two years in ADHD

G. DOSING AND KINETICS [1, 5]

Initial Dosing/Titration

- HTN: start at 1 mg PO qhs, may increase to 2 mg PO qhs after three to four weeks
- ADHD (Tenex) (6–17 year olds): 27–40.5 kg start 0.5 mg PO qhs, then may increase by 0.5 mg/day q week
- ADHD (Tenex) (6–17 year olds): 40.5–45 kg start 0.5 mg PO qhs, then may increase by 0.5 mg/day q week up to 1.5 mg/day, then increase by 0.5 mg/day q 2 weeks
- ADHD (Tenex) (6–17 year olds): >45 kg start 1 mg PO qhs, then may increase by 1 mg/day q week up to 3 mg/day, then increase to 4 mg/day after two weeks
- Opioid withdrawal: 3–4 mg/day PO divided TID
- Migraine headache prophylaxis: 1 mg PO QD
- Tourette syndrome: start 0.5 mg PO QD titrate slowly

Half-Life

- Guanfacine (IR) in individuals with normal renal function, the average elimination half-life is approximately 17 hours (range 10–30 hours). Younger patients tend to have shorter elimination half-lives (13–14 hours) while older patients tend to have half-lives at the upper end of the range
- Guanfacine (ER): 18 hours

Bioavailability

- Oral bioavailability of guanfacine is about 80%
- Do not administer ER formulation guanfacine with high-fat meals as this increases exposure

Adjustment for Hepatic Dysfunction (by Child-Pugh Criteria)

- Not defined. Caution advised. Consider decrease of usual dose if significant impairment

Adjustment for Renal Dysfunction

- When prescribing for patients with renal impairment, the low end of the dosing range should be used. Patients on dialysis also can be given usual doses of guanfacine hydrochloride as the drug is poorly dialyzed

CNS Depressants (e.g. phenothiazines, barbiturates, benzodiazepines)

- Increased sedation may occur when guanfacine is given with other CNS-depressant drugs

cyp 3A4 Inducers (e.g. carbamazepine, phenobarbital, phenytoin, rifampin, St. John's Wort)

- cyp 3A4 inducers lower guanfacine plasma levels

cyp 3A4 Inhibitors (e.g. nefazodone, fluvoxamine, fluoxetine and ketoconazole)

- cyp 3A4 inhibitors increase guanfacine plasma levels

Valproate

- Guanfacine combined with valproate may increase valproate plasma levels

Warnings

- Rebound: abrupt cessation of therapy with orally active central α-adrenergic agonists may be associated with increases (from depressed on-therapy levels) in plasma and urinary catecholamines, symptoms of "nervousness and anxiety" and, less commonly, increases in blood pressure to levels significantly greater than those prior to therapy
- Patients should be advised not to discontinue therapy abruptly. Taper over four to seven days
- Do not substitute IR and ER tablets on a mg-per-mg basis as they have different pharmacokinetic properties
- ER tablets should not be crushed, chewed or broken as this could alter the controlled-release properties
- Exercise caution when operating dangerous machinery or driving motor vehicles until it is determined that there is no drowsiness or dizziness from the medication
- Tolerance for alcohol and other CNS depressants may be diminished
- Excessive heat (e.g. saunas) may increase side effects such as dizziness and drowsiness

2.85 Guanfacine (Continued)

- Guanfacine has been found to be effective in children and adults.
- ER guanfacine is approved for ADHD in children aged 6–17 years old.
- No known abuse potential. Not a controlled substance.
- Non-stimulant option to treat ADHD, though not well studied in adults.
- May be used as monotherapy or in combination with stimulants for oppositional behavior in children with or without ADHD.

- Guanfacine can also be used to treat tic disorders, including Tourette's syndrome.
- Guanfacine and clonidine are both α_2 adrenergic agonists, but guanfacine is relatively selective for α_{2a}-receptors, whereas clonidine binds $\alpha_{2a, b, and c}$ receptors and imidazoline receptors, causing more sedation, hypotension and side effects than guanfacine.

References

1. Arnsten, A. F., Scahill, L., Findling, R. L. (2007). Alpha2-adrenergic receptor agonists for the treatment of attention-deficit/hyperactivity disorder: emerging concepts from new data. *J Child Adolesc Psychopharmacol*, 17, 393–406.
2. Posey, D. J., McDougle, C. J. (2007). Guanfacine and guanfacine extended release: treatment for ADHD and related disorders. *CNS Drug Rev*, 13, 465–474.
3. Amneal Pharmaceuticals LLC. (2019). *Guanfacine HCl Package Insert*. Bridgewater, New Jersey.
4. Sallee, F. R., Lyne, A., Wigal, T., et al. (2009). Long-term safety and efficacy of guanfacine extended release in children and adolescents with attention-deficit/hyperactivity disorder. *J Child Adolesc Psychopharmacol*, 19, 215–226.
5. Sallee, F. R., McGough, J., Wigal, T., et al. (2009). Guanfacine extended release in children and adolescents with attention-deficit/hyperactivity disorder: a placebo-controlled trial. *J Am Acad Child Adolesc Psychiatry*, 48, 155–165.
6. Biederman, J., Melmed, R. D., Patel, A., et al. (2008). Long-term, open-label extension study of guanfacine extended release in children and adolescents with ADHD. *CNS Spectr*, 13, 1047–1055.
7. Spencer, T. J., Greenbaum, M., Ginsberg, L. D., et al. (2009). Safety and effectiveness of coadministration of guanfacine extended release and psychostimulants in children and adolescents with attention-deficit/hyperactivity disorder. *J Child Adolesc Psychopharmacol*, 19, 501–510.

Appendices

3.01 Appendix Optimal Antipsychotic Plasma Concentration Ranges [1–4]

Medication	Minimum Response Threshold	Point of Futility
Aripiprazole expected level = 12 x oral dose (mg/d)	150 ng/ml	550 ng/ml
Clozapine male nonsmoker – expected level = 1.08 x oral dose (mg/d) female nonsmoker – expected level = 1.32 x oral dose (mg/d)	350 ng/ml	1000 ng/ml
Fluphenazine nonsmoker – expected level = 0.08 x oral dose (mg/d)	0.8 ng/ml	4.0 ng/ml
Haloperidol expected level = 0.78 x oral dose (mg/d)	2 ng/ml	18 ng/ml
Olanzapine nonsmoker – expected level = 2.0 x oral dose (mg/d)	23 ng/ml	150 ng/ml
Paliperidone expected level = 4.7 x oral dose (mg/d)	28 ng/ml	112 ng/ml
Risperidone + 9-OH Risperidone expected level = 7.0 x oral dose (mg/d)	28 ng/ml	112 ng/ml
Perphenazine expected level = 0.04 x oral dose (mg/d)	0.8 ng/ml	5.0 ng/ml

• See also Chapter 1.02 "Use of Plasma Levels in Antipsychotic and Mood Stabilizer Treatment".

References

1. Meyer, J. M. (2014). A rational approach to employing high plasma levels of antipsychotics for violence associated with schizophrenia: case vignettes. *CNS Spectr*, 19, 432–438.
2. Meyer, J. M., Cummings, M. A., Proctor, G., et al. (2016). Psychopharmacology of persistent violence and aggression. *Psychiatr Clin North Am*, 39, 541–556.
3. Meyer, J. M. (2018). Pharmacotherapy of psychosis and mania. In *Gilman: The Pharmacological Basis of Therapeutics* (eds.). New York: McGraw-Hill.
4. Schoretsanitis, G., Kane, J. M., Correll, C. U., et al. (2020). Blood levels to optimize antipsychotic treatment in clinical practice: a joint consensus statement of the American Society of Clinical Psychopharmacology and the Therapeutic Drug Monitoring Task Force of the Arbeitsgemeinschaft für Neuropsychopharmakologie und Pharmakopsychiatrie. *J Clin Psychiatry*, 81(3), 19cs13169.

3.02 Appendix Optimal Mood Stabilizer Plasma Concentration Ranges [1, 2]

Mood Stabilizer	Plasma Concentration of Mood Stabilizer	
	Acute Mania	**Maintenance**
Lithium	1.0–1.4 meq/l	0.8–1.2 meq/l (see #2 under "Mood Stabilizers")
Divalproex Valproic acid	100–120 mcg/l	80–120 mcg/l
Carbamazepine	9–12 mcg/ml	6–12 mcg/l

- See also Chapter 1.02 "Use of Plasma Levels in Antipsychotic and Mood Stabilizer Treatment".
- **IMPORTANTLY**, chronic exposure to maintenance lithium plasma concentrations >1.0 meq/l may increase the long-term risk of renal insufficiency.

 ### References

1. Castro, V. M., Roberson, A. M., McCoy, T. H., et al. (2016). Stratifying risk for renal insufficiency among lithium-treated patients: an electronic health record study. *Neuropsychopharmacol*, 41, 1138–1143.
2. Meyer, J. M. (2018). *Gilman: The Pharmacological Basis of Therapeutics. Pharmacotherapy of Psychosis and Mania.* New York: McGraw-Hill.

3.03 Appendix Formulas for Correcting QT Interval [1, 2]

The most commonly used ECG machine formula, Bazett's formula, for correcting the QT interval (repolarization) rapidly becomes inaccurate as heart rate increases. At tachycardic (BPM >100) heart rates, Bazett's formula substantially overestimates the QT interval. The normal upper thresholds for QTc are 450 ms in men and 470 ms in women. Risk of cardiac arrythmia (Torsades de Pointes) begins to significantly increase at QTc intervals >500 ms. Below are three formulas that more accurately calculate QTc.

Formula Name	Formula
Fridericia	QTc = QT/(RR^0.33)
Framingham	QTc = QT + 0.154(1 − RR)
Hodges	QTc = QT + 1.75(HR − 60)

• A web-based calculator is available at https://www.mdcalc.com/Corrected-qt-interval-qtc
• RR intervals are in seconds
• Examples on how to use each formula (HR 80 BPM, RR = 0.75 sec, QT uncorrected = 400 ms or 0.4 sec)
a. Fridericia: .400 sec/(0.75)1/3 = 0.440 sec = 440 ms
b. Framingham: .400 sec + 0.154(1 − 0.75) = .439 sec = 439 ms
c. Hodges: .400 sec + 0.175(80 − 60) = .435 sec = 435 ms

 ## References

1. Beach, S. R., Celano, C. M., Noseworthy, P. A., et al. (2013). QTc prolongation, Torsades de Pointes, and psychotropic medications. *Psychosomatics*, 54, 1–13.
2. Trinkley, K. E., Page, R. L., 2nd, Lien, H., et al. (2013). QT interval prolongation and the risk of Torsades de Pointes: essentials for clinicians. *Curr Med Res Opin*, 29, 1719–1726.

3.04 Appendix Common Cytochrome P450 Inducers and Inhibitors [1, 2]

Circa 75% of medications are catabolized via the cytochrome P450 enzyme system in the liver. Inducers and inhibitors of these hepatic enzymes may substantially decrease or increase medication plasma concentrations, respectively. That is, they may cause medications to become subtherapeutic or toxic.

Enzyme	Inducers	Inhibitors
1A2	Omeprazole Phenytoin* Rifampin*	Ciprofloxacin* Fluvoxamine*
2C9	Carbamazepine* Rifampin*	Fluconazole*
2D6	None	Bupropion* Fluoxetine* Paroxetine*
3A	Carbamazepine* Modafinil Nudafinil Phenytoin* Phenobarbitone* Rifabutin Rifampicin St. John's Wort	Azole antifungals Fluconazole* Itraconazole Ketoconazole* Voriconazole Cimetidine* Ciprofloxacin* Grapefruit juice Macrolides Clarithromycin* Erythromycin* Protease inhibitors Indinavir Ritonavir* Saquinavir

* Classified as a potent inducer or inhibitor and/or noted to be frequently involved in significant drug-drug interactions

References

1. Day, R. O., Snowden, L., McLachlan, A. J. (2017). Life-threatening drug interactions: what the physician needs to know. *Intern Med J*, 47, 501–512.
2. Voigt, N., Ort, K., Sossalla, S. (2019). Drug-drug interactions you should know!. *Fortschr Neurol Psychiatr*, 87, 320–332.

3.05 Appendix Management of Constipation [1, 2]

A frequent adverse effect of psychopharmacological treatment, especially with some medications such as clozapine, is constipation with risks of developing fecal impaction, paralytic ileus or bowel obstruction. Thus, for many patients, an effective bowel regimen is critically important.

Treatment Step	Treatment Intervention
Step 1	Applies to anyone with a constipation history or who is started on potentially constipating medications. Give docusate 250 mg BID at the beginning of treatment (e.g. when starting clozapine), with rescue PRN medication (e.g. magnesium citrate 150 ml or magnesium hydroxide 30 ml q two days PRN lack of bowel movement).
Step 2	If step 1 isn't adequate, then **add one** osmotic laxative, e.g. polyethylene glycol 17 grams QAM or lactulose 30 ml BID. Polyethylene glycol 3350 (Miralax®) is generally superior to lactulose. (Lactulose is reserved for the treatment of hyperammonemia.)
Step 3	If steps 1 and 2 aren't adequate to alleviate constipation, then **add one** stimulant laxative. Options include sennosides starting at 17.2 mg qhs (max 34.4 mg BID) or bisacodyl starting at 5 mg qhs (max 30 mg per day).
Step 4	If steps 1–3 fail to adequately control constipation, then **add one** secretogogue (see table below). If the secretory laxative is effective, it may be possible to taper off the stimulant laxative and then the osmotic laxative.

- **IMPORTANTLY,** bulk laxatives, e.g. psyllium, must be avoided during treatment with drugs that substantially increase bowel transit time, e.g. clozapine, as bulk laxatives add to the risks of fecal impaction and bowel obstruction under these circumstances.

Name	Mechanism	Starting Dose	Max Dose	Comments
Lubiprostone (Amitiza®) (US)	Prostaglandin E1 analog	8 mcg BID	24 mcg BID	**Give with food and water.** No drug interactions. (Adverse effects can include nausea, abdominal pain, distention, diarrhea, dehydration and rectal bleeding.)
Linaclotide (Linzess®) (US)	Guanylate cyclase-C agonist	145 mcg QD	290 mcg QD	**Give >30 minutes before first meal.** No drug interactions. (Adverse effects can include diarrhea, dehydration, hypokalemia and rectal bleeding.)
Plecanatide (Trulance®) (US)	Guanylate cyclase-C agonist	3 mg QD	3 mg QD	No drug interactions. (Adverse effects can include diarrhea, dehydration, hypokalemia and rectal bleeding.)
Prucalopride (Motegrity®) (US)	$5HT_4$ agonist	2 mg QD	2 mg QD	No drug interactions. (Adverse effects can include headache, abdominal pain, nausea, diarrhea, abdominal distention, dizziness. Monitor for worsening depressive symptoms or emergence of suicidal thoughts/behavior.)

References

1. Wald, A. (2015). Constipation: pathophysiology and management. *Curr Opin Gastroenterol*, 31, 45–49.
2. Prichard, D. O., Bharucha, A. E. (2018). Recent advances in understanding and managing chronic constipation. *F1000Res*, 7, 1640.

3.06 Appendix Child-Pugh Hepatic Function Scoring [1, 2]

item	Score = 0	Score = 1	Score = 2
Bilirubin	<2.0 mg/dl	2–3 mg/dl	>3 mg/dl
Serum albumin	>3.5 g/dl	2.8–3.5 g/dl	<2.8 g/dl
INR	<1.7 s	1.7–2.3 s	>2.3 s
Ascites	None	Mild or controlled medications	Moderate to severe or refractory
Hepatic encephalopathy	None	Grade I–II	Grade III–IV

- Child-Pugh Score = sum of all points
- Some variants substitute INR or PT and direct bilirubin for total bilirubin
- Interpretation: Category A = 5–6 points; Category B = 7–9 points; Category C >9 points
- Category A does not require adjustment of medication doses or avoidance of hepatically catabolized drugs. Category B may require dose reductions of 30% to 50% to avoid elevated drug concentrations in a limited number of drugs. Category C may require dose reductions of 80–90% or avoidance of drugs requiring extensive hepatic catabolism.

References

1. Hofmann, W. P., Radle, J., Moench, C., et al. (2008). Prediction of perioperative mortality in patients with advanced liver disease and abdominal surgery by the use of different scoring systems and tests. *Z Gastroenterol*, 46, 1283–1289.
2. Tsoris, A., Marlar, C. A. (2020). Use of the child Pugh score in liver disease. In *StatPearls* (eds.). Treasure Island, FL: StatPearls Publishing LLC.

3.07 Appendix Loading of Lithium and Valproic Acid [1–3]

In acutely mania or psychomotor agitation, it may be desirable to achieve therapeutic plasma concentrations of lithium or valproic acid efficiently. The table below outlines loading of lithium and valproic acid.

Medication	Loading Strategy	Comments
Lithium	• Calculate lithium 30 mg/kg to the nearest available dose • Using lithium extended-release (ER), give the total calculated dose in three divided doses over a six-hour time span on the first day at 4:00 pm, 6:00 pm and 8:00 pm • Obtain a lithium plasma concentration at about 8:00 am the following morning • If the lithium level is <1.0 meq/l, then prescribe lithium immediate-release 1500 mg q bedtime • If the lithium plasma concentration is >1.0 meq/l, then prescribe lithium immediate-release 1200 mg q bedtime • Re-measure the lithium level after five days and fine tune the dosing aiming for a level of up to 1.4 meq/l in acute mania or 0.8–1.0 meq/l for maintenance	• The ER formulation is used for loading to minimize the risk of post-dose peak nausea • The ER formulation is used only for loading, as once per day immediate-release lithium carries the least renal risk • The total daily loading dose should exceed 3000 mg only with caution • If the immediate-release (IR) lithium is not tolerated, then switch to ER while keeping the dosing all at bedtime to minimize renal adverse effects • Some have advocated limiting the loading dose to a total of 2000 mg; however, this is not supported by data
Valproic Acid	• Calculate 20–30 mg/kg and give the nearest available dose as valproic acid tablets or divalproex DR tablets in two divided doses using a BID schedule • After three days, obtain a trough plasma concentration (12 hours post-dose) and fine tune dosing to achieve a plasma concentration of 80–120 mcg/ml	• If divalproex ER is used, increase the estimated dose by 10–15% • If valproic acid liquid is used, then increase the estimated dose by 30–50%

References

1. Kook, K. A., Stimmel, G. L., Wilkins, J. N., et al. (1985). Accuracy and safety of a priori lithium loading. *J Clin Psychiatry*, 46, 49–51.
2. Hirschfeld, R. M., Baker, J. D., Wozniak, P., et al. (2003). The safety and early efficacy of oral-loaded divalproex versus standard-titration divalproex, lithium, olanzapine, and placebo in the treatment of acute mania associated with bipolar disorder. *J Clin Psychiatry*, 64, 841–846.
3. Tohen, M., Ketter, T. A., Zarate, C. A., et al. (2003). Olanzapine versus divalproex sodium for the treatment of acute mania and maintenance of remission: a 47-week study. *Am J Psychiatry*, 160, 1263–1271.

3.08 Appendix Treatment of Prolactin Elevation [1–3]

Prolactin (PRL) synthesis and secretion by the anterior pituitary gland is inhibited by dopamine in the tuberoinfundibular tract via pituitary D_2 receptors. Dopamine antagonist antipsychotics increase prolactin by blocking these receptors. Elevated prolactin secretion may lead to acute symptoms such as amenorrhea, galactorrhea, erectile dysfunction, gynecomastia, acceleration of prolactin-sensitive breast cancer, and, rarely, pituitary adenoma. Risperidone and paliperidone (9-hydroxy-risperidone) are especially provocative, as they are actively pumped out of the brain at the blood-brain barrier by P-glycoprotein directly onto the pituitary. Thus, pituitary concentrations of these drugs may be higher in the pituitary than in the brain. The goals of treatment are to reduce prolactin to alleviate prolactin-related symptoms and/or to maintain prolactin plasma concentrations at <100 ng/ml.

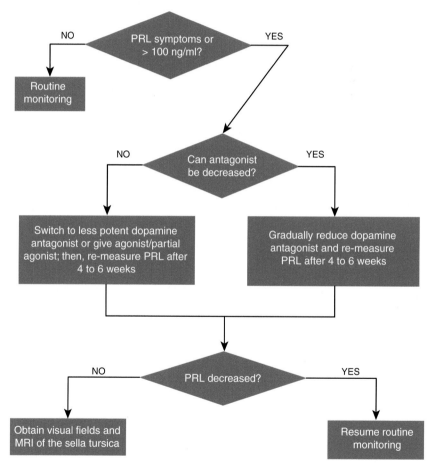

3.08 Treatment of Prolactin Elevation (Continued)

Medications Used to Suppress Prolactin		
Medication	Dosing	Comments
Aripiprazole	2–5 mg per day	Higher doses will supplant dopamine antagonist antipsychotics due to very high binding affinity for D_2 dopamine receptors (K_i = 0.3 nM)
Bromocriptine	1.25–5.0 mg BID	Requires titration. May cause sedation and post-dose nausea. Available as 1.25, 2.5 and 5.0 mg tablets
Pramipexole	0.125–2.0 mg q bedtime	Initiate at 0.125 mg q bedtime and double every two to three days to tolerance/effectiveness (usually 1–2 mg q bedtime). If post-dose nausea occurs, an ER formulation also is available. Immediate-release is supplied as 0.125 mg, 0.25 mg, 0.5 mg, 0.75 mg, 1.0 mg and 1.5 mg tablets

References

1. Bakker, I. C., Schubart, C. D., Zelissen, P. M. (2016). Successful treatment of a prolactinoma with the antipsychotic drug aripiprazole. *Endocrinol Diabetes Metab Case Rep*, 2016, 160028.
2. Grigg, J., Worsley, R., Thew, C., et al. (2017). Antipsychotic-induced hyperprolactinemia: synthesis of world-wide guidelines and integrated recommendations for assessment, management and future research. *Psychopharmacology (Berl)*, 234, 3279–3297.
3. Gonzalez-Rodriguez, A., Labad, J., Seeman, M. V. (2020). Antipsychotic-induced hyperprolactinemia in aging populations: prevalence, implications, prevention and management. *Prog Neuropsychopharmacol Biol Psychiatry*, 101, 109941.

3.09 Appendix A Select List of Foods High in Tyramine [1–5][a]

	Maximal tyramine content per kg or l	Serving required to ingest 25 mg of tyramine
Cheeses		
Highly aged artisanal cheeses	1000 mg	25 g (0.88 oz)
Aged feta	250 mg	100 g (3.5 oz)
Commercial cheeses and cheddar	200 mg	125 g (4.4 oz)
Grana padano, pecorino, provolone, ripened goat cheese, emmentaler, taleggio, bel paese	200 mg	125 g (4.4 oz)
Parmigiano reggiano	150 mg	167 g (5.9 oz)
Edam	120 mg	208 g (7.3 oz)
Gouda, gruyere	100 mg	250 g (8.8 oz)
Dried aged sausages		
Various, from Europe (primarily)	200 mg (rare reports up to 600 mg)	125 g (4.4 oz) (if 600 mg: 42 g; 1.5 oz)
Sauces, spreads, vegetables, wine, beer		
Fermented yeast (Marmite, Vegemite)	300 mg	75 g (2.64 oz)[b]
Specialty soy sauce	940 mg	27 g (0.94 oz)[c]
Fish sauce (e.g. Nam-pla, etc.)	500 mg	50 g (1.8 oz)[c]
Commercial soy sauce	200 mg	125 g (4.4 oz)[c]
Sauerkraut	200 mg (rare reports up to 900 mg)	125 g (4.4 oz) (if 900 mg: 28 g; 0.98 oz)
Kimchi	120 mg	208 g (7.33 oz)
Wines	none exceeded 10 g/l	>2.5 l
Beers	majority <10 g/l (rare 30–100 mg/l)	>2.5 l (if 30–100 mg: 250–833 ml)

[a] For an exhaustive list, see: psychotropical.com/maois-diet-drug-interactions/ (last updated February 2020)

[b] 1 oz = 28.35 g; 100 g = 3.53 oz; 3.53 oz = 0.22 lb

[c] Usual serving: 5 g (5 ml)

Comments

1. Emphasize to patients that only a small number of highly aged cheeses, foods and sauces contain high quantities of tyramine, and that even these foods can be enjoyed in small amounts [5].
2. All patients prescribed an MAOI should purchase a portable blood pressure (BP) cuff for rare instances when a dietary lapse occurs, and a headache ensues within one to two hours after tyramine ingestion. Most reactions are self-limited and resolve over two to four hours [4].

3.09 A Select List of Foods High in Tyramine (Continued)

3. Patients who ingest ≥100 mg of tyramine should be evaluated by a physician. Under no circumstances should a prescription be given for nifedipine or any agent that abruptly lowers BP, because this may result in complications, including myocardial infarction [1, 2].
4. Counsel patients to remain calm. Low-dose benzodiazepines (equivalent of alprazolam 0.5 mg) can facilitate this, and also lower BP. An emergency room study of patients with an initial systolic BP ≥160 mm Hg or diastolic BP ≥100 mm Hg without end-organ damage noted that alprazolam, 0.5 mg, was as effective as captopril, 25 mg, in lowering BP [3].

References

1. Marik, P. E., Varon, J. (2007). Hypertensive crises: challenges and management. *Chest*, 131, 1949–1962.
2. Burton, T. J., Wilkinson, I. B. (2008). The dangers of immediate-release nifedipine in the emergency treatment of hypertension. *J Hum Hypertens*, 22, 301–302.
3. Yilmaz, S., Pekdemir, M., Tural, U., et al. (2011). Comparison of alprazolam versus captopril in high blood pressure: a randomized controlled trial. *Blood Press*, 20, 239–243.
4. Meyer, J. M. (2017). A concise guide to monoamine oxidase inhibitors: part 1. *Current Psychiatry*, 16, 14–16.
5. Gillman, P. K. (2020). Monoamine oxidase inhibitors: a review concerning dietary tyramine and drug interactions. PsychoTropical Commentaries, PsychoTropical Research, Bucasia, Queensland, Australia. Available at: psychotropical.com/maois-diet-drug-interactions (last accessed November 13, 2020).

3.10 Appendix Medications That Present Risk for Serotonin Syndrome When Combined with Monoamine Oxidase Inhibitor [1–7]

Medication Class[a]	Examples
Tricyclic antidepressants	Imipramine, desipramine, amitriptyline, nortriptyline, clomipramine
SSRI antidepressants[b]	Citalopram, escitalopram, fluoxetine, fluvoxamine, paroxetine, sertraline, trazodone, vilazodone, vortioxetine
SNRI antidepressants[b]	Duloxetine, levomilnacipran, milnacipran, O-desmethylvenlafaxine, venlafaxine
Antipsychotics	Ziprasidone, lumateperone[c]
Specific cold products	Dextromethorphan, chlorpheniramine
Synthetic analgesics	Fentanyl, meperidine, tramadol
Migraine medications	Almotriptan, eletriptan, frovatriptan, naratriptan, rizatriptan, sumatriptan, zolmitriptan
Antibiotics	Linezolid
Other[c]	Methylene blue
Drugs of abuse	MDMA, LSD

[a] Before commencing an MAOI, medications that present risk for serotonin syndrome must be stopped for 14 days or five half-lives, whichever is greater. In particular, fluoxetine has an active metabolite, norfluoxetine, with a half-life of one to two weeks, and must be discontinued for eight to ten weeks before starting an MAOI. After discontinuing an MAOI, 14 days should elapse before medications that present risk for serotonin syndrome can be started.

[b] Neither bupropion (a norepinephrine and dopamine reuptake inhibitor) nor mirtazapine (a serotonin $5HT_{2A}$, $5HT_{2C}$ antagonist, with presynaptic $alpha_2$-adrenergic antagonism) are serotonergic agonists or serotonin reuptake inhibitors and can be combined with MAOIs [1–3].

[c] The affinity of lumateperone for the serotonin transporter (SERT) is moderate (Ki 33 nM), but greater than that for ziprasidone (Ki 53–112 nM) [4, 7]. Lumateperone peak SERT occupancy at the dose approved for schizophrenia (42 mg/day) is low at 30%, but the safety of combining this medication with an MAOI has not been established.

References

1. Gillman, P. K. (2003). Mirtazapine: unable to induce serotonin toxicity? *Clin Neuropharmacol*, 26, 288–289; author reply 289–290.
2. Gillman, P. K. (2006). A systematic review of the serotonergic effects of mirtazapine in humans: implications for its dual action status. *Human Psychopharmacol*, 21, 117–125.
3. Quante, A., Zeugmann, S. (2012). Tranylcypromine and bupropion combination therapy in treatment-resistant major depression: a report of 2 cases. *J Clin Psychopharmacol*, 32, 572–574.
4. Davis, R. E., Vanover, K. E., Zhou, Y., et al. (2015). ITI-007 demonstrates brain occupancy at serotonin 5-HT(2)A and dopamine D(2) receptors and serotonin transporters using positron emission tomography in healthy volunteers. *Psychopharmacology (Berl)*, 232, 2863–2872.
5. Meyer, J. M. (2018). A concise guide to monoamine oxidase inhibitors: part 2. *Current Psychiatry*, 17, 22–33.
6. Meyer, J. M. (2018). *Gilman: The Pharmacological Basis of Therapeutics. Pharmacotherapy of Psychosis and Mania.* New York: McGraw-Hill.
7. Meyer, J. M. (2018). Pharmacotherapy of psychosis and mania. In Brunton, L. L., Hilal-Dandan, R., Knollmann, B. C. (eds.). *Goodman & Gilman's The Pharmacological Basis of Therapeutics*, 13th ed. Chicago, IL: McGraw-Hill, pp. 279–302.

3.11 Appendix Selected Treatment of Psychomotor Agitation Algorithm [1–36]

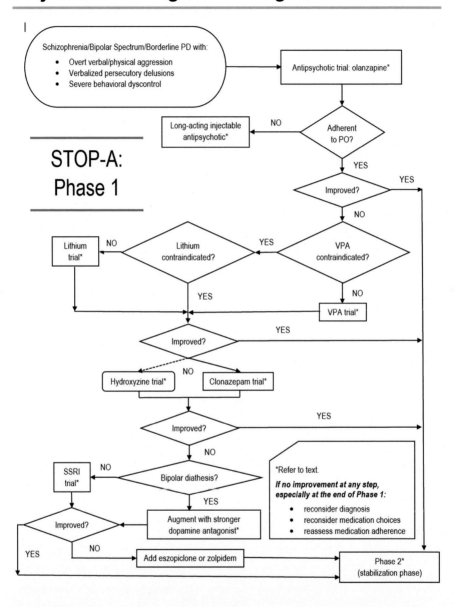

Introduction: Imaging studies have indicated overactivity of the amygdala complex in persons exhibiting hypervigilance, paranoia and proneness to psychomotorically agitated violence. Brain injuries resulting in either irritative lesions in the anterior temporal lobe, e.g. temporal lobe epilepsy, or loss of prefrontal cortical inhibition of the amygdala also have pointed to the role of the amygdala in producing psychomotorically agitated violent behavior [1]. Similarly, electrophysiological and imaging studies have reflected hypofrontality and increased temporal lobe/amygdala hyperactivity as common in the pathophysiology of schizophrenia spectrum disorders [2, 3]. Similar, but less pronounced, patterns of disturbed physiology have been described in bipolar spectrum disorders, as well as borderline personality disorder [4].

Individual Selection: Many of the recommended treatment measures described below carry increased risks of adverse effects that are counterbalanced against the increased risks of injury or death imposed by persistent agitated and violent behavior. Individuals selected for this algorithm should exhibit many of the following features [5, 6].

A. Overt psychomotor agitation, e.g. frequent pacing, yelling, screaming, etc.
B. Current or recent violent behavior toward objects
C. Verbalized ideas of being watched, followed or harmed by others
D. Verbalized or gestured threats to harm others without apparent rational cause
E. Attempts to harm others without apparent rational cause
F. Battery of others without apparent rational cause
G. History of recurring violent behavior which appears derived from persecutory perception, severe mood lability or psychotic disorganization
H. Presence of enhanced observation needs due to severe behavioral dyscontrol

Algorithm Overview: This algorithm is divided into three phases and the duration of each phase should be flexible and based on the response of the patient to treatment. One of the principle reasons for pursuing psychopharmacological treatment is to help the individual become mentally available for additional forms of psychosocial treatment. The goal of the first phase of treatment is to decrease the individual's level of psychomotor agitation and acute risk of violence. The focus of the second phase of treatment shifts to stabilization of the underlying mental disorders so that additional rehabilitation and psychotherapeutic modalities may be employed to help further reduce the risk of violence and promote normative socialization. The third phase is focused on simplifying and adjusting effective medications to provide continuing stabilization of the patient's mental disorders [7].

While specific medications and doses are provided, the prescriber should attend to relevant individual indications, contraindications, precautions and monitoring requirements. For example, suggested doses for older or medically fragile individuals should typically be decreased by 30% to 50%. Moreover, in selecting medications within this algorithm, the clinician should develop an evolving clinical hypothesis about the origins of the observed psychomotor agitation and violence (e.g. psychotically driven violence, impulsive violence or predatory violence) that will help to effectively apply recommended psychopharmacological measures or inform alternative treatment approaches [8].

ALGORITHM
Phase 1 (Acute Intervention)

The following measures should be effective within one to three weeks, as measured against overall level of psychomotor agitation and frequency of threatened or completed violence. If substantial improvement is not seen by week three, re-evaluation of the initial diagnoses and medication choices is necessary.

Antipsychotics are the initial cornerstone of pharmacological treatment. Based on the CATIE trials and subsequent meta-analyses, olanzapine beginning at a dose of 20 mg PO BID to 20 mg TID is recommended [7]. Olanzapine 10 mg IM can be given for refused oral doses. Note that the first expected change is reduced ability of the psychotic, manic or mood lability signs and symptoms to compel behavior and drive psychomotor agitation, rather than a change in the frequency or content of the signs and symptoms themselves.

If there is minimal response by the end of week one, add risperidone 2 mg qhs and increase by 2 mg every other day to a target of 6 mg qhs. Alternatively, haloperidol or fluphenazine 5 mg can be substituted for risperidone 2 mg [9]. If the individual is uncooperative with oral antipsychotic treatment, choose treatment with fluphenazine decanoate, haloperidol decanoate or paliperidone palmitate. Each medication requires a different loading dose strategy to overcome its unique pharmacokinetics in order to achieve effective plasma concentrations within a reasonable time period [10]. Please see the subsequent section on long-acting injectable (LAI) antipsychotics. Valproic acid or lithium can be helpful adjuncts in further decreasing limbic firing rates and the activity level of the amygdaloid nuclei in psychomotorically agitated individuals suffering from a primary psychotic disorder [11, 12].

If not contraindicated, give valproic acid at an initial dose of 20–30 mg/kg in divided doses rounded to the nearest available dose (if using tablets). When using valproic acid for acutely manic or agitated states, the optimal VPA serum concentration range is 100–120 mcg/ml and for maintenance the range is 80–120 mcg/ml. Above 80 mcg/ml the proportion of free drug available to enter the central nervous system (CNS) increases at a greater than linear rate due to saturation of plasma proteins. For example, at a serum concentration of 40 mcg/ml, the free fraction is about 10% of the VPA level (4 mcg/ml), while at 130 mcg/ml, the free fraction is about 18.5% of the VPA level (24 mcg/ml). The beneficial effects and toxicities of valproic acid (VPA) are mediated by free valproate levels with a therapeutic range: 7–23 mcg/ml (toxic: >30 mcg/ml) [13–15].

Alternatively, begin lithium carbonate (or the liquid citrate) at 600 mg qhs and increase by 300 mg every other day to a target of 900 mg to 1200 mg qhs. Note that once per day dosing helps spare renal functioning by providing a maximum plasma trough period, while the brain half-life is about 25 hours [16, 17]. Extended-release forms of lithium are not necessary due to the long CNS half-life of the lithium ion, but can be used if there is a complaint of gastrointestinal upset. Also note that when used as an adjunctive medication, lithium serum concentrations do not correlate well with clinical effectiveness, but should be at least 0.6 meq/l. For bipolar mood disorder, optimal serum concentrations are thought to be 0.8–1.2 meq/l. The maximum recommended serum concentration during acute mania is 1.4 meq/l [18].

If neither valproic acid/divalproex nor lithium can be safely given, then give clonazepam beginning at a dose of 1 mg TID to QID. Doses can then be adjusted to 0.5 mg to 2 mg TID to QID, depending on clinical response. Note that at very low doses, disinhibition is a risk, however, this risk tends to be overridden by limbic GABAergic inhibition at higher doses. Excessively high doses carry a risk of inducing delirium [19, 20]. An alternative for anxiolysis and sedation is hydroxyzine given in a range of 25 mg to 100 mg BID PO or IM with adjustment and then tapering as the patient stabilizes. Importantly, hydroxyzine, unlike diphenhydramine, does not add to anticholinergic burden [21].

Except for people with a bipolar component to their illness, selective serotonin reuptake inhibitor (SSRI) antidepressants can assist in increasing limbic serotonin concentrations, which has been associated with decreased irritability, impulsive violence and impulsive suicide [22]. Conversely, SSRI antidepressants have been reported to increase irritability and violent behavior in individuals suffering from autism spectrum disorders, intellectual disability, and in some cases of brain injury [22]. Note that the US FDA has warned of possible QT interval prolongation and cardiac arrhythmia at citalopram doses above 40 mg per day [23]. Paroxetine is less favored due to increased sedation and anticholinergic effects [24]. Avoid the combination of fluvoxamine and olanzapine because fluvoxamine inhibits cytochrome P450 1A2 which may increase olanzapine plasma concentrations to a toxic level [25].

If hypomania or mania are driving psychomotor agitation and violent behaviors, sleep promotion is vital to mitigate the antidepressant and destabilizing effects of sleep deprivation. A trial of zolpidem at 10 mg qhs is recommended. If zolpidem does not maintain sleep due to its relatively short half-life, then switch to eszopiclone beginning at 4 mg qhs. Note that eszopiclone has a broad dose range of 1–8 mg qhs [26]. The antihistamine diphenhydramine can fragment sleep and cause an idiosyncratic activation in some individuals [27]. Also note that IM doses of diphenhydramine >50 mg may induce seizures by lowering the seizure threshold abruptly [28]. Phase 1 treatment usually requires pro re nata (PRN) medications to control breakthrough episodes of psychomotor agitation, especially in the first few days of treatment. Recommended medications include: haloperidol 5 mg PO/IM, fluphenazine 5 mg QID, chlorpromazine 100 mg PO or 25 mg IM, olanzapine 10 mg IM, or ziprasidone 20 mg IM. Note that since oral olanzapine requires six to nine hours to reach peak plasma concentration, it is an ineffective treatment for acute psychomotor agitation. Also note that chlorpromazine should be avoided if orthostatic hypotension is a substantial risk.

Regardless of the PRN agents chosen, smaller doses at increased frequency to mitigate the possibility of breakthrough psychomotor agitation that increases substantially before the next PRN dose is available are recommended. A sample order would be haloperidol 5 mg plus hydroxyzine (not anticholinergic) or diphenhydramine 25 mg PO or IM every two hours PRN psychomotor agitation associated with threatening, attempted or actual violent behavior, **not to exceed six doses in 24 hours.**

In general, orders for PRN medications to treat neurological side effects should also be written but should not automatically be included in the order for psychomotor agitation to avoid the risk of anticholinergic adverse effects or toxicity. For recurring dystonia, parkinsonism or akathisia give amantadine 100 mg QAM to 200 mg BID. Akathisia may respond better to propranolol 10–30 mg BID to TID or to mirtazapine 15 mg qhs [7, 29, 30, 31, 32].

Phase 2 (Stabilization)

With a sustained decline in the level of psychomotor agitation and associated frequency of threatening or violent behavior, the most common clinical errors are persisting with Phase 1 treatment too long or moving too quickly toward more typical medication doses and strategies. The first error can result in unnecessary adverse medication risks and the latter can lead to relapse.

Phase 2 typically lasts from 12 to 26 weeks before shading into Phase 3. The first step is to consolidate the oral antipsychotic dosing schedule. For example, if the individual was prescribed olanzapine 20 mg TID, consolidate the dose to 20 mg QAM and 40 mg qhs. If stability was maintained over four weeks, the dose could be gradually reduced, beginning with the morning dose at a rate of 5 mg/week. Before beginning a gradual taper, a measurement of plasma concentration may be helpful to rule out rapid metabolism. Some data have suggested that refractory psychosis is more likely to respond at concentrations of 120 ng/ml to 200 ng/ml, i.e. at dopamine D_2 receptor occupancies >80%.

While acute treatment of psychomotor agitation with fluphenazine may require plasma concentrations of up to 4.0 ng/ml, the more typical therapeutic plasma concentration range for fluphenazine is 0.8–2.0 ng/ml. Similarly, plasma haloperidol levels can help guide oral or depot dosing adjustment in a range of 5–30 ng/ml weighed against tolerance and benefits with any further benefit clearly trailing off by circa 30 ng/ml due to receptor saturation. Treatment should be approached via gradual change, e.g. a decrease in dose not faster than 10–15% per month.

The modal dose for paliperidone palmitate is 117 mg every 28 days, but it should be noted that in the average individual, a monthly dose of 234 mg provides the risperidone oral equivalent of 4–5 mg/day. Dose should change gradually, i.e. not more than one dose level per 28 days.

Valproic acid or divalproex should be dosed BID due to the risk of seizure induction during trough plasma concentrations. Conversely, divalproex extended-release (Depakote ER) should be given once per day from the outset, as it provides constant absorption across 22 of 24 hours. Lithium should be started as a single HS dose to spare renal function. If clonazepam was dosed TID to QID, the goal is to taper and consolidate to a BID schedule with the aim of tapering off completely in Phase 3. For example, if prescribed 1 mg QID, consolidate this to 2 mg BID and then to decrease by 0.5 mg at each dose point per month. SSRIs are typically dosed once/day and if the SSRI is deemed unnecessary, it is best to taper off over two to four weeks to avoid a withdrawal syndrome. This is not an issue for fluoxetine, as its active metabolite exhibits a half-life of nine to 14 days.

If there is reduced breakthrough psychomotor agitation, the PRN order can be adjusted accordingly. For example, if currently prescribed haloperidol 5 mg with diphenhydramine 25 mg PO or IM every two hours PRN not to exceed six doses in 24 hours, this might be changed to haloperidol 5 mg with diphenhydramine 25 mg PO or IM PRN every four hours. Determine the need for continuation of either zolpidem or eszopiclone [33, 34].

Phase 3 (Maintenance)

The goals are to fine tune medications to provide long-term stability with the least risk exposure and to identify clinical targets for which either other medications or additional treatment modalities may be beneficial. The overriding goal is to simplify and optimize beneficial medications at the lowest effective dose to enhance long-term psychosocial functioning. Note that long-term treatment adherence shows a strong inverse correlation to dosing frequency and once daily dosing is optimal when the pharmacokinetics of the medication permit.

By this phase of treatment, psychotropic PRN medications not used in the previous 30 days should generally be discontinued [35, 36].

 References

1. Smith, D., Smith, R., Misquitta, D. (2016). Neuroimaging and violence. *Psychiatr Clin North Am*, 39, 579–597.
2. Davidson, L. L., Heinrichs, R. W. (2003). Quantification of frontal and temporal lobe brain-imaging findings in schizophrenia: a meta-analysis. *Psychiatry Res*, 122, 69–87.
3. Hill, K., Mann, L., Laws, K. R., et al. (2004). Hypofrontality in schizophrenia: a meta-analysis of functional imaging studies. *Acta Psychiatr Scand*, 110, 243–256.
4. Sripada, C. S., Silk, K. R. (2007). The role of functional neuroimaging in exploring the overlap between borderline personality disorder and bipolar disorder. *Curr Psychiatry Rep*, 9, 40–45.
5. McDermott, B. E., Holoyda, B. J. (2014). Assessment of aggression in inpatient settings. *CNS Spectr*, 19, 425–431.
6. Poldrack, R. A., Monahan, J., Imrey, P. B., et al. (2018). Predicting violent behavior: what can neuroscience add? *Trends Cogn Sci*, 22, 111–123.
7. Stahl, S. M., Morrissette, D. A., Cummings, M., et al. (2014). California State Hospital Violence Assessment and Treatment (Cal-VAT) guidelines. *CNS Spectr*, 19, 449–465.
8. Meyer, J. M., Cummings, M. A., Proctor, G., et al. (2016). Psychopharmacology of persistent violence and aggression. *Psychiatr Clin North Am*, 39, 541–556.
9. Morrissette, D. A., Stahl, S. M. (2014). Treating the violent patient with psychosis or impulsivity utilizing antipsychotic polypharmacy and high-dose monotherapy. *CNS Spectr*, 19, 439–448.
10. Cummings, M. A., Proctor, G. J., Arias, A. W. (2019). Dopamine antagonist antipsychotics in diverted forensic populations. *CNS Spectr*, in press, doi: 10.1017/S1092852919000841
11. Citrome, L., Volavka, J. (2011). Pharmacological management of acute and persistent aggression in forensic psychiatry settings. *CNS Drugs*, 25, 1009–1021.
12. Correll, C. U., Yu, X., Xiang, Y., et al. (2017). Biological treatment of acute agitation or aggression with schizophrenia or bipolar disorder in the inpatient setting. *Ann Clin Psychiatry*, 29, 92–107.
13. Levy, R. H., Friel, P. N., Johno, I., et al. (1984). Filtration for free drug level monitoring: carbamazepine and valproic acid. *Ther Drug Monit*, 6, 67–76.
14. Keck, P. E., Jr., McElroy, S. L., Bennett, J. A. (1996). Health-economic implications of the onset of action of antimanic agents. *J Clin Psychiatry*, 57 13–18.
15. Leppik, I. E., Hovinga, C. A. (2013). Extended-release antiepileptic drugs: a comparison of pharmacokinetic parameters relative to original immediate-release formulations. *Epilepsia*, 54, 28–35.
16. Plenge, P., Stensgaard, A., Jensen, H. V., et al. (1994). 24-hour lithium concentration in human brain studied by Li-7 magnetic resonance spectroscopy. *Biol Psychiatry*, 36, 511–516.
17. Castro, V. M., Roberson, A. M., McCoy, T. H., et al. (2016). Stratifying risk for renal insufficiency among lithium-treated patients: an electronic health record study. *Neuropsychopharmacol*, 41, 1138–1143.
18. Malhi, G. S., Gessler, D., Outhred, T. (2017). The use of lithium for the treatment of bipolar disorder: recommendations from clinical practice guidelines. *J Affect Disord*, 217, 266–280.
19. Chouinard, G. (2004). Issues in the clinical use of benzodiazepines: potency, withdrawal, and rebound. *J Clin Psychiatry*, 65, 7–12.
20. Amodeo, G., Fagiolini, A., Sachs, G., et al. (2017). Older and newer strategies for the pharmacological management of agitation in patients with bipolar disorder or schizophrenia. *CNS Neurol Disord Drug Targets*, 16, 885–890.
21. Liu, J., Chan, T. C. T., Chong, S. A., et al. (2019). Impact of emotion dysregulation and cognitive insight on psychotic and depressive symptoms during the early course of schizophrenia spectrum disorders. *Early Interv Psychiatry*, 14(6), 691–697.
22. Walsh, M. T., Dinan, T. G. (2001). Selective serotonin reuptake inhibitors and violence: a review of the available evidence. *Acta Psychiatr Scand*, 104, 84–91.
23. Beach, S. R., Kostis, W. J., Celano, C. M., et al. (2014). Meta-analysis of selective serotonin reuptake inhibitor-associated QTc prolongation. *J Clin Psychiatry*, 75, e441–449.
24. Sanchez, C., Reines, E. H., Montgomery, S. A. (2014). A comparative review of escitalopram, paroxetine, and sertraline: are they all alike? *Int Clin Psychopharmacol*, 29, 185–196.
25. Chiu, C. C., Lane, H. Y., Huang, M. C., et al. (2004). Dose-dependent alternations in the pharmacokinetics of olanzapine during coadministration of fluvoxamine in patients with schizophrenia. *J Clin Pharmacol*, 44, 1385–1390.
26. Asnis, G. M., Thomas, M., Henderson, M. A. (2015). Pharmacotherapy treatment options for insomnia: a primer for clinicians. *Int J Mol Sci*, 17, 1–11.
27. Ozdemir, P. G., Karadag, A. S., Selvi, Y., et al. (2014). Assessment of the effects of antihistamine drugs on mood, sleep quality, sleepiness, and dream anxiety. *Int J Psychiatry Clin Pract*, 18, 161–168.
28. Jang, D. H., Manini, A. F., Trueger, N. S., et al. (2010). Status epilepticus and wide-complex tachycardia secondary to diphenhydramine overdose. *Clin Toxicol (Phila)*, 48, 945–948.
29. Tonda, M. E., Guthrie, S. K. (1994). Treatment of acute neuroleptic-induced movement disorders. *Pharmacotherapy*, 14, 543–560.

30. Ogino, S., Miyamoto, S., Miyake, N., et al. (2014). Benefits and limits of anticholinergic use in schizophrenia: focusing on its effect on cognitive function. *Psychiatry Clin Neurosci*, 68, 37–49.

31. Praharaj, S. K., Kongasseri, S., Behere, R. V., et al. (2015). Mirtazapine for antipsychotic-induced acute akathisia: a systematic review and meta-analysis of randomized placebo-controlled trials. *Ther Adv Psychopharmacol*, 5, 307–313.

32. Morkunas, B., Porritt, K., Stephenson, M. (2016). Experiences of mental health professionals and patients in the use of pro re nata medication in acute adult mental healthcare settings: a systematic review. *JBI Database System Rev Implement Rep*, 14, 209–250.

33. Maiocchi, L., Bernardi, E. (2013). Optimisation of prescription in patients with long-term treatment-resistant schizophrenia. *Australas Psychiatry*, 21, 446–448.

34. Remington, G., Addington, D., Honer, W., et al. (2017). Guidelines for the pharmacotherapy of schizophrenia in adults. *Can J Psychiatry*, 62, 604–616.

35. Patterson, T. L., Leeuwenkamp, O. R. (2008). Adjunctive psychosocial therapies for the treatment of schizophrenia. *Schizophr Res*, 100, 108–119.

36. Deutschenbaur, L., Lambert, M., Walter, M., et al. (2014). Long-term treatment of schizophrenia spectrum disorders: focus on pharmacotherapy. *Nervenarzt*, 85, 363–375.

Index

Locators in **bold** refer to tables; those in *italic* to figures

MAOIs (monoamine oxidase inhibitors); *see also specific drugs*
  dietary restrictions **499–500**
  drug interactions risking serotonin syndrome **501**
MATRICS Consensus Cognitive Battery (MCCB) 81
maximum response thresholds *see* point of futility
MDMA (methylenedioxymethamphetamine)/ ecstasy
  drug interactions **501**
  urine sampling **88–89**
  use in children/adolescents **65**, 66–67
measurement instruments *see* screening tools
medication *see* psychopharmacological approaches
medication-related psychosis, children/ adolescents **67–68**
melatonin **58**, **393**
  art of psychopharmacology/pearls **396**
  dosages and kinetics **395**
  drug interactions **395**
  initial workup/laboratory tests **394**
  mechanisms of action **393**
  neurotransmitters/receptors **393**, **397**
  plasma concentrations **394**
  schizophrenia spectrum disorders 57, **57**
  treatment monitoring **394**
  treatment response and side effects **394**
memantine **465**
  art of psychopharmacology/pearls **468**
  dosages and kinetics **467**
  drug interactions **467**
  geriatric patients **7**
  initial workup/laboratory tests **466**
  mechanisms of action **465**
  plasma concentrations **466**
  treatment monitoring **467**
  treatment response and side effects **466**
metabolic disorders, psychosis in children/ adolescents **68–69**
methadone **94**
methamphetamine
  children/adolescents **65**, 66–67
  and risk of psychotic illness 86
  treatment approaches 95
methylphenidate **421**
  art of psychopharmacology/pearls **426**
  dosages and kinetics **424**
  drug interactions **425**, **438**, **444**
  initial workup/laboratory tests **423**
  mechanisms of action **422**
  plasma concentrations **422**
  treatment monitoring **424**

  treatment response and side effects **422**
migraine
  drug interactions 501
  induced psychosis in children/adolescents **68–69**
  medication *see* guanfacine; valproic acid; venlafaxine
minimal response thresholds, plasma concentrations 12–13, **12**
mirtazapine **295**
  anxiety in schizophrenia patients 52
  art of psychopharmacology/pearls **298**
  dosages and kinetics **297**
  drug interactions **297**
  initial workup/laboratory tests **296**
  mechanisms of action **295**
  medication-related psychosis **67–68**
  plasma concentrations **296**
  treatment monitoring **297**
  treatment response and side effects **296**
mixed amphetamine salts **427**
  art of psychopharmacology/pearls **433**
  dosages and kinetics **430**
  drug interactions **431–432**
  initial workup/laboratory tests **429**
  mechanisms of action **428**
  plasma concentrations **428**
  treatment monitoring **430**
  treatment response and side effects **428**
moclobemide **331**
  art of psychopharmacology/pearls **333**
  dosages and kinetics **333**
  drug interactions **333**
  initial workup/laboratory tests **332**
  mechanisms of action **331**
  plasma concentrations **332**
  treatment monitoring **332**
  treatment response and side effects **332**
modafinil **440**
  art of psychopharmacology/pearls **445**
  cytochrome P450 induction/inhibition **492**
  dosages and kinetics **443**
  drug interactions **444**
  initial workup/laboratory tests **442**
  mechanisms of action **440**
  plasma concentrations **441**
  treatment monitoring **443**
  treatment response and side effects **441**
molindone, children/adolescents **73–74**
mood stabilizers; *see also* lithium; valproic acid
  plasma concentrations 13, **14**, **490**
  positive psychotic symptoms **8**
  SAD-BT patients – acute manic phase 42–45, **45**
  SAD-BT patients – maintenance phase 45–47

Printed in the United States
by Baker & Taylor Publisher Services